Choices in Healing

MICHAEL LERNER

The MIT Press
Cambridge, Massachusetts
London, England

Choices in Healing

INTEGRATING THE

BEST OF CONVENTIONAL

AND COMPLEMENTARY

APPROACHES TO CANCER

Seventh printing, 2000
First MIT Press paperback edition, 1996
© 1994 Michael Lerner

This book was set in Adobe Perpetua and Frutiger by DEKR Corporation and was printed and bound in the United States of America.

Library of Congress Cataloging-in-Publication Data

Lerner, Michael, 1943–
    Choices in healing : integrating the best of conventional and complementary approaches to cancer / Michael Lerner.
        p. cm.
    Includes bibliographical references and index.
    ISBN 0-262-12180-8 (HB), 0-262-62104-5 (PB)
    1. Cancer—Treatment. 2. Cancer—Alternative treatment.
3. Cancer—Popular works. I. Title.
RC270.8.L47 1994
616.99′406—dc20   93-39913
                                                              CIP

This book is dedicated to Jenifer Altman, Brendan O'Regan, and Max Lerner.

Jennifer Altman was a participant in the Commonweal Cancer Help Program and subsequently a Senior Research Associate at Commonweal.

Brendan O'Regan was Vice President for Research at the Institute of Noetic Sciences.

Max Lerner, my father, was an observer of American civilizations, and a public intellectual.

Each faced a life-threatening illness with courage.

Each lived, as it happened, far beyond what others thought was the appointed time.

Each was a true friend.

Contents

Foreword

A diagnosis of cancer can be so overwhelming, and our health care system so bewildering and impersonal, that one often doesn't know where to turn or whom to trust. Many people, sensibly, want to know all their options, only to discover that cancer and its treatment, conventional and otherwise, is a universe in itself, and a rather intimidating one at that, especially for the cancer patient who has at most a layperson's knowledge of science and medicine. Cancer and cancer treatment has a history, a politics, a mainstream, a lunatic fringe. There are a multitude of choices and treatment decisions to be made even within the mainstream culture of medicine. Then there are other potentially valuable treatment avenues outside of the mainstream. Some people will want to at least become informed about them and consider them in their decision-making process. Some are specific to cancer, others are adjunctive or palliative. Some support generalized health and healing. Each has potential risks and benefits which need to be weighed according to the specifics of the disease, one's life situation and personal values, the time frame involved, and of course, the latest research findings, which are usually incomplete and more suggestive than definitive. While medical and surgical oncology specialists know their own fields well and are in an excellent position to explain certain risks and benefits to their patients, they are frequently ignorant and sometimes scornful of other views or approaches, even if they are intended to be complementary or adjunctive to more mainstream approaches.

So it is not unusual for the person with cancer and his or her family to wind up feeling isolated and on their own in trying to decide what to do.

How then to make sense of this universe of cancer for oneself, at least enough to make informed choices, decisions that might well affect the deepest aspects of one's life? Where to turn? What to do? What not to do? Whom to believe? What to ask? What is known? What is not known? How to decide? What to combine? What order to do things in? What about the mind and inner well-being? What about nutritional approaches? Chinese medicine? Stress reduction? Yoga? What about my family? My fears? What about the meaning of all this in my life?

Even if you stay completely within the mainstream of conventional medical approaches, opinions and recommendations can differ considerably in critical areas such as diagnosis, prognosis, and treatment among different physicians and surgeons, different subspecialists, and in different countries. Then, if you wanted to know about alternatives of any kind, until now you had to start from scratch, research things for yourself, find the right people to see and elicit advice from, then weigh things and come to reasonable conclusions on your own, and this at a time of great stress, turmoil, and vulnerability.

With the advent of this book, a great deal of the information a person with cancer or people supporting a person with cancer might want to consider has been gathered together in one place. *Choices in Healing* gives people both a starting point and a method to follow in gathering information and pondering choices. It is sorely needed and will be put to immediate use by many people who presently feel adrift in their quest for a framework for understanding different approaches to the disease. Its arrival will be celebrated by many and perhaps criticized by some as well who may, wrongly, see it as advocating voodoo or quackery. In this regard, it is significant that MIT Press has published this book. Perhaps this signals an acknowledgment that such material, controversial as much of it is, merits serious scientific scrutiny and debate.

Its arrival is timely. A study recently published in the *New England Journal of Medicine* (Eisenberg et al., 328:246, 1993) reports that one third of Americans seek out and use nontraditional medical alternatives, frequently without informing their mainstream doctors. Alternative medical therapies now constitute a multibillion dollar industry in the United States alone. Yet there are few places that anyone can turn to which serve as knowledgeable and dispassionate clearinghouses to guide people in their decision making. This book is a major contribution in this area.

In another recent development, the National Institutes of Health recently funded an Office of Alternative Medicine to support research of alternative approaches, since ultimately, we cannot know the value of a therapy until it has been tested experimentally according to the standards of scientific scrutiny, but a scrutiny that does not ignore psychological, social, nutritional, environmental, possibly even spiritual factors which might significantly influence health and disease processes.

Choices in Healing had a vigorous life for several years even before it achieved its final form as the book you hold in your hands. In various incarnations, it was available from Commonweal in bound manuscript form. I was given a copy when I visited there for the first time in late 1992.

When I got home and started reading it, I found myself moved to get ahold of additional copies right away so I could give them to the people I knew who had cancer. Here was something, I felt, that might be extremely useful as well as comforting. And indeed, the feedback I have gotten is that the book is a true gift to people trying to figure out what to do as they face cancer and its aftermath.

One young lawyer dealing with an episode of recurrence of breast cancer said that she felt caring on every page she read, to the point that she was often in tears, and that this deeply human tone made the technical material much more accessible to her and helped her develop her own framework for analyzing various treatment options, some of which she went on to pursue. It also helped her become more aware of a deep yearning she had for a "magic bullet" alternative, and to avoid the problems that such an attitude often results in when evaluating treatment options, frequently "hyped" by their proponents, and making choices.

To read this book is an education in itself. It is far more than a catalogue of resources; it is nothing less than a highly intelligent guide to the universe of cancer. In tone and perspective, it is warm and caring, personal and supportive, compassionate and wise. Michael Lerner the person does comes through on every page, as my friend observed. One feels held, cared for, acknowledged, not alone. Michael's voice is present as a companion, an ally. People feel uplifted when they use this book. And this book is to be *used,* not simply read. It is food for thought. It is not meant to replace the advice of doctors and specialists. It is a complement to their recommendations, and perhaps a source for developing hard questions to ask of them to help in making hard decisions. And it provides an additional source of nourishment and strength when it comes to wrestling with those often life-wrenching decisions.

It does not have to be read from cover to cover. It can serve as something of a wise and knowledgeable friend, to be consulted, read, and reread as needed, a reference library in itself. It is encyclopedic in scope, yet totally accessible to the layperson. It offers up-to-date and hard-to-find information relevant to making decisions about conventional as well as unconventional therapies. It also encourages the interested reader to develop his or her own expanded ways of looking not only at various treatment options, but also at the whole of his or her life as it is colored by the experience of having one form or another of the disease we call cancer.

Michael gives us the science and the politics of cancer and of various cancer therapies, as well as the medicine, in a compelling narrative. He presents evidence where it is available, tells us what is known and what is not known in both conventional and complementary medicine, and frames the whole discussion in such a way that the reader feels supported in at least knowing the lay of the entire landscape and not just the part his or her oncologist, surgeon, friends, or family happens to know or approve of. He points out the pros and cons and the areas of uncertainty. By describing the state of our scientific knowledge, such as it is, by citing references to the medical literature that people might consult for further details, by recounting his own explorations and conversations with doctors and scientists, he gives readers an opportunity to grasp what is going on within the various fields of research and inquiry and draw their own conclusions.

The format blends technical detail with an appreciation for the inner life of mind and spirit, human relationship and meaning. Discussions are buttressed by literary as well as medical citations. Some chapters contain practical advice and resource listings. This structure allows for virtually limitless on-going explorations according to one's personal inclinations and the circumstances of the disease.

The book provides a map of a certain territory, some of which is now coming to be called mind/body, or integrative, or complementary medicine. As with any map, people can do with this one what they like, including ignore it or criticize it, or use it as maps are most commonly used, to chart an itinerary that visits some places but not others. In this world, the territory is constantly changing as we learn more about cancer and effective treatments for it, and as we learn more about the mind/body connection. So the map, too, will have to change as new knowledge is acquired. But at least it is available now for those who would like to explore an expanded range of possible attitudes and approaches toward cancer and healing.

I believe this book will also be valuable to health professionals in the field of cancer. The sympathetic, hopeful, and respectful tone could serve as an example to us all in our communications with people with cancer. We might also gain some respect for at least some alternative/complementary approaches that we may have been unaware of before. Practicing oncologists frequently know surprisingly little of even the psychosocial oncology literature, where the scientific basis for a major role in adjunctive therapy is perhaps most compelling.

None of the alternatives presented here, as Lerner emphasizes, provides in any sense a definitive cure. But at the very least, the reader can gain a new vantage point from which to look at cancer and at possible ways to approach treatment decisions and the question of alternative therapies. At the same time, the reader can take comfort in Michael's reassuring tone and the wisdom of his own deeply personal as well as professional inquiry into what is "out there" in the way of treatment approaches and what is "in here" in the way of different attitudes and disciplines one might explore for facing questions of health and illness, mind and body, diet, pain, death and dying.

This book provides a framework for the reader to contemplate, perhaps for the first time, that your own mind and body might shelter deep inner resources for healing and for coping. You might be interested to learn that *how* you approach your illness might make a big difference in your quality of life and in your relationships, and that even the course of the disease itself and its response to treatment might potentially be affected. Strong recent evidence suggests the possibility that sharing feelings in a group and practicing stress reduction exercises as a complement to more traditional treatments might extend periods of remission and positively influence survival (see, for example, Spiegel et al., *Lancet* 2:888, 1989; Fawzy et al., *Arch. Gen. Psychiatry* 50:681, 1993).

The informed pursuit of treatment options, including disciplines such as meditation and yoga which may help us as human beings to mobilize the full range of our resources for healing, can also influence how we encounter our own mortality. Perhaps inner peace, freedom and meaning, even health lie embedded within the very pain, fear, and uncertainty we frequently experience as we face illness and engage with it as full participants along the road we call our life.

A full professor at a prestigious university, who had struggled mightily with his doctors and insurer to develop and pay for the treatment plan he felt he needed, commented in class in our clinic one day that his leukemia and the impending bone marrow transplant he faced had brought him into what he called "this community of the afflicted" where he felt more at home, in a funny way, than with his colleagues. Pain and life-threatening illness frequently create a separate reality and the potential for a consciousness all its own. When we explore this reality, as people do in the Commonweal Cancer Help Program, in our clinic, and in many other places, remarkable new openings often occur for people. In his case, an insight came to him while riding on the subway that the people sitting on either side of him might very well be suffering every bit as deeply as he was or that the other people in the class were. He saw that the community of the afflicted potentially extends to everybody. So what started as a feeling of separation blossomed into a deeper feeling of inclusion and unity, one from which he took considerable satisfaction since it was in resonance with his deepest values.

As Michael reminds us, affliction can itself become a powerful teacher and augur a turning point in one's life. While there may be few or no reliable cures at this time, profound healing is possible. It usually requires active participation on the part of the person with the disease. The illness may become an occasion for a deep looking into life itself, an acknowledgment of what is really important, a falling away of a certain automaticity or mindlessness, a blindness which frequently ignores or takes for granted that which is most fundamental and dearest to us. Often, the change appears as a subtle "rotation in consciousness," a shift in perspective arising out of a careful observing of the activity of mind and body without judging or condemning what it is that one sees and is feeling. This is the inner work of on-going human development that is the domain of meditation and yoga, which are mentioned and discussed at various points throughout the book as options and vehicles for exploring healing and inner well-being.

I believe that the more options we have in dealing with distress and crisis, the healthier we will be psychologically, and the more we will feel like an important if not crucial participant in what is happening in our lives, with at least some degree of influence and control. Michael's simile of the cancer patient in the role of policymaker rather than cancer researcher is entirely accurate. It explains why the message of the entire book is aimed just where it ought to be, namely, at making realistic, hopeful, and uniquely personal choices under time pressure and on the basis of incomplete evidence and partial understanding of an extremely complex disease, where nobody has the last word or a magic bullet, and many approaches can be complementary to one another.

Little is fixed while we are alive. As things unfold, as we see how the body responds to a chosen course of treatment, as our understanding and our experience grow and deepen, as circumstances change, we might want to change course, make new choices, pursue other options. This book makes the journey that much richer for those seeking information and alternatives as they grope, fight, and grow toward wholeness. I wish all who come to this book well, on their unique paths of healing.

Jon Kabat-Zinn, Ph.D.
Associate Professor of Medicine
Director, Stress Reduction Clinic
University of Massachusetts Medical Center
Worcester, Massachusetts
January 3, 1994

Preface

Dear Reader:

This book is written for you—someone with cancer who wants to understand the many choices available to you in both conventional medicine and alternative therapies. It is also for your family members, friends, and health care professionals, but primarily it is for you. It is a book about how to find your way through the unfamiliar and often frightening territory that you face when you are diagnosed with cancer.

I believe that the experience of a person who is given a cancer diagnosis is similar to that of a soldier who is given orders by his officers to parachute into a jungle war zone without a map, a compass, or training of any kind. No military expert would claim that it is only the officers who need training. And yet, in medicine, physicians often assume that only the medical team that sends patients into the battlefield of treatment needs training. Physicians often assume that the patient needs to know nothing except how to follow medical advice.

In recent years, this assumption has begun to change for medical treatment in general. For example, patients are now encouraged to get more than one opinion about their treatment. Laws now require that patients be given extensive information about treatment options and effects. Particularly in cancer, the discussion of treatment options has reached the point where some patients feel that, rather than being given too few choices, they face too many.

Although some cancer patients encounter physicians who still fail to explain treatment options to them, the more common problem facing most cancer patients today is not that there are no choices but rather *the absence of credible maps—and training in reading these maps—when actually trying to traverse the forbidding landscape of cancer diagnosis and treatment.*

The central problem, in brief, is that we have not yet recognized the need for systematic education and training for cancer patients when facing the tremendous and traumatic changes that occur after a diagnosis of cancer.

Choices in Healing is a book designed for the cancer patient who wants to have a comprehensive overview of what his choices are—both in treatments and in living with cancer. It describes the maps of choice which I have developed in over a decade of studying informed choice in both conventional and complementary (or unconventional) cancer therapies. But it does *not* say that you should automatically trust *my* maps. Rather, it is a book that illustrates some of the rudiments of the *process* of mapmaking in charting the course you will want to set for yourself.

I wish I could tell you that the maps of informed choice in cancer treatment and life with cancer were simple and straightforward. Like much of the rest of modern life, they are frustratingly ambiguous and complex. After more than 10 years of study, I am no closer to simple recommendations for what roads a person diagnosed with cancer *should* travel than I was at the start. What has changed is my knowledge of the terrain. I believe I have learned some useful things about informed choice in both conventional and complementary cancer therapies and about what the choices in cancer look like for the hundreds of people I have cared deeply about who have faced a diagnosis of cancer.

The experience of cancer contains a whole "life cycle," starting with the shock of diagnosis, then the immediate decisions about conventional therapies, subsequent decisions about complementary therapies, the process of going through therapy, the period of recovery from therapy, and then the prospect of living life with the ever-present possibility of recurrence.

Among the hundreds of friends I have known with cancer, the extraordinary reality is that *the cancer is not always the most difficult part of their lives.* Even in the face of a cancer diagnosis, other, greater difficulties may exist in relationships, at work, or in dealing with scars and traumas from the past. In these situations, the major work of healing may not address the cancer directly. Instead, it may be directed at problems of living that are related only tangentially to cancer.

On the other hand, some problems of living with cancer *are* directly related to the illness. One set of challenges is financial and work-related. People lose their jobs, or they are treated badly at work, or they cannot leave a job they detest because they depend on their insurance policy, or they cannot find new employment because of their history of cancer.

A second set of challenges is in relationships. Husbands stop having sex with wives who have had mastectomies. Friends do not know how to relate to a person with cancer. A mother with life-threatening cancer is as torn by the grief over the future of her child as she is by her own struggle with the illness.

A third set of challenges occurs when the person with cancer undergoes—as a result of the diagnosis—a process of rapid inner growth and reevaluation of what is important in his or her life. The cancer patient may conclude that his work situation or relationships no longer fit with the new phase he is moving into. The problems are not those of being rejected by a mate or friend, or of rejection at work, but rather of increasingly vivid recognition that old relationships or old jobs no longer meet emerging and vitally important inner needs.

This Is Not a Simple Book

Many inspirational books for people with cancer are available. There are also some excellent books about choice in (primarily) conventional cancer treatment that have been honed into simple language to make them easily readable. *Choices in Healing* is not a simple book, although I have done everything that I can to provide accessible summaries of the main points in each chapter.

Because *Choices in Healing* is often charting territory that most people with cancer and many physicians and other health care practitioners are unfamiliar with, I felt a need to ground it extensively in scientific studies of the many and diverse areas we discuss. As a result, this is the kind of book that a cancer patient might take to his oncologist to ask if he has reviewed the studies it cites in an area of special interest.

My approach also has meant that there are numerous direct quotations from scientific or related studies in the text. While these quotations make the reader's job a little more difficult, they have the advantage of directly providing the reader with many key findings that he might otherwise need to look up in the medical literature.

A note about my use of the masculine pronoun. It is deeply regrettable that the English language does not have a singular pronoun that refers to both men and women. I use the pronouns *he*, *him*, and *his* generically to refer to men *and* women.

Hope, Doubt, and the Uses of Science

One of the great difficulties in writing a book that covers so many different areas of research is that it is impossible for any individual to have personal expertise in each of these areas. While I have benefited from the comments of the many expert reviewers of this book, their comments have made me aware of the many deficiencies in individual chapters that I simply do not have the depth of knowledge to remedy. It is beyond the scope of this book, for example, to consider the methodological shortcomings of some of the studies discussed.

In this book, I will help you begin to learn how to think critically about choice in complementary and unconventional therapies, just as I have suggested ways of thinking critically about choice in conventional therapies. The word *education* comes from a Latin word that means "to lead out." Again, I do not ask you to accept the maps I have drawn of informed choice in conventional or complementary cancer therapies, but I hope that the experience of mapmaking that you see me engaged in will help you as you undertake the challenge of living with cancer.

In doing this, I am consciously using scientific research differently from the way most cancer researchers use it. Cancer researchers, like all scientists, often do their work best by a constant process of doubting whether promising results from a new study are actually correct or not. That healthy process of doubt leads them to check and recheck every study. They have nothing to lose and everything to gain by living in a research culture that emphasizes the primacy of doubt. Their goal is to contribute to the formulation of lasting true statements about the biomedical nature and treatment of cancer.

People with cancer are fundamentally in a different situation. To begin with, the time perspective of cancer patients is different. They are more interested than cancer researchers in treatment possibilities that offer *some* hope during the time defined by their particular disease. In some ways, a cancer patient is like a policymaker faced with choices for a nation which is facing a mortal national emergency that involves complex decisions about scientific issues. In the policy world, scientific advisors to policymakers must help the policymakers decide questions with inadequate or incomplete scientific information. In fact, the management of scientific information and scientific uncertainty to meet the special and urgent needs of policymakers has become a social science of its own. It is considered legitimate that the policymaker use scientific data differently than the scientist's colleagues would. The scientist advises the policymaker of what he knows, what he does not know, what would clearly, in view of current knowledge, be a disastrous course of action, and what levels of risk are associated with other courses of action. The policymaker then decides on a course of action based on considerations that are often entirely extraneous to the scientific argument. The policymaker decides for the nation just as the cancer patient must decide for himself.

The clinician who treats cancer patients also differs from the scientific researcher in the way he uses science. However, he is often more *inclined* than a policymaker would be to evaluate treatment options the way the scientist would *because he is trained as a scientist*. He is frequently not trained in what effects the treatments that he recommends might have on the inner world of the cancer patient. He does not always give the same legitimacy to the need of the cancer patient to make his own choices—choices that meet the demands of his patient's inner *polity*—that the policymaker's scientific advisor would. And yet, medical ethics clearly recognizes the right of every person to determine what medical treatments will be used on his body. This is a fundamental principle of medical ethics. Not only is the physician rarely trained to understand the inner-choice process of a patient but the cancer patient himself is rarely trained to give his inner inclinations and feelings about treatment serious attention. Yet these inner feelings and inclinations deserve the most respectful attention, for the patient and his family are the ones who will profoundly experience the consequences of both the illness and the treatment.

Cancer patients also differ from cancer researchers in another way. They have a fundamentally different set of relationships to the clinical uses of hope and the scientific uses of doubt. This is not a hypothetical observation. Imagine again a soldier parachuting into a jungle war zone behind enemy lines. The chances of his survival may be slight, but unless he *hopes* for survival, his chances are slighter still. If he has no hope, he will not try to save himself. Among the hundreds of cancer patients I have known well, hope has been important to the large majority.

Jimmie Holland, M.D., a pioneering psychooncologist at Memorial Sloan-Kettering Cancer Center in New York, put it well when she said that, in the face of a life-threatening cancer, the mind often operates on two tracks. At one level the patient is aware of the "reality" as his oncologist has described it. If the prognosis is grave, he is aware of the fact and of the low probability that the treatments offered—or others that he may choose on his own—will be effective. On another level, Holland suggests, the patient continues to hope that he or she will have the exceptional experience of recovery from a difficult cancer. Then, if that hope slips away, the patient's hope naturally shifts toward other goals: to live long enough to achieve something important; or to die without too much pain; or to die with dignity. In chapter 1 you will find a fuller description of what I believe to be the enormous value of hope.

I am in no way a simplistic purveyor of unrealistic hopes about complementary cancer therapies. After more than 10 years of study in the field, I have seen no documented cure for cancer among the complementary cancer therapies—in the sense of a treatment that regularly and reliably reverses any form of cancer.

On the other hand, I believe that people who are inclined to fight for life with cancer using whatever combination of conventional and complementary cancer therapies that makes sense to them are wise to do so. I am certain that some of the complementary cancer therapies I discuss in this book enhance quality of life. I am equally certain that some of the complementary cancer therapies, given sufficient time to work, help people become healthier cancer patients—that is to say, physically, mentally, and emotionally healthier people who happen to have cancer. It seems to me reasonable—and many oncologist friends agree—that healthier cancer patients often do better with arduous conventional therapies because their greater physical and mental strength makes them more resilient, both to treatment and in some instances to the disease itself. I believe—though I cannot prove—that the improved physical and mental health of people who engage in intelligent integration of conventional and complementary cancer therapies may in some cases help shift the balance toward improved outcomes in a notoriously unpredictable group of diseases.

On Not Recommending Complementary Therapies to the Disinclined

Given how little we know about most of the complementary therapies, I believe that, with few exceptions, they should not be *recommended* to patients who are disinclined to use them. When relatives call me asking me to help them convince a parent or a spouse to use some complementary therapy, I vigorously refuse. I suggest instead that the relative recognize that, if he develops cancer, he can choose his own course, but that the most truly *healing* approach to his parent, spouse, or child is to inquire gently what that person would find most helpful. It may be something as simple as help with shopping or doctor visits, or more time together at home. It can be a very touching shift in perspective as the genuinely caring son realizes that Mom does not have to try a macrobiotic diet, and may actually do better with her cancer if her son is able to make a few more visits home.

Thus, the reader will find in this book an unusual combination of a *critical* approach to both conventional and complementary cancer therapies juxtaposed with a *hopeful* approach toward both types of therapies wherever the scientific data indicate that hope is reasonable. I am as hopeful about the continued progress of new treatments in conventional cancer care as I am that useful adjuncts to the *judicious use* of conventional therapies will continue to emerge from among the complementary therapies. Some researchers in conventional medicine doubt the probability of progress in *both* conventional and complementary cancer therapies. I respect their doubts because I understand that doubt is the way they progress as scientists. But I am not a scientist. I am an educator who works with people facing life-threatening illnesses. I understand their need for hope as clearly as I understand the scientists' need for doubt. What is more important, I understand that for the cancer patient—as for the policymaker—there is a place for hope in the uses of science that is as valid as the place for doubt.

Finally, I suggest that as you read this book, *avoid reading any section that does not currently interest you or draw your attention*. You can start reading anywhere and finish anywhere. Every section is self-contained and self-explanatory.

It is my greatest hope that this book may be of some help to you.

PART ONE

Paths of Hope and Ways of Healing

On Never Giving Up Hope:
Three Stories

Wrestling with the Angel

This chapter is about the uses of hope in cancer. A wise man once said to a group of cancer patients in the Commonweal Cancer Help Program: "Above all, never give up hope." The truth in those simple words has stayed with me through the years. It is hard to live without hope. Hope is truly therapeutic. There is always something worth hoping for in the face of a difficult illness.

I will tell you three stories about hope in cancer. The first is about my father. In 1980 my father, Max Lerner, was diagnosed with cancer. His physician told him he might have 6 months to live. He was 77. Six months earlier he had suffered a deep disappointment about a book project he had been working on. "I felt like my gut was just torn out of me," he told me as we talked about the diagnosis in his cluttered book-lined study. Six months later, a non-Hodgkin's lymphoma was diagnosed in his abdomen. Later, his physician found prostate cancer that had metastasized to his lung. Intuitively, my father felt certain that there was a connection between the deep sense of loss he had felt and the appearance of the cancer in his gut.

If anyone I have ever known loved life, my father did. Born in a Russian-Jewish community near Minsk, he came to the United States with his parents when he was age 3. He fought his way up from the slums of New York and New Haven into a life as a public intellectual that suited him perfectly. He lived almost entirely absorbed in a world of ideas, delighting in what life brought him every day. So the depression caused by his disappointment was uncharacteristic of him, and, in the light of a life-threatening cancer, that loss now seemed trivial to him. He wanted, above all, to live and live and live. He wanted to live for all the unwritten books he felt he still had in him. He wanted to live for the sheer joy he felt in life.

As we talked that day, it became clear that his fundamental question was whether or not he should undergo chemotherapy, which held no clear promise of recovery. My mother was for it. I was inclined against it. If chemotherapy offered any real certainty of recovery, I would have favored it. But with a poor prognosis, even with chemotherapy, I wondered if he should visit that additional suffering on himself.

My father underwent the chemotherapy. He suffered greatly. His hair fell out, he lost weight, and he was terribly fatigued. He had been a very youthful 77-year-old before the chemotherapy. He seemed to age 5 years in the passage of a few months. We thought he might die. As for myself, I found it incredibly difficult to watch this wonderful, rambunctious, Rabelaisian lover of life so reduced by the ravages of cancer and chemotherapy.

But my father did not die. He fought with tenacity for life. He survived the chemotherapy and very slowly began to heal. He found a remarkable doctor, James Holland, who shared his literary frame of reference and supported his strong desire to keep his male equipment intact in the face of recommendations from other physicians that his testicles be removed. "Don't let them do an Abelard on you, Max," Holland said. The allusion was to the medieval theologian and philosopher Abelard, who was castrated for secretly marrying his pupil, Héloise after she bore him a child. Holland proved to be the physician for my father—a physician absolutely meticulous in his physical examinations (which reassured my father greatly) who shared his love of ideas. Holland recommended a hormonal therapy that was then in use in Canada but which had not yet been released for general use in the United States—a hormonal therapy less feminizing in its side effects than the standard hormonal treatment for prostate cancer.

On this regimen, my father continued to recover. Then one summer day he suffered a heart attack and again we thought we might lose him. So heart medication was added to the cancer medications. And he fought on.

Notre Dame University offered him a university professorship. I am convinced that this public mark of esteem and the opportunity to continue his teaching, which at 77 he still loved, was a fundamental force in his recovery. He accepted the offer. He had to be well in order to go to Notre Dame, and this further reinforced his determination to live.

And so, bit by bit, year by year, he recovered. Until he was 89, he continued to write a newspaper column about world events twice a week. Until he was 87, he flew regularly from New York to California to teach a course at one of the few universities that does not discriminate against vibrantly alive 87-year-old men. His 1990 book about his experience with cancer and heart disease, *Wrestling with the Angel,* was greeted by the *New York Times* as "the best of the illness memoirs." Dozens of cancer patients have told me how important the book was to them in their lives.

No one can know for certain why my father recovered from two such serious cancers. He unquestionably made some wise choices about medical treatment. He improved his diet and health habits moderately. He quickly surrendered all concern with the professional disappointment he had suffered and recovered his tremendous appetite for life.

Significantly, however, he never chose to undertake any of the alternative or adjunctive cancer therapies that I had begun to investigate at the time of his diagnosis to see if I could find anything of value for him. Medically, he used only conventional and conventional-experimental therapies. Psychologically, he came to recognize the survival potential of his enormous will to live and to recognize his wisdom about how to navigate the frail yet still seaworthy physical vessel of his life, but he had no interest in undertaking psychotherapy or joining a cancer support group. To me, his recovery was a joyful confirmation of my belief that every human being must find his own unique path in the effort to recover from cancer.

Above all, my father instinctively made one of the wisest choices a person with cancer can make. He never gave up hope. Even in the face of what sometimes seemed insurmountable odds and terrible suffering, he struggled on, nursing and protecting the hope that somehow he would survive.

There is an epilogue. At the age of 89, my father finally died of a stroke and a third cancer, a cancer of the pancreas. Was he reconciled to his dying? Not at all. He fought death every last inch of the way. There was for him no consoling belief in a life after death. He fought because he believed that every wonderful thing about life was contained in the life we know: the life between birth and death. He died surrounded by his family, a man who had lived fully and who had understood the uses of hope.

The Uses of Hope

If I could say only one thing to cancer patients who want to live (not everyone does), I would repeat the words of the wise man who spoke to the cancer patients in the Commonweal Cancer Help Program. Never give up hope. You can fight for your life, even in the face of tremendous odds. Give yourself permission to hope, even in the face of all the statistics that physicians may present to you. Statistics are only statistics. They are not you. There is no such thing as false hope. I saw the truth of this in my father's experience, and in the experience of many other people with cancer who have far outlived their prognosis.

William Buchholz, M.D., is an oncologist in Palo Alto, California, who has thought and written about the "therapeutic uses of hope" in cancer treatment. He consciously uses hope as a treatment tool. In ancient times, when medical technologies were more limited, the physician's appreciation of the therapeutic uses of hope was much more refined than it is today. I have seen people days away from death who continued to hope for recovery, and this hope for recovery was an essential element in how some of those people chose to cope with this ultimate life experience. I know many other cancer patients who were years away from death, who had no fear of death, and some who even looked forward to death with curiosity, interest, relief, or the hope of being reunited with people they loved. But although they had no difficulty accepting the prospect of death, they also had hopes: hope of a death without too much suffering; hope of a death with dignity, a death that did not impose too much on family members; hope of a death that did not impoverish the family; or a death that reunited them with a husband or wife who had died before.

I rarely if ever intervene to change the object of the hope of a cancer patient. I am much more likely to encourage family members to understand exactly what the true hopes and beliefs of the person with cancer are, and to support the patient in the ways he seeks to realize or hold these hopes, rather than pressing upon him the hopes or beliefs that family and friends wish he had. I try to support people with cancer in whatever it is that they are hoping for, knowing that their hopes will shift toward other goals in alignment with their own inner clock.

Physicians, as I have said, are trained both as scientists and as clinicians. As scientists, they are part of a culture that thrives through the inculcation of doubt. As clinicians they are part of a much more ancient culture of healing that thrives through the inculcation of hope. Often they are not aware of this dual role. They do not know the damage they do when they thoughtlessly dash the hopes of a patient facing a difficult cancer. Fortunately, there are physician-scientists who have begun to work consciously with the therapeutic uses of hope. They are practitioners of the high art of combining honesty about what they know as scientists with humility and hopefulness about what they do not know as clinicians. In the now well-known words of Bernie Siegel, M.D., *"in the absence of certainty, there is nothing wrong with hope."* If a patient with a serious cancer *hopes* to be the one person in a hundred or in a thousand to overcome the cancer, it is not correct for the physician to propose that this is a false hope. It may be a slender hope, but that slender hope may still provide light as the cancer patient goes through the inner work of learning to live under new and difficult circumstances. The difficult issue of how to balance scientific doubt with clinical hope was one that I wrestled with throughout this book.

What Do I Have to Lose?

Kim and Sarah Brown also discovered the uses of hope. They were both 37 when they enrolled in one of the week-long workshops we offer at Commonweal for people with cancer. They looked and acted like a storybook couple. Kim had been an artist ever since he was 8, when his grandmother gave him a supersize box of 136 crayons and he said "Thank you, Grandma, I'm going to be an artist," and drew until the crayons were worn down to tiny stubs. He was an "Air Force brat," growing up at Air Force bases all over the world, switching schools every few years, feeling like a character out of Star Trek being beamed up and down as his father's orders moved the family from base to base.

In Southern California, during a period of stability, he met Sarah Brown, who just coincidentally had the same last name. Sarah had been born in New York but moved to California with her mother when she was 3 after her parents divorced. "I realized by the time I was 6 that my father was dead for me—he just wasn't there for me at all. And then my mother married another man who was terrifically negative about everything I tried to do. So the way I survived was by thinking: 'Oh yeah? You think I can't do that? I'll show you.' It was a great survival tool, but it was probably a double-edged sword—I could push myself too hard proving that I could do things."

Kim and Sarah dated through high school and college, then married, and soon Sarah had established a promising career in government administration, while Kim's work as an artist thrived. When Sarah was offered a job in Connecticut, they moved from California to New York. But Sarah's new job proved an excruciating experience: "I was the first woman hired for a top management position and the company was run by an 'old boys' club. I tried too hard for years to make it right. Finally, I had to give up." Sarah was then offered a top management position with a New York bank. She was working as a vice president at the bank doing some of the most creative and interesting work of her life when she was diagnosed with a life-threatening refractory anemia and leukemia. Her body was refusing to make the blood cells that she needed to survive.

Sarah was given 2 months to live. She sat at home waiting to die. One physician recommended ara-C, or cytosine arabinoside, a chemotherapeutic agent used for leukemia. Because her bones were fibrotic, she would not have benefited from a bone marrow transplant and, in any case, a suitable bone marrow donor could not be found. Her physician recommended monthly blood transfusions to keep her alive, but warned that there was no cure and that she would probably soon die of an infection. Sarah asked if anyone had survived her condition. The answer was no. Gradually, Sarah decided that she wanted to try to be the first person to recover from this obscure refractory anemia. Still receiving her monthly blood transfusion, she decided to go on a macrobiotic diet. "I was very skeptical, but I figured, 'What do I have to lose?'"

A macrobiotic diet is a strict regimen that requires considerable dedication. Kim and Sarah read *Recalled by Life,* by Anthony J. Sattilaro, M.D., a book about a physician who recovered for many years from a life-threatening testicular cancer while on the macrobiotic diet.[1] She decided she wanted to try the same thing. "The diet was a godsend for me," said Kim. "I had tried all our life together to protect Sarah, but now that she had the cancer, all I was doing was taking her to places where physicians hurt her. With the macrobiotic diet, there was something I could do. I became the cook. . . . Sarah called me the 'enforcer.'"

Sarah and Kim found, to their surprise, that the diet made them both feel much better. Sarah's recurrent chronic headaches and menstrual cramps disappeared. Kim lost 30 lbs and returned to his college weight. They both felt light and energetic. Sarah also started getting shiatsu massage, a form of Oriental pressure point treatment, and began to practice meditation, imagery, and yoga. She read about the healing power of crystals and started wearing a crystal around her neck. Much to her physician's surprise, Sarah did not develop the infections that he thought would soon end her life. In fact, she felt extraordinarily healthy except when she went to the physician's office and received reconfirmation that her body was still not producing the cells she needed to live. So she continued getting the blood transfusions and started an experimental procedure to rid her body of the iron buildup that was caused by the death of the red blood cells she received every month.

Long after her doctors expected her to die, Sarah finally did die. But the spirit and hope with which she and Kim fought for her life transformed their lives. They lived with wonder at the beauty of life and the preciousness of their lives together. The experience of the cancer deeply changed their values, reconnecting them—they both said—with an idealism about life that they last felt in their early twenties. From their own experience they learned the difference between "healing" and "curing." A cure is a medical procedure that reliably helps you recover from an illness. Healing is an inner process through which the human organism seeks its own recovery—physically, mentally, emotionally, and spiritually. I talk more about this in the next chapter.

Sarah reached that exceptional stage that some people with cancer discover where the question of whether she actually succeeded in her quest to become the first survivor of this cancer—while tremendously important—was not *the* most important thing for her. What became most important to her were the transcendental insights into life and meaning that she found through the fight for physical recovery. Kim subsequently became deeply convinced that Sarah's spirit survived her death. But that is a story I will save for a later chapter.

The experience of Sarah and Kim is important because it is a vivid example of the redeeming value of hope in the face of the most difficult cancer prognosis. Not everyone would choose to fight for life in these circumstances or to make such drastic lifestyle changes. I have known others—often older people—who also want to fight for recovery but who feel at the same time that they have already had long and full lives.

Hope and Dignity

Sandra Simmons, age 65, from Taos, New Mexico, attended the same Commonweal Cancer Help Program retreat as Kim and Sarah. She also wanted to live, in the face of a difficult prognosis, but her greatest hope was that, when the time came for her life to end, she would not be an invalid in a hospital room connected to dozens of tubes. Sandra's husband had died of cancer of the liver after going through chemotherapy and prolonged hospitalization, which she believed only added to his suffering. She had a friend, a retired military doctor, who supported her desire not to undergo chemotherapy. "Let nature take its course," he counseled her. So even though chemotherapy might have extended her life, she decided *for the time being* (her decision was not irrevocable) against it. She developed a personal recovery program of nutritional supplements, herbal remedies, and Reiki healing—a kind of spiritual healing practice—which she and several friends practiced with one another on a weekly basis. But note that Sandra, too, did not give up hope. She continued to hope that she might somehow overcome this cancer and live as her parents did, into her eighties or nineties. If this was not to be, she hoped to die a death of dignity without too much suffering.

With all four of these very different people—my father, Kim and Sarah, and Sandra—hope against the odds was fundamental to the quality of their lives.

My belief is that hope is fundamental to achieving the best possible quality of life with cancer. I also happen to believe, although I cannot prove this to be true, that hope helps some people who are fighting for life to achieve life extension and, occasionally, the remission of the cancer.

Reference

1   Anthony J. Sattilaro, *Recalled by Life* (Boston: Houghton Mifflin, 1982).

Healing and Curing:
The Starting Point for Informed Choice

Healing Goes Beyond Curing

There is a fundamental distinction between healing and curing that lies at the heart of all genuinely patient-centered approaches to cancer treatment and care. This is not some "flaky" New Age distinction, but one rooted in the greatest and oldest continuous traditions of medicine. It is a distinction yet to be fully recognized and honored in mainstream American medicine today. But while the distinction between curing and healing is widely recognized, the *significance* of these two complementary approaches to recovery from cancer is rarely explained to people with cancer.

As the term is generally used, a *cure* is a successful medical *treatment*. In other words, a cure is a treatment that removes all evidence of the disease and allows the person who previously had cancer to live as long as he would have lived without cancer. A cure is what the physician hopes to bring to the patient. Curing is what the doctors hope to do, the external medical process of effecting an outcome in which the disease disappears.[1]

Healing, in contrast, is an inner process through which a person becomes whole. Healing can take place at the physical level, as when a wound or broken bone heals. It can take place at an emotional level, as when we recover from terrible childhood traumas or from a death or a divorce. It can take place at a mental level, as when we learn to reframe or restructure destructive ideas about ourselves and the world that we carried in the past. And it can take place at what some would call a spiritual level, as when we move toward God, toward a deeper connection with nature, or toward inner peace and a sense of connectedness.

Although curing and healing are different, they are deeply entwined. For any cure to work, the physical healing power of the organism must be sufficient to enable recovery to take place. When a physician sets a bone or prescribes an antibiotic for an infection, he is doing his part for recovery by offering curative therapy. Yet when the inner healing power of the organism is insufficiently strong, the bone will not knit or the infection will not subside. Healing is thus a *necessary* part of curing—a fact with profound implications for medicine, since the authentically holistic physician is deeply aware of the essential role his patient's recuperative powers play and will do everything he can to encourage the patient to enhance those recuperative powers.

Healing, however, goes beyond curing and may take place when curing is not at issue or has proved impossible. Although the capacity to heal physically is necessary to any successful cure, healing can also take place on deeper levels whether or not physical recovery occurs. I have had many friends with cancer for whom curative treatment ultimately proved impossible. Yet, even as their disease progressed, the inner healing process—emotional, mental, and spiritual—was astonishingly powerful in their own lives and in those of their families and friends.

That you *can* participate in the fight for life with cancer—by working to enhance your own healing and recuperative resources—is a profoundly important discovery for many people. Cancer patients often experience themselves as losing all control of their lives. They become the passive objects of all kinds of decisions and treatments by their medical teams. They feel they must do what their physicians tell them. They may feel that they can do nothing to help themselves. Often, no one has offered them the opportunity to consider the distinction between healing and curing.

It is not yet known *scientifically* how much difference personal efforts at healing can mean in terms of *life extension*. However, it is *clinically* known by most psychotherapists who work with cancer that a patient engaged in personal healing work can make a transformative difference in his *quality of life*. An ever-increasing body of scientific evidence now suggests that a strong desire to live—a willingness to engage in the struggle for life—and a continuous movement toward a healthy relationship with life, do help some people in their fight for physical recovery. Conversely, long-term chronic depression, hopelessness, cynicism, and similar characteristics tend to diminish resilience and increase physical vulnerability.

Interestingly, the successful fight for life is not necessarily waged best by the person with an excessive attachment to the outcome. As we shall see, the shamans in traditional systems of medicine around the world found that if they sought first to safeguard the soul, rather than the body, the body tended to respond better. Similarly, a boxer who is angry at his opponent is usually less skillful and more likely to lose the fight. Surgeons do not operate on their wives or children because they know that their attachment to the outcome would lessen their skills. Soldiers in desperate battlefield situations know that to be trapped in fear of death may doom them: they need clear heads, courage, and hope, against all odds, to survive.

In Europe, mountain climbing stories have been meticulously collected from climbers who survived life-threatening falls, and these stories may illustrate the complexity of the healing response. As the fall begins, the climber does not scream as falling people do in the movies. Instead, time slows down enormously—as it does for many people just before a car accident. Everything seems to be taking place in slow motion. The survival benefit of this slowing down of time is that the falling climber has every opportunity to notice lifesaving possibilities—handholds or shrubs that might be grasped to break the fall. But if the opportunities for active self-preservation disappear, the faller then enters a state not of panic but of deep peace. He may experience the often-reported process of life recall, with his life flashing back before his eyes. He may hear celestial music. Hitting the ground is usually experienced without pain—he only hears the impact. Hearing is the last sense to disappear into unconsciousness.

By analogy, the healing response that takes place as we go into the "free fall" of a cancer diagnosis seeks every opportunity to maximize the possibilities for physical life recovery. Intelligence and intuition may be brought together in choices of treatment, hospital, doctor, and of complementary therapies or the paths of self-exploration, health promotion, and self-care. The very process that maximizes the opportunities to recover also prepares us to make the best of a long life with cancer, or the best use of whatever time we have available.

Thus the starting point for informed choice in both mainstream and complementary cancer therapies is the patient's recognition that he can play a crucial role in the fight for his life. The recognition of the unique role that each of us can play in our own healing reaches beyond choices about therapy to choices about how we intend to live each day for the rest of our lives.

Universal, Common, and Unique Conditions of Healing

How do we set about healing ourselves? One of the best analogies Rachel Naomi Remen, M.D., uses is that of becoming a gardener of ourselves. We cannot grow ourselves in our garden by simple, direct volition. But we can create the conditions of growth, or the *conditions of healing,* by nourishing, nurturing, and tending within us that which we value and wish to help grow.

Obviously, there are many different kinds of conditions for healing: physical conditions such as diet, exercise, relaxation, clean air, good water, and time spent in nature; social conditions for healing, such as work that is meaningful, friends that you care about, and a loving family; and emotional, mental, and spiritual conditions.

It is useful to differentiate between universal, common, and unique conditions of healing. For example, inner peace is an almost universal condition of healing. A deep experience of love is also almost universally healing. (By contrast, anger or hate is a less common condition of healing; yet there are those cases of people who have recovered physically from the most life-threatening conditions out of an intense desire for revenge or sheer negative cussedness—the "too mean to die" phenomenon.)

There are many common conditions of healing. Many of us are healed by attention and care from our friends and family, by finding work that we deeply enjoy, by laughter, by music that moves us, by great art. But some of the most important conditions of healing are the *unique* conditions of healing. William Blake said that any man who would help another must do so in "minute particulars." He was talking about helping another person by assisting him in the minute particulars—the unique way—that is most meaningful to him.

One of my favorite experiences of the discovery of a *unique* condition of healing was with a renowned elderly pediatrician—whom I will call William Sawyer—who attended the Commonweal Cancer Help Program with advanced prostate cancer after his wife had died a very difficult death with amyotrophic lateral sclerosis (sometimes called "Lou Gehrig's disease"). He had nursed her throughout her illness, and had developed cancer while she was ill. Rather than have the curative surgery that was available to him during his wife's final months, which would have required that he leave his wife alone, Bill chose palliative treatment so that he could be with her. After his wife died and his cancer spread, he flew across the country to attend our Cancer Help Program.

Bill made it very clear to us that he was not at all certain why he had come to Commonweal. Others, he said, wanted to live. He was not sure he did. Although he had never believed in life after death before, since his wife had died he had an increasing sense that he would join her when he died. And he looked forward to that prospect. It was not, he said, his cancer that distressed him. It was his depression over his wife's death.

I had no inclination to try to talk him out of his authentic experience of grief and his sober encounter with reality. So I spent the week with him listening. Listening, by the way, is one of the greatest ways we can help others heal—one of the greatest ways to create conditions of healing. Most people back away from great pain that others are suffering, or rush in with suggestions for how to "fix it." At Commonweal, we do not back away and we do not try to fix it. We listen.

I acknowledged the truth of what Bill was telling me. But since he was alive for the time being, I wondered what gave him any kind of enjoyment. And Bill began to talk about the birds that he fed outside his home in rural Massachusetts. He loved birds deeply. He had also always loved cats—he had a special capacity to communicate with cats. I asked if he had a cat. No, he said, he did not have a cat because if he got a cat he would worry about what would happen to the cat if he went into the hospital or if he died.

So Bill and I spent the rest of the week working on whether or not he could have a cat. I said that I would help find people to take care of the cat if he went into the hospital. I said that I would be honored to take his cat if he died. Since my wife liked Siamese cats, I suggested that perhaps we should get him a Siamese that we might inherit one day. But Bill did not want a Siamese cat. He had taken care of poor, forgotten, and mistreated children all of his life. What he wanted was to go to the ASPCA and get a cat that had been abandoned—perhaps hurt—and nurse it back to health.

Bill left at the end of the week and went home. A few weeks later I got a call. Bill had found a mongrel kitten at the ASPCA that had been thrown from a moving car and had broken many bones. He was now nursing it back to health. At regular intervals until Bill's death we received cards and letters signed "William and the Cat."

I tell Bill's story because it is a perfect example of a person with cancer who needed to discover for himself a *unique* condition of healing. We could have talked to Bill forever about diet, exercise, imagery, and other common conditions of healing that have, in fact, been relevant for many other people on the Cancer Help Program. We could have urged him to fight for his physical recovery. If we had, we would have missed completely the opportunity to help him find his true condition for healing: giving himself permission to have a cat. But note that not just any cat would do. He had to rescue a wounded and abandoned cat, as he had helped rescue wounded and abandoned children all of his life. It was a way that he could continue to express the love in his great heart, a way that he could continue to give.

One day years later Rachel Naomi Remen remarked to me that Bill's struggle over whether or not he could have a cat might have had a deeper significance. He might have been struggling, she suggested, with whether he was permitted to love again. Here was a man who had lost a wife whom he had deeply loved for many decades. He did not seek another wife, but he did seek another companion with whom he had deep communication.

Although his struggle with cancer continued, reinforced by many other ailments of old age, Bill lived on for many years. And through the struggle, the company of a cat that he rescued and nursed back to health remained a deep source of solace.

Biomedicine and Biopsychosocial Medicine

Cancer patients should be aware that a great debate is now taking place today as to what role, if any, modern medicine should play in helping patients with their healing processes.

On one side of this debate are proponents of biomedicine, who honestly and straightforwardly believe that the physician-scientist is a technician who should offer the patient his technical skills, and stay out of psychological and spiritual issues. This is a clean and reasonable position, not to be mocked.

On the other side of the debate are proponents of what George Engle has named "biopsychosocial" medicine. Biopsychosocial medicine recognizes that disease takes place in a psychological and social context, that these psychosocial contexts influence both the cause and the course of many diseases, and that the physician interested in the most effective curative processes must also be concerned with healing in the psychosocial context.[2]

Professional interest in biopsychosocial medicine has grown over the past few decades as popular and professional interest has increased in "mind-body" medicine and such emerging scientific disciplines as psychoneuroimmunology. Psychoneuroimmunology is an interdisciplinary field of study that proposes that the mind, the neurological system, and the immune system are a deeply interrelated single system. In psychoneuroimmunology and allied fields of behavioral medicine and health psychology, a growing body of research has indicated that it often *matters* to the physical course of disease what is happening in the emotional and mental processes of the patient. Hence George Engle, Norman Cousins, and numerous others have argued that the physician truly *ought* to concern himself with healing as well as curing.

Further thought about the distinction between biomedicine and biopsychosocial medicine has led to distinctions that can be genuinely useful for the cancer patient. Consider the following relationships:

Biomedicine (Science)	Biopsychosocial Medicine (Human Experience)
Disease	Illness
Pain	Suffering
Curing	Healing

Biomedicine is legitimately concerned with the physical processes of *disease.* Biopsychosocial medicine is concerned both with the physical process of *disease* and with the *human experience of disease,* which is *illness.*

Biomedicine is legitimately concerned with the relief of *pain.* Biopsychosocial medicine is concerned with the relief of *pain* but also with the *human experience of pain,* which is *suffering.*

Biomedicine is legitimately concerned with the physiological process of *curing.* Biopsychosocial medicine is concerned with physiological process of *curing* but also with *the human experience of whatever is physically, mentally, emotionally, and spiritually possible in the face of illness,* which is *healing.*

It is very important—and not adequately considered in the popular cancer literature—that medicine has a language that distinguishes biomedicine from biopsychosocial medicine, disease from illness, pain from suffering, and curing from healing. Within the vast biomedical-industrial complex that modern society has created, it is worth knowing that many great physicians have thought long and hard about these issues, and recognize that our modern sophistication with biomedical technology is matched on the negative side by an often shocking lack of sophistication or interest in helping patients become aware of and participate in their own healing process.

How to Begin Your Own Healing

How can you participate in your own healing process? Many great physicians and healers through the ages have given this question a great deal of thought, and have produced many answers—answers that usually take the form of questions. Here are a few:

> *If you could do (or be) absolutely anything in the world that you wanted during the rest of your life,* what would you truly want to do (or be)?

This is the question that the pioneering psychotherapist Larry LeShan asks in *Cancer as a Turning Point.* "What is the unique purpose of your life, the unique song that you were put on earth to sing?," LeShan often asks. Some people know the answer instantly. Others discover it after a time of living with the question. Still others have to work long and hard for the answer. It is a great question, and a great guide on the path to healing, for if you discover the answer, LeShan's next question is: "Under the present circumstances, what would be the first steps you need to take to begin moving toward living this life?" Embarking on this path can bring great healing.

Another such question might be:

> *Since you have been diagnosed with cancer, what do you find has become important to you, and what that previously seemed important do you discover you are ready to let go?*

A cancer diagnosis can thus lead to a profound transformation of values. Things that used to seem important often become less salient, while other values to which you may have given little thought take priority. This sorting process can go on throughout your life—What do I want to hold on to? What do I choose to let go of? and, more painfully, What that I care about am I able to hold onto? What that I care about do I need to let go of?

You might also ask yourself:

> *Within the circumstances of the cancer diagnosis, what would I optimally choose in every area of my current life? What kind of mainstream and complementary therapies should I undertake? What kind of relationships? What kind of work? What forms of relaxation or meditation? What forms of exercise or recreation? What kind of diet? What rhythms of daily life? What studies or activities? What kinds of support and response do I want from family and friends? What are some of the unique things—very personal to me—that would give me special delight and pleasure each day?*

This is an exercise in making yourself aware of what feels authentic to you. It is surprising how many people with cancer have never given much thought to what *they* would actually like. Clinicians often report the impression that many cancer patients have been "givers" for much of their lives, subordinating awareness of their own needs to awareness of the needs of others. Learning to be aware of and to articulate what *you* would like can sometimes be a new and even frightening prospect. But discovering the little (and big) activities that give you special pleasure is both fulfilling and healing. One way of exploring this question is to divide your life into different areas of inquiry. What are the specific physical, emotional, mental, and spiritual conditions that could support healing for you?

Healing and Psychosynthesis

For cancer patients who want a more explicit map of the human psyche, one of the most interesting schools of transpersonal psychology is psychosynthesis. Founded by an Italian psychoanalyst, Roberto Assagioli, who had studied with both Jung and Freud and who was a close student of Eastern as well as Western spiritual traditions, psychosynthesis offers some helpful perspectives on the nature of healing.

Psychosynthesis recognizes with Freud that many people struggle with impulses coming up from their lower unconscious—impulses related to basic drives and appetites. But it also recognizes with Jung that some people also struggle with repressed impulses from their upper unconscious, or superconscious, and that one can be as neurotically miserable seeking to be *less than one is* in order to conform as one can be seeking to be *more than one is* in order to conform.

Psychosynthesis convincingly organizes much of our experience of the world into various personality substructures it calls "subpersonalities." Most people are able, if asked, to make a list of at least some of the subpersonalities that we unconsciously move in and out of all day. A typical list of subpersonality structures of a professional woman with cancer might include physician, mother, wife, daughter, friend, cancer patient, jogger, spiritual seeker, frustrated circus performer, etc.

The goals of psychosynthesis include becoming aware of the various subpersonalities, acknowledging that they are part of us, learning to *identify* and *disidentify* with them—how to step in and out of each subpersonality—and then gradually to synthesize and integrate them. The relevance of this to a cancer patient is that, if healing is a process of self-discovery, a process of becoming aware of and interested in our own process of self-actualization, then psychosynthesis provides one interesting map for coming to know ourselves.

I have described healing as a process of becoming whole on many different levels through increasing awareness of the conditions of self-actualization and personal evolution.

Imagery, Rachel Naomi Remen says, is the language that the unconscious speaks in its efforts to communicate with us. Imagery is an extraordinarily powerful tool for communicating with the vast universe within ourselves that we are not aware of in ordinary states of consciousness. Imagery takes many forms: visual, tactile, olfactory, intuitive. We can see, feel, sense, touch, smell, or intuit a communication from within. We can discover imagery through meditation, prayer, hypnotherapy, guided imagery techniques, art, poetry, dreams, journal writing, music, or movement, to name only a few of the methods.

People with cancer often have very potent imagery close to the surface of consciousness. The enormous upheavals in their lives have brought this material into a range of ready access. Yet they may live for months or years without communicating with these extraordinarily powerful constellations of experience within themselves. Getting in touch with one's inner world through imagery can be an astoundingly powerful route to healing.

Creativity is closely related to imagery. W.H. Auden wrote some famous lines about cancer, in which a country physician ruminates about how curious cancer is:

> *Childless women get it*
> *And men when they retire—*
> *It's as though they needed some outlet*
> *For that foiled creative fire.*[3]

Many cancer patients resonate to these lines, and come to experience to what a degree they had shut down their own creativity and wholeness in the service of fitting into the lives they have constructed. All the questions about finding one's unique song in life, deciding how one wants to live now, and getting in touch with powerful inner constellations of energy by imagery are processes of reconnecting with that inner creativity, that "foiled creative fire."

We are not in the land of science here—we are in the inner imagic landscape. We should *not* assume that any of the things we have said in passing about some cancer patients—that they are often "giving" people, that they may have subordinated their own needs to the needs of others, that they may have lost some contact with their own creativity—are true for all or even most cancer patients. And I surely do not mean to suggest that these characteristics *caused* the cancer. I simply want to give the reader a few key ideas about what is involved in the journey of inner healing. (I will discuss the subject of imagery further in chapter 10.)

Healing and Spirituality

The healing process not only has a tendency to bring people closer to an appreciation of who they uniquely are and what their unique purpose is in this world. It also brings them closer to God, spirit, inner peace, connectedness, or whatever we choose to call that which is great and mysterious.

The longer I have considered this fact—the fundamental connection between healing and psychological development—the more I think it one of the most remarkable signatory details left to us by the architect of human consciousness, whoever that may be. Consider how truly *elegant* the design process is that created us so that in the face of the most difficult times of our lives, there is the possibility—not the certainty but the possibility—of access to states of awareness and experience that enable us to cope with these crises better than we otherwise could. And consider how remarkable it is that these states of awareness make many people say that they feel more alive and more whole with cancer than they ever felt before. Consider how curious it is that many people come to acknowledge, in the face of the pain, shock, and suffering of cancer, that there also can be gains of immense personal value.

A central tenet of all the great spiritual traditions is that pain and suffering, loss and sorrow, carry within them keys that unlock gates of spiritual experience that often had been closed before. How extraordinary that we should be designed in this way. What does it mean? What does it imply? (I will discuss spirit and healing further in chapter 9.)

I place such emphasis on the significance of healing with cancer because I believe that awareness of the power and process of healing is the key to informed choice in all areas of cancer: choice in mainstream therapies, choice in complementary therapies, choice in life with cancer, choice in response to pain and suffering, and choice in living and dying.

There is no single *right* way to respond to any of the choices, large or small, that cancer brings. You will certainly experience pressures from physicians, family, and friends to choose one course over another. Physicians will offer you the best conventional medical wisdom about therapies. Family and friends may urge you to try alternative therapies, or conversely urge you not to try them. People may expect you to continue to live the way you did before, to continue to respond to them in the same ways. Or they may urge new ways of life on you.

At every turn there are bewildering arrays of choices, and often there is no adequate external guidance that you can count on. So when all the information is before you, consider turning inward to discover from as deep a source as possible *what makes sense to you*.

Information can help us develop maps of informed choice. But the healing process can be the inner compass by which we read these maps. Healing helps us discover "which way is up"—*for us*. Healing encourages us to move upward, toward higher and more integrated levels of awareness, toward courage, toward *expansion*—if not always toward *extension*—of life, and toward becoming more deeply the person we want to be.

Notes and References

1   Five-year cancer-free survival is often considered a "cure" with many cancers for statistical purposes, but this is a dubious use of the term. A truly "cured" cancer patient should live as long as he would have without cancer.

2   George L. Engel, "The Need for a New Medical Model: A Challenge for Biomedicine," *Science* 196:4286 (8 April 1977).

3   W.H. Auden, *Collected Shorter Poems 1927–1957* (New York: Random House, 1966), 111.

PART TWO

Choice in Conventional Cancer Therapies

More often than not, cancer patients believe that their choices for therapy are dictated by the findings of pure biomedical science. Cancer patients also tend to believe that biomedical science is a monolith—a huge body of knowledge that dictates what an individual must do with a specific kind of cancer—and that all the information generated by this monolithic science is funneled into the brains of the first physicians they consult. Neither belief is accurate.

Physicians are not handicapped by these illusions when members of their own families develop cancer. Characteristically they get several opinions from different physicians before they make a choice of treatments. What the physician knows—and what is rarely articulated to the cancer patient—is that there are markedly different *cultures of cancer therapy* within mainstream American medicine. With the word "culture" I refer to the nonscientific assumptions and approaches that physicians bring to the design, direction, and emphasis of cancer treatment.

There are very different cultures of mainstream cancer therapy at the international, national, and professional specialty levels. To make a sound decision on treatment, the cancer patient needs to understand the different approaches undertaken by these cultures. Such knowledge helps cancer patients create a comprehensible *map* of choice in cancer treatment. Mapping cultures of choice in cancer is a powerful antidote to anxiety about what appears to be a bewildering array of treatment options. We can identify three principal cultures of cancer therapy, each with its own set of options:

1. Cancer therapy within mainstream American medicine. Large differences in treatment exist between surgeons, oncologists, and radiation therapists, with each group naturally tending to favor the contribution of its own specialty.
2. Cancer therapy among complementary approaches to cancer, both in the United States and abroad: treatment varies widely among the practitioners of nutritional therapies, practitioners of psychological approaches, and practitioners of immunological approaches to cancer, to name just a few of these subcultures. (I discuss this area in later chapters.)
3. Cancer therapy among advanced technological-industrial societies. Remarkable differences exist in the way cancer is treated in England, in France, in Germany, in Japan, and in the United States.

The key point is how profoundly culture affects *all* approaches—even bio-medical systems of cancer treatment. In this section, I explore the choices available to cancer patients within mainstream American medicine. But cancer patients should know that many physicians and scientists in other technologically advanced nations regard American cancer therapy as extraordinarily *aggressive,* using surgery, chemotherapy, and radiation therapy far more extensively than physicians and researchers abroad believe the evidence warrants.

Our exploration begins, therefore, with international differences in the treatment of cancer, and then in chapters 4 and 5, we turn to the options and choices in mainstream American treatment. In these chapters, I mean to draw your attention to three main points: that American cancer treatments are generally at the "aggressive" end of mainstream cancer care when looked at from an international perspective; that within the community of conventional cancer care, there is an intense debate about the gains achieved through chemotherapy and radiation therapy; and that there are important "cultural" differences among different medical specialties and the treatments offered by different types of hospitals in the United States.

three

The Crucial Difference: International Variations in Conventional Cancer Therapies

One of the most important pieces of medical information for cancer patients seeking to make truly informed choices among cancer therapies is the high level of variation in the cancer therapies offered by physicians in the different advanced industrial nations. *Mainstream cancer therapies differ profoundly in England, France, Germany, Japan, and the United States.* Cancer patients should let the significance of this fact sink in. It is not some abstract finding by medical sociologists.

These five nations are all advanced scientific societies. The physicians in each country have access to the same world scientific literature. Yet in each country, doctors treat cancer patients very differently. And *American* cancer medicine stands out among the rest in one key respect: cancer therapy in America is *consistently the most aggressive.* This chapter traces the strong evidence that the differences in conventional cancer therapies in advanced industrial nations reflect *cultural beliefs* more than *scientific certainties.* Understanding these facts is a crucial step in a cancer patient's journey to genuine informed choice.

Lynn Payer, a leading medical journalist, has written a book, *Medicine & Culture: Varieties of Treatment in the United States, England, West Germany, and France*[1] that provides the best single guide to the international cultures of medicine in the United States and Europe. Much of this chapter draws directly on her research. Mark Lipkin, Jr., M.D., director of primary care at New York University School of Medicine, says that Payer's work "forcefully documents that while practitioners regard themselves as the servants of science, they are often prisoners of belief and custom. . . . This [book] will inspire patients *to examine and trust their own experience and preferences even if they must go beyond their national borders to see what is possible* [emphasis added]."[2]

Scientific findings in medicine, Payer argues, are necessarily *evaluated* in different countries through different cultural prisms:

> Consider, for example, a study that shows that giving chemotherapy to elderly patients with cancer prolongs their lives by an average of a few months but also causes them severe, intractable, drug-induced vomiting. [*Not* true for *all* chemotherapies.] If one believes that length of life is the most important criterion, this study would indicate that such patients should be given chemotherapy; if one believes quality of life is more important it might indicate that chemotherapy should not be given.

> In fact, the American authors of this particular paper felt the added months justified a recommendation of chemotherapy; Englishmen who commented on it in the *BMJ [British Medical Journal]* felt this recommendation was off base. *In neither commentary did the authors recommend that patients be asked how they felt about the matter* [emphasis added].[3]

French Aesthetics and the Preservation of Sexual Organs

Payer was first deeply impressed by the role of culture in medicine at a meeting in Strasbourg, France, in 1972 on nonmutilating treatments for breast cancer.

> The meeting got off to a roaring start with its organizer, Professor Charles Gros, giving a slide show on the breast and breast cancer in the history of art, referring to the breast as "man's pleasure" and "woman's narcissism." The exhibitors seemed to enjoy the theme—there were breasts everywhere in the exhibition area, including one entire wall of plastic breasts so pointed it seemed that anyone who accidentally pushed against it would receive major puncture wounds. By the third day everyone was booing slides that showed a bad cosmetic result, which seemed as appropriate a response as any in that setting.[4]

French medical culture, Payer goes on to show, is deeply influenced by the French admiration for thought as a guide to action; a deep concern with the aesthetics of the human body; a strong commitment to the preservation of sexual organs and fertility wherever possible; an obsession with the role of the liver in health; a strong belief in the importance of the vitality of the inner *terrain* in repulsing illness and the value of "inoculating" exposure to dirt as a way of keeping the *terrain* robust; and a national commitment to holidays and health spas as ways of rejuvenating the *terrain* and sustaining health.

As a result of this perspective, the French moved toward lumpectomies and partial mastectomies in breast cancer long before the Americans. Says Payer: "Men, too, are likely to find their sexual and reproductive organs are treated more gently in France than elsewhere. In the United States, for example, cancer of the prostate is often treated by prostatectomy and castration. In France, it is more likely to be treated by radiation therapy and low-dose estrogens or chemotherapy instead of castration."[5]

The French concern with aesthetic outcomes was shared, one French physician told Payer, by patients from other Latin countries: "The Latin patients seem to feel that they are not whole as a person after amputation of a hand or a finger," the physician told her. "It is important for them to have a complete body. But people from the northern countries don't have the same feelings. They are more interested in being functional than aesthetically pleasing."[6]

The French have a deep concern with the *terrain*—with the vitality of the inner field of the body—a belief that "skews consumption away from antibiotics, which fit the English and American concept of disease as invader, toward tonics, vitamins, and 'modifiers of the *terrain*'. . . . It favors treatments such as rest and stays at France's spas as ways to build up the *terrain*. . . . It makes the French leaders in fields that concentrate on shoring up the *terrain,* such as immunotherapy for cancer."[7] "If the *terrain* is more important than the disease, it becomes less important to fight the disease 'aggressively' and more important to shore up the *terrain*. While American doctors love to use the word 'aggressive,' the French much prefer *les médecines douces,* or 'gentle therapies.'"[8]

This preference for gentle therapies leads the French into much wider use of nonallopathic medicines, notably homeopathy, in which infinitesimally dilute remedies are believed to be increasingly potent as the dilution becomes greater. The French also generally use lower doses of mainstream drugs. "Even the strongest types of drugs may be weaker in France," says Payer. "The shah of Iran was prescribed chlorambucil for his cancer by his French doctors, and Americans were surprised that he had not been given a stronger drug. . . . A belief in the *terrain* also undoubtedly plays a role in the fact that fewer invasive procedures are used in intensive care units in France than in the United States—with patients doing equally well in both countries."[9]

Germany: An Open Medical System with Strong Conventional and Complementary Medical Traditions

Germany is one of the great innovators in the field of alternative and adjunctive approaches to cancer, with strong traditions of naturopathic, herbal, homeopathic, and spiritual approaches to medical care. German cancer patients have, perhaps, a wider choice of cancer therapies than patients in any other modern industrialized country.

While the French are obsessed with the state of their livers, the aesthetic shape of their bodies, and the vitality of the inner *terrain,* the Germans are obsessed with their hearts, both physically and spiritually. Payer quotes Novalis: "The heart is the key to the world." And Goethe: "He seems to value my mind and my various talents more than this heart of mine, of which I am so proud, for it is the source of all things—all strength, all bliss, all misery. The things I know, every man can know, but, oh, my heart is mine alone!"[10]

West Germans use six times as many heart drugs per capita as the French and the English. And while outsiders see Germans primarily as authoritarian and efficient, "Germans themselves tend to see their chief characteristic as emotionalism." Says Payer:

> The West German health care system accommodates both the efficient and the romantic aspects of the German character by including both high-tech medicine, such as electrocardiograms and CAT scanners, and "soft" medicine based on the healing power of nature, such as homeopathy and spas. The West German health care system, in fact, accommodates practically everything. . . . "There are 120,000 different drugs on the market in Germany," Dr. M.N.G. Dukes, then of the Dutch drug regulatory agency, informed me when I interviewed him, "as compared to 1,180 in Iceland. . . ."[11]

Still another legacy of romanticism to German medicine is the healing power accorded to nature, whether it be in the form of long walks in the forest, mud baths, or herbal medicine.

The medical use of spas is even more widespread than in France, and plants are more widely used for their healing powers. . . . About one fifth of German M.D.'s practice either homeopathy or anthroposophic medicine, as well as *Phytotherapie,* or plant therapy. These forms of therapy are recognized under the West German health system. . . . Under recent drug laws, *the alternative medicines will have to be shown to be harmless, but there is no requirement that they be shown to be effective, and their continued use will be decided by commissions composed of practitioners of the particular alternative therapies* [emphasis added] . . .[12]

The contrast with American medicine is obvious. In the United States, in theory, new medicines must be proved both safe and effective. In practice, however, there are many controversies over how well this system works. On the one hand, the American system offers considerable protection that Germans do not have against ineffective and sometimes tragically unsafe medicines such as thalidomide. On the other hand, the German cancer patient has extraordinary access to a wide range of cancer therapies that Americans can only explore by traveling to Germany. The German physician, moreover, has authority to use a wide range of cancer drugs in his medical practice, is easily reimbursed for this wide-open medical practice, and can follow clinically the effectiveness of innovative drugs in his practice.

Nowhere, perhaps, is the beauty of German cancer medicine more visible than in its anthroposophical hospitals. Briefly, anthroposophy is a tradition founded by the Austrian philosopher Rudolf Steiner, a Christian mystic, philosophical follower of Goethe, and a student of Eastern, as well as Western, spiritual traditions, which has deep roots in central European folk medicine. Steiner's followers created a network of schools, hospitals, and homes for the elderly and the retarded throughout Europe and the United States. In America, anthroposophy is best known for its "Waldorf schools" for children.

The anthroposophical hospitals I visited in Germany and Switzerland combine an efficient and effective use of conventional medicine for cancer with intensive use of naturopathic, homeopathic, and anthroposophical remedies. The anthroposophical hospitals are widely known and admired in Germany, and are frequently used by Germans with life-threatening cancer diagnoses. The hospitals are aesthetically beautiful; there is a strong emphasis on treatments that will enable the patient to make the best possible use of his life; and nursing and medical care are strikingly humane by American standards.

Great Britain: Economy, Empiricism, and Freedom for Complementary Medicines

At the Strasbourg meeting on breast cancer that Payer attended

> . . . one of the British surgeons present pointed out that lumpectomy would tend to be favored by British surgeons for a reason other than its aesthetic results: it's an easier operation. While an American or French surgeon gets more money for more difficult operations, and would therefore be better paid for performing a radical mastectomy than a lumpectomy, the British surgeon receives the same salary no matter how he treats the disease.

Payer continues:

> The most striking characteristic of British medicine is its economy. The British do less of nearly everything. . . . Should the doctor decide that surgery is necessary, the surgery itself will probably be less extensive: there will be no lymph node dissection for testicular cancer, for example, which Professor Michael Baum of King's College Hospital referred to as "an antique, barbarous custom."[13]

While the French pride themselves on the scope and brilliance of their medical thinking, and take a special pride in the aesthetics and vitality of the body, the English, Payer finds, come from an empirical tradition of focus on details, a public school tradition that taught denial of the body, and a stoic "stiff upper lip" tradition that accustomed them to minimalist medical interventions. "Compared to the French and the Germans," she says, "the English deemphasize *terrain,* preferring to place the cause of disease outside their body, or, failing that, in the intermediate position of their bowels. Unlike the French, British doctors do not seem to believe much in building up the resistance, and there is almost a total lack of prescription of vitamins, tonics, cures at a spa, etc."[14]

While the British spend a little more than *half* of what Americans spend on health care, their emphasis is more on relieving and comforting than on cure.

Britain is generally recognized to be ten to fifteen years ahead of Canada and the United States in geriatric medicine. . . . Kindness can also be seen in the different interpretation often given to medical studies by the English. Not only are they more skeptical about whether medical treatment is actually doing any good; they are more sensitive to the "soft" side effects that may affect a patient's quality of life more than the hard ones. . . . A British reviewer of a book on cancer chemotherapy noted that in the six hundred-page book there "is too much uncritical listing of drugs found to be 'active' (this so-called activity sometimes achieving very little of real benefit to the patient) and too little discussion of what side effects may mean to the patient and his family, especially psychological effects. The quality of life is hardly mentioned."

The lesser belief in medicine's ability to prolong life and the greater belief in medicine's role in making life nicer are undoubtedly the reason that hospices for the dying grew up first in Britain, not in America. To accept the idea of hospice, one must accept the fact that people die. [Wrote one physician], "in the UK we strive less officiously to keep alive. This is not callousness but stems from a different attitude toward death. American physicians seem to regard death as the ultimate failure of their skill. British doctors frequently regard death as physiological, sometimes even devoutly to be wished."[15]

While Payer restricted her study to conventional medicine, Britain is also characterized in the field of complementary therapies by strong traditions of vegetarianism, naturopathic medicine, homeopathy (which she mentions), spiritual healing, and a social tolerance that far exceeds that in the United States for the practice of these and other alternative approaches to cancer.

The United States: An Aggressive Culture and an Aggressive Medicine

"Even as Europeans were developing the simple mastectomy and the lumpectomy as less mutilating ways to treat breast cancer," Payer writes, "American doctors were advocating the superradical mastectomy and prophylactic removal of both breasts to prevent breast cancer."

American medicine is aggressive. From birth—which is more likely to be by cesarean than anywhere in Europe—to death in the hospital, from invasive examination to prophylactic surgery, American doctors want to *do* something, preferably as much as possible. . . .

American doctors perform more diagnostic tests than doctors in France, West Germany, or England. They often eschew drug treatment in favor of aggressive surgery, but if they do use drugs they are likely to use higher doses and more aggressive drugs. . . .

Surgery, too, besides being performed more often, is likely to be more aggressive when it is performed. This seems to be particularly true when surgery on or near the sex organs is performed. An American woman has two to three times the chance of having a hysterectomy as her counterpart in England, France, or West Germany, and foreign doctors joke about American "birthday hysterectomies," perhaps without realizing how young the birthday is: over 60% of hysterectomies in the United States are performed in women under forty-four. Besides the policy of some doctors of taking out uteruses routinely in healthy women around the age of forty, often with removal of the ovaries, too, a policy approved by the 1975 edition in one of the leading gynecologic textbooks, many U.S. doctors consider hysterectomy the treatment for many precancerous conditions treated less radically in Europe. When cancer is found, the surgery will be more radical. Prostate surgery will be performed more often than in Europe . . . on both younger and older men.[16]

Payer suggests that this medical aggressiveness reflects the aggressiveness of the American character, and my observations in medicine and in other fields of American endeavor suggest that she is right. Aggressive action is part of the American ethos: football is the most aggressive of national sports; the rate of violent crime is far higher in America than in any of the other industrial democracies; and the rate of incarceration of Americans far exceeds that of any other industrial democracy, rivaling those of the former Soviet Union and the Union of South Africa. Nor does the violence come only from the high violent crime rate of the American underclass. The existence of the underclass reflects American social policies that are startlingly less supportive of its citizens than those of any of the other industrial democracies. In medical insurance, in education, in pregnancy benefits and leave, in job training or retraining, in housing, and in virtually every other field except higher education, the United States does less to take care of its citizens than any other advanced industrial democracy. From the European perspective, much of our foreign policy mirrors the aggressiveness and the "cowboy" mentality that they see reflected in so many aspects of American life.

This is not to say that Europeans are entirely critical of American culture. Many Europeans feel hemmed in by their population densities and the myriad regulations that go hand in hand with their strong systems of social support. They are fascinated by the freedom they see in American society, by a culture where people are free to make or lose everything, and where life seems to take place on a dangerous high wire without a safety net.

But the main point here is that, from the perspective of most educated Europeans, the aggressiveness of American medicine in general, and American cancer medicine in particular, is a perfect reflection of one of the major themes in American culture and the American national character. So they would be loathe to accept automatically an American oncologist's recommendation of an aggressive course of therapy without comparing these recommendations with those of a cancer specialist at home. And they would also see the trend toward even more aggressive therapies in experimental cancer research as a further expression of this American obsession.

Payer traces aggressiveness in American medicine back to Benjamin Rush, physician and signer of the Declaration of Independence, who opposed an "undue reliance upon the powers of nature in curing disease." The early medical texts echoed Rush with observations that "desperate diseases require desperate remedies" and that "mildness of medical treatment is real cruelty."[17] Incidentally, these are explicitly the views of the mainstream of American oncologists today.

According to Payer, this aggressiveness in medicine was found in surgery, where "frontier surgeons" pioneered radical operations "which, they bragged, Europeans had been too sensitive and timid to perform. . . . American surgeons attributed their successes in part to a frontier stoicism lacking in effete Old World practitioners; European critics denounced the American practice as an example of frontier barbarism and cruelty."[18]

It is not difficult to argue that the aggressiveness of American medicine has found its purest expression in cancer therapy. However, some elements of aggressiveness in cancer therapy have peaked. The hemicorporectomies of the 1950s, pioneered in the United States, in which patients were cut in half to save their lives, are no longer performed. Radical mastectomies in general have given way to less radical surgeries for breast cancer. As a clinical and research issue in cancer, a greater interest is arising in quality of life, and an increasing number of studies compare shorter chemotherapy treatments with older and more arduous ones.

So the picture is complex. But, at the same time that some of the most aggressive approaches to cancer have peaked or begun to subside, other extraordinarily aggressive treatments have arisen to take their place. The growing application of bone marrow transplants together with total body irradiation is an example. This is a set of procedures in which the patient is given a combination of therapies that are essentially lethal, and then aggressive efforts at rescue are made.

I am not passing judgment on the efficacy of the quintessential American aggressiveness in cancer therapy. Aggressive therapies can undoubtedly save lives in some cases. But I have found an international perspective on cancer treatment to be of real value to thoughtful patients seeking to evaluate their options.

Cancer in Japan: The Denial of Cancer, Germ Phobia, Constitutional Theories of Causation, and the Alliance of Conventional and Complementary Medicine

Cancer patients in Japan are rarely told of their diagnosis by their physician. The physician, instead, tells the family, which decides whether or not to tell the patient and, in most cases, elects not to. A leading Japanese physician explains: "Human beings react very strongly to the notion of death. We should let the patients spend the rest of their short lives without anxiety; we therefore should not inform the patient of the cancer verdict." This particular doctor sees the American practice of telling cancer patients their diagnosis as caused largely by the American physicians' fear of malpractice suits.[19]

Even when medical school faculty members develop cancer, their colleagues do not give them the diagnosis. Moreover, patients at the National Center for Cancer Research in Tokyo and at regional cancer centers are not told. Emiko Ohnuki-Tierney recounts: "A doctor at the National Center for Circulatory Diseases told me that patients believe that, whereas all other people there may be cancer patients, I am somehow an exception."[20]

These observations come from a gem of anthropological research by Ohnuki-Tierney, called *Illness and Culture in Contemporary Japan: An Anthropological Perspective*. As in Europe, medical pluralism is much more widely and deeply sanctioned in Japan than in the United States, so that biomedicine exists side by side with a rich array of traditional forms of health care—notably the folk medical tradition of *kanpo,* and the great religious and spiritual traditions of Shintoism, Buddhism, Confucianism, and shamanism. These traditions penetrate and deeply influence the biomedical systems of allopathic care in Japan.

Unlike the French—and like the Germans and Americans—the Japanese have a deeply phobic response to germs and dirt, but they carry it further than anyone else. When Japanese children come into the house after playing outside, they take off their shoes, wash their hands, and frequently gargle. Many Japanese adults wear a kind of surgical mask when outside, especially in winter, to protect themselves from germs. In public libraries, stickers inside book covers state, "Before and after reading, wash your hands well," and "Do not lick your finger to turn pages." *At Japan's National Institute for Cancer Research, all books returned by cancer patients are wiped with alcohol before others can use them.* Some Japanese leave used books in the sun so that sunshine will kill the germs. The Japanese are reluctant to use secondhand clothing for fear that it may carry germs.

From these and others observations, Ohnuki-Tierney builds a powerful picture of the Japanese germ theory that permeates both Japanese culture and its medical institutions. She persuasively locates this theory in the Japanese tradition of protecting the purity of inner space (the inner self or private home), while expecting and often accepting a dirty and impure exterior space (the world outside the home).

But if germs carry disease, the more fundamental cause of illness, the Japanese believe, is a series of imbalances created by changes in the weather or seasons, or by exposure to cold foods. In this view, the Japanese occupy an intermediate position between the French and German concern with the vitality of the *terrain* and the English tendency to minimize concern with the body. Essentially, the Japanese are concerned with inner vitality, but they see that vitality as being deeply affected by outer, natural influences.

At the same time, Americans see the Japanese as having amazingly little interest in the psychological factors of disease, in general, and of cancer, in particular. Instead, the Japanese see the inner cause of illness in terms of *taishitsu,* the constitution with which one was born, and *jibyo,* the "carrying illness" that goes along with this constitution and which may become acute on aggravation. As Ohnuki-Tierney points out, the focus on physical as opposed to psychological sources of illness performs a social function in "eliminating the possibility of blaming another person for misfortune."[21]

Japanese have a very high incidence of abdominal cancer, a fact that is generally attributed to certain aspects of their diet—and there is certainly reason to believe their diet is a major contributing factor. But it is also interesting to note that "in terms of illness the greatest attention by far is given to the abdomen, including the stomach and intestines." Traditionally, the abdomen, or *hara*, is considered the seat of the soul (recall that, for Germans, it is the heart). The *haramaki* is a long piece of material traditionally wrapped around the abdomen to protect it. Ohnuki-Tierney lists many Japanese expressions that involve the abdomen: "To heal the abdomen" means to wreak one's anger on someone; "the worm in the abdomen is not satisfied" means that one is angry; "to read the abdomen" means to read someone's thoughts; and "to show the abdomen" means to be candid with someone.[22]

Kanpo, the Japanese traditional folk medicine, was introduced in Japan from China in the sixth century. It uses acupuncture and moxibustion (burning small cones of mugwort on different parts of the body), and plants and animal medicines. It was suppressed once in the nineteenth century and again by the occupation forces at the end of World War II. Today, its use is growing. Ohnuki-Tierney describes her personal experience with *kanpo*:

> Before I left for fieldwork in Japan in 1979, I was told by my gynecologist that I had multiple fibroids requiring "immediate surgery." . . . In Japan, I decided to be a participant observer and asked Dr. I [a skilled practitioner of *kanpo*] to prescribe herbs for me, although I was not a believer in *kanpo*. I took his medicine, consisting of twenty herbs, for three months. Upon my return to the United States I surprised my doctor, who found none of the fibroids. Even if we take into account other factors that may have contributed to the disappearance of the growths, it would be hard to deny the real "medical efficacy" of the treatment.[23]

Ohnuki-Tierney then goes on to report that *Dr. I rarely prescribes surgery, even with cancer, because, in his view, the shock to the body increases the imbalances and the operation may spread the cancer.*[24]

The critical point about the use of *kanpo* in Japanese medicine is that it is widely seen as *complementing* biomedicine, while in the United States, as

Ohnuki-Tierney points out, alternative medicine largely operates in opposition to biomedicine. Thus biomedicine in Japan is seen as more effective with pathogen-specific, organ-specific, and acute conditions, while *kanpo* is more effective with a wide range of chronic conditions.

Finally, a profound difference exists between the experience of illness in Japan and that in the United States. Many Japanese still choose a hospital because it is in a favorable direction from their house. The average hospital stay is 42.9 days, as compared with 8 to 16 days in the United States and Europe. The hospitalized patient wears his own nightclothes. A prominent physician told Ohnuki-Tierney that requiring hospital nightclothes would cause legal suits "against this abrogation of human rights, and it would be in all the newspapers." Family members help with the patient's care and frequently cook the meals: "One doctor stated emphatically: 'We certainly cannot expect a sick person to eat the hospital food, which is not edible even for a healthy person.'"[25]

Thus the hospitalized patient keeps his identity in many important ways, and is surrounded by a network of caring family members and friends. Says Ohnuki-Tierney,

> In the United States, where the sovereignty of the individual is sacred, the patient role ironically denies individualism, at least symbolically. . . . In sharp contrast, the patient role in Japan reinforces individual identity. . . . For both men and women, there is an implicit and sometimes explicit expectation on the part of the patient, approved by family members and doctors, that hospitalization is a form of "vacation," a reward for hard work.[26]

Is One National Approach to Cancer Better than Others?

Approaches to cancer therapy in all five countries are remarkably different from one another, and would lead to very different personal experiences of cancer. For the American cancer patient, the bottom line is that the system of cancer therapy in the United States is by far the most aggressive of any advanced technological nation. This aggressiveness cannot be attributed to science, which is equally accessible to biomedical cancer specialists in the four other countries.

Does the aggressiveness of American cancer therapy extend life for some cancer patients at an acceptable cost in terms of its effect on the quality of life? For some cancer patients, it certainly does. For others, it equally certainly does not. Very few studies accurately assess the difference in outcomes among these five nations for specific cancers. In general, there is no known difference between the efficacy of one national medicine and another.

Quite apart from the differences between nations in cancer care, it is important to realize that no other industrialized nation has separated conventional biomedicine from other practices to the extent that the United States has. In the early part of the century, biomedicine achieved an overwhelming hegemony in the United States that has effectively marginalized—and often criminalized—other systems of cancer care. In Europe and Japan, biomedicine never achieved a similar level of complete hegemony, with the result that medical pluralism flourishes more widely abroad. This means that a wider range of choices are available for cancer patients elsewhere, as well as a greater freedom for physicians to experiment with integrating therapies from different traditions, if they so choose.

References

1 Lynn Payer, *Medicine & Culture: Varieties of Treatment in the United States, England, West Germany, and France* (New York: Holt, 1988). Copyright © 1988 by Lynn Payer. Quotations reprinted by permission of Henry Holt and Co., Inc.

2 Ibid., back cover.

3 Ibid., 31.

4 Ibid., 35–6.

5 Ibid., 53.

6 Ibid., 54.

7 Ibid., 62.

8 Ibid., 65.

9 Ibid., 66.

10 Ibid., 74.

11 Ibid., 77–8.

12 Ibid., 96–7.

13 Ibid., 101–2.

14 Ibid., 118.

15 Ibid., 120–1.

16 Ibid., 124–6.

17 Ibid., 128–9.

18 Ibid., 129.

19 Emiko Ohnuki-Tierney, *Illness and Culture in Contemporary Japan: An Anthropological View* (New York: Cambridge University Press, 1984), reviewed by Michael Lerner in *Advances* 2(2):77–80 (Spring 1985). This and all following quotes are from the review.

20 Ibid., 77.

21 Ibid., 78.

22 Ibid., 78.

23 Ibid., 78.

24 Ibid., 78.

25 Ibid., 79.

26 Ibid., 79.

four

The Debate over Conventional Cancer Therapies

There is an important difference between a conventional cancer therapy that has proven efficacy in achieving cures or significant life extension at acceptable cost in terms of quality of life and a conventional therapy that does not have such a clearly superior track record. This difference, as we saw in chapter 3, is well recognized in England, where much of medical opinion is on the side of more conservative, less aggressive, and less toxic treatments. Yet even though American cancer medicine is far more aggressive, an intense debate over the efficacy of mainstream cancer treatments continues within the United States. This chapter is about that debate.

The American cancer establishment today is seriously divided between those who believe that aggressive therapies are overutilized without adequate scientific evidence and those who believe that aggressive treatments have begun to yield superior results which will be upheld by future studies, even if they have not been demonstrated effective so far.

In November 1985, an eminent Harvard researcher, John Cairns, published an article in *Scientific American* entitled "The Treatment of Diseases and the War Against Cancer." His article signaled an intensification of the ongoing debate over the efficacy of conventional cancer therapies. Cairns described how, since World War II, cancer registries have been set up in a number of American states and several nations that chart changing trends in cancer incidence and mortality. "These registries yield a rather precise picture of the natural history of cancer, and that is a necessary starting point for any discussion of treatment."

> A group of patients can be considered cured of their cancers if they die at about the same rate as the general population, which they would if, thanks to their treatment, they had been returned to the common pool. . . . The survival rate of Norwegian women who have colon cancer, for instance, has been compared with the survival rate of the general population of women. . . . Most of the patients die rather soon after diagnosis, but a sizeable minority, about 30%, die at the same rate as the general population (that is, behave as if they had been cured). . . . About a third of all Norwegian cancer patients suffered no loss of life span as a result of their disease.[1]

The Norwegian statistics, Cairns noted, came from the 1950s and 1960s: "We are looking at the results of treatment by surgery, occasionally backed up by X-irradiation when the primary tumor was inaccessible to surgery. It is the picture of what used to happen before the advent of screening programs, chemotherapy and numerous clinical trials." He notes that "the major ancillary aids to surgery, such as blood transfusions, antibiotics, and improved forms of anesthesia" had already been developed and disseminated. The deciding issue, for nearly every cancer patient, then, was "the extent of spread of the cancer at the time of surgery."[2]

Cairns explores the advantage that early screening programs had brought for cancer prevention. He found different results for different cancers. For breast cancer, he found that about a fourth of total mortality could be prevented if all women over 50 were offered a free breast examination every 1 to 3 years. For cervical cancer, while the Pap (Papanicolaou) smear, as Cairns explains, has never been fairly evaluated since it was introduced in the United States at a time when cervical cancer had begun its marked decline—"presumably because during this period the average levels of hygiene, affluence, and education have gone up"—available population comparisons indicate that "the decline in mortality from cervical cancer invariably accelerated at the time testing became widespread," although the causal connection is disputed by many authorities. For lung cancer, on the other hand, a large-scale trial of its early diagnosis "indicated that no great benefit comes from having the disease detected by chest X-rays before it has produced any symptoms. . . . To summarize, screening programs for earlier diagnosis sometimes bring benefits and sometimes do not."[3]

Cairns then turns to the subject of adjuvant therapies—hormonal therapies, x-irradiation, and chemotherapy: "It remains a depressing truth that fewer than 50 percent of cancer patients can be cured by surgery. A tremendous effort has therefore gone into discovering adjuvant forms of treatment that can be given following surgery."[4] For a number of cancers, he concludes, impressive gains have been made in the use of adjuvant therapies. Hormonal treatment has been beneficial for some cancers of the breast and prostate. And, according to the National Cancer Institute (NCI), radiation therapy has been particularly useful in the treatment of Hodgkin's disease, for which mortality has fallen 61% between 1950 and 1985, accompanied by a doubling of the 5-year survival rate. New chemotherapeutic techniques hold out the promise of even further improvements in the treatment of Hodgkin's disease in coming years.[5] Radiation treatment has also brought about improved survival in cervical cancer and in one kind of testicular cancer, and in combination with other modalities it has become one option in breast cancer.

Advances in chemotherapy have contributed to gains in overall survival rates for leukemia, from 10% for those diagnosed in the period from 1950 to 1954, to 32% for patients diagnosed between 1979 and 1984. Among the various leukemias, patients with acute lymphocytic leukemias experienced the most dramatic increase in 5-year survival, from virtually zero for those diagnosed in the period from 1950 to 1954 to a high of 54% for those diagnosed in 1977 and 1978. Five-year survival rates among children with acute lymphocytic leukemia similarly jumped 73% between 1950 and 1978. Slight declines in the survival rates in subsequent years were attributed by the NCI to the use of less aggressive therapies after the late 1970s.[6]

Most of the gains achieved by adjuvant therapies, according to Cairns, have come with cancers normally occurring in children or young adults:

> With suitable combinations of chemotherapy it is now possible to cure many kinds of childhood cancer that would otherwise be rapidly fatal . . . The reduction in the annual mortality of older children and young adults has been less spectacular, with the following notable exceptions. Hodgkin's disease used to be inevitably fatal, but now most patients can be cured. . . . About 35 percent of testicular cancers were fatal before chemotherapy, but now roughly a third of these deaths can be prevented. . . . Finally, choriocarcinoma, a rare cancer of the placenta . . . can now be cured by chemotherapy. [Most oncologists would add non-Hodgkin's lymphoma to this list of potentially chemotherapy-curable malignancies.]

Despite this improvement, Cairns nevertheless concludes that overall, "the gains [from the use of chemotherapy] have been limited." Under the age of 30, the gains have been substantial: "The latest figures for the U.S. show about 7,000 deaths per year from cancer under the age of 30, compared with the 10,000 we would have expected if the death rate had remained unchanged since the 1950s."[7]

However, and this is a key point, Cairns points out that only 2% of cancer patients in the United States are under 30. "For the vast majority of cancers, which arise in older patients, the results of chemotherapy are much more controversial. . . . Apart from the success with Hodgkin's disease, childhood leukemia and a few other cancers, *it is not possible to detect any sudden change in death rates for any of the major cancers that could be credited to chemotherapy* [emphasis added]."

> Those who organize cancer centers and supervise the many clinical trials of chemotherapy look for ways to circumvent these relentless statistics. Sometimes they explain away the unchanging statistics for mortality by pointing out that the national statistics are inevitably a few years behind the times and therefore do not reflect the most recent advances in treatment. Although this point is absolutely correct, it has been made repeatedly in the past 10 years but has never been vindicated by national statistics when these eventually became available. For the most part, however, the organizers disregard the figures for mortality and simply point out that the fraction of patients who are alive five years after diagnosis has been steadily increasing for nearly every kind of cancer. They attribute this increase in five-year survival to steady improvements in methods of treatment.[8]

Cairns explores the origins of this increase in 5-year survival, and argues that it is due to more accurate classification and not to actual treatment. In prostate cancer, for example, it turns out that a quarter of all American men who die over age 70 show, on postmortem examination, evidence of small prostate cancers, but only 10% of these cancers ever produce symptoms and a still smaller percent prove fatal. The increase in 5-year survival in prostate cancer, he finds, appears to be due largely to intensified surveillance. "The survival rate has therefore increased not because fewer men are dying from prostate cancer but because more men are being classified as having prostate cancer . . . Similar artifacts probably affect the survival rates for many other types of cancer, particularly cancer of the breast."[9]

"The role of chemotherapy in the treatment of the other major cancers of adults is much less well documented," Cairns says. Ovarian cancers sometimes respond to chemotherapy. Chemotherapy and irradiation can shrink cancers at inaccessible sites, such as certain areas of the head and neck. "Overall, however, in terms of duration of survival, the results have been more often negative than positive." Then Cairns renders his considered, powerful, and unforgettable judgment:

> In spite of these rather sobering findings several cytotoxic drugs are now commonly employed. The Connecticut Cancer Registry, for instance, reports that about a fourth of all cancer patients are recorded as having some form of chemotherapy during their initial stay in the hospital. The National Cancer Institute estimates that more than 20,000 patients receive chemotherapy in the U.S. each year. *For a dangerous and technologically exacting form of treatment these are disturbing figures, particularly since the benefit for most categories of patients has yet to be established. Furthermore, the number of patients who are cured can hardly amount to more than a few percent of those who are treated* [emphasis added].[10]

In the end, Cairns holds to his judgment. He estimates that adjuvant treatments may avert "perhaps 2% or 3% of the 400,000 deaths from cancer that occur each year in the U.S." He then puts his conclusion in a broader context:

> These are very real gains and a fitting memorial to the many thousands of patients who took part in the early trials of chemotherapy. The fortitude and altruism of these patients have not, however, been matched by any comparable sense of responsibility on the part of those who determine national policies. By the 1960s, cigarette smoking had been established as the major cause of lung cancer . . . Unfortunately, there are huge financial incentives for nations to sit back and do nothing. The cigarette is a readily taxable commodity; in the U.S. it provides the Federal government with about $6 billion a year. More important (at least for the British government, and possibly also in the eyes of the U.S. Government), smoking cuts down the bill for old age benefits because it reduces life span. At the price of a slight increase in costs for health care, the current smokers in the U.S. on the average each have saved the U.S. Government about $35,000 in Social Security payments . . . The loss of life span represents a total saving of some $10 billion a year over the next half century or so. Some countries have banned all tobacco advertising, and this has had an almost instant effect on tobacco sales. *The failure of the U.S. Government to take such a step far outweighs all the advances made in the treatment of cancer since the advent of modern surgery* [emphasis added].[11]

In conclusion, Cairns notes, "It seems bad cost-accounting for the Federal Government to subsidize chemotherapy through research and not to subsidize the screening of women for breast cancer. Worse, it is surely an act of folly to pour hundreds of millions of dollars every year into giving a growing number of patients chemotherapy while doing virtually nothing to protect the population from cigarettes."[12]

The Debate Intensifies

One would have thought that such an extensive and careful critique of cancer therapies published in *Scientific American* would receive some substantial response. That it did not says a great deal about the politics of medical and scientific journals. It was not until May 8, 1986, that a remarkably similar critique, this time published in the *New England Journal of Medicine,* initiated a major public debate. The article, "Progress Against Cancer?," was written by Cairn's Harvard colleagues John C. Bailar III and Elaine M. Smith.

There is "no evidence that some 35 years of intense and growing efforts to improve the treatment of cancer have had much overall effect on the most fundamental measure of clinical outcome—death," Smith and Bailar wrote. In fact, the age-adjusted annual rate of cancer deaths *increased* in recent decades from 170 per 100,000 in 1962 to 185 per 100,000 in 1982, an age-adjusted rise of 8.7%. "We are losing the war against cancer, notwithstanding progress against several uncommon forms of the disease, improvements in palliation and extension of productive years of life." The authors conclude: "Some thirty-five years of intense effort focused largely on improving treatment must be judged a qualified failure."[13]

The Bailar and Smith article provoked a tremendous scientific and public debate. Vincent T. DeVita, Jr., then Director of the NCI, criticized the "glaring weakness" of using "age-adjusted mortality as the sole measure of progress." This, he said, led to the "erroneous view" that the war on cancer was being lost.[14] Another critic, Ezra M. Greenspan of Mount Sinai Medical Center in New York, noted that most oncologists treating breast cancer, for example, were still using

> the mild convenience regimen consisting of cyclophosphamide, methotrexate and fluorouracil (CMF) for premenopausal women and less than 35% employ

the more aggressive (Cooper-type) regimen consisting of cyclophosphamide, methotrexate, fluorouracil, vincristine, and prednisone or regimens containing doxorubicin. . . . I estimate that 10,000 lives could be saved by the early aggressive use of polychemotherapy in breast cancer, as compared with the negligible number of lives, perhaps several thousand, now being saved. . . . Before condemning current treatment as futile one needs to examine the extent to which improved treatments are actually being employed."[15]

Lawrence Garfinkel of the American Cancer Society took a different tack: "There's no doubt that the reason the overall death rate continues to go up is because of lung cancer. If you take away lung cancer, instead of having an 8 percent increase, you have a 13 percent decrease," he said.[16] "That only proves my point," Bailar responded.

Most every lung cancer death could be avoided if people quit smoking. We know how to prevent lung cancer deaths and we're not doing enough to prevent them. We should not build a long-range research program on the assumption we'll find fully effective cures. We gave that a good shot, and now it's time to get serious about another approach—prevention. If we can convince the American people that their hope lies in preventing the disease [through reducing diet, lifestyle, and environmental risks] we will save more lives than any of these drugs ever will.[17]

One more important criticism was leveled at the Bailar-Smith analysis by Lester Breslow and William Cumberland writing in the *Journal of the American Medical Association:*

The problem with reliance on a single measure of progress is that the impression conveyed can vary dramatically when the measure is changed. For example, another view of cancer's impact over the years, and one that paints a different picture from that given by Bailar and Smith, may be obtained by determining years of potential life lost (YPLL) due to cancer mortality . . . The YPLL tend to emphasize reduction in cancer mortality in younger age groups, while the age-adjusted statistic counts a death at age 75 years essentially the same as a death at 5 years. . . . How much the picture will change if we use YPLL rather than age adjusted mortality can be seen from the following calculations. In 1980, cancer was responsible for 1.824 million lost years of potential life in the United States to age 65. If, however, the cancer mortality rates of 1950 had prevailed, 2.093 million years of potential life would have been lost . . . We are not advocating replacing the age-adjusted mortality with YPLL; rather, our purpose in making these calculations is to indicate how sensitive one's conclusions are to the choice of measure.[18]

The debate over the Bailar-Smith assertion that the war on cancer was a qualified failure and that the national policy emphasis should turn toward prevention was so important for public policy that U.S. House member Ted Weiss of New York asked the General Accounting Office (GAO) to prepare a report on the extent of progress in cancer treatment for the Congress. The results of the GAO study were summarized in the *Journal of the American Medical Association*:

> The (congressional) General Accounting Office has just presented a similar [to Bailar-Smith's] dismal view, evidently based largely on Bailar and Smith's analysis. It said that "Of the three major empirical indicators—incidence, mortality, and survival rates—the only indicator that improved since 1950 was the survival rate." The General Accounting Office then attributed the reported improvement in survival largely to a statistical artifact [e.g., the fact that cancers were being diagnosed earlier and that the net of diagnosis was being broadened to include more nonfatal or slower-growing cancers].[19]

This debate indicates how deeply the question of whether or not there has been any meaningful progress in cancer therapy since the 1950s cuts to the heart of the concerns of the mainstream medical community and national policymakers. It is important for cancer patients facing choices about toxic adjuvant therapies to be aware of the intensity of the debate *within* the medical mainstream.

This much can be concluded. The great victories since the perfection of surgery in the 1950s have been in adjuvant treatment for the cancers of childhood and Hodgkin's disease, which afflict a very small proportion of the population. For the common cancers of adult years—lung, breast, colon, and prostate cancer—adjuvant therapies have a mixed and more controversial record. Some, such as Cairns, would argue that chemotherapy in particular is widely and disturbingly overused, with great cost in quality of life and little gain in cancer cure. Others argue that more rigorous chemotherapies are being demonstrated to convey additional survival advantage, and that the major problem is that practicing oncologists are not moving quickly enough to provide their patients with the gains to be achieved with more rigorous chemotherapies.

References

1   John Cairns, "The Treatment of Diseases and the War Against Cancer," *Scientific American* 253(5):52–3 (1985). Copyright © 1985 by Scientific American, Inc. All rights reserved.

2   Ibid., 53.

3   Ibid., 54–5.

4   Ibid., 56.

5   United States Department of Health and Human Services, Public Health Service, National Institutes of Health, National Cancer Institute, *1987 Annual Cancer Statistics Reviews* (Bethesda, MD, February 1988), II.149.

6   Ibid., 174–5.

7   Cairns, "The Treatment of Diseases and the War Against Cancer," 57.

8   Ibid.

9   Ibid.

10 Ibid., 59.

11 Ibid.

12 Ibid.

13 J.C. Bailar III and E.M. Smith, "Progress Against Cancer?" *New England Journal of Medicine* 314:1226–32 (1986).

14 Vincent T. DeVita, Jr., letter to the editor, *New England Journal of Medicine* 315(15):964 (1986).

15 Ezra M. Greenspan, letter to the editor, ibid., 963.

16 "Time for New Tactics Against Cancer," *Harvard Magazine* July-August, 1986:7–8.

17 Ibid.

18 Lester Breslow and William G. Cumberland, "Progress and Objectives in Cancer Control," *Journal of the American Medical Association* 259(11):1690–1 (1988).

19 Ibid., 1690.

five

American Cultures of Conventional Cancer Therapy

The most obvious divisions within American conventional cancer therapies are the differences in views between surgeons, radiation therapists, and oncologists (who provide chemotherapies, hormonal therapies, and related therapies). Historically, great battles have been waged in medical practice and in the medical journals between these three professional groups in regard to the relative efficacy of the treatments each offers for cancer. For example, surgeons committed to the use of radical mastectomy for breast cancer were skeptical of the benefits of lumpectomy combined with radiation therapy. The surgeons were equally skeptical of using nonsurgical approaches to prostate cancer.

These battles involve not only a very human economic conflict between these specialties for control of cancer treatment fees, but also reflect the strong tendency of almost every specialty to believe in the benefits of its own skills and instruments in contrast to those of other specialties. The debate among the armed services as to the relative merits of the Army, Air Force, and Navy is an obvious parallel.

What this means for cancer patients is simple but fundamental: If the first person you see about your cancer is a surgeon and he recommends immediate surgery, you may want additional opinions not only from other surgeons but also from oncologists and radiation therapists. This comparative approach is entirely obvious to physicians and others familiar with the reality of divergent medical cultures, but it is rarely spelled out to patients who want to obtain a second or third opinion.

Aggressive versus Conservative Treatment

In all three disciplines—surgery, oncology, and radiation therapy—doctors vary in their predisposition to aggressive or conservative approaches to treatment. An aggressive oncologist faced with a metastatic breast cancer in a young woman may, for example, be inclined to recommend autologous bone marrow transplant in combination with very high-dose chemotherapy and radiation therapy. In this procedure, the patient is given a lethal dose of chemotherapy and radiation and then a combination of increasingly effective "rescue" therapies that include replacing the bone marrow destroyed by the treatment with a store harvested from the patient in advance of the therapy.

This therapy is tremendously difficult, painful, and expensive, and is not reimbursed by most insurance plans. Further, as I write in 1993, no clear evidence yet exists that this protocol has demonstrated benefit in breast cancer treatment, although there is evidence of its benefits for Hodgkin's disease and other lymphomas. Nonetheless, aggressive oncologists who believe in pushing the frontiers of aggressive treatments to the very limits of human tolerance present this protocol to many women with metastatic breast cancer as their "only hope."

Conservative oncologists—such as Craig Henderson, M.D., at the University of California, San Francisco School of Medicine—are inclined against such aggressive recommendations when there is no clear evidence of their benefit. Henderson fought a similar battle in recent years when the National Cancer Institute issued a special bulletin recommending chemotherapy for all women with primary breast cancer, even for those with no positive nodes. Henderson and many other oncologists with a conservative clinical orientation believed that the evidence was not sufficient to justify this recommendation.

Similar stories can be told of differences between aggressive and conservative surgeons and between aggressive and conservative radiation therapists. Each specialty naturally believes in its own professional skills and tools, but within each specialty there are those who wield them cautiously and those who wield them more aggressively.

Rachel Naomi Remen, M.D., speaks of these differences in aggressive or conservative approaches to cancer as different personal styles of relationship to risk. She believes that a patient may wish to seek out a physician who has—or at least can accommodate—a style of relationship to risk that is similar to the patient's own.

Cultures of Cancer Therapy in Different Hospitals

Profound differences in medical cultures also exist among different kinds of hospitals. Some patients instinctively want to find "the best doctor in the field," whom they define as the chairman of a department at a major teaching hospital that is "on the cutting edge of research" in their particular disease. Nothing is wrong with the instinct to find the "top man" at a research institution, provided you have a clear understanding of what often happens when you seek a physician in that position.

First, your physician will be at a *teaching* hospital, and therefore you will be subjected to the ministrations of medical students, interns, and residents who are there in order to learn by practicing on you.

Second, your physician will be a leading academic who has made his reputation doing *research,* and his institution is oriented toward research. This necessarily means that, when he sees you, he sees a possible candidate for a research study. Most good research studies are randomized, controlled, clinical trials in which patients consent to be in the trial and then are randomly assigned to one of several "arms" of the research study. Patients are given one of the several treatments that are being compared with one another, and they *are not allowed to choose* which treatment they want. Whenever possible, the study is "blinded," meaning that neither the patient nor the physician knows which treatment the patient is receiving. Finally, the physicians and research staff try to keep each recruited patient in the study if at all possible, which means adhering as closely as possible to the protocol which has been set up for all patients in that wing of the study.

It is, of course, heroic and commendable for patients to decide, in the face of a serious cancer, that they wish to participate in a research study in order to contribute to knowledge that may help save future cancer patients. I have known some patients who chose to enter a clinical trial for just those reasons. But most patients I have known who have entered clinical trials have done so not out of heroism but because *a physician they trusted recommended the programs to them,* or because only through the trials could they *potentially* receive (depending on the study design and randomization) treatments they believed held promise.

Oncologists and other cancer specialists know well that different patients may respond to the same chemotherapy or other treatment in profoundly different ways. Some patients sail through a particular course of chemotherapy with minimal side effects; others become very sick. So it is no trivial matter that, in the culture of a teaching hospital, a patient in a controlled clinical trial will be under more pressure to stay with the protocol—even if he is suffering greatly—than he would be if he were treated by an oncologist in private practice. Whether affiliated with a teaching hospital or a private hospital, oncologists in private practice are free to design any treatment program that they wish (within broad limits) for their patients. They can modify the treatment in accordance with the patient's response far more easily than can a research oncologist committed to a research protocol.

The difference between cancer treatment in teaching hospitals and in private practice is well-known among oncologists. "We're here to try to cure cancer," one leading oncologist in a teaching hospital told me. "I often think that in private practice the most popular oncologists are the ones whose patients have the least symptoms simply because they are getting the smallest doses of chemotherapy." He was suggesting that oncologists in private practice may get more patients by giving lower-dose chemotherapy that may be less curative. Health Maintenance Organizations, or HMOs, which offer prepaid health services that can be delivered only through their hospitals and physicians, present a different set of cultural demands. The goal of an HMO is to provide a high standard of medical care while controlling medical costs as rigorously as possible. The amount of time the patient spends with a physician represents one major cost and medical procedures represent a second. So while the oncologist in private practice is often paid in proportion to the number of patient visits and procedures he undertakes, the HMO physician is encouraged to ration time and procedures as much as he reasonably can.

For the cancer patient, HMOs often mean a very restricted choice of physicians, longer waits to see doctors, less personal relationships with the doctors, and very brief doctor visits. But HMOs also mean far less pressure for potentially unnecessary medical procedures—and a heightened risk that some procedures that might be helpful will be missed.

Cultures of Care, Cultures of Competence

Cancer treatment specialists also differ widely from one another in their capacity to provide competent treatment and in their capacity to care deeply about their patients.

Speaking about his specialty, one of my closest oncologist friends said that, in his experience at his teaching hospital, there were a handful of oncologists who were extremely competent and very committed in the care they provided for their patients. Then, he said, there was a larger middle group in which care and commitment were more hit-or-miss, depending on the patient and the day. Finally, he said, there was a third group whose patients he was very concerned about because their doctors had neither sufficient competence nor commitment. Of course, such differences in competence and commitment are present in every profession: a minority at the top who are exceptionally capable; a large middle group possessing varying capacities; and a group at the bottom end whose clients are at serious risk.

But my oncologist friend added another note: some of those whom he would assign to the third group (medically incompetent and uncommitted) were heads of departments or famous in their specialty fields. Fame and position, in his view, were neither necessary nor sufficient evidence of competence in oncology practice.

Choice in Conventional Cancer Treatment

As I explained earlier, I have used the term *culture* broadly to describe differences of many kinds among conventional cancer treatment specialists. Let me summarize what these differences can mean to you as you begin to map choices in your own conventional cancer treatment:

- Be aware that American cancer treatments are generally at the "aggressive" end of mainstream cancer care when looked at from an international perspective. Know that less aggressive treatment choices are more widely sanctioned in other advanced industrial countries.
- Be aware of the debate within conventional cancer medicine on how greatly advances in chemotherapy and radiation therapy have contributed to cancer survival, with strong differences of opinion between those favoring more aggressive treatments and those taking more conservative positions.
- Be aware of the cultural differences in American cancer medicine—starting with the differences between surgeons, oncologists, and radiation therapists; the differences between aggressive and conservative orientations in each of these specialties; the differences among hospital cultures of cancer treatment; and the differences in competence and commitment among individual physicians.

So if you decide that you would like a second or third opinion, you are only doing what virtually every physician would do if he or a member of his family had cancer. With these maps of the cultures of cancer therapy, you may be better able to sample the kinds of second and third opinions that can be of most use.

six

Choosing Conventional Physicians, Hospitals, and Therapies

After 10 years of listening to hundreds of cancer patients tell their stories, I have concluded that many patients choose an oncologist, surgeon, or radiation therapist with less care and less comparative shopping than they would put into the choice of a new car.

How you choose a new car and how you choose physicians is not as far-fetched an analogy as it may seem. Most of us do not know a lot about the technology of automobiles. But when we decide to buy one, we usually go to considerable lengths to try to identify the best car for us. We read the *Consumer Reports* comparison of the different makes and models. We talk with friends who own the car we are considering and ask about their experience. We may talk with a mechanic about his opinion. We may rent the car to see what it is like to drive. Or we may simply test-drive the car at the dealer and visit some other dealers to test-drive other cars we are considering. For an informed car buyer, purchasing a new car may take a number of weeks, if not several months. This is entirely reasonable: it is a major purchase and you will be living with the car for some time.

Consider, then, the process by which the same person chooses a surgeon, oncologist, or radiation therapist. Apart from being in shock from a cancer diagnosis, a patient is often overcome by a sense of personal incompetence in making the pressing medical decisions. Obviously, he is making a choice that is *far* more important than choosing a new car, and yet all his confidence in his capacity to assess technologies that he does not understand deserts him. Culturally, Americans have what might be called a pattern of *learned helplessness* when it comes to choosing physicians and treatments. We sense that it is somehow illegitimate and embarrassing to shop for quality medical care with the same attention that we shop for a new car.

Even my father—an assertive and highly intelligent man, with boundless curiosity—had trouble in the early days after his diagnosis finding his own balance in the doctor-patient relationship. In his book *Wrestling with the Angel* he writes: "Few patients have more than an inkling, on their own, of the knowledge and experience needed for intelligent decisions. Most, like me, start as medical illiterates. The traditions of the profession call for the specialist or internist to deliver the verdict and recommend the decision, and the patient to accept it."[1]

He then comments on the implications of these traditions for the patient and for himself:

> The let-the-doctor-do-it model relieves the patient of incentive and responsibility. When we leave all the decisions to the doctor we surrender part of our fighting faith in our survival and healing. We may do it because we are awed by expertise, or because we think we don't know enough, or because we lack the courage to engage in a doctor-patient dialogue. But this model assumes a passivity on the patient's part which was alien to me. Within the larger frame of the doctor's medical authority I sought a measure of patient autonomy.
>
> There can be no grandiose role here. It would be *hubris* for me (my parents would have called it *chutzpa*) to place myself above specialists who have devoted their lives to clinical practice and are in touch with current research, and to substitute my own judgements for theirs. No, the province of autonomy I sought was more modest, quite simply to inform myself—by every available means—to play whatever role came to me, because it was my life and my death.
>
> Reading over my journals I am struck by how long it took me to assert this role. The torment of choice was pretty much what every patient with a dangerous illness endures. I had to learn how to resolve the often conflicting advice from my array of doctors and consultants, including my doctor son in Boston and my "behavioral son" in Bolinas. At each crisis point they all became sources of "input" to balance against each other when there was a conflict

between them. Nor did I mind if they didn't pull their punches. "If I want to hear someone's opinion," said Goethe, "it must be expressed positively; I have ambiguity enough in myself." I was in the realm of conflicting judgements and values. I needed the input to resolve my own ambivalence and end in decisive outcomes.

Once I had the assessments and recommendations of my consortium of doctors, I was the one who had to take charge. When a difficult choice had to be made, no one else could assume its burden. I had to carry it, not because of knowledge or experience but for the existential reason that my life was at stake.

My doctors recognized how much it meant to me to have the chance to disagree, as well as agree, with them. They knew also that a patient who becomes part of the decision process thereby becomes part of the healing process as well.[2]

How to Choose a Physician

One of the best resources on how to choose a cancer care doctor is a book called *Choices: Realistic Alternatives in Cancer Treatment* by Marion Morra and Eve Potts. Chapter 2, "Deciding on Your Doctor and Hospital," provides a comprehensive checklist and encourages patients to recognize that they do not have to remain with the physician they currently have. The authors recommend choosing (a) a cancer specialist who practices in a one-specialty group or hospital; (b) a cancer specialist affiliated with a hospital; and (c) someone who is board-certified in his specialty. They provide equally good checklists on assessing a doctor's manner with patients, how his office is run, his personality, his willingness to discuss fees, his accessibility, and the insurance arrangements he makes.

The authors present a similar checklist for hospitals and recommend (a) a "comprehensive cancer center" designated by the National Cancer Institute (NCI), if there is one in your area; (b) hospitals that have cancer programs accredited by the American College of Surgeons; and (c) hospitals directly or closely affiliated to medical schools. They note that a quarter of American hospitals are not accredited at all; that care at government-supported hospitals ranges from excellent to poor; that, with a few exceptions, for-profit hospitals frequently have limited services; and that larger hospitals usually have more services.[3]

Choices and similar books are widely available, and I highly recommend that you read at least one of them.

Informal Networks: Allies in Choosing Cancer Specialists

Formal medical advice on how to choose a cancer specialist in your community usually suggests you contact the American Medical Association (AMA) and ask for a listing of cancer specialists; ask the NCI for access to a similar listing; or contact the chief of a department of surgery, oncology, or radiation therapy at the most prestigious cancer treatment center in your area and ask for his advice. This is not bad advice, but the AMA and NCI can usually give you only alphabetical lists of specialists, and the chairman of the department is often under considerable political constraints about telling you whom he would choose for care.

I find it striking that conventional advice about choosing a physician rarely points cancer patients toward some of the most skillful approaches: the use of informal networks of people who really know which cancer specialists in a given community are the best. For example, in choosing a surgeon, the best people to ask would include (a) other surgeons, (b) anesthesiologists who work with surgeons every day; (c) operating room nurses or physician's assistants; and (d) cancer patients who have undergone surgery. In choosing an oncologist, the best people to ask would include (a) other oncologists, (b) surgeons and radiation therapists who work with oncologists, (c) oncology ward nurses or physician's assistants, and (d) cancer patients. In choosing a radiation therapist, the best people to ask would be (a) other radiation therapists, (b) surgeons and oncologists who work with radiation therapists, (c) radiation therapy service nurses or physician's assistants, and (d) cancer patients.

Physicians as a Resource

Physicians can tell you what the professional reputations of their fellow practitioners are. This can be very valuable advice. However, the primary problem with accepting their advice alone is that they have never been under treatment with the physicians they are recommending, and they rarely work directly alongside them (the exceptions are anesthesiologists, who work with surgeons). Also, many cancer specialists have regular relationships with specialists in other cancer treatment disciplines. They refer their patients to a colleague who reciprocates by sending patients their way. This practice of "trading material," as it is sometimes irreverently known, can be the result of great mutual respect for each other's skills. But it may also have a financial motivation. So the referral of a cancer specialist is not always the best way of identifying the most suitable physician for you.

You can identify physicians to help you either through the formal approach described above or through your personal contacts with family doctors or physician friends, asking whom they know who would be able to advise you. Often a family physician or internist who does not specialize in cancer can serve as an ongoing trusted advisor as you make your way through these complex choices. Engaging your family doctor—or some physician you trust—to serve as treatment coordinator for you has an additional advantage: it may spare you the common experience of modern or "fractionated" cancer treatment, with no doctor providing continued human contact and long-term evaluation.

Nurses and Physician's Assistants

The advice of nurses and physician's assistants is invaluable and underutilized. They work directly with the surgeons, oncologists, and radiation therapists, either in the hospital or in outpatient offices. Hospital nurses, particularly, have no vested interest in the choice that the patient makes among physicians.

An experienced operating room nurse knows a great deal about the surgeons in his hospital—from their technical skills to their human skills. Equally important, an experienced operating room nurse has less constraints on giving you his honest opinion about *whom he would choose if it were a member of his family* than a physician. The same holds true for the advice of experienced radiation therapy nurses about radiation therapists.

The evaluation of an oncologist by nurses and physician's assistants is somewhat more difficult because the skills of the oncologist are more variegated than a surgeon's or radiation therapist's skills. Here, the nurse can tell you how careful an oncologist is, how committed he is to his patients, how humane he is, and so forth. It is more difficult to evaluate his choice of chemotherapy protocols.

It is usually easy to reach an experienced nurse who can be of assistance. You may know a nurse who knows a nurse who knows someone who works in one of the cancer specialty services, and this nurse in turn might either be able to help you or could identify the most experienced nurses in his service. The same holds true of physician's assistants, except that they are fewer in number.

Cancer Patients

Cancer patients are also a good source of information. No better place exists to get a lot of information quickly about which physicians are respected by cancer patients than at an independent cancer support center in your community. Cancer patients may also be able to point you toward physicians who helped them choose cancer specialists and toward nurses who may be helpful in making these choices. Obviously, cancer patients cannot readily evaluate some areas of medical skill, but being on the receiving end of these services they know a great deal that is invaluable.

Networking Skills

Some people with cancer are skilled networkers in other areas of their lives. They may also have the closely related skill of moving effectively through bureaucracies. Once they realize that these information-finding and bureaucratic skills are applicable to the choice of a medical care team, they need little guidance to apply these skills. But other cancer patients need help with networking and bureaucratic maneuvering. In this instance, a willing family member or friend who has these skills can be of *inestimable* assistance in identifying good doctors, hospitals, and therapies and ensuring delivery of good care.

Take Time to Make the Right Choice

If you adopt the above strategies of choosing a physician, you will find that the names of certain physicians begin to recur. Using both formal and informal networks, it should take no more than a week or 10 days of concentrated effort to make an informed choice. Taking a week or two to choose the right physician will very rarely jeopardize your treatment or your health. Most physicians would agree that taking time to find the right doctor may be one of the best investments you can make.

Establish a Working Relationship with Your Doctor

Once you have found a doctor who looks promising, how do you establish a good relationship?

Harold Benjamin, Ph.D., founder of The Wellness Community in Santa Monica, California—one of the most successful independent support programs for cancer patients in the United States—has developed a written pledge for cancer patients and their physicians (see figure 6.1), Benjamin has strong support from most oncologists in the Los Angeles area. The pledge is a productive approach to clarifying communications between patients and physicians. I recommend considering it, and possibly bringing it with you to an early meeting with your doctor, explaining that it is a cosignatory pledge agreed to by many patients and oncologists in Los Angeles and elsewhere and asking if it might serve as a basis for an understanding between you and him.

Choosing Treatments

Once you have found the right physician and established a working relationship, you then face the choice of treatment. Different patients have different preferences about whether they want (a) their physician to make the choice of treatments essentially without consulting them; (b) the physician to play the primary role in choosing therapies but to do so in close consultation with them; or (c) to make the primary choices themselves, using their physicians as consultants only. Be clear with your doctor about which of these three

The Wellness Community Oncologist-Patient Statement

The effective treatment of serious illness requires a considerable effort by both the patient and the physician. A clear understanding by both of us as to what each of us can realistically and reasonably expect of the other will do much to enhance the outlook. I am giving this "statement" to you as one step in making our relationship as effective and productive as possible. It might be helpful if you would read this statement and, if you think it appropriate, discuss it with me.

As your physician I will make every effort to:

1 Provide you with the care most likely to be beneficial to you.

2 Inform and educate you about your situation, and the various treatment alternatives. How detailed an explanation is given will be dependent upon your specific desires.

3 Encourage you to ask questions about your illness and its treatment and to answer your questions as clearly as possible. I will also attempt to answer the questions asked by your family; however, my primary responsibility is to you, and I will discuss your medical situation only with those people authorized by you.

4 Remain aware that all major decisions about the course of your care shall be made by you. However, I will accept the responsibility for making certain decisions if you want me to.

5 Assist you to obtain other professional opinions if you desire, or if I believe it to be in your best interests.

6 Relate to you as one competent adult to another, always attempting to consider your emotional, social, and psychological needs as well as your physical needs.

7 Spend a reasonable amount of time with you on each return visit unless required by something urgent to do otherwise, and give you my undivided attention during that time.

8 Honor all appointment times unless required by something urgent to do otherwise.

9 Return phone calls as promptly as possible, especially those you indicate are urgent.

10 Make available test results promptly if you desire such reports.

11 Provide you with any information you request concerning my professional training, experience, philosophy and fees.

12 Respect your desire to try treatment that might not be conventionally accepted. However, I will give you my honest opinion about such unconventional treatments.

13 Maintain my active support and attention throughout the course of the illness.

I hope that you as the patient will make every effort to:

1   Comply with our agreed-upon treatment plan.

2   Be as candid as possible with me about what you need and expect from me.

3   Inform me if you desire another professional opinion.

4   Inform me of all forms of therapy you are involved with.

5   Honor all appointment times unless required by something urgent to do otherwise.

6   Be as considerate as possible of my need to adhere to a schedule to see other patients.

7   Attempt to make all phone calls to me during the working hours. Call on nights and week-ends only when absolutely necessary.

8   Attempt to coordinate the requests of your family and confidants, so that I do not have to answer the same questions about you to several different people.

Figure 6.1

The Wellness Community Oncologist-Patient Statement. (Courtesy of Harold Benjamin, Richard Steckel, Laurence Heiftez, Daniel J. Lieber, Fred Rosenfelt, and Michael Van Scou-Mosher, The Wellness Community, Santa Monica, Calif.)

models you wish to work with. Such an understanding is very helpful for establishing a good working relationship.

For choosing conventional therapies, some excellent resource books are available about both choice in cancer in general and specific choices for specific cancers. *Choices* by Morra and Potts, which I discussed above, is one of the bibles in this field and includes some discussion of complementary cancer therapies as well. The book covers diagnosis, deciding on a physician and hospital, understanding cancer, diagnostic tests, all forms of conventional treatments, investigational treatments and unproven methods, all the major cancers, coping with recurrence, living with cancer, and where to get help. The section on where to get help is one of the most complete available.

Another valuable resource available to patients is the NCI's 1-800-4-CANCER phone line that provides a wealth of primary information on therapy choices. Numerous booklets are also available from the NCI and the American Cancer Society that provide patients with basic information about treatment choice.

Also, the R.A. Bloch Cancer Foundation, created by H&R Block, Inc. co-founder Richard Bloch, operates a computerized cancer information network called Cancer Forum through which patients can communicate free of charge with each other or with volunteer researchers. The foundation also operates the Cancer Hot Line at 816–932–8453, which provides newly diagnosed cancer patients with the opportunity to talk with people who have had cancers similar to their own.

The Power of Information: Understanding Cancer Treatments as Physicians Understand Them

Some cancer patients have both the skills and the desire to develop a basic understanding of choices in cancer treatment by reading the same literature that their physicians refer to. This is not as difficult to do as many patients fear. Other patients may assign this task to a family member or friend. If there is someone—yourself or a support person—who is willing and able to read the medical literature, it can make a *profound* difference in your ability to make informed choices. Often, it will also change the relationship between your doctor and yourself.

Here are some simple approaches to getting medical literature:

- Go to a medical library—at a medical school or cancer treatment center—and ask for the most widely used cancer textbook, *Cancer: Principles and Practice of Oncology*, edited by Vincent T. DeVita, Jr. (Philadelphia: J.B. Lippincott Co., 1989). It is a two-volume bible on all the cancers and all the major phases of treatment. Look up the chapter on your cancer. Make a photocopy of the chapter (the chapters are often 50 pages long) so you can take it home with you.
- Consider buying a medical dictionary if the medical vocabulary is a problem for you. A number of medical dictionaries explain in simple English the meaning of most medical terminology.
- Find a way to obtain three to five of the most recent review articles discussing your specific cancer and the treatment options. A "review article" is an article in which one of the leading specialists in your type of cancer reviews all the recent studies and summa-

rizes what is known about treatment. If you have a cancer in which there are significant treatment choices—such as the choice between surgery and radiotherapy—ask for review articles by specialists in both fields, since the surgeons will have a different bias than the radiotherapists and you want to understand both perspectives. Asking your doctor if he can help you obtain the most recent review articles on your cancer—after having told him that you have read the chapter on your cancer in DeVita's textbook—will signal to him the kind of patient you are. The review articles can be obtained by your physician, a reference librarian at a medical library, a number of the medical consulting services, and possibly through the NCI hot line.

• If you have a rare cancer or want to go even deeper into technical treatment choices—or if you have more obscure questions about specific cancer therapies—find a friendly person who has a computer with a modem hooked into one of the medical databases, such as BRS Colleague. (Medical reference librarians can do this.) With his computer and phone link, he has access to the entire cancer literature of the world, and with a few simple search words he can track down in seconds the articles on your obscure or difficult subject. He can then display the titles of these articles on his screen. He can print these titles out, look at them, and circle the titles for which you want to read the brief abstracts. He can go back into the database and ask for these abstracts, which he can print out for you. You can read the abstracts and then order the full text of any article you want from the service. In some instances, the database has the full text available for immediate printout through the computer.

• The same computer database also gives you access to two NCI databases: the PDQ database on treatment choice for patients and the PDQ database for physicians on current clinical trials involving your type of cancer. The PDQ physician database is more interesting, and you can access it. It lists all current clinical trials for your type of cancer, including complete details about who can qualify, what the investigational therapy is, possible side effects, etc. It gives the name of the chief investigator and his phone number.

With all of this information, it is possible for you or a member of your family to reach a very sophisticated level of understanding of available cancer treatments. But even if you only take the first step—reading the chapter in *Principles and Practice of Oncology* about your specific type of cancer and options, you will have moved much further into understanding your cancer *as your physician sees it.*

Avoiding Serious Mistakes and Getting the Best out of Large Medical Institutions

One thing everyone wants to avoid is needless and sometimes life-threatening 'iatrogenic' ("physician-caused") complications from treatment. These mistakes are, unfortunately, increasingly common as medical treatment becomes more aggressive, more complex, and more bureaucratic. Large complex bureaucratic systems are intrinsically prone to error; hospitals or busy medical practices are no exception. To avoid potentially serious treatment errors, you or your support person should consider monitoring your treatment carefully so that you are more likely to catch mistakes your medical team may make. Monitoring can also help you to catch mistakes that *you* make through misunderstanding treatment recommendations.

There is more to obtaining quality treatment than monitoring to avoid mistakes. Large institutions, such as hospitals, are intrinsically more likely to deliver quality treatment to people with skills in extracting better outcomes from these institutions than to people who quietly put themselves at the mercy of the system. So it becomes very important to be an effective advocate for your own quality care.

The need to monitor treatment often begins before the first exploratory surgery. It is often a good idea, for example, to engage an oncologist *in advance* of surgery, so that he can help you with the choices a surgeon may not fully explain. Oncologists may bring out important choices for the patient that may alter plans for surgery in significant ways.

After surgery, if you need chemotherapy or other adjuvant treatment, you need to keep an eye on what the oncologist or radiation therapist is recommending and whether he is providing you with all the information you need. Oncologists and radiation therapists—good ones especially—are often tremendously busy, and they rarely keep your situation constantly on their minds. Many independent cancer support groups play a critical role in facilitating the exchange of information on subjects like surviving chemotherapy, which allows you to piece together information from various physicians that your own doctor may have failed to provide.

In critical periods of hospitalization, ask someone else to monitor your medications and other procedures so that mistakes in medication are avoided, unnecessary procedures eliminated, and necessary procedures utilized. In the hospital every day, this friend may also be the most effective advocate for getting your needs met.

Sooner or later, most cancer patients come to realize that the medical profession as organized today rarely does an adequate job of tracking and coordinating all aspects of treatment and of minimizing errors of omission or commission. The sooner you realize this, the less likely you are to suffer from iatrogenic health problems.

References

1   Max Lerner, *Wrestling with the Angel* (New York: Touchstone, 1990), 68.
2   Ibid., 68–9.
3   Marion Morra and Eve Potts, *Choices: Realistic Alternatives in Cancer Treatment* (New York: Avon Books, 1987).

PART THREE

Choice in Unconventional Cancer Therapies

Unconventional cancer therapies include some of the best and some of the worst treatments available. I have come to this conclusion after over 10 years of studying unconventional therapies, visiting over 50 centers throughout the world that use them, and interviewing hundreds of health care professionals and patients involved with these therapies.

The best unconventional treatments are generally those that enhance quality of life, promote general health, and engage the patient in his own treatment in psychologically and sometimes physically beneficial ways. The worst treatments are those cynically undertaken for financial gain by unscrupulous people. Between these two extremes, there are many therapies that represent puzzling admixtures of positive and negative qualities. How can patients, doctors, and policymakers evaluate unconventional therapies? How can you decide which of these therapies seems valid and which will be appropriate for you with your own particular values and preferences and your particular cancer?

In the next chapter, I discuss the acrimonious debate between proponents of mainstream and unconventional therapies in the United States. In the chapter that follows, I describe a framework within which to analyze the unconventional cancer therapies. In later chapters, I discuss some of the different approaches, as well as some of the most important unconventional cancer therapies, in detail.

To begin, it is useful to indicate how I use the many—and often confusing—terms associated with unconventional therapies: "adjunctive," "alternative," "complementary," "unorthodox," and "unconventional." What does each mean specifically?

Proponents and opponents of unconventional cancer therapies argue frequently about these terms. In common usage, the terms used relate primarily to the degree of "acceptability" that a particular therapy enjoys within the medical establishment. "Mainstream" or "conventional" cancer therapies consist of those forms of cancer treatment widely practiced in major American cancer centers today: surgery, chemotherapy, and radiation, and, increasingly, other pharmacological and biological therapies. "Unconventional" cancer therapies, by contrast, are those approaches to the diagnosis, treatment, and care of cancer that fall outside conventional cancer treatments. I use the term "complementary" frequently to describe these therapies because I believe that, at their best, unconventional cancer therapies *complement* the *intelligent* use of conventional approaches scientifically demonstrated to be efficacious.[1]

Complementary cancer therapies are also called "unorthodox" and "unconventional." The term "unconventional" is perhaps the best neutral term available, so I use it frequently. I use the term "complementary" and "unconventional" interchangeably in referring to these therapies. I use the term "alternative" when referring to unconventional therapies that are further outside the mainstream culture of cancer treatment, although this says nothing about their objective merits or deficiencies. I use the term "adjunctive" to refer to those approaches closer to mainstream respectability, mostly, and notably, psychosocial approaches, such as support groups, psychotherapy, hypnosis, and imagery.

The cultural differences among the unconventional cancer therapies are often as great as the cultural differences among the conventional cancer therapies. For example, in psychological approaches to cancer, there is a continuum from practitioners who believe only in psychological palliation to those who believe that visual imagery, psychotherapy, or affirmations regularly cause dramatic cancer recoveries. And among nutritional therapists, there is a continuum from those who offer palliative nutritional support, to scientists who are documenting the complex effects of nutrients on cancer, to alternative therapists who believe that nutritional therapies reliably reverse cancer. Similar continua could be described in other areas of unconventional cancer therapies.

Among the many subcultures of unconventional therapies that could be identified, seven stand out for most American patients as popular cultures of unconventional cancer treatments with distinctive characteristics:

1. Adjunctive psychological approaches to cancer, whose practitioners have maintained (despite some very vigorous disagreements) communication with mainstream medicine. This group generally sees itself as offering an *adjunctive,* as opposed to alternative, approach to cancer. They offer individual psychotherapy, imagery, group therapy, or cancer support groups.
2. Macrobiotics—a subculture unto itself—whose practitioners offer the most popular current nutritional approach to cancer, supported by a spiritual perspective on how to live.

3. A whole range of "nutritional-metabolic" programs that involve a combination of vegetarian diet and nutritional supplements. These therapies are usually offered by physicians, naturopaths, or chiropractors who specialize in such programs.

4. Traditional Chinese medicine, whose practitioners offer a combination of acupuncture and Chinese herbal remedies as an adjunctive approach to treating cancer and, significantly, alleviating side effects of chemotherapy and radiation.

5. The group of "great men and women" who offer unique and often closed or partially closed pharmacological therapies for cancer. This group includes Emanuel Revici in New York, Stanislaw Burzynski in Texas, the late Virginia Livingston in San Diego, the late Lawrence Burton in the Bahamas, and Gaston Naessens in Canada.

6. Healers—religious and spiritual—who through prayer or laying on of hands seek to assist the patient in actively recovering from cancer.

7. The cluster of clinics and practitioners in Southern California and along the Mexican-California border that offer a wide range of options, such as laetrile, Hoxsey herbs, nutritional-metabolic therapies, and immunosupportive therapies.

In the United States, most cancer patients seeking to combine conventional and unconventional cancer therapies characteristically find themselves integrating some combination of therapies from these seven subcultures with a judicious use of mainstream therapies. While there are some overlaps, many of these cultures of unconventional therapies differ greatly and are often mutually hostile.

These are the unconventional cancer therapies one hears the most about, but in reality tens of thousands of American cancer patients make use of unconventional cancer therapies that are part of folk and traditional medical systems belonging to their ethnic cultures. Latin American, Caribbean, Asian, African, and other immigrants have brought their native folk medical traditions with them to the United States. Patients with cancer from these groups often consult their traditional healers. But because these patients are for the most part people with low incomes and no health insurance, and because they consult their healers quietly and do not challenge the hegemony of the medical system, their widespread use of unconventional therapies attracts almost no attention.

Note

1   Robert Houston, one of the most knowledgeable analysts of unconventional cancer therapies to be found in the alternative cancer therapy community, provides a different definition of "complementary": "According to Dr. Andrew Stanway, a founder of the Institute for Complementary Medicine in London, the term originally was based on the dictionary sense of 'complement' as 'something that serves to make whole' and referred to therapies promoting wholeness of health. He notes that the common use of 'complementary' as supplementary to standard treatment is unrealistic, for 'they are often at loggerheads.' Used in the latter sense, the term would be most applicable to adjuvant chemotherapy and radiation."

seven

The Debate over Unconventional Cancer Therapies

It is impossible to evaluate how unconventional cancer therapies are treated legally and socially in the United States without first understanding how these therapies are treated legally and socially in other nations. Over hundreds or thousands of years, most of the world's cultures have evolved pluralistic systems of medicine within which the allopathic, or the currently "mainstream" system, of medical treatment has come to coexist with other systems of medical care in a balance that most patients and health professionals accept as normal. Germany, England, France, and Japan, as we saw earlier, are four diverse examples of advanced technological-industrial nations that have established pluralistic systems of medicine in which conventional and unconventional systems of cancer therapy exist side by side. This is not to say that there are no controversies among proponents of the various cancer therapies in these countries. But allopathic medicine has never developed the political power in these countries to force leading unconventional cancer therapies outside the framework of legal and accessible health care.

In the United States, for historical reasons, allopathic medicine developed a degree of control over the medical marketplace that has restricted medical pluralism to a much greater extent than in Germany, England, France, or Japan. This hegemony of allopathic medicine in the United States has pushed many of what Richard Grossman has aptly called "the other medicines" to the outer boundaries of mainstream medicine or over those boundaries into illegality.[1] As a result of this mainstream medical restriction—particularly in the field of cancer therapies—any U.S. medical practitioner who wishes to explore unconventional cancer therapies does so at risk to his career, his reputation, and even to his medical license.

The logical consequence of this is that health professionals who do offer these therapies in the United States often have the educational, social, and personal characteristics of people who are attracted to therapeutic, scientific, or legal frontiers. These frontiers, by their nature, are not well regulated. They offer opportunities for creative cancer therapies and also dark corners for misguided or even cynically exploitative treatments. The unregulated medical frontier therefore attracts both the most and the least ethical of practitioners.

The central question posed by the current regulatory system governing unconventional cancer therapies in the United States is whether it represents the best policy for American citizens who have a cancer that cannot be cured by a scientifically demonstrated conventional therapy. This is not an easy question, and it cries out to be addressed thoughtfully and carefully. On the one hand, it is an important function of government to protect citizens from health fraud. On the other hand, the right of patients in free societies to determine what they will do with their own bodies is one of the first and best-established principles of medical ethics.

Further tension exists between the consumer protection function of government and the important freedom of physicians to practice the medicine they believe in. The hegemony of allopathic medicine in the United States has also had a chilling effect on the development of mainstream research into the most promising unconventional cancer therapies. At present, any researcher investigating these therapies does so at high professional risk to his reputation and career. Funding is largely unavailable for such endeavors.

Is there a skillful means to reconcile these important social, medical, scientific, and legal values so as to protect the interests and personal liberties of American patients, physicians, and researchers alike? To answer this question, the United States needs to study carefully the advanced technological-industrial cultures where conventional and complementary cancer therapies are allowed greater freedom to compete in the medical marketplace.

If we overlook these working systems of pluralistic medicine in other countries, I believe we impoverish our chances to achieve a balanced view of personal, clinical, and policy options. This is not to say that, in societies that have more pluralistic medical systems, one finds that complementary cancer therapies have achieved any decisive triumphs over conventional cancer therapies—far from it. Conventional therapies are in ascendance in every country with a pluralistic medical system, in part because of their demonstrably superior efficacy in treating many forms of disease, including some cancers. I am suggesting only that legitimizing a wider range of complementary cancer therapies, and holding all medical therapies to similar legal standards, produces a higher quality of complementary cancer therapies than pushing these therapies out of the regulatory structure and beyond to the boundaries of legality. Moreover, the citizens of the advanced societies that sanction these complementary therapies seem reasonably satisfied with their pluralistic but regulated medical marketplace.

But cross-cultural comparisons do not substitute for the urgently needed studies of the costs and benefits of medically pluralistic cancer treatments in the United States. I do not agree with proponents of unconventional therapies who believe that "freedom of choice in cancer therapy" is an unmixed policy blessing. Such a position does not deal with the real problems of cancer quackery. What I am proposing is that our health policy goal as a nation should be to develop skillful regulatory policies that open the doors to the best aspects of complementary therapies in general—and cancer therapies in particular—while doing all that we can to create powerful disincentives for their exploitative use. Instead of trying to reinvent the wheel, we should look carefully at how more pluralistic medical systems work.

The United States Debate over Unconventional Cancer Therapies

I do not include in this book the details of the acrimonious political conflict over unconventional cancer therapies in the United States which has gone on for over 50 years. My goal is to *raise the level of dialogue* about these therapies, and an immersion in the lengthy, bitter, and contested history of this conflict does not necessarily contribute to this end. But just as I described the debate over conventional cancer therapies in chapter 4, I must also outline, at least, the debate over unconventional cancer therapies. Here I will discuss *primarily* the more explicitly *alternative* cancer therapies—those farthest out from the mainstream medical networks.

For decades, the debate over these therapies has been vituperative. Critics have characteristically dismissed the alternative therapies as quackery. Some critics, seeing themselves as the defenders of scientific medicine and the protectors of consumers against health fraud, have worked systematically and often effectively to discredit the unconventional therapies and, where possible, to disbar or "defrock" physicians and other practitioners who use alternative therapies. The "Quack Busters," as they call themselves, include a loose national network of physicians, researchers, and attorneys. They are powerful, feared, and often despised opponents of the practitioners of alternative cancer therapies, many of whom have faced legal prosecution, lengthy trials with high legal expenses, suspension or loss of their license to practice medicine, and sometimes jail terms. To continue their practices, some have moved to other, less restrictive states, or even to Mexico or the Bahamas.

Opposing the Quack Busters is a coalition of proponents of alternative cancer therapies. The National Health Federation, the International Association of Cancer Victors and Friends, and support groups for specific alternative treatment programs are among the key participants in this coalition. The coalition consists primarily of cancer patients, relatives of patients, aficionados of alternative therapies, researchers, writers, journalists, lawyers, lobbyists, publicists, and organizers. While some members of the coalition are moderate in tone, others use harsh language and tactics. Opponents of alternative therapies have been seriously compared to Nazis. Conventional therapies such as surgery, radiotherapy, and chemotherapy are denounced as "cut, burn, and poison." Just as a persistent belief exists in parts of the black community that the acquired immunodeficiency syndrome (AIDS) virus was engineered as part of a genocidal program aimed at blacks, a similar persistent view exists among some advocates of unconventional cancer therapies that there is a high-level conspiracy in mainstream medicine to suppress alternative cancer "cures" because they threaten to undercut the profits of the cancer industry.

While for many years the Quack Buster coalition held the advantage in this vociferous conflict, a significant shift in the balance of societal forces has occurred in the last 10 years, so that conditions are now somewhat more favorable to the proponents of alternative therapies. Several factors have been responsible for this shift:

First, the meteoric rise of interest in personal health has played a crucial role. What began as a New Age interest in organic foods, vegetarian diet, and a wide range of psychospiritual approaches to health and self-actualization gradually entered the mainstream as health promotion, behavioral medicine, mind-body medicine, and an enthusiasm for fitness and medical self-care. Since many of the alternative cancer therapies were loosely or tightly allied with these New Age endeavors, they also tended to move toward respectability.

Second, the media played a critical role in portraying alternative cancer therapies to good advantage. Since cancer is one of the most feared diseases, controversial new "cures" for cancer make excellent copy, and stories about them sell newspapers and magazines and increase ratings on radio and television shows. The rise of magazines and newspapers targeted to New Age audiences reinforced this trend, but lengthy articles favorable to alternative therapies also appeared repeatedly in magazines such as *Penthouse* and on major television and radio programs. The Quack Busters were often called upon to respond, but in media terms they were on the defensive.

Third, a declining faith in virtually all mainstream institutions in the United States over the past 20 years gradually fragmented the once strong consensus that had supported the War on Cancer, the American Cancer Society, and the vigilant use of legal sanctions against any approach to health not endorsed by this consensus. The investment of over $20 billion in the War on Cancer proclaimed by President Nixon failed to produce the expected "breakthrough" in cancer treatment, and even some mainstream researchers have called the War on Cancer "a qualified failure."[2] Americans became intellectually freer to explore choices in cancer therapy. Increasing numbers of U.S. citizens traveled abroad and became more sophisticated about the realities of medical pluralism.

Finally, a phenomenon closely related to the declining faith in institutions was the breakdown of mass markets throughout American society (mainstream cancer therapies had represented a mass market) and the increasing segmentation of markets to which specific products had to be targeted. Alternative cancer therapies represented, in effect, a set of health products and services that could be effectively targeted to a growing market segment of health care consumers. While this growing market was diverse, it was politically crucial to the increasing respectability of these therapies in that it included disproportionate numbers of politically, economically, and culturally advantaged individuals and groups. The fact that at least some alternative therapies appealed strongly to informed, educated, and often influential people was a powerful factor in shifting the balance of social factors in their favor.

A Boost from the AIDS Activists

The rise of the AIDS epidemic and the debate over AIDS treatment has had a profound effect on the national debate over unconventional cancer therapies. While a small minority of patients with life-threatening cancers had an interest in alternative therapies, a much larger proportion of AIDS patients were interested in alternative approaches. Unlike the vast majority of cancer patients, who had for decades quietly accepted the status quo in cancer treatment, a large proportion of gay men with AIDS were to prove militantly unwilling to accept the status quo denial of access to promising experimental or unconventional AIDS treatments.

Even more significant, many top researchers and policy officials in AIDS research tended to agree with the goals, if not the tactics, of the militants. Some of these officials stated publicly that the AIDS militants were making a fruitful contribution to science and science policy. As a result, alternative cancer therapies, which are often similar to or identical with some alternative AIDS therapies, became more broadly disseminated and more culturally acceptable while riding the slipstream of unconventional AIDS treatments.

One of most significant specific victories of the AIDS coalition was a change in Food and Drug Administration (FDA) regulations designed to allow AIDS patients to bring into the country small amounts of non-FDA approved drugs for personal use. These regulations also apply to patients bringing in similar drugs for cancer. "Buying clubs," set up by AIDS support networks to purchase legal and illegal pharmaceuticals for people with AIDS, sometimes offer drugs that are used for alternative cancer therapies as well. Further, community-based clinical trials for new, unproven AIDS remedies were set up by AIDS physicians, researchers, and patients when they became dissatisfied with the official clinical trials. While criticized by some researchers, they have been endorsed by others. They represent a model of ethical low-cost community-based research, which advocates of unconventional cancer therapies may at some point emulate. In addition, support services for people with AIDS in gay communities—most notably San Francisco—have created extraordinary models of compassionate caring for people with life-threatening illnesses. It is a model of psychosocial, community-based support that people with cancer (and others with life-threatening illnesses) could benefit by studying.

What all this means is that people with AIDS, faced with a new disease with a lethal prognosis, rapidly created a model of multifaceted integration of conventional and unconventional treatment modalities, exceptional community-based psychosocial support, innovative research, and effective policy advocacy to change those aspects of the treatment and research systems that they found objectionable. In fact, AIDS activists essentially co-opted almost all the major elements through which a much smaller proportion of people with cancer had sought to integrate conventional and unconventional cancer therapies. In doing so, people with AIDS did a much more effective job of organizing, articulating, and meeting their needs than people with cancer—or any other disease—had ever done in modern medicine. Whatever else one may think about the AIDS epidemic, the response of the AIDS community in reshaping health care to fit its needs was unquestionably a brilliantly creative act. It expanded treatment options, accelerated research processes, built support systems, and made public health institutions more responsive to the people suffering from the disease. Because cancer patients—and those suffering from all other chronic and degenerative illnesses—could all benefit from similar changes, the initial response of people with AIDS to this global epidemic represents a milestone in public health.

Politics of Mainstream versus Alternative Therapies

Although societal forces contributed significantly to a shift in the balance of power from the Quack Busters toward the proponents of unconventional cancer therapies, the extent of the shift can be overstated. The Quack Busters still have strong institutional influence with the mainstream medical profession—particularly with oncologists, the American Medical Association, state medical societies, the National Cancer Institute, and key state and federal officials and lawmakers. Thus, despite increasing public support for unconventional cancer therapies, the Quack Busters often have the institutional advantage in the critical areas of legal and professional sanctions against practitioners of unconventional cancer therapies. With every physician whose license to practice medicine is revoked for the practice of unconventional cancer therapies, a clear message is sent to hundreds of other physicians who might have considered exploring the integration of conventional and complementary therapies. Physicians who do integrate conventional and complementary therapies, or who offer primarily unconventional cancer therapies, do so with a constant sense of anxiety that they may be the next to face legal or professional sanctions. To the Quack Busters and their supporters, this is exactly as it should be: they are upholding the standards of scientific medicine and the law, and protecting consumers against dangerous and fraudulent therapies. To the proponents of unconventional therapies, the Quack Busters are trampling on the fundamental constitutional and ethical rights of patients facing cancer and of the practitioners who serve them.

An intriguing fact about the politics of unconventional cancer therapies is that the lines of battle cut straight across the political spectrum. Proponents and practitioners of unconventional cancer therapies include numerous conservatives and considerable numbers of physicians on the far right, some actually members of the John Birch Society. They regard mainstream organized medicine as a logical extension of creeping liberal socialism, and they *bitterly* resent the intrusion of the state on their freedom to practice medicine as they choose. Other conservatives sympathize with their standpoint, which is essentially a free-market position. The far-right conservatives have found that some of their closest allies in the fight for "freedom of choice in cancer therapy" are New Age cultural left-wing radicals, who equally abhor the restrictive powers of organized medicine. What is fascinating is that over the years, the strength of the common cause has been so powerful that the relationship between the two groups has become much more than a temporary alliance of convenience. Similarly, on the other side of the argument, political conservatives and liberals make common cause to combat unconventional cancer therapies in the name of medical science and consumer protection.

While the bitter war between the advocates and the opponents of the more explicitly alternative cancer therapies (a relatively small proportion of all unconventional therapies) continues unabated in the courts and in the media, a growing number of health professionals and cancer patients are moving toward convergence. They are seeking to define a middle ground on which those professionals and patients sincerely committed to the objective evaluation and exploration of these therapies could convene. They envision the development of a disciplined field that would encourage rigorous scientific study of alternative therapies. They envision the crafting of state and national policy positions on unconventional therapies that would protect patients from the real threats of fraud, while providing opportunities for licensed health professionals and fully informed patients to work together in the face of life-threatening illnesses. This search for a middle ground is signaled by, but not limited to, a growing consensus that a constructive dialogue is possible about the possible benefits of psychological, nutritional, and immunosupportive approaches to cancer treatment. The Office of Alternative Medicine at the National Institutes of Health in Washington is an institutional expression of the burgeoning interest in scientific evaluation of these therapies.

References

1   Richard Grossman, *The Other Medicines* (Garden City, NY: Doubleday & Co., 1985).
2   J.C. Baillar III and E.M. Smith, "Progress Against Cancer?" *New England Journal of Medicine* 314:1226–32 (1986).

eight

A Framework for Evaluating Unconventional Cancer Therapies

In the course of my investigations of unconventional cancer treatments, I have reached several conclusions that seem to have stood the test of time:

- To date, I have seen *no decisive and scientifically documented cure* for any type of cancer among the complementary cancer therapies.[1]
- Relatively little scientific evidence exists for most therapies on which to evaluate questions of whether these therapies sometimes result in *survival advantage, life extension,* or *improved quality of life.*
- However, significant anecdotal or case evidence indicates that some people have recovered from life-threatening cancers or lived for an unexpectedly long time while using many of these therapies, and that some of these therapies do enhance quality of life.
- The old stereotypes that describe unconventional cancer therapies as the domain of cynical "quack" practitioners catering to ignorant, credulous patients are largely (but not entirely) erroneous.
- While the hostilities between the most vocal proponents and opponents of some of the *alternative* cancer therapies continues unabated, there is also cautious movement by thoughtful people on both sides of the "war over cancer therapies" toward a middle ground with respect to ethical, spiritual, psychological, nutritional, herbal, traditional, and immunosupportive approaches to cancer.

The following sections discuss these findings in more detail.

No Scientifically Documented Cure

I have seen no systematic cure for any form of cancer among the therapies currently described as "unconventional." This is an important finding. Conventional therapies, for all their real shortcomings, are capable of curing a number of cancers reliably. When I say I have seen no *systematic* cure for cancer among the unconventional therapies, this does *not* mean that I have seen no *individual* cures among people who have used unconventional therapies. In fact, there are well-documented examples of people who have recovered from "terminal" cancers using various unconventional cancer therapies. But these examples of individual recoveries from terminal cancers are not frequent enough to form a pattern that would allow me to say that there is a *cure* for any cancer among the unconventional therapies. There are therapies, as we shall see, which appear *possibly* to *extend survival* with specific cancers—such as hydrazine sulfate for non-small cell lung cancer, or psychosocial support for metastatic breast cancer and malignant melanoma. And there are many complementary therapies which definitely contribute to enhanced quality of life. These therapies that enhance quality of life may, I propose, confer *some* survival advantage by enhancing physical and psychological general health.

I emphasize the absence of any *decisive cure* as my first finding about these therapies because some of the alternative cancer literature suggests that there *are* cures for cancer among unconventional cancer therapies which are being suppressed by a medical-industrial conspiracy because these "cures" would cut into its profits. Certainly, the medical establishment disapproves of many unconventional cancer therapies, and certainly there are powerful structural forces at work to delegitimize them and sometimes punish their practitioners. But there is no documented *cure* for cancer among the unconventional cancer therapies known to me.

Relatively Little Scientific Evidence

Relatively few scientific studies have been made of most unconventional cancer therapies, although some therapies do have significant scientific documentation. Scientific studies are urgently needed to determine if some of these therapies might extend survival or enhance quality of life for patients who integrate them with the judicious use of conventional therapies.

For a few therapies, notably psychological treatments, scientific studies do document quality of life and some possible survival advantage for patients using them. Moreover, unconventional cancer therapies *do* occasionally cross the line into mainstream medical practice. It is more than a rhetorical point made by proponents of unconventional cancer treatments that chemotherapy, radiotherapy, and hyperthermia (raising a patient's body temperature to abnormally high levels) all started out as unconventional cancer therapies, with hyperthermia being the most recent therapy to cross the line. It is equally important to note, as opponents of unconventional therapies do, that such cases of the subsequent legitimization of unconventional cancer treatments represent the rare exceptions, not the rule.

Psychological treatments for *possible* survival advantage, as well as *demonstrated* quality-of-life benefits, appear to be the most plausible candidates to cross over next into mainstream medicine. I anticipate that medically supervised nutritional support—drawing extensively on some of the tenets of the unconventional nutritional therapies—may follow psychological treatments across the line in the next few decades.

At present, the possibilities that Stanislaw Burzynski in Texas is getting is getting good results with some brain tumors (see chapter 21) and that hydrazine sulfate may extend life with some lung cancers (see chapter 22) are based on preliminary, though intriguing, findings. Thus, the field of unconventional cancer therapies is, by definition, continuously stripped of the most notable examples of scientifically and clinically demonstrated treatments.

Reliable Case Evidence

Case evidence and anecdotal evidence have demonstrated that some cancer patients have recovered from life-threatening cancers while using current unconventional cancer therapies, whether or not one chooses to attribute the recoveries to the use of the unconventional treatment. Rarely, however, are there reliable data on how common these recoveries are. The number of patients who have undertaken the same unconventional therapy that were associated with the well-publicized recoveries without achieving exceptional recovery is simply not known. More important, given the high probability that most unconventional cancer therapies—like most conventional cancer therapies—will at best usually extend survival rather than "cure" cancer, we do not have reliable data for most unconventional cancer therapies that enable us to assess their contributions to life extension rather than cure.

Evidence of individual cases of recoveries from metastatic (or other life-threatening) cancers, and of the correlation between the use of unconventional treatments and length of life, could be gathered by practitioners of these therapies at relatively low cost. Unfortunately, few practitioners of unconventional therapies are committed to careful record keeping, or even rudimentary assessment of outcomes. This is a serious shortcoming in the field.

The work of people with AIDS and the physicians and researchers supporting them in organizing community clinical trials of unconventional AIDS therapies provide a fine example of what is possible in terms of evaluating unconventional cancer therapies. Such initial studies need not be either extremely expensive or extremely difficult to design and execute. For those concerned with unconventional cancer therapies, collaborative work to design and initiate such clinical studies is critically important. Until this happens, most of what even the best-informed clinicians and researchers can tell patients about these therapies is highly subjective and of relatively little value for facilitating informed choice.

Old Stereotypes of Patients and Practitioners

For almost 50 years, mainstream opponents of unconventional cancer therapies successfully portrayed unconventional therapies to the American public as practiced largely by unethical "quack" practitioners, cynically exploiting the fears of patients for personal profit. The patients who used these therapies were portrayed as desperate and credulous people too ignorant to make informed choices. These stereotypes have proved to be highly inaccurate.

The studies of Barrie Cassileth, Ph.D., and my own more journalistic surveys, suggest that, for the most part, unconventional therapies in the United States are offered by licensed physicians or other credentialed health care practitioners who believe in the therapies they offer, who are not charging excessive fees for treatment, and who are treating patients of above-average education. These patients are likely to be more deeply engaged than the average patient in their fight for recovery. In the large majority of cases, these patients also, significantly, choose to remain under the care of a mainstream physician.[2]

In my experience, patients generally leave mainstream medicine *completely* only because their doctors told them they had "nothing more to offer them," or because they had shockingly poor experience with mainstream medicine, or because they weighed the risks and benefits of what mainstream medicine offered and decided to explore other options.

The vast majority of cancer patients do not see conventional and unconventional therapies as an either-or proposition. Rather, they seek to make informed, personal choices about how to *integrate* what conventional therapies offer them and what unconventional therapies offer them. It is also important to recognize that the problem of *impaired physicians* is as real in conventional medicine as the problem of quack practitioners is in unconventional medicine. It is my opinion, based entirely on my own personal experience, that unethical and impaired practitioners probably represent a somewhat larger proportion of unconventional than of conventional practitioners, largely because the field of unconventional therapies is unregulated and, given its socially marginalized position, probably attracts disproportionate numbers of both highly committed ethical practitioners and unethical quack practitioners.

Unconventional cancer therapies also have the problem, which conventional medicine does not have, of attracting well-intentioned but poorly informed "true believer" practitioners who may do cancer patients as much harm as the unethical quacks, out of ignorance and incompetence. It is true that many mainstream oncologists are also true believers in conventional treatments and are poorly informed about ethical, legitimate complementary approaches to cancer care. But at least they have extensive training in cancer treatment, which some of the most dangerous unconventional practitioners lack entirely. Legalization and intelligent regulation of ethical complementary cancer therapies, on the German model, for example, could help to minimize the serious problems presented by quacks and true believer practitioners.

Types of Unconventional Approaches

Because relatively few scientific studies have been made of many of the unconventional cancer therapies, some system for analyzing these divergent approaches to cancer treatment is necessary. The typology I present here—which was adapted in part by the Office of Technology Assessment in framing its report on unconventional cancer therapies—is entirely flexible, and other people may wish to add or subtract elements from the typology. However, in my experience, this typology represents a useful map with which to explore the otherwise confusing terrain of unconventional, alternative, adjunctive, and complementary cancer therapies. Many unconventional cancer therapies combine several of the following 12 elements. The 12 elements in my typology of unconventional cancer therapies are:

1. Spiritual approaches
2. Psychological approaches
3. Nutritional and dietary approaches
4. Physical and psychophysiological approaches
5. Traditional medicines
6. Pharmacological approaches
7. Herbal approaches
8. Electromagnetic approaches
9. Unconventional uses of conventional therapies
10. Esoteric and psychic approaches
11. Unconventional instruments, apparatuses, and diagnostic tests
12. Humane approaches

Spiritual Approaches

A spiritual response is undoubtedly one of the most common human reactions to cancer. The fact that spiritual support in the treatment and care of people with cancer is considered *unconventional* today, or at best the marginal province of the hospital chaplain, is a testament to how alienated from core human needs the conventional medical system has become. Spiritual approaches to cancer, some going back to the dawn of human history, include prayer, laying on of hands, and many forms of spiritual imagery or inner dialogue designed to help align the patient with higher forces in himself or the guiding spirit of nature or the universe, however he defines it.

Prayer and Therapeutic Touch are two of the areas in which exciting early research suggests that extraordinary fields may open up for both physical and psychospiritual healing. The growing scientific literature on "near death experiences" is another area in which research tends to corroborate—although it has not and perhaps cannot "prove"—some of the most ancient human teachings about the immortality of the human soul.

Spiritual approaches to cancer partially overlap religious approaches, but should be clearly differentiated from them. Many cancer patients with negative religious experiences or associations from childhood find to their surprise that they are drawn toward a spiritual response to the "spiritual emergency" of cancer that is authentic and very different from the religious experiences that disappointed them earlier in life. Conversely, many cancer patients access powerful spiritual experiences directly through their fulfilling religious traditions. My own view is that, in future scientific studies, spiritual approaches will be shown both to enhance quality of life—a fairly obvious proposition— and also to extend life for some patients with some cancers. However, spiritually based "cures" will remain the rare exception rather than the rule.

But neither physical recovery nor life extension is the test of the value of spiritual approaches to cancer. The test is in the effect they have on the living experience of the person involved.

Psychological Approaches

Numerous psychological approaches to cancer—both ancient and modern— are now available, and many of these approaches have crossed the line into mainstream respectability. The approaches that are now widely *respectable* within the medical mainstream—although relatively rarely *practiced*—include individual psychotherapy, group therapy, support groups, imagery, psychoeducational programs, guided self-exploration, biofeedback, and hypnosis. They are used variously for:

- Support in recovering from the shock of diagnosis.
- Reducing the anxiety and stress of having cancer.
- Reducing the stress of cancer treatment.
- Minimizing side effects and enhancing recovery from surgery, chemotherapy, and radiotherapy.
- Controlling pain, nausea, sleeplessness, and appetite loss.

- Facing and grieving over losses associated with cancer.
- Exploring possible areas of life enhancement.
- Learning to live a full life with cancer or the threat of recurrence.
- Facing the shock of diagnosis of a cancer recurrence.
- Learning to live with a cancer for which cure is unlikely or for which there is no known cure.
- Facing death and dying from one's own perspective and that of one's family.

The *only* major hypothesis about psychological approaches to cancer on this list that remains genuinely *controversial* is the hypothesis that psychological interventions may extend survival with cancer. Several well-designed studies support the life extension hypothesis, as we shall see in chapter 10, but the scientific jury will not reach a definitive conclusion for another 10 years. My own estimate is that well-designed future studies will show that psychological approaches to cancer—in addition to enhancing quality of life, protecting against the side effects and enhancing the effects of treatment—will, indeed, prove to extend life for some patients with some cancers, and prevent recurrence of cancer for other patients, often to a degree sufficient to make these interventions an important adjunctive treatment option. I believe equally firmly that "cures" of metastatic cancer using psychological approaches will remain rare, individual exceptions rather than the rule.

Nutritional and Dietary Approaches

The dietary and nutritional approaches to cancer therapy are as numerous as the psychological approaches. Diet is now well recognized by scientists to play a *major* role in lowering the risk of some types of cancer, including some of the most common cancers, such as colon, prostate, and breast cancer. The possibility that a diet known to *prevent* a specific cancer could play a role in slowing, stopping, or reversing the development of an established cancer of that type, or indeed in preventing or slowing the *recurrence* of such a cancer, remains highly controversial, with plausible arguments on both sides. Some unconventional practitioners believe that one or another of these unconventional therapies can offer full or partial cures for some cancers. Among the best known of the nutritional and dietary approaches are the macrobiotic diet, the Gerson diet, the Hippocrates wheat-grass diet, the Kelley-Gonzalez nutritional program, and the Livingston-Wheeler nutritional program.

One heavily neglected area of mainstream research is in the role of nutritional interventions in enhancing outcomes for patients who have had chemotherapy, surgery, or radiotherapy. The scientific reports that vitamin E may prevent hair loss for patients treated with doxorubicin (Adriamicin), and possibly protect against cardiac damage as well, are one example of a promising nontoxic use of nutritional supplements as an adjunct to conventional therapy.[3] I expect that adjunctive programs of intensive nutritional support will follow the adjunctive psychosocial approaches into medical mainstream respectability in cancer treatment. I think that in the future diet and nutrition will play a significant role in enhancing the response to and controlling the side effects of conventional therapies. I further believe that well-designed future studies will show that, in addition to improving quality of life, diet and nutrition may extend life for some patients with some cancers, and that diet and nutrition work best when used synergistically with other currently unconventional approaches to healing, including spiritual, psychological, and physical approaches.

Physical and Psychophysiological Approaches

The wide range of physical and psychophysiological approaches to cancer includes exercise, movement therapies, massage therapies, chiropractic and osteopathic treatments, progressive relaxation, breathing practices, yoga, and an element of traditional Chinese medicine called qi gong. These therapies are occasionally recommended as potentially curative in themselves, but far more frequently are offered as adjuncts to conventional treatment or to other complementary treatments. Just as mainstream medicine ignores spiritual, psychological, and nutritional adjuncts to conventional treatments, so, to a lesser degree, even *mainstream* physical therapies are often overlooked or underemphasized as key elements in recovery from common cancer treatments, particularly mastectomies. Thus conventional physical therapy must paradoxically be included as "unconventional" because it is so frequently ignored in mainstream protocols, although its role in recovery from mastectomy and other cancer treatments is well documented. I feel quite certain that physical and physiological approaches to cancer will join nutritional approaches in following the psychological approaches into the medical mainstream. I believe they will be found to contribute to quality of life, symptom control, minimizing side effects of treatment, enhancing effects of treatment, and life extension for some patients with some cancers. Definitive "cures" attributable to them will remain the rare exception rather than the rule.

The Vital Quartet

At this point, I pause in the discussion of the 12 common elements in unconventional cancer therapies to make a crucial point about the first four common elements described above. Spiritual, psychological, nutritional, and physical approaches to cancer represent a quartet of ethical approaches to improving health that have benefited many cancer patients. When a cancer patient takes the time to undertake a system of intensive multimodal health promotion that includes these four elements—and which makes sense to him—the general result is that he becomes a healthier cancer patient. The effects of such a regimen on quality of life, symptom control, and controlling side effects of treatment are fairly obvious. But it is also reasonable that becoming a healthy cancer patient *may* help extend life. I believe the effect on life extension of intensive multimodal efforts to improve quality of life by becoming a healthier person with cancer will someday be demonstrated to significantly extend life or prevent recurrence for some patients with some cancers. I believe it will also prove true that sometimes, but not always, integrating these four approaches will have a synergistic effect on life extension that exceeds the effect of using only one approach. Therefore, these four intrinsically health-promoting therapies could be described as categorically distinct from the other eight elements I describe below. Without any question, research on the effects of intensive spiritual, psychological, nutritional, and physical health promotion in cancer treatment should become an integral part of the mainstream agenda.

Traditional Medicines

The World Health Organization (WHO) designates "traditional medicine"—as opposed to "conventional" or "allopathic" medicine—as those practices which come from the great medical traditions of the world, such as traditional Chinese medicine, Tibetan medicine, Ayurvedic medicine from India, naturopathic and homeopathic medicine from Europe, and the eclectic modern folk medicines practiced in many countries. WHO recognizes traditional medicines as the legitimate and often efficacious providers of medical care to a large part of the world's people.

The traditional medicine most commonly used by American cancer patients is Chinese medicine, which includes acupuncture, herbal therapies, moxibustion (the burning of a herbal paste over key acupuncture points), and often recommendations on diet and changes in mental state. Western patients widely report that traditional Chinese medicine offers considerable relief from the side effects of chemotherapy and radiation, as well as being a nonpharmacological method of pain control. Ayurvedic medicine from India, Tibetan medicine, and homeopathic medicine also have their adherents among American cancer patients and health practitioners.

Relatively few of the traditional medicines claim to be able to cure cancer on a regular basis. But some have treatments that seem to help with symptom control, the side effects of mainstream treatments, and quality of life. In some instances, the potential for achieving unexpected recoveries is also recognized. The great traditional medicines tend to concur with the informed consensus regarding the possible benefits of an integrated therapy using spiritual, psychological, nutritional, and physical approaches to cancer—all of which are often incorporated in their treatments. They also often use specific herbal remedies, which in in vitro research tests have been found to have anticancer effects.

Pharmacological Approaches

A vast range of pharmacological approaches to cancer includes pharmacological use of nutritional supplementation, herbs, and hundreds of other unconventional pharmaceutical agents, new and old. Laetrile, vitamin C, the mistletoe extract Iscador, and hydrazine sulfate are examples of a few of these pharmacological treatments. Pharmacological approaches are among the most common unconventional cancer treatments.

Herbal Approaches

Herbal therapies for cancer are largely derived from traditional ethnomedicines from hundreds of different medical traditions. Pau D'Arco tea from South America, the Hoxsey herbs from the United States and Mexico, the Canadian treatment Essiac, and the herbal remedies used in traditional Chinese medicine are a few of the best-known herbal treatments. Fortunately, a respected scientific literature is available on laboratory tests of the anticancer effects of herbal remedies that patients, physicians, and researchers can consult. However, there are few rigorous studies for most of these remedies as actual treatments for human cancer. This category of herbal approaches overlaps significantly with the pharmacological category above.

Electromagnetic Approaches

Electromagnetic approaches to the diagnosis and treatment of cancer are now making significant claims on scientific attention—most notably the work of Bjorn Nordenstrom at the Karolinska Institute in Sweden.[4] There is also a growing scientific literature on electromagnetic hazards in everyday life associated with increased incidence of some cancers.[5]

Unconventional Uses of Conventional Treatments

Unconventional uses of conventional treatment modalities go beyond the normal range of "variations in medical practice" that are found within mainstream medical research and treatment facilities. Wolfgang Scheef, Dr. med., at the Janker Klinik in Bonn, Germany, is a clinician offering unconventional use of conventional or experimental cancer treatments which have attracted many American cancer patients. In Canada, Rudy Falk, M.D., former Chief of Surgical Oncology at the Toronto General Hospital, also uses conventional and experimental agents in unconventional ways.

Esoteric and Psychic Approaches

Esoteric approaches to the prevention, diagnosis, and treatment of cancer often overlap the spiritual approaches and those of the various systems of traditional medicine. Psychic diagnosis of cancer, psychic surgery as practiced by some healers from the Philippines, and the use of crystals in healing are examples of esoteric approaches.

Psychic diagnosis and psychic recommendations for treatment seem extraordinarily far-fetched to most people in the medical mainstream. Yet, as research in psychic phenomena has become more scientific, more researchers and clinicians have become interested in the possible continuum between psychic phenomena—such as clairvoyance and "remote viewing" capacities with respect to diagnosis and treatment—and the common intuitive experiences of many clinicians and patients in which one or the other "knows" when the cancer is active, or in remission, before diagnostic tests confirm this intuitive knowledge. The role of intuition in diagnosis and treatment and its relationship to increasingly well-studied psychic phenomena are certainly likely to attract more attention in coming decades.

Unconventional Instruments, Apparatuses, and Diagnostic Tests

Some unconventional instruments and diagnostic tests are blatantly and cynically fraudulent, others intriguing. Special microscopes for the diagnosis of cancerous and precancerous conditions are some of the most intriguing diagnostic tools. Virginia Livingston-Wheeler, M.D., in San Diego, made unconventional use of mainstream dark-field microscopes for the study of live blood for the purposes of refined cancer diagnosis. Gaston Naessens in Quebec has an unconventional microscope that he designed and built himself—but will not allow others to replicate—with very high magnification powers that he uses to study live blood for refined diagnosis of cancer and other conditions. Royal Rife also developed a microscope in the 1930s in San Diego for which unusual diagnostic potential has been claimed. Many clinicians involved in unconventional cancer treatments who have used dark-field microscopes have confirmed that intriguing phenomena seem to show up in live blood that seem well correlated to cancerous conditions. These diagnostic tools, according to these practitioners' theories, allow the clinician to track the response of the blood to unconventional cancer treatments and so guide their progress.

Humane Approaches

A pervasive theme in many unconventional cancer therapies is the emphasis on humane treatment. Obviously, practitioners of conventional cancer therapies are often equally concerned with humane care. Equally obviously, many complementary practitioners are inhumane in their delivery of unconventional treatments. Nevertheless, an emphasis on the humane, compassionate, and sensitive treatment of the patient is one of the major themes that runs throughout the literature on complementary cancer therapies, and some of the best of these treatment systems—notably the anthroposophical hospitals founded in Germany and central Europe by the followers of Rudolf Steiner— do achieve systematically more humane levels of treatment for cancer patients than mainstream hospitals in the United States and Europe usually do. In their focus on humane treatment, practitioners of unconventional cancer therapies come to conclusions similar to the growing number of advocates of "patient-centered" or "humanistic" medicine in the United States medical mainstream.

Evaluating the Therapy, the Practitioner, and Service Delivery

This completes our brief review of the 12 elements often found in various combinations among the hundreds of unconventional cancer therapies used by cancer patients. But how can we begin to approach the practical evaluation of these therapies? Given that valid scientific evidence for evaluating unconventional cancer therapies is often so sparse, there are three categorical distinctions that have proved useful to me in assessing these therapies. I believe that patients, clinicians, and researchers assessing an unconventional cancer therapy should differentiate clearly between (a) the therapy itself, (b) the practitioner offering the therapy, and (c) the quality of the service delivery. (These three categories are, incidentally, equally valuable in assessing a conventional therapy.)

In order to evaluate the *therapy,* the following questions are useful: Can you assess whether the therapy is probably harmless, possibly dangerous, or plausibly helpful in some significant way? Does it operate according to known or plausible principles? Most important, is there any significant scientific literature that supports the use of this therapy?

A further very crucial distinction in evaluating therapies can be made between "open" and "closed" (or "partially closed") therapies. An open therapy is one where all the information regarding the therapy is publicly available. This is usually true of the spiritual, psychological, nutritional, and physical therapies, as well as the traditional medicines. A closed therapy is one in which the practitioner, wittingly or unwittingly, acts so that the critical information is unavailable. A closed therapy inevitably raises suspicion about the motives of the practitioner. The most important closed therapies are, significantly, pharmacological.

Important commonalities, as well as important differences, exist between closed unconventional therapies and "proprietary" therapies of major pharmaceutical companies. The commonality is that—particularly during the development stage of a new mainstream pharmacological remedy—the ingredients of the treatment may be kept a secret. The difference is that the mainstream closed or proprietary formulas must be registered with the FDA and undergo extensive scientific evaluation.

One line of defense for closed unconventional therapies is that the use by physicians of secret or mysterious treatments has an ancient history and an undeniable psychological pedigree in terms of its potential to augment a placebo healing power. For some patients, the mystery of a closed therapy contributes to the numinous quality of the remedy. This may help explain why, although 90% of unconventional cancer therapies may be open, some of the closed or partially closed therapies have traditionally attracted the greatest patient interest both in the United States and abroad. Lawrence Burton's immuno-augmentative therapy in the Bahamas is perhaps the frankest and best-known example of a closed and proprietary unconventional therapy. The Essiac herbal therapy in Canada is a widely used partially closed herbal therapy whose formula the practitioners have not disclosed, although it has been analyzed by herbal research specialists.

An almost mythological quality seems to infuse the story of why closed therapies remain closed. The mythological tale often runs like this: The practitioner discovered a cure for cancer outside the establishment. More and more patients came to be successfully treated. Mainstream authorities approached the practitioner, or the practitioner approached mainstream authorities, to discuss the new therapy. The practitioner offered to share the secret with the world if the mainstream authorities guaranteed that it would be made freely available, or available at low cost. But the mainstream authorities wanted to control the treatment, either in order to make large profits or to suppress it because they are part of a conspiracy to continue the profitable cancer industry. The practitioner resolutely refused this bargain with the forces of darkness and underwent long persecution as a result, only to emerge victorious in the end. This archetypal story of the "hero's journey" will be familiar to students of mythology. It often appears incredible to the mainstream worldview, but it is highly credible to many patients oriented toward alternative cancer therapies. It is interesting to note that the "hero's journey" undertaken by the practitioner of a closed therapy is often paralleled by many patients in their own journey, in which they partially or fully break with the mainstream system, undergo many hardships along the way, and arrive to find themselves in a community of believers where they are treated with the precious and mysterious substance. This is a psychologically potent process with *significant* placebo potential which may arguably enhance prospects for recovery, irrespective of the pharmacological action of the therapy itself.

Having evaluated the *therapy,* a second useful set of criteria may be applied to evaluating the *practitioner.* What is his training? What is his reputation within his own social network? For example, what do other unconventional practitioners, who may have referred patients to him, think of him? Most important, what is the experience of other patients who have gone to see him, especially patients with a type and stage of cancer similar to that of the inquiring patient? What are his claims regarding outcomes? Is he willing to make data available to open-minded investigators, or to provide (with their permission) contact with other cancer patients with the same kind of cancer that the inquiring patient has? Does he encourage patients to reject conventional therapies when these therapies offer scientifically documented evidence of cure or significant life extension at acceptable cost in terms of quality of life? Finally, *and very important,* does he appear to be a person of psychological balance and integrity worthy of your trust?

The quality of the *service delivery* is the third important factor in assessing the usefulness of an unconventional therapy. What is the cost and quality of the service? What do other patients say about the service delivery? Do most patients who have completed the treatment program believe (whether or not the treatment was effective) that the service was reasonably related to the cost? I have seen instances where the therapy is probably either harmless or potentially beneficial, and the practitioner ethical and devoted to his work, but where the delivery of the service is severely flawed and potentially dangerous to the patient's health. Costs also vary widely, from reasonable fees—or even free services—to staggeringly expensive fees. Of course, the same questions regarding service delivery hold for the delivery of conventional cancer therapies.

These three areas—the quality of the therapy, practitioner, and service delivery—are critical both for the patient and for the analyst committed to objective evaluation, since so much of the debate over unconventional cancer therapies indiscriminately mixes analysis on each of these three points. You cannot have a legitimate evaluation process for an unconventional therapy unless you distinguish clearly whether you are evaluating the treatment itself, the practitioner of the treatment, or the service delivery.

Curing, Healing, and Intensive Health Promotion

As I indicated in chapter 2, it is also essential to distinguish between "curing" and "healing" in evaluating unconventional cancer therapies. Recall that a "cure" generally refers to a medical treatment that reliably relieves the patient of the disease. "Healing" is recognized as referring primarily to an internal process of becoming whole, which can take place simultaneously or differentially at the physical, psychological, and spiritual levels.

Obviously, the capacity of either mainstream or unconventional therapies to be curative depends in part on the availability of the patient's inner resources for physical healing and recovery. But beyond that, it is also entirely possible for someone to be "cured" of breast cancer by a mastectomy, chemotherapy, or radiation, yet never "heal" or feel whole again. It is also possible for conventional therapies to *fail* in their efforts to "cure," yet for profound "healing" to take place spiritually and psychologically nonetheless. It is also quite possible—probable in my view—that the psychospiritual "healing process" may augment access to an interior biophysiological potential which will maximize the response to potentially "curative" therapies. In this view, efforts at psychospiritual and physiological healing represent a win-win strategy: the patient wins if he achieves physical recovery, and he also can enhance profoundly the quality of his life if physical recovery is impossible.

The most ancient traditions of medicine understood this point far better than mainstream medicine does today. They placed their primary emphasis on psychospiritual healing—on safeguarding the human soul—rather than on curing. The ancient shamans believed that if deep psychospiritual healing took place, whatever energies were available for physical recovery would be released. "Seek ye first the Kingdom of God, and everything else will be added unto you" is a pithy summary of this psychospiritual truth.

The ancient shamans also often practiced what we have identified as *intensive health promotion,* integrating spiritual, psychological, nutritional, and physical approaches to enhancing the conditions of healing. This combination of support for the inner and outer "conditions of healing" characterizes, as I have said, some of the best unconventional cancer therapies. Many cancer diagnoses give the patient months, if not years, of opportunity to enhance general health. Many cancer patients routinely succeed in enhancing general health through intensive health promotion while they have cancer.

One of the most important unanswered clinical and research questions is whether these efforts at intensive physical and psychospiritual health promotion in unconventional cancer therapies do more than manifestly improve quality of life with cancer, that is, whether they might actually lead to improved "functional status" for people with cancer. According to William Buchholz, M.D., a Los Altos, California oncologist with a strong interest in working with cancer patients who actively collaborate in their own care, "functional status is an independent predictor of survival in almost all cancers, as well as an independent predictor of response and survival for most chemotherapies."[6] Thus there is good reason to believe that intensive health promotion may extend survival in those cancers where the functional status of the patient is a significant predictor of survival.

Most "healing" therapists also know that psychospiritual healing can take place as the patient is losing physical ground, or even as he enters the dying process, and that such psychospiritual healing can be of enormous importance to the patient, to the family, and to all others involved. From my own experience, I want to add that efforts at physical as well as psychospiritual healing can be extremely helpful to the quality of life in people with advanced progressive cancer. The value of health-promoting activities even for people who are near death is, in my view, often overlooked. In cancer, often a limited number of organs are involved, and the person may still be able to work gently to enhance physical as well as psychospiritual health, sometimes with surprisingly positive quality-of-life results.

Controlling Versus Curing

It is also profoundly important to recognize that practitioners of some unconventional cancer therapies propose that they cannot "cure" but may be able to "control," or "partially control," some cancers. They offer the analogy of the use of nutritional, behavioral, or pharmacological approaches to the control of asthma, hypertension, angina, or diabetes, or the use of behavioral and psychospiritual approaches to the control of alcoholism and drug addiction. This is an important point, because many of the unconventional cancer therapies, when they work, do appear to function by controlling rather than curing. The evidence for this is that, on the occasions when an unconventional therapy appears to be working, the control often fails when the treatments or health-promoting practices are discontinued or, more important, when another psychological or physical life stress upsets the delicate balance that previously favored control.

Improved Quality of Life and Control of Symptoms

Many benefits beyond curing, healing, and control of the disease are offered by proponents of unconventional cancer therapies. As suggested above, many practitioners of the spiritual, psychological, nutritional, and physical therapies, who essentially offer a variety of forms of intensive, multimodal health promotion, report that patients achieve higher quality of life, respond better to most conventional cancer therapies, experience fewer side effects of treatment and fewer symptoms of the disease, control pain better with less need for medication, experience more lasting or partial remissions and, if and when they die, experience better deaths. Such reports also come from practitioners of other unconventional cancer therapies, such as practitioners of traditional Chinese medicine. Proponents of many of these therapies also say that their treatments are more humane, although the record on humane delivery of services in unconventional therapies is as mixed as in conventional therapies.

In the chapters that follow, I discuss in detail the five most significant categories of unconventional cancer treatment: spiritual, psychological, nutritional, physical, traditional, and pharmacological therapies.

Notes and References

1   Robert Houston, a leading authority on unconventional cancer therapies, challenges this statement. He says, "This sets up a strawman. Rarely do scientific proponents claim a 'cure.' The question is, are there promising and beneficial therapies among the alternative approaches? There most certainly are."

2   Barrie R. Cassileth and Helene Brown, "Unorthodox Cancer Medicine," *Cancer Journal for Clinicians* 38(3):182–3 (1988).

3   K.N. Prasad et al., "Vitamin E Enhances the Growth Inhibitory and Differentiating Effects of Tumor Therapeutic Agents on Neuroblastoma and Glioma Cells in Culture," *Proceedings of the Society for Experimental Biological Medicine* 164(2):158–63 (1980). See also L. Wood, "Possible Prevention of Adriamicin-Induced Alopecia by Tocopherol," *New England Journal of Medicine* 312:1060 (1985).

4   Bjorn E.W. Nordenstrom, *Biologically Closed Electric Circuits: Clinical, Experimental and Theoretical Evidence for an Additional Circulatory System* (Stockholm: Nordic Medical Publications, 1983).

5   D.A. Savitz et al., "Case-Control Study of Childhood Cancer and Exposure to 60-Hz Magnetic Fields," *American Journal of Epidemiology* 128(1):21–38 (1988). See also A. Ahlbom, et al. "Biological Affects of Power Line Fields: New York State Power Lines Project Scientific Advisory Panel, Final Report," New York State Department of Health, Albany, NY. Available from: National Technical Information Service, Springfield, VA (1988).

6   William Buchholz, M.D., personal communication with author, 28 November 1990.

nine

Spiritual Approaches to Cancer

Cancer means facing the certainty of illness, the probability of pain, and the possibility of death. For many people, these encounters evoke profound shifts in consciousness that *may* be called "spiritual." For some, the use of prayer, meditation, contemplation, and a review of how they are acting in the world—and how they choose to act under these new circumstances—comes easily. For others, who may never have considered the possibility that they have a spiritual nature, the encounter with these deep shifts in consciousness brings them into unknown territory. They may have had no previous reason to sort out the differences between religion—which they may have had difficulties with—and personal spirituality. They may not have considered the relationship between spirituality and the opportunities for healing. They may not have considered how spirituality is often evoked—sometimes for the first time—by a deep wound such as cancer.[1]

My father, Max Lerner, had just such an experience with cancer. In his book, *Wrestling with the Angel*, he wrote:

> In earlier years, while teaching seminars on selfhood and its components, I would move from soma to brain to mind to psyche, elaborating on what differentiated and connected them. During my healing phase, as I stood at the blackboard for another go at the same question, I found myself, after psyche, adding spirit and soul. I had not planned it, yet somehow, having written the

added words, I knew that after the experience I have described I could do no other. In a different way each stage moves through what physiology, neurology, logic, and psychology study, to a realm that transcends them but remains an important component of the total person.[2]

On Definitions of Spirit, Spirituality, and Spiritual Healing

What is spirit? What is spirituality? What is spiritual healing? A superb symposium in *Advances*, the journal of mind-body health published by the Fetzer Institute, discussed the issue of spiritual healing in unusual depth. David Aldridge wrote:

> The natural sciences base of modern medicine that, in turn, influences the way in which modern medicine is delivered, often ignores the spiritual factors associated with health. Health invariably is defined in anatomical or physiological, psychological or social terms. Rarely do we find diagnoses that include the spiritual concerns of patients.
>
> The descriptions we invoke as clinicians or researchers to characterize disease have implications for the treatment strategies we suggest and the ways we believe people can be encouraged to become healthy or to maintain the state we regard as "health." We need to recognize that patience, grace, prayer, meditation, hope, forgiveness and fellowship are as important to many of our health initiatives as medication, hospitalization, incarceration or surgery. The spiritual elements of experience help us to rise above the matters at hand such that in the face of suffering we can find purpose, meaning and hope.[3]

Aldridge quotes a definition of the spiritual in medicine by Hiatt, a psychiatrist: "Spirit refers to that noncorporeal and nonmental dimension of the person that is the source of unity and meaning, and spirituality refers to the concepts, attitudes and behaviors that derive from one's experience of that dimension. Spirit can be addressed only indirectly and inferentially, while spirituality can be understood and worked with in psychologic terms."[4]

It is a very critical point that spirit is that which *some people* experience as a source of unity and meaning, while spirituality refers to the experience of that dimension that we are able to talk about. The distinction is critical because while all human beings—perhaps all beings—may be said to be one in spirit, as soon as we begin to talk about spirituality we inevitably use concepts that have the potential to disrupt the unity to which we refer, and to divide us.

It is useful to think of spirit, spirituality, and religion as different points on a continuum. Spirit is the source dimension behind every personal or collective experience of spirituality. It is also the source dimension behind every religion. Spirituality can be considered closer to the source dimension than everyday religion that has moved far from the experience of spirit and primarily serves social and moral purposes. Spirituality can be found both within religious frameworks, by people who have stayed close to or recovered the source dimension of their religion, and outside of religious frameworks. But since any discussion of spirituality, in order to talk about spirit, necessarily uses concepts and proposes attitudes regarding that experience, it already has the makings of divisiveness, and indeed the potential structures of a religion, within it.

Spirit is said, then, to be a realm that unites us. When we talk about spirit, and therefore enter the realm of spirituality, we have seen how concepts and attitudes that divide us begin to enter the dialogue. This is particularly true when we begin to address the question of whether any kinds of spiritual energies or spiritual realities exist beyond what we see or what is scientifically demonstrable. For example, claims that prayer or laying on of hands can be physiologically healing begins to bring us into this realm.

Spiritual and Psychological Approaches to Cancer

Spiritual and psychological approaches to cancer are deeply interrelated, yet distinct. The mind, the subject of psychology, is one of the approaches to the spirit, but not the only one. The very word "spiritual" repulses many people, particularly people who were forced into religious systems in their childhood that thwarted or even denied the authentic voyage of inner self-discovery that spiritual life represents. In fact, only in the face of cancer do some patients discover that there can be a profound difference for some people between being religious and being spiritual. One can be spiritual without being religious, and one can be religious without being spiritual. For people who are fortunate enough to have had families or religious teachers who did not destroy their religious tradition for them, the great religions are often safe and known paths into the life of the spirit. For others, the distorted presentation of these traditions has turned them away from the spiritual quest for inner knowledge.

There are still others who recoil from the word "spiritual" because it evokes for them ways of relating to life that they find inauthentic for reasons that may have nothing to do with early childhood experience. Many cancer patients have told me that they cannot relate to the concept of a spiritual reality, but that they can relate deeply to nature, mankind, friends and family, art and music, or science and reason. At the heart of all great spiritual traditions is a clear recognition that all forms of dedication to what is worthy in human experience are ultimately spiritual. In this sense, the spiritual quest is the search for the life path on which we explore the highest potential each of us was given in this life. The spiritual quest can be undertaken as completely by an atheist or agnostic, or a worshiper of nature, family, mankind, art, music, or science, as by a believer in an explicitly religious or spiritual tradition.

For the cancer patient engaged in an intense search for healing and recovery, these considerations are not abstract theological issues. Like a soldier in a trench under bombardment who suddenly discovers prayer, or a prisoner in a forgotten cell awaiting execution, the person with cancer often has urgent reason to reflect on ultimate questions: the meaning of his life; what has true value for him; what happens when he dies; how he should live from now on. If he immerses himself in books about alternative cancer therapies, he will read about many spiritual approaches to cancer. But he may feel blocked and frustrated because he does not consider himself a religious or spiritual person, or because the kinds of spiritual experiences that the books describe seem foreign to him. For such a person, the fundamental distinctions between spirit, spirituality, and religion may never have been made clear. Without these distinctions, he may not see—or give himself permission to explore—the path to the realm of spirit that *for him,* as a unique human being, would be authentic, life-enhancing, and perhaps lifesaving.

Spirituality and the Perennial Philosophy

Aldous Huxley, the great British writer and thinker, died of cancer. When his first wife died of cancer before him, he sat beside her as she died and whispered in her ear the sacred instructions from the *Tibetan Book of the Dead,* reminding her—as many great spiritual teachings do—to follow the light as her soul gradually separated from her body. Huxley also was one of the great early ethical experimenters with lysergic acid diethylamide (LSD). He wrote a book about his experience called *The Gates of Perception*. When his own death came near and he sensed its nearness, he wrote his second wife a note asking her to ask his physician to give him an intramuscular injection of LSD. His physician complied. After the injection, Huxley grew still and seemed to turn inward. "Interesting" was the last word he said before he died.

During World War II, Huxley wrote a beautiful book called *The Perennial Philosophy*. The book was an anthology of passages that Huxley had selected from the great religious and spiritual traditions of the world. His purpose was to demonstrate that there was a central unchanging teaching—a perennial philosophy—at the core of all the great spiritual traditions, and that all traditions represent different paths to that teaching. As the *Rig Veda,* one of the most ancient of spiritual texts, puts it:

> *Truth is one: sages call it by various names.*
> *It is the one Sun who reflects in all the ponds;*
> *It is the one water which slakes the thirst of all;*
> *It is the one air which sustains all life;*
> *It is the one fire which shines in all houses.*
> *Colors of the cows may be different, but milk is white;*
> *Flowers and bees may be different, but honey is the same;*
> *Systems of faith may be different, but God is one.*

. . .

> *As the rain dropping from the sky wends its way toward the ocean,*
> *So the prostrations offered in all faiths reach the One God, who is*
> *supreme.*[5]

Because most ancient religions grew out of tribal traditions where the religion played the dual role of a spiritual guidance system and a social boundary system, many religions—including Christianity and Judaism—have teachings that seem to say that they are the only true way to God. While this was a natural stage in the evolution of spiritual consciousness, most great spiritual teachers in the ages since humans have emerged from tribal consciousness have recognized the teaching that religious and spiritual traditions represent, as Huxley believed, different approaches—suited to different peoples and different temperaments—to cultivating the life of the spirit.

This recognition of the huge variety of spiritual paths that ultimately lead toward the same essential self-realization is important to cancer patients because it further liberates them to find a spiritual path that has vitality for them. This is more than theory for the person with cancer. Hugh Prather and Gerald Jampolsky, M.D., reflect on the importance of this truth for those in crisis:

> It has been assumed that although the perennial wisdom remains the same, it is really a mental plaything for the comfortably situated and is partially, if not wholly, impractical for those who struggle and suffer and even for those whose lives contain a common measure of hardship. . . . We have seen that, on the contrary, the more desperately these concepts are needed and the more wholeheartedly they are turned to, the more enormous is their potential for delivering a growing sense of peace and even glimpses of a higher reality.[6]

Achieving deeper levels of self-realization can unquestionably transform the experience of cancer, deeply lessening unnecessary stress and anguish. And the psychobiological correlates of achieving inner peace, of regaining inner tranquility and joy in life, may transform the biological environment in which the cancer developed. There are those, myself included, who believe that in some cases this inner quest may have an important effect on the course that the cancer takes.

Yoga and Meditation

One example of the distinction between spirituality and religion is the relationship between yoga and the religious tradition which gave birth to it as a spiritual path. Yoga is only one manifestation of the Perennial Philosophy, but one which is very accessible for people in the West and which can accommodate within its range people of all backgrounds, tastes and temperaments. Meditation, the stilling of mind, is at the heart of yoga. But yoga is only one of many paths to learning meditation. I have a personal prejudice in favor of yoga that the reader should be aware of. I believe that yoga probably saved my life and helped me in a transition from a highly stressful period to a much more fulfilling way of living.

What is yoga? The word means, among other things, "union," which is taken to mean "union with the Higher Self" or whatever we designate as sacred or meaningful that is greater than our individual selves. Yoga originated as one of the religious schools of Hinduism. Hinduism is, as Arnold Toynbee described it, the oldest of the six principal surviving "higher religions." The list includes Hinduism, Judaism, Zoroastrianism, Buddhism, Christianity, and Islam. The higher religions (many would argue whether or not "higher" is a correct description) differed from their predecessors, according to Toynbee, in that their principal purpose was "to enable human beings to enter into a direct personal relation with a trans-human presence in and behind the Universe, instead of being introduced to this ultimate spiritual reality only indirectly, through the medium of the civilization or the pre-civilized society that is the individual's social setting."[7]

Hinduism, Judaism, and Zoroastrianism, the oldest of the principal religions, retained a kind of double line of thinking that straddled the division between sectarian religious thought and universal religious thought: they conceived of God as universal but, according to Toynbee, "they went on thinking of him at the same time as being the peculiar local god of the society or community in which he had originally been worshipped as such . . . It has never been feasible to be converted to the Hindu, the Jewish or the Zoroastrian religion without at the same time having to become a member of the Hindu, Jewish, or Zoroastrian society."[8]

In contrast says Toynbee:

> Buddhism, Christianity and Islam have each been—or become—whole-heartedly universalistic. Each of these three religions has set out to convert the whole of Mankind . . . Each has succeeded in converting whole continents, embracing the regional domains of a number of different civilizations. . . . This missionary prowess has been the reward of Buddhism's, Christianity's and Islam's relative success in disengaging themselves from the irrelevant legacy of their historical origins. . . . Unlike Christianity and Islam, Buddhism has usually coexisted amicably with other faiths. It is surely not just a coincidence that Buddhism has been the most successful of the three missionary religions.[9]

While it is unquestionably correct that Hinduism never extricated itself from its origins, it is also true that Hinduism made space within its bounds for a general tolerance and sometimes endorsement of a remarkable range of religious experiences. But the critical point here—my reason for this digression into the history of religions—is that while Hinduism did not disengage itself from its historical antecedents, *yoga did.* Yoga as an international psycho-physiological discipline and spiritual path to a direct personal relationship with God, Nature, or whatever we choose to call the Greater Reality, detached itself from the historical circumstances of its birth, where its mother religion could not. Yoga went on to become, at least in the teachings of many of its adherents, a profoundly ecumenical approach to spiritual life, which values equally every religion and spiritual path. It does not seek, moreover, to *replace* the mother religions of its practitioners, but simply to serve as a kind of complementary "operations manual" for achieving higher states of consciousness, thereby enabling the practitioner to appreciate more deeply the teachings of his or her mother religion—and the teachings of the mother religions of all other peoples as well.

Yoga is best known as a set of physical practices that include gentle stretches, breathing practices, and progressive deep relaxation. These physical practices are intended to ready the body and mind for meditation as well as for a meditative perspective on life. These meditative practices also follow a sequence. First developed is the capacity to withdraw the senses from focus on the outer world, then, the capacity to concentrate on a meditative subject—a candle flame, a sacred or uplifting word or image, or the movement of the breath. Finally, and for most of us only occasionally, the concentration leads into a wordless and timeless experience of inner peace. The yoga masters describe various subtleties among these states of inner peace, but most of us, at best, achieve moments of this experience from time to time.

Yoga also includes, for those who wish to go beyond the physical and meditative practices, a set of ethical imperatives similar to the Ten Commandments and the moral precepts of the other great spiritual traditions, as well as a set of recommendations for clean and healthy living. Finally, yoga offers a set of spiritual scriptures including the *Bhagavad Gita,*[10] perhaps the greatest of Hindu spiritual texts, and Patanjali's *Yoga Sutras,* which are specifically devoted to the description of yoga. The *Yoga Sutras* begin with the statement that "Yoga is the stilling of the mind-stuff." Patanjali then explains that when the mind-stuff is quiet, the busy images and concepts with which we identify our "selves" subside and we can recognize the true inner self, the place from which we watch (and mistakenly identify ourselves with) the busy activities of our daily lives.[11]

One of the greatest sutras (sutra means "string of thought") introduces the third book of the Yoga Sutras. Patanjali writes: "The acceptance of pain as an aid to purification, the study of great scriptures, and complete surrender to the divine being constitute yoga in practice."[12] This idea, that pain is an aid in purification, is central, Aldous Huxley believed, to the perennial philosophy of all the great spiritual traditions. It is a difficult concept to embrace, but for anyone facing pain and illness, one well worth contemplating.

Another aspect of yoga deeply related to healing is its recognition that every person has his own personal way to self-realization (or healing), but that there are some major highways of the spirit that have proved useful to accelerating these inner processes. *Hatha yoga*, for example, represents the physical poses, breathing, and related practices: some people need a major emphasis on these *physical* practices to heal. *Karma yoga* is the yoga of work: healing is achieved by working in the world—through art, through service, through education or an exciting or worthwhile business—with full commitment to the work but without any personal attachment to praise or blame for the outcome. *Bhakti yoga* is the yoga of achieving inner peace or healing by emotional devotion to God or a spiritual teacher: this is the path of passionate devotion and prayer. *Jnana yoga* is the yoga of achieving inner peace or healing through wisdom, through understanding scriptures and spiritual teachings: this is the way of the person who absorbs books, audiotapes or videotapes, and information, and who seeks to move from information to understanding to wisdom to the transcendence of mind by the power of mind. *Raja yoga* is the yoga that integrates these and other forms of yoga as a balanced whole: *raja yoga* means the "kingly yoga," and the name is a recognition that the yoga that integrates, according to the individual's needs, physical practices, work practices, prayer and devotion, and wisdom, is the greatest yoga—or path to union—of all. The recognition that different people are psychophysiologically and culturally suited to different paths to self-realization is one of the most fundamental precepts of yoga.[13]

The specific relevance of yoga and meditation to *cancer patients* is clear and profound. Inasmuch as the physical, mental, and spiritual practices of yoga that lead to inner transformation can help us heal at many levels, the cancer patient is advised by the most fundamental teachings of yoga that *there is no single right way to do this.* The Bible contains many similar scriptural admonitions: "In my Father's house are many rooms . . ."[14] Yoga is simply one of the clearest statements of the fundamental ecumenicism of this perennial truth. Meditation, common to virtually all religious and spiritual traditions, teaches us the profound benefits of sitting still.

Shamanism and the Perennial Philosophy of Healing

In societies all over the world, the ancient human art of guiding sick people through life-threatening illness, either back to recovery or through the dying process, has through the millennia of human history been conducted by medicine men and women known as *shamans.* Shamanism has more recently become something of a fad in holistic healing circles. Purists decry the abuses and romanticism of this modern neoshamanism; advocates celebrate its contribution to the understanding of healing. The abuses are real, but I will focus on the benefits of the neoshamanic metaphor.

Scholars of shamanism, such as Micrea Eliade and Michael Harner, have noted the striking similarities of shamanism in otherwise wholly dissimilar tribes and cultures. Harner came to the conclusion that the central healing traditions of shamanism were—like the incest taboo—among the very few human teachings that are *culturally invariant.* He suggested that shamanism was, perhaps, culturally invariant because, as a human response to illness, shamanism was somehow rooted in a bedrock of human experience. The shamans were not only healers of the sick. They were also spiritual leaders. So the fact that shamanism was to a surprising degree culturally invariant leads us back to the idea of a common core in all spiritual traditions.

What were some of the elements at the core of shamanism? One of the deepest teachings of shamanic healers was that the shaman, *in order to be of the greatest possible assistance to the patient,* should be less concerned with the maintenance of physical health and more concerned with safeguarding the patient's soul. The shaman went into trance and ventured down into the underworld to see if he could find the secret to helping this soul that had become lost, or that had—as Rachel Naomi Remen has so beautifully put it—entered into the illusion of having become lost. The shaman was there to help bring the soul back into this life, if that was God's will, or, if this life were passing, to conduct the soul safely into the next world.

How similar this shamanic teaching—to safeguard the soul above all—is to one of the central traditions of what Huxley called the perennial philosophy at the heart of all spiritual traditions. In Christianity, this teaching says: "Seek ye first the kingdom of God, and everything else will be added unto you." And how fundamentally similar this shamanic teaching is to the most important insight of psychotherapists who work with cancer: that if, as Lawrence LeShan says, the patient looks for his own "unique song," his own unique way of being in the world—if the patient is true to his deepest self, which is to say his soul—he may maximize his potential for physical survival.[15]

So shamanism, the perennial philosophy, and contemporary wisdom on healing seek to help the physician, patient, and family *create the conditions under which whatever healing is possible—physical, emotional, mental or spiritual—may take place.* And if physical recovery is no longer possible, the search for the spiritual heart of life may extend life or bring a peaceful and dignified death.

It is interesting to contrast the shamanic tradition of healing with contemporary medical care. The shaman had no modern medical tools. But he understood that, in the face of illness, the inner healing force was at its strongest when the patient was attended by an experienced spiritual midwife—someone familiar with, and unafraid of, the frontier between life and death. The shaman was, as we have seen, almost always one who had been near death himself. His lack of fear, his hope for the possibility of recovery, his certainty that the journey through the portals of death could be taken safely, his capacity to communicate with powers that maximized the chances for recovery—all of these things made the patient feel safe and cared for, come what may.

The modern medical doctor, equipped with every instrument for technical care, usually has not been trained as a shaman. More often than not, he has not been near death himself. He is often afraid of death; it is something he may not have explored. Frequently, he feels obliged not to reinforce hopes for recovery so that the patient "doesn't develop false hopes." He feels ill-equipped to communicate with the deep inner powers. Recruited for his skills in mathematics and science, he is commonly unfamiliar with the world in which the patient with serious illness lives. And frequently, he feels that the death of a patient is a personal and professional failure on his part.

A physical wound naturally evokes the physical healing response. But some physical wounds, as well as some emotional and spiritual wounds, are so deep that they evoke psychospiritual, as well as physical, healing responses. Cancer is often such a wound.

The ancient shamans were, almost without exception, people who became shamans as a result of life-threatening illnesses. In the course of coming to the frontier between life and death, they arrived at a state of awareness in which it became clear to them that, if they recovered, they would devote the rest of the life that they had been given to helping others traveling the same perilous passage. They lost all fear of death; they were unafraid in the presence of death; and it was, in part, this fearlessness that prepared them to help others to fight for life when the margins were thin.

The psychoanalytic pioneer C.G. Jung considered shamans to be representative of one of the greatest archetypes of human experience. He called this archetype the "wounded physician" of Greek myth. "It is his own hurt that gives the measure of his power to heal."[16] This archetype is now widely known as the "wounded healer."

Rachel Naomi Remen suggests that many of us have within us the capacity to be wounded healers. The wound in us—and we are all at some level wounded—evokes the healer in those who care about us. The wound in those we care for evokes the healer in us. "My wound evokes your healer. Your wound evokes my healer. My wound enables me to find you with your wound where you have the illusion of having become lost," she says.

It is certainly a common experience of cancer patients who attend the Commonweal Cancer Help Program that they have had their own versions of the shamanic awakening. Their experiences with cancer have often led them into deep places and encounters with the ultimate realities of life that they never experienced before. Some refer to these encounters as "the gift" of the cancer experience. Many come away from these encounters with a certainty that, if they recover, they want to devote at least a part of their time to helping others with cancer.

In reality, I believe it is an illusion to think that you have to *recover* from cancer to offer others spiritual assistance. The healing that takes place among people with ongoing cancer is often beyond any words. It is not an accident that some of the deepest healing work in the course of the week-long Cancer Help Programs is not initiated by the staff but takes place among the participants. Many people come to the Cancer Help Program saying that their primary reason for being there is to be with others who are "in the same boat." They instinctively recognize how *healing* it would be for them to be able to share their experience of cancer with others who are having a similar experience.

The Creative Force in Illness

Many have recognized the creative role of illness in helping us find our true selves—in moving us forward on our life paths. A little known biographical work called *Creative Malady* by George Pickering describes the essential role of illness in forming or consolidating the lifework of Charles Darwin, Florence Nightingale, Marcel Proust, and others. The wound in each evoked the special genius of the life force. "He was cracked," Dame Edith Sitwell once said of William Blake, "but it was through the crack that the light came through." A wound, Rachel Naomi Remen reminds us, is also an opening.

The role of illness and suffering in spiritual growth is one of the central teachings of the perennial philosophy. The diaries of early Christian saints record that they welcomed suffering for its known benefits for spiritual clarification. This dual nature of painful events—as both causes of suffering and also possible deliverers of great wisdom—is noted by Howard Brody, M.D., when he says that "suffering is produced, and alleviated, primarily by the meaning that one attaches to one's experience."[17]

In modern Western civilization, we often see only the obvious negative side of pain and suffering. We have forgotten the ancient teachings about their possible benefits. Most of the great spiritual traditions emphasize that you need not seek out pain and suffering. In fact, they counsel that "the wise learn by observation, the rest by experience." So, if you have the wisdom and the discipline, you can avoid a great deal of needless pain. But even if you avoid needless pain, pain and suffering will still come. If the benefits of pain seem hypothetical or even ridiculous to you, ask yourself whether you have learned the most and grown the most during the easy times in your life, or whether the quantum leaps toward self-discovery have taken place in times of adversity. Most of us recognize that it is in adversity that we tend to grow most quickly.

"Illness," someone said, "is the meditation of Western man." Another way to put it is that, in a society that has forgotten how to meditate while healthy, many people are guided to deep contemplation of the meaning of life only by illness.

Healing and the Sense of Connection

Many of the elements of spirituality as it relates to healing—the search for "union" in yoga, the wisdom of the shaman, and the bedrock of truth of the perennial philosophy—are summed up by Joan Borysenko, Ph.D., a cell biologist and author of *Minding the Body, Mending the Mind*.[18] Borysenko is in the forefront of biologists and psychologists whose work is converging with that of healers from the spiritual traditions. She maintains that healing is fundamentally about connectedness—connectedness with our deepest nature, with other humans in community, or with the transpersonal realities. Such moments of connectedness—whether attained through meditation, inspiration, or human intimacy—are what Abraham Maslow calls "peak experiences." These are, according to Borysenko, moments of profound peace and healing, both emotionally and physically.

Borysenko maintains that we fall away from the sense of deeper connection in our day-to-day lives by identifying with a "false self," resulting in feelings of isolation, loneliness, and unworthiness. After being born into this world as "balls of radiance," we gradually abandon parts of ourselves to the "shadow self" that Jung describes, in the belief that we need to do so in order to gain the love and acceptance that, as children, we needed above all else. We come to identify with the false self which we feel will be more acceptable to those we depend upon for love and care. The false self isolates us not only from other people, but from our own authentic natures as well. In doing so, it stands in the way of our true healing.

So the healing process, according to Borysenko, is in large part the rediscovery of our connection with self, with community, and with the transpersonal. At same time, healing involves disidentification with the false self. Times of adversity and serious illness can also be times of great personal growth because the false self and its way of being in the world serve us so poorly in times of difficulty. With little energy to spare, we realize the true difficulty of maintaining the artificial facade. In turn, the necessity to accept who we really are can open us to the healing power of connectedness.[19]

Results obtained in studies of more routine levels of social contact and measures of physical well-being provide a glimpse of the significance of profound connection. In a series of studies with rabbits in 1977 and 1978, Robert Nerem and colleagues at the University of Houston demonstrated that the social environment of the animals had a dramatic effect on diet-induced aortic atherosclerosis. Animals that were regularly handled, stroked, talked to, and played with had significantly lower levels of arterial disease than controls. Though the authors did not speculate about the possible mechanisms responsible for this effect, they did point out that the magnitude of the result was large enough that careful consideration must be given to social factors in the design of future studies of atherosclerosis interventions.[20]

Conversely, human studies show that feelings of isolation and loneliness have a detrimental effect on physical well-being, as measured by immune function. Ronald Glaser at the Ohio State University College of Medicine found in a study with medical students that those who scored high on the UCLA Loneliness Scale displayed significantly higher levels of immunosuppression as measured by changes in antibody levels in response to herpesvirus compared with students who scored low in the scale.[21] Similarly, Janice K. Kiecolt-Glaser at the Department of Psychiatry at Ohio State University found that among students who scored high on the UCLA Loneliness Scale, significantly higher levels of Epstein-Barr viruses were required to transform B lymphocytes into plasma cells, which in turn make and secrete antibodies.[22]

Prayer

One can think about the data reported in the preceding section in either psychological or spiritual terms. There are no assumptions of any special "spiritual" energy or force in those studies. But at the start of this chapter we identified the question of whether spiritual energies exist as one of the divisive issues that this field raises.

In chapter 18, we review the extraordinary literature on Therapeutic Touch and report that researchers have found that a practitioner trained in this technique can raise hemoglobin levels without touching the patient. Even more remarkable, working under randomized blind conditions, a researcher showed that Therapeutic Touch could make experimental wounds heal faster than controls. This and a series of other studies of the capacity of healers to affect growth of plants, healing in animals, and enzyme activities in laboratory solutions, point to the existence of energies we do not yet know how to measure. As Aldridge sums up the situation: "Most of the studies have fallen by the wayside because of poor research design. Nonetheless, there appears to be material evidence for an intentional healing effect. At the same time it must be said that the energetic correlates of that effect remain elusive to measurement in both the laboratory and the clinic."[23]

Can prayer by others reverse or mitigate physical illness? The most frequently cited research study on this subject was carried out by Randolph Byrd, M.D., at San Francisco General Medical Center in 1982–83. Byrd wanted to determine whether intercessionary prayer—prayer for a patient by others—made any measurable difference in outcomes in the coronary care unit where he worked. The results of the study, entitled "Positive Therapeutic Effects of Intercessionary Prayer [IP] in a Coronary Care Unit Population," was published in the *Southern Medical Journal* in July 1988.

Byrd enrolled a total of 393 patients in his study—192 in the intervention group and 201 in the control group. The patients were watched over a 10-month period from August 1982 to May 1983. Byrd had asked all 450 patients who came through the coronary care unit over the 10-month period to participate. Fifty-seven (14.5%) patients declined. The patients who enrolled were told the purpose of the study and signed informed consent forms. They were then randomly assigned to the study group or the control group. Byrd then chose "intercessors" who were "born again Christians (according to the Gospel of John 3:3) with an active Christian life." These Christians, who were to pray for the participants in the study group, were randomly assigned a patient for whom they prayed daily.

Byrd found that six conditions improved significantly more for the study group than for the control group. They were (1) the need for intubation or ventilation, (2) the need for antibiotics, (3) the incidence of cardiopulmonary arrest,

(4) the incidence of congestive heart failure, (5) the incidence of pneumonia, and (6) the need for diuretics. There was a general tendency for the study group—those who were prayed for—to have better physical outcomes than those who were not prayed for.[24]

The study was summarized as follows in the *Journal of the American Medical Association:*

> The therapeutic effects of intercessionary prayer (IP) to the Judeo-Christian God, one of the oldest forms of therapy, has had little attention in the medical literature. To evaluate the effects of IP in a coronary care unit population, a prospective, randomized, double-blind protocol was followed. . . . While hospitalized, the [study] group received IP by participating Christians praying outside the hospital; the control group did not. An . . . analysis revealed no statistical difference between the groups. After entry, all patients had follow-up for the remainder of admission. The IP group subsequently had a significantly lower severity score ($P < .01$). Multivariate analysis separated the groups on the basis of outcome variables ($P < .0001$). The control patients required ventilatory assistance, antibiotics, and diuretics more frequently than patients in the IP group. These data suggest that IP to the Judeo-Christian God has a beneficial therapeutic effect in patients admitted to a coronary care unit.[25]

This study appears to me to be one of the most important—if not the most important—empirical study of prayer ever to be undertaken. I do not regard the study as conclusive. The question is far too important to be assessed with a single study. Byrd's study should be replicated and prayer studied in many different ways.

It would have been far less surprising if a study had shown that patients who *pray for themselves* had better outcomes. Although this would be an important and powerful finding—and such studies should be done—it could be explained as a simple placebo effect. However, Byrd's finding that patients with a life-threatening illness who were prayed for *by others* did significantly better under randomized, controlled, double-blind conditions is a far more provocative finding in terms of our basic belief systems. There are only four or five possible explanations: (a) the data were not correctly reported, (b) the data were correctly reported but not correctly analyzed, (c) the data were correctly analyzed but represented a fluke (against high odds!) and the findings would not be replicated by other studies, (d) the study demonstrates that transpersonal healing effects can be obtained by "intercessors" with a strong Judeo-Christian healing belief system, but "God" has nothing to do with it, or (e) the study demonstrates that transpersonal healing effects can be obtained by "intercessors" with a strong Judeo-Christian belief system and points to the transpersonal reality called "God." Explanations (d) and (e) may be essentially equivalent.

Aldridge comments as follows on the Byrd study and the frequency with which it is cited in the *Advances* symposium on spiritual healing:

> We see a touching faith in science in the way in which several commentators have echoed my example of the Byrd study (1988). While the study is well constructed, and a fine example of medical research that highlights a healing phenomenon itself defying modern science, it is based on statistical inferences that are essentially flawed, or at least, open to interpretation. Belief in mathematic abstraction is an act of faith.[26]

If Byrd's findings are correct and replicable under different conditions, they represent in my judgment an advance in medicine of the greatest importance; and in terms of empirically demonstrable outcomes, the convergence of the technologies of biomedicine and the technologies of the sacred. I assume, for example, that prayers to God in His or Her many other forms would be equally efficacious. But if Byrd's findings *cannot* be replicated, that does not disprove the significance of intercessionary prayer. Rather, it could indicate that the results achieved by intercessionary prayer cannot be counted by any empirical calculus: that what we achieve by intercessionary prayer is too uniquely individual in terms of improved outcomes to be researched in this way.

Aesthetically and intuitively, it is not obvious to me that the efficacy of prayer *should in principle* be scientifically demonstrable. Or, if its efficacy is partially demonstrable, we should bear in mind what a tiny proportion of the benefits of prayer may be demonstrated. For prayer, like love, like creativity, like dedication to a life of service, is one of the great paths into the life of the spirit. If, 10 years from now, a review article finds that intercessionary prayer made an average contribution of approximately 15% to 25% in improvements in selected measurable outcomes for a wide range of health conditions, we would have to consider the possibility that the result might be the smallest glimpse of the true significance of prayer.

It should be noted, however, that an agnostic could accept the possible reality of healing phenomena such as those associated with intercessionary prayer or Therapeutic Touch, and the possible explanation that undiscovered energies of some kind account for these phenomena, without accepting any of the metaphysical explanations that the spiritually or religiously inclined use for these phenomena. The same would even be true if the existence of energetic bodies, as described in many religious and spiritual traditions from around the world, were identified surrounding the human body. Scientists could go a long way down the road of demonstrating the reality of various psychic and energetic phenomena that appear in religious and spiritual accounts without changing the fundamental terms of the debate over whether there is meaning and purpose in the universe or not.

Different Approaches to Prayer

"More things are wrought by prayer than this world dreams of," wrote Alfred Lord Tennyson. Reasonable people differ on whether or not this is true. But for those who have cancer and are exploring prayer for the first time, I offer some examples of the rich variety of prayers related to healing.

The simplest and most obvious prayer is a request to God that the adversity end and that one be restored to health. Such prayers often involve "affirmations." There is a considerable psychological literature on the healing power of affirmations, and many cancer patients use them. Here is a beautiful Navajo prayer that uses affirmation:

> *O you who dwell*
> *In the house made of the dawn,*
> *In the house made of the evening twilight . . .*
> *Where the dark mist curtains the doorway,*
> *The path to which is on the rainbow . . .*
> *I have made your sacrifice.*
> *I have prepared a smoke for you.*
> *My feet restore for me.*
> *My limbs restore for me.*
> *My body restore for me.*
> *My mind restore for me.*

My voice restore for me.
Today, take away your spell from me.
Away from me you have taken it.
Far off from me you have taken it.

Happily I recover.
Happily my interior becomes cool.
Happily my eyes regain their power.
Happily my head becomes cool.
Happily my limbs regain their power.
Happily I hear again.
Happily for me the spell is taken off.
Happily I walk.
Impervious to pain, I walk.
Feeling light within, I walk . . .
In beauty I walk.
With beauty before me, I walk.
With beauty behind me, I walk.
With beauty below me, I walk.
With beauty all around me, I walk.
It is finished in beauty.
It is finished in beauty.
It is finished in beauty.[27]

A prayer by an American Confederate soldier seriously disabled in the Civil War is a beautiful example of the depths of discovery of the gifts of suffering that a wound can bring:

I asked God for strength, that I might achieve,
I was made weak, that I might learn humbly to obey.
I asked for health, that I might do great things,
I was given infirmity, that I might do better things.
I asked for riches, that I might be happy,
I was given poverty, that I might be wise.
I asked for power, that I might have the praise of men,
I was given weakness, that I might feel the need of God.
I asked for all things, that I might enjoy life,

I was given life, that I might enjoy all things.
I got nothing that I asked for—but everything I had hoped for.
Almost despite myself, my unspoken prayers were answered.
I am, among all men, most richly blessed.[28]

One of the most powerful and most universal of all forms of prayer is a prayer seeking to be awakened to the inner light. Lao-tzu wrote:

See the small and develop clear vision.
Practice yielding and develop strength.
Use the outer light to return to the inner light,
And save yourself from harm.[29]

An Inuit Indian who had known adversity wrote this:

I think over again my small adventures,
My fears,
Those small ones that seemed so big,
For all the vital things
I had to get and reach.
And yet there is only one great thing,
The only thing,
To live to see the great day that dawns
And the light that fills the world.[30]

"The Lord is my light and my salvation; whom shall I fear?" begins a psalm of David. Many prayers and visualizations of healing involve surrounding yourself, or the person you pray for, with light. Reading prayers from around the world develops our knowledge of how fundamental prayer has been to human experience.

Conclusion

Spirit and spirituality are meaningful categories of experience for me. But I have family members and friends for whom the categories are without meaning, and they seem to me every bit as "spiritual" as those for whom these categories have meaning.

We live in a time in which concepts of spirituality are becoming more and more popular in many parts of American culture. While this increasing popularity of spirituality may bring benefits for some, religious and spiritual revivals have historically been a sharp and double-edged sword. For spiritual and religious revivals have great collective psychic power that invites corruption and abuse, and may attenuate the collective commitments to reason, tolerance, and law that Western civilization developed at such great cost as an antidote to the religious and spiritual passions of the past.

So my friends for whom spirit and spiritual are not useful categories have a strong case that they can make with respect to the dangers of the spiritual perspective, just as I, acknowledging the dangers, also see its value. If spirit is what unites us, then true spirit must embrace equally these two ancient antipodes of human experience. Thus any spirituality that divides us is too far along the track toward religious sectarianism for my personal taste.

We have seen that the experience of cancer opens many people up to spiritual experience in ways that were often completely unexpected. But there are others for whom cancer brings no such opening to spiritual experience. They must be equally—not grudgingly—honored. Are they missing something?

If a person for whom spirit has no meaning experiences himself as missing something—if he feels that he would like to open himself to spiritual experience but cannot—that is one thing. It is legitimate to help him try to find what he feels he is missing. But often such a person feels no sense of missing something. To the contrary, he may be actively deepening his connection to another one of the great pathways to the highest meanings in life. Skepticism, said Santayana, is the chastity of the intellect. That chastity—that integrity—may have been a lifelong friend for a lover of nature, family, friends, art, music, science, reason, or animals. Someone who sees mind as an epiphenomenon of the brain and nothing more; who sees humanity as a lonely species in the universe finding only such meaning as it assigns to its journey; and who values the courage to face these realities without what he regards as the narcotic comforts of religion or spirituality—such a man or woman is, for me, as close to spirit as I am.

Whether spirit has meaning beyond the psychological and social significance we assign to it is one of the greatest questions of our time. I believe it does.

Watching the opening of many people with cancer to spirit and spirituality in their lives has strengthened that belief. But I have watched others, equally "spiritual," live and face death without any wish to move toward the use of spiritual language or categories. The spirit to which I pay homage is the one that equally embraces us all.

Notes and References

1 This chapter owes a special debt to Rachel Naomi Remen, M.D., because my thinking about healing and spirituality has borrowed so much from her lifetime study of this question.

2 Max Lerner, *Wrestling with the Angel* (New York: Touchstone, 1990), 109.

3 David Aldridge, "Is There Evidence for Spiritual Healing?," *Advances* 9(4):4 (1993).

4 J. Hiatt, "Spirituality, Medicine and Healing," *Southern Medical Journal* 79(6):b 736–43, quoted in Aldridge, *ibid.*, 5.

5 *Lotus Prayer Book* (Buckingham, VA: Integral Yoga Publications, 1986), 189.

6 Hugh Prather and Gerald Jampolsky, foreword to Arnold R. Beisser, *Flying Without Wings: Personal Reflections on Loss, Disability, and Healing* (New York: Bantam Books, 1990), vii.

7 Arnold Toynbee, *A Study of History* [illustrated abridged] (New York: Weathervane Books, 1972), 333.

8 Ibid.

9 Ibid., 336.

10 Sri Swami Satchidananda, *The Living Gita: The Complete Bhagavad Gita* (Buckingham, VA: Integral Yoga Publications, 1988).

11 Sri Swami Satchidananda, *Integral Yoga: The Yoga Sutras of Patanjali* (Buckingham, VA: Integral Yoga Publications, 1988), 3–7.

12 Ibid., 93.

13 Swami Rama, *Lectures on Yoga* (Honesdale, PA: The Himalayan International Institute of Yoga Science and Philosophy, 1979), 10–12.

14 John 14:2.

15 Lawrence LeShan, Ph.D., *Cancer as a Turning Point: A Handbook for People with Cancer, Their Families, and Health Professionals* (New York: E.P. Dutton, 1989), 22.

16 C.G. Jung, *The Practice of Psychotherapy: Essays on the Psychology of the Transference and Other Subjects* translated by R.F.C. Hull, Bollingen Series XX, The Collected Works of C.G. Jung, volume 16, edited by William McGuire, et al. (Princeton, NJ: Princeton University Press, 1966), 116.

17 Howard Brody, *Stories of Sickness* (New Haven: Yale University Press, 1987), 5.

18 Joan Borysenko, *Minding the Body, Mending the Mind* (Reading, MA: Addison-Wesley Publishing Company, Inc., 1987).

19 Joan Borysenko, Jean Waldman Memorial Lecture, University of California, San Francisco, 26 November 1990.

20   Robert M. Nerem, Murina J. Levesque, and J. Fredrick Cornhill, "Social Environment as a Factor in Diet-induced Atherosclerosis," *Science* 208(27 June):1475–6 (1980).

21   R. Glaser, "Stress, Loneliness, and Changes in Herpesvirus Latency," *Journal of Behavioral Medicine* 8(3):249–60 (1985).

22   J.K. Kiecolt-Glaser, "Stress and the Transformation of Lymphocytes by Epstein-Barr Virus," *Journal of Behavioral Medicine* 7(1):1–12 (1984).

23   Aldridge, *op. cit.*, 15.

24   Randolph C. Byrd, "Positive Therapeutic Effects of Intercessionary Prayer in a Coronary Care Unit Population," *Southern Journal of Medicine* 81(7):26–9 (1988). For critical review, see Kent Harker, "Onward Christian Healers," *Basis: Bay Area Skeptics Information Sheet* 8(July 1989). For positive review, see "Cardiologist Studies Effect of Prayer on Patients," *Brain-Mind Bulletin* 11(25 March 1986).

25   Byrd. Abstracted in *Journal of the American Medical Association* 261(3):372 (1989).

26   Aldridge, *op. cit.*, 83.

27   *Lotus Prayer Book,* 95–6.

28   Ibid., 7.

29   Ibid., 26.

30   Ibid., 39.

ten

Psychological Approaches to Cancer

Psychoneuroimmunology

Our current blindness to the importance of mental hygiene in cancer is all the more astonishing because of the fast-emerging and fascinating field of psychoneuroimmunology—the academic study of the new-found body-mind connections between psychological states and the neurological, endocrine, and immune systems. Psychoneuroimmunology, or PNI, is an even younger field than psychooncology. The first major text in the field, *Psychoneuroimmunology*, edited by Robert Ader and his colleagues, was published in 1981 and came out in a second edition in 1991. The authors describe the evolution of their field:

> The neurosciences and immunology developed and matured without seriously considering that there might be communications networks between these systems that could mutually influence their respective functions. . . . Although it still may not be a universally accepted conceptualization, research conducted over the past ten years has made it increasingly apparent that there are complex interrelationships among behavioral, neural, endocrine and immune processes.[1]

In simpler terms, it is now beginning to appear that mind-body interactions are so ubiquitous that it may no longer be possible to refer to body and mind as separate entities but only as bodymind. For psychology, this means that emotional states of mind and behavioral patterns may profoundly affect not only our symptoms but also the progress of our disease itself. Most dramatically, PNI research by and large supports—though not conclusively so—the controversial position that psychosocial factors, including psychosocial interventions, may contribute to the extension of life with cancer.

Often, people with cancer who are interested in psychological approaches to their illness fail to look at the scientific evidence offered by PNI or psychooncology research. They turn instead to the ever-increasing collection of inspirational books—Bernie Siegel's *Love, Medicine and Miracles,*[2] Larry LeShan's *Cancer as a Turning Point,*[3] O. Carl Simonton, Stephanie Matthews Simonton, and James Creighton's, *Getting Well Again,*[4] or Joan Borysenko's *Minding the Body, Mending the Mind.*[5] Cancer patients often wonder why the psychological approaches to cancer they read about in these books are not more a part of mainstream medicine.

In fact, psychological approaches to cancer have emerged in mainstream medicine, most decisively in the past 20 years. While these certainly have limitations from the perspective of a cancer patient who is seeking what the inspirational popular books have to offer—strong affirmations of the possibility that he can participate actively in the struggle not only for quality of life but also for recovery and life extension—nonetheless they are based on a wealth of scientific studies and firmly grounded clinical observations focused primarily on coping with cancer. Let us now look at what psychooncologists have to offer.

Psychooncology

Coping with cancer as a goal is sometimes denigrated by advocates of psychological work with life extension as a goal. But in fact, coping with cancer is a large part of the psychological work of every cancer patient, whether he also believes it may be possible to extend his life through psychological practices or not. Psychooncology research focused on coping also provides a framework for a balanced evaluation of the sometimes unbalanced claims of some of the inspirational popular books about psychological and spiritual approaches to cancer. For these reasons, psychooncology is worthy of careful study.

Psychooncology is a young field. Jimmie C. Holland, M.D., of Memorial Sloan-Kettering Cancer Center in New York, one of the founders of psycho-oncology, has traced its evolution. In the 1950s, Holland writes, interest in psychosomatic medicine led to clinical studies that sought to link personality with a predisposition to cancer. These studies were primarily anecdotal yet led to hypotheses about the relationship of personality to cancer that remain viable to this day. This led to studies in the 1960s of psychological issues that patients and physicians confronted in responding to life-threatening illnesses including cancer. In the 1970s, the field of "consultation-liaison psychiatry" began to have a greater impact on cancer patients as psychiatrists were asked to help oncologists with the problems that cancer patients—especially children and their families—faced in the course of medical treatment. The 1970s also saw the first conferences bringing together psychosocial researchers concerned with cancer. That decade also brought the development of funding for psychosocial research in cancer by the American Cancer Society and other institutions. This led to the emergence of the subspecialty called psychosocial oncology, or psychooncology.[6]

Just as there is a classic text on the medical treatment of cancer (DeVita's *Principles and Practice of Oncology)*, there is now a classic text on psychooncology. It is the *Handbook of Psychooncology* edited by Holland and Julia H. Rowland, Ph.D. The most useful thing for cancer patients about the *Handbook of Psychooncology* is that it contains an enormous wealth of research reports and clinical recommendations across the entire spectrum of problems that patients face. None of the inspirational psychospiritual books on cancer can match the range of practical, research-based findings that the *Handbook* offers.

Holland and Rowland introduce the field of psychooncology by proposing that there are three overarching elements that influence the psychological adaptation of patients to cancer: the sociocultural context, the medical context, and the individual psychological context. The sociocultural context refers to individual and collective beliefs about cancer; the medical context refers to the type and stage of cancer that the patient has and the treatments being used; and the individual psychological context refers to the issues that the patient faces and the resources he brings to coping with these issues.

Focusing on the third—or psychological—context, Rowland proposes that the three core issues for a cancer patient are: (1) What stage of the life cycle are you in when you develop cancer?, (2) How do you tend to respond psychologically to major developments in your life such as cancer?, and (3) What resources—both interpersonal (such as family, friends, and other social support) and concrete (such as money and health insurance)—are available to you to deal with this crisis?[7]

The first question is a particularly critical one. Since the fundamental psychological tasks of each stage of life are different, cancer represents a different set of challenges in every developmental period. But, whatever stage of life we are in, Rowland suggests that there are five common disruptions to the pursuit of our life goals that are caused by cancer. She refers to these five common disruptions informally (this is where the language of psychooncology is less than inspirational in its tone!) as the "five D's." They are:

1. *Distance*, or changes in interpersonal relationships that bring about shifts in emotional distance—either closer or farther apart—between you and family members, friends, business colleagues, and others.
2. *Dependence*, or changes in the dependence on or independence from family, friends, and others.
3. *Disability*, or disruption in developmental tasks, personal goals, and meaningful activities, both now and in the future.
4. *Disfigurement*, or changes in body image, sexual function, and physical integrity.
5. *Death*, or facing the existential issues that every life-threatening illness brings.

In an invaluable chapter, Rowland traces for each stage of life the common developmental tasks, the common cancers of that age, and the common disruptions created by a cancer diagnosis.[8]

Rowland then addresses intrapersonal issues, or what she calls "coping resources." Early psychological studies of cancer focused primarily on the stress of the disease and the patient's reflexive ego defenses. More recently, she says, there has been a "shift away from a view of human beings under siege . . . to an adaptational view of human beings in which life's stresses are seen as challenges or tasks to be mastered." Rowland makes a distinction between the "reflexive" ego defenses—such as denial—and the "reflective" capacities we develop to face the "difficult and unusual" qualities of the new situation, which can be summarized as "coping style," and success in meeting these new challenges, which can be described as "mastery."[9]

Rowland then turns her attention to interpersonal resources, or what she characterizes as "social support." Social support includes: people who can help the patient mobilize his inner resources to face the illness; people who share tasks that the patient must carry out; and people or institutions that provide tangible forms of support such as health insurance, financial support, and information.[10]

Social support is, as we shall see, one of the most important and interesting categories which psychooncologists address. In discussing the benefits of social support, Holland and Rowland mention for the first time studies that show that cancer patients with stronger social support systems may actually *live longer* than patients with weaker social support systems. You will recall that it has been highly controversial in psychooncology to suggest that *psychological interventions* might extend life with cancer. But it has not been controversial to point out that *social support* may extend life with cancer. If the psycho-oncologists suspect that social support may extend life with cancer, we might very well ask why, then, do not psychooncologists place a high priority on studies to determine whether or not *psychological interventions that enhance social support* might extend life with cancer?

"The degree of social support is positively associated with both better adjust-ment and longer survival," says Rowland. She cites, among others, studies by A.D. Weisman and J.W. Worden in 1975 in which patients with varied cancers who had "good interpersonal relationships" lived longer than those who did not. A second important study by D.P. Funch and J. Marshall in 1983 followed 208 women with breast cancer and assessed social support based on total number of acquaintances and relatives, number of religious and nonreligious meetings attended, and marital status. The study found that for women younger than 46, those with higher social involvement lived longer.[11] I return to research on social support later in this chapter when I describe David Spiegel's dramatic findings that women with metastatic breast cancer who participated in a support group lived longer than women in a control group who did not. The crucial point is that, while research into psychological interventions that extend life with cancer has until recently been professionally risky, it was both possible and necessary for psychooncologists to report those interesting "experiments of nature" that showed that social support was positively correlated with survival. Nor was this life extension only true for people who had more physical resources such as income and health insurance (it is well known that survival with most diseases, including cancer, goes up with income and concrete support). The studies Rowland presented were studies where enhanced *psychosocial support alone* was the key correlate of extended survival.

Holland and Rowland describe the psychological issues that people with cancer face at every stage of cancer development. In an invaluable discussion for patients and health professionals, Holland discusses the psychological issues and useful interventions for each major phase of cancer and cancer treatment: diagnosis, prognosis, treatment, remission or recovery, recurrence, renewed treatment, and progression of the disease. This is followed by chapters about psychological dilemmas that arise for cancer survivors and the issues for patients undergoing each of the major forms of cancer treatment: surgery, radiotherapy, chemotherapy, endocrine therapy, immunotherapy, and bone marrow transplantation.

Holland and Rowland also describe the problems related to the specific type of cancer a patient may have. They devote a chapter to each of the major cancers. They also present chapters on pain, sexual problems, nausea and vomiting, and anorexia. Another section in the book discusses the wide range of psychotherapeutic interventions used with cancer patients: psychotherapy, pharmacological management of psychological problems, behavioral techniques such as progressive relaxation and hypnotherapy, and support groups. Overall, the *Handbook of Psychooncology* covers what mental health professionals working inside cancer treatment institutions have learned over the last several decades. Holland notes that practitioners of psychooncology have worked in settings which characteristically give "low status" to psychosocial issues. In her characteristically understated way, she says: "The need to try to 'sell' the importance of these issues to some staff members who are not interested creates a sense of devaluation of the work that can be felt personally."[12] From my own experience, I vividly recall one of the most rigorously scientific and best-respected researchers in psychooncology, who holds a distinguished position at a major teaching institution, telling me how a senior surgeon asked him about his work and, after listening briefly, had said to him: "You don't really believe all this bullshit, do you?" "Low status" is a gentle word for the welcome psychooncology has been afforded in much of the biomedical community.

If there is a major shortcoming in psychooncology, it derives in large measure from the defensive position that psychooncology has occupied in relation to other specialties in mainstream cancer treatment centers. Institutional constraints have made it difficult for psychooncologists to push into the most exciting frontiers of clinical practice and research—most notably to determine whether or not psychological interventions can extend the life of cancer patients. In order to minimize conflict with the cancer treatment specialists, until very recently practitioners of psychooncology have presented themselves almost exclusively as the facilitators of patients' better adaptation to cancer, cancer treatment, cancer progression, or cancer survival. For many years, most psychooncologists strongly disclaimed any suggestion that their methods might actually contribute to life extension or the likelihood of cure. As research findings began to support the idea that psychological methods might contribute to life extension, practitioners of psychooncology did not seize on these hints and move forward vigorously with a strong research agenda for the life extension hypothesis. They remained extremely cautious. This caution is strikingly in contrast to the aggressive research agendas of specialists in other fields of cancer treatment who were seeking life extension using techniques such as bone marrow transplantation, endocrine therapy, and immunotherapy.

But in the midst of a popular culture in which excessive claims about psychologically based cures for cancer are often made in the inspirational cancer literature, it is refreshing to read in the *Handbook of Psychooncology* about the modest and careful descriptions of psychological problems and useful interventions. With its sometimes excessively conservative approach, psychooncology balances the popular literature with its excessively optimistic claims. For cancer patients, the truth probably lies somewhere between these two poles.

Therapies That Reduce the Stress of Cancer

One of the most important findings by psychooncology researchers is that progressive muscle relaxation training, imagery, hypnotherapy, and other stress reduction techniques can reduce the side effects of cancer treatment and some syndromes associated with cancer, such as sleeplessness, pain, and weight loss. Rene Mastrovito, in a chapter on behavioral techniques in the *Handbook of Psychooncology*, reports that:

> The last two decades have seen a dramatic rise in the use of behavioral therapies for control of symptoms. . . . Particularly in cancer, they are now extensively applied to control psychological distress and pain. . . . The behavioral techniques, encompassing hypnosis, meditation, autogenic training, progressive relaxation, and biofeedback, are also called by some cognitive-behavioral, holistic, and alternative modes of therapy. All are forms of self-regulating therapies, a more comprehensive and appropriate term. Such therapeutic interventions generally are characterized by two basic stages in which the patient is first guided through a primarily cognitive activity that creates the second stage, an altered state of consciousness. . . . By far the most widely used technique in cancer is relaxation therapy, which promotes an altered state of awareness through reducing distressing emotions and producing a physiologically quiescent state in which there is selective awareness of specific sensory stimuli to the exclusion of others.[13]

Behavioral interventions to diminish anticipatory nausea and vomiting represent one of the most rigorously documented and effective uses of these approaches. William Redd, Ph.D., a leading authority in this field, notes that 25% to 65% of patients in protracted chemotherapy report nausea in anticipation of treatment. "For some patients," says Redd, ". . . any event or stimulus that is repeatedly associated with post-treatment side-effects becomes an elicitor of anticipatory reactions. . . . Clearly the most potent stimulus for the chemotherapy patient is the smell of the rubbing alcohol used to clean the skin in preparation for an infusion. After four or five infusions, the nurse's perfume, the handsoap the doctor uses, and the odor of coffee may elicit it."[14]

After reviewing the literature, T.G. Burish and colleagues report that behavioral relaxation techniques, including hypnosis, progressive muscle relaxation training, electromyogram (EMG) biofeedback, and systematic desensitization, "alleviate some conditioned side effects of chemotherapy including nausea, vomiting, and negative emotions such as anxiety and depression. These behavioral techniques are generally inexpensive, easily learned, and have few if any negative side effects."[15]

Redd reviews a series of studies by different investigators who used hypnosis with imagery, progressive relaxation with imagery, biofeedback with imagery, systematic desensitization, and cognitive or attentional distraction to relieve anticipatory nausea and vomiting:

> The consistency of the positive results obtained in the group of studies just reviewed is remarkable, because clinically significant reductions in ANV [antici-patory nausea and vomiting] were achieved despite wide variations in the type of cancer, stage of disease, and chemotherapy protocol . . . by separate groups of investigators using different research methods. . . . Behavioral techniques clearly appear to have a place as an adjunctive treatment in the care of many cancer patients.

The question of whether these techniques are helpful in posttreatment nausea and vomiting, Redd reports, is more complex. Most research has not focused in this area. Some patients report that relaxation tapes themselves become aversive stimuli in situations where there is severe posttreatment nausea, especially with protocols that include cisplatin. But "Burish and colleagues consistently report reductions in post-treatment reactions when their patients use self-relaxation and distraction with protocols that do not incorporate cisplatin. Although posttreatment nausea is not eliminated, significant reductions are observed."[16]

Other significant uses of behavioral therapies are less well known but equally important. Campbell and colleagues reported that progressive muscle relaxation training promoted normal food consumption and weight gain for cancer patients.[17] Cannici and colleagues found progressive muscle relaxation training reduced insomnia that is often found in people with cancer. Fifteen patients trained in the technique reduced the time they spent trying to get to sleep from 124 minutes to 29 minutes, while 15 participants in the control group experienced almost no reduction. The training had a lasting effect, with the differences between the two groups continuing 3 months later.[18] To have an adequate appetite, to gain weight, and to go to sleep in half an hour instead of 2 hours are no small accomplishments in living with cancer. Who is to say they are not crucial building blocks in the fight for life extension as well?

Mastrovito reviewed a series of studies on hypnosis, especially with pediatric patients whose "easy suggestibility and readiness to engage in imaginative ventures" made them especially good candidates. A number of studies showed that children undergoing bone marrow aspiration experienced less pain when prepared for the procedure with hypnotherapy or imagery.[19] It is shocking that these simple procedures are not universally used for children undergoing these painful procedures.

Mastrovito also states that progressive relaxation is particularly useful (for adults as well as children) in oncology units and clinics "in situations that provoke fear and apprehension, such as painful diagnostic and treatment procedures (e.g., bone marrow aspiration, lumbar puncture, and chemotherapy infusions)." The unique assets of progressive relaxation, Mastrovito says, are that it can be done in almost any quiet place, is widely accepted by patients, has very rare adverse effects, is neither time-consuming nor expensive, and can even be applied in "emergency situations." Mastrovito correctly notes that very occasionally progressive relaxation may increase anxiety rather than diminish it and, equally rarely, it can lead to hypnotic trance states—not at all necessarily negative in themselves—that the practitioner should be prepared to respond appropriately to.[20]

Does Stress Make Tumors Grow?

One of the best research summaries of the effects of stress on tumor growth is contained in an important book by Daniel P. Brown and Erika Fromm, *Hypnosis and Behavioral Medicine*. Brown is Director of Behavioral Medicine at the Cambridge Hospital and a member of the Harvard Medical School Faculty. Fromm is Professor of Psychology at the University of Chicago. According to Brown and Fromm:

> Numerous studies have shown that animals in which tumors have been induced (by means of chemicals, transplantations, or radiation) and were then exposed to acute stressors (electrical shock, bright lights, extreme temperatures, rapid rotation, immobilization, isolation, overcrowding, confrontation with other—feared—animals) suffered from immunosuppression. *Rapid tumor growth was facilitated in the stressed animals. The accumulated data for humans, although not so extensively documented, are similar and suggest that acute stressors result in immunosuppression or tumor facilitation in humans* [emphasis added].[21]

This conclusion is supported by PNI research on the effects of stress in animals, summarized in a number of chapters in the bible of this field, *Psychoneuroimmunology*. One of the authors in this text, Yehuda Shavit, writes:

Reviewing the literature on stress and tumors in animal studies reveals a picture similar to that relating stress and infection. Stress can alter the incidence and development of experimental tumors in animals. In general, stress appears to enhance tumor induction and development, although stress-induced retardation of tumor growth has also been reported.

PNI research has found that the relationship between stress, tumor growth, and immunity is highly complex. Shavit describes three major areas where stress, immunity, and tumor development have been explored: acute stress is generally more likely to depress immune function and enhance tumor growth than chronic stress; giving animals a capacity to control stress enhances immunity and diminishes tumor development in contrast to situations where stress is inescapable; and housing conditions affect stress, with both loneliness and overcrowding having deleterious effects.[22] In humans, the most distinctive difference is that chronic psychological stress appears to continue over time to be immunosuppressive.[23]

A second vital area of PNI research has focused on opiates (such as morphine) and "opioid peptides," or opiate-like peptides. Within the body, stress can induce analgesia or pain control by different biochemical mechanisms, one of which involves opioid peptides and the other a nonopioid system. This is important because, when a stressor induces pain control with an opioid peptide, the presence of that peptide more often than not may enhance tumor development, just as morphine may support tumor development. Shavit writes:

> There is growing evidence implicating opiates in the regulation of the immune system. Opiate addicts are known to be highly susceptible to bacterial, viral and fungal infections and, in fact, to have deficits in immune function. Acute and chronic morphine administration in experimental animals and humans usually produces immunosuppression. . . . Opiate agonists and antagonists [substances which, respectively, enhance or retard the effects of opiates] have also been implicated in tumor development. For example, morphine enhances the rate of pulmonary metastases in rats. . . . On the other hand, opiates and opiate antagonists were shown to retard tumor growth.[24]

PNI animal research has also identified critical immunosurveillance mechanisms against both viral infections and cancer that are differentially affected by stress. The two primary mechanisms considered in this research to date are cytotoxic T lymphocytes and NK [natural killer] cells. Acute stress in animal research often markedly reduces NK cell activity, and research that exposed animals to the specific kinds of stress that bring opioid peptides into play also suppressed NK cell activity. Morphine has also shown a dose-related capacity to suppress NK cell activity in animals.[25] Shavit writes:

> Although there are obvious differences between rats and humans in response to narcotic drugs, our results nonetheless indicate that the effects of high-dose narcotic drugs on the immune system should be studied in humans. Surgical stress, including anesthesia, has been shown to increase tumor metastasis, perhaps owing to tumor embolus [tissue fragments] dissemination during the surgery. The impairment of NK cells at the time of surgery may contribute to tumor implantation, and our findings suggest that this NK suppression is attributable, at least in part, to narcotic agents.[26]

In human studies, PNI researchers have found specifically that bereavement, divorce, depression, chronic stress, and academic stress (exams, etc.) may all depress immune function. Janice R. Kiecolt-Glaser and Ronald Glaser are two leading researchers in this field and summarized the research in *Psychoneuroimmunology*. They cite a "large and relatively consistent literature" suggesting that stressful life events, specifically "major negative life changes," put people at greater risk for a variety of diseases. Interestingly, these events only account for about 10% of the variance in most studies. But the effects are "remarkably consistent across populations and different kinds of events. In particular, events associated with the loss of important personal relationships appear to put individuals at greater risk."[27]

Among the major life stressors, bereavement and divorce have been carefully studied. The Glasers cite studies showing that bereaved people have higher mortality in general and a higher incidence of cancer in particular than controls do. (Holland, in contrast, interprets the most recent studies to show higher mortality but not an elevated incidence of cancer.) Divorce, the Glasers report, has even greater health risks associated with it than bereavement.[28] But in general, while there is good evidence of an increase in morbidity and mortality associated with major negative life events, there is not a large body of robust evidence that these events result in a disproportionate increase in the incidence of cancer in particular.

Personality and Social Support as "Buffers" Against Stress

Personality may have a strong influence on how we experience stress. Recent research by S.R. Maddi and S.C. Kobasa, Holland reports, "found that the 'hardy' personality (viewing stress as a challenge, attempting to control stressful situations, and exercising a strong sense of commitment), had fewer physical illnesses, complaints and psychological distress than those who lacked these qualities."[29]

As we have seen, social support is another potential antidote to stress. As Rowland writes, "One of the most important 'buffers' against the harmful effects of the stress of illness is the presence or availability of persons in the patient's environment with whom the experience can be shared. . . . Research indicates that *the presence of positive social support not only diminishes the psychic distress of cancer, but may be important in modulating survival as well* [emphasis added]."[30]

This passage covers a point of *vital* importance to people who are considering some form of psychological work on themselves in hopes of extending their lives. Holland and Rowland explicitly endorse the view that the presence in a cancer patient's life of people *"with whom the experience of cancer can be shared"* not only softens the psychological impact of cancer *but may 'modulate' survival as well.*

Personality and social support probably interactively modulate the psychological and biological stressors that may be related to both the incidence and progression of some cancers. Evidence for this proposition now also comes from research in PNI. Sandra Levy and her colleagues (1985, 1987) examined psychological and biological variables in women with breast cancer. The studies measured their psychosocial condition and immunological status at the time of their mastectomies and 3 months later. They found that NK cell status was a significant predictor of how many positive axillary nodes the women had. (The number of positive nodes, it should be recalled, is a significant predictor of the likelihood of recurrence of the disease and of survival.) Levy et al. also found that 51% of the variance in NK cell activity was accounted for by three "distress indicators": lack of adjustment, lack of social support, and fatigue and depressive symptoms. In other words, if you had difficulty coping with cancer, had few social supports, and felt tired and depressed, the NK cell component of your immune system would be lower and you would be likely to have more positive nodes. This is an intriguing example of personality and social support apparently affecting the biological and psychological response to the stress of cancer with specific implications (the number of positive nodes) for survival. Jimmie Holland comments:

> The Levy studies are of particular interest because of the findings from studies of Kiecolt-Glaser and colleagues that NK activity is negatively perturbed in physically healthy individuals under the stresses of examinations (1984), and loneliness (1986) in medical students. . . . Their reports are also important in that NK-cell activity is important in response to tumors of viral origin, such as herpes virus and cervical cancer.

> The affective state described as "helplessness-hopelessness" as an outcome predictor in human cancer has received considerable attention, in part because of animal studies (Sklar and Anisman, 1981). Animals that lacked control over environmental stress (such as inescapable shock) had shorter survival from tumors than animals that could control it. Cox and Mackay (1982) have used these studies to hypothesize that helplessness is associated with depletion of catecholamines; in turn adrenocorticotrophic hormone (ACTH) release stimulates the release of corticosteroids, which suppress immune function. The intense need to regain control of events in patients with cancer has led to extrapolation of these concepts to the clinical area. Regaining a sense of control has been seen as not only promoting coping but also enhancing host resistance to tumor growth. Clearly, it is an intriguing hypothesis that needs further testing.[31]

Another very important set of studies, similar in concept to those of Levy, have been performed by Lydia Temoshok, Ph.D., and her colleagues who conducted pioneering studies of psychosocial variables related to prognosis in malignant melanoma. Temoshok, now principal scientist with the Henry M. Jackson Foundation for the Advancement of Military Medicine in Bethesda, Maryland, found an elegant way to compare "repressive coping reactions— defined as the discrepancy between reported anxiety and that reflected in electrodermal activity [a physical electrical response of the skin to anxiety]— in melanoma patients, cardiovascular patients, and disease-free controls." She found that the melanoma patients were significantly more "repressed" in terms of expressing their anxiety than the heart patients or the healthy control group.

Temoshok then studied whether two specific clinical variables significantly correlated with the progression of melanoma. (The progression of melanoma, incidentally, varies greatly from patient to patient.) These two variables were the rate of mitosis of the tumor (the speed with which it divides and grows) and the number of lymphocytes (cells attacking the tumor) at the tumor site. Temoshok found that the patients who could express sadness and anger—rated from videotaped interviews—had a higher "protective host-response" (as measured by lymphocytes) and those who had a difficult time expressing sadness and anger had a higher mitotic rate and therefore more quickly growing cancers.

Temoshok then matched patients who had died or who were experiencing disease progression with others who had no evidence of progression of the disease. In this study, in apparent contrast to the preceding one, the patients who died or had disease progression had, in earlier testing, expressed more anxiety and distress than those who had no evidence of disease progression. Temoshok argued that these two findings could be reconciled as follows:

> The following logic is offered to reconcile these findings with the ones in the preceding study, in which greater emotional expressiveness was associated with enhanced host response factors and diminished mitotic rate (which are, in turn, associated with favorable outcome): a high degree of consciously perceived stress, subjectively experienced as anxiety, distress, and/or dysphoric emotion, contributes significantly to melanoma progression. . . . It is possible that coping with this stress by *expressing* the emotion will buffer these otherwise negative effects.

Temoshok then suggested that both the negative effects of *experiencing* stress and anxiety—and the positive effects of *expressing* these feelings—are mediated by cellular immune factors. "To the extent that the course of malignant melanoma is influenced by the host's immune response, these psychosocial factors will have an indirect, but significant effect on disease progression."[32]

The role of stress in enhancing some kinds of tumor growth (and therefore affecting survival) is a key concept that cancer patients should know about. Stress probably affects different types of cancer differently. It is probably modulated by personality and coping style, social support, and other factors. With all these caveats in mind, what are the implications? A diagnosis of cancer and every subsequent experience connected with cancer are for most people inherently stressful. At each stage, the stress can be consciously and skillfully diminished by an effective collaboration between the patient, his family, his health professionals, and his friends. There are four things cancer patients can do for themselves about stresses that feel unhealthy to them:

1. Find a way to reduce or remove stresses that feel genuinely unhealthy to you, either in your medical treatment or your personal or work life. This applies not only to stress you experienced *after* your diagnosis but also to stresses *before* that time.
2. Practice stress reduction techniques that feel genuinely nurturing to you (a key criterion) such as progressive muscle relaxation, meditation, hypnosis, or imagery.
3. Join a support group where you feel free to *express* your feelings—especially sadness and anger—about your situation.
4. Consciously cultivate paths of personal development that may lead you to a new perspective on life in which situations that were once stressful to you are no longer as stressful. In many spiritual traditions, the work on ourselves that transforms stress in this way is sometimes called the path to inner peace. The capacity to grow toward this inner peace is based on a fundamental reevaluation of what matters to us in our lives. Many people find that this reevaluation comes to them quite naturally in the course of facing cancer.

Psychological Approaches to Extending Life with Cancer

Many individual cases and uncontrolled studies have reported life extension as a result of psychological interventions. In 1984, Alastair Cunningham, Ph.D., of the Ontario Cancer Institute, Toronto, reviewed the studies on whether or not psychological interventions could change the course of cancer. As Locke summarizes Cunningham:

> Can psychological treatments ameliorate cancer? Alastair J. Cunningham, who recognizes the methodological deficiencies of the clinical studies but who is concerned that their claims may nonetheless be "both true and important," maintains that another standard should be used to weight the findings—a standard that might be called the principle of cross-study consistency. Cunningham argues that the results of the clinical studies are consistent with each other

and also with the results of prospective studies correlating personality factors with cancer and animal studies investigating the effects of stress on tumor growth. This broad consistency, he suggests, points to a possible core of validity. It indicates, at the very least, that the clinical claims should not be dismissed on methodological grounds and that the time has come to subject the claims to "properly controlled clinical trials."[33]

One example of the uncontrolled studies that Cunningham reviewed can be found in the work of a remarkable Australian psychiatrist, the late Ainslie Meares. Meares worked with cancer patients using a form of meditation "characterized by extreme simplicity and stillness of the mind." He published specific cases of regression of cancer of the rectum, remission of "massive metastasis from undifferentiated carcinoma of the lung," regression of a recurrence of carcinoma of the breast at the mastectomy site, and regression of a metastasized osteogenic sarcoma (bone cancer). Of the last case, he wrote: "It would seem that the patient has let the effects of the intense and prolonged meditation enter into his whole experience of life. His extraordinarily low level of anxiety is obvious to the most casual observer. It is suggested that this has enhanced the activity of his immune system by reducing his level of cortisone."[34] (The patient in this extraordinary recovery was Ian Gawler, founder of the Australian Cancer Patients Foundation and author of a spell-binding account of his recovery entitled *You Can Conquer Cancer.*)

In summarizing his work with 73 patients who had attended at least 20 sessions of intensive meditation, Meares found that

> Nearly all such patients should expect significant reduction of anxiety and depression, together with much less discomfort and pain. There is reason to expect a ten per cent chance of quite remarkable slowing of the rate of growth of the tumor, and a ten per cent chance of less marked but still significant slowing. The results indicate that patients with advanced cancer have a ten per cent chance of regression of the growth. There is a fifty per cent chance of greatly improved quality of life and for those who die, a ninety per cent chance of death with dignity.[35]

Meares's method calls for the systematic use of a wordless meditation closely related to progressive relaxation. His findings show how enhancement in quality of life for all patients may go hand in hand with slowing of tumor growth for some and a regression of a tumor for a few.

Similarly, O. Carl Simonton, M.D., and Stephanie Matthews Simonton, Ph.D., developers of the most popular of imagery techniques for cancer, reported with T.F. Sparks that "a preliminary study of the effects of psychological intervention in the treatment of advanced cancer [showed that] patients so treated survived up to twice as long as would have been expected based on national averages."[36] Bernauer Newton also has reported—as we shall see in a later section—a study of hypnotherapy with cancer patients that showed at least a doubling of survival for patients who received "adequate" hypnotherapy as opposed to those who were "inadequately" treated. Both studies have serious methodological problems but they exhibit the "cross-study consistency" Cunningham noted in calling for controlled clinical trials. These studies are particularly interesting as precursors of David Spiegel's randomized prospective clinical trial which also found a doubling of average survival in women with metastatic breast cancer who participated in a support group as compared with women who did not. Cunningham summarizes a study investigating psychological interventions aimed at reversing cancer:

> A randomized control study with positive results has . . . been published by Grossarth-Matticek *et al.* (1984). They tested . . . the effects of both chemotherapy and 20–30 individual sessions of psychotherapy based on teaching problem-solving, examination of beliefs and expectations, relaxation and positive suggestion. *The life span of randomly assigned metastatic breast cancer patients was recorded as prolonged by approximately six months on average in those receiving the psychotherapy. There was an additive effect with chemotherapy: patients receiving both treatments lived about a year longer than those getting neither* [emphasis added].[37]

This and other similar studies by Grossarth-Matticek, while intriguing, remain highly controversial. This research has been widely questioned by researchers in the field despite its apparent methodological rigor. The accuracy of the data itself has been questioned.

The Turning Point for Life Extension Research: David Spiegel's Study of Women with Metastatic Breast Cancer

In May 1989, a watershed event took place in the field of psychooncology. A Stanford Medical School associate professor of psychiatry and behavioral sciences, David Spiegel, M.D., told the annual meeting of the American

Psychiatric Association of a very unexpected finding. He and his colleagues had studied 86 women with metastatic breast cancer who had been randomized into two groups: One group received standard medical treatment alone; the other group received standard medical treatment plus weekly group therapy sessions and lessons in self-hypnosis to help control pain.

The 10-year study found that the women in the intervention group had *twice the survival time* of women in the control group. At the 10-year point, 83 of the 86 women in the study had died. But the women who received group therapy lived an average of 36.6 months after entering the program, while the participants in the control group lived an average of 18.9 months. And all three long-term survivors were in the group therapy program.

"I must say I was quite stunned," said Spiegel. He told the *Los Angeles Times* that he "undertook the study expecting to refute often overstated notions about the power of mind over disease, which he said he had found clinically as well as theoretically irritating, as well as destructive to many of my patients." The science writer for the *Los Angeles Times* reported:

> The 10-year study of women with metastatic breast cancer . . . is believed to be the first to examine in a scientifically controlled manner the effect of psychological and social supports on cancer patients' survival. . . . The women in the support group experienced fewer mood swings and less phobia and pain than their counterparts [in addition to surviving for an average of twice as long].
>
> Previous studies suggest that social support may influence the survival of sick people and the elderly, perhaps by serving as a buffer against stress. The opportunities to express feelings, as in group therapy, can also counter the sense of social isolation in some patients and perhaps contribute to survival, other studies suggest.
>
> Spiegel also theorized that the group therapy might have nourished a sense of hope, enabling the women to comply better with medical treatment or perhaps improve their diet. Finally, he pointed to developing theories that the emotions may influence the immune system.
>
> The group therapy the women received lasted one-and-one-half hours a week and centered on expressing fears, anger, anxiety and depression. The women were encouraged to confront their physical problems, to be assertive with their physicians and to grieve the loss of friends in the group who died.

"They came to feel that they were experts in living," Spiegel said. "As a result of their foreshortened lives," he said, "the women felt they had learned lessons about living . . ."

Other researchers called Spiegel's findings marvelous and provocative—but in need of replication by other teams. Cautioned Dr. Troy Thompson, a professor of psychiatry at Jefferson Medical College in Philadelphia, "When something seems too good to be true, often it is. . . . This is a marvelous study, a surprising study to me as well. I would have bet the mortgage of my home that it would not have come out this way."[38]

Interestingly, Spiegel did *not* report the kinds of dramatic and systematic patterns of regression of tumors that Meares reported in 10% of his patients, although the fact that three women in the support group were alive 12 years after the study is of great interest. He reported a doubling of survival time for the women in the treatment group (36.6 months vs. 18.9 months for the control group). He also found a significant increase in time from first metastasis to death: 58 months for the intervention group vs. 43 months for the control group. And he found that there was a "dose-effect" curve: people who had been placed in the intervention group but attended rarely if at all lived a shorter time than those who attended regularly.

In terms of quality of life, Spiegel found that mood disturbances for the intervention group grew better during the intervention while mood disturbances for the control group grew worse. The intervention group was also taught pain control through a combination of self-hypnotic imagery and relaxation. During the course of the program experiences of pain increased in the control group and decreased in the intervention group. The frequency and duration of pain attacks remained the same for both groups, but the intervention group had learned to manage pain with less distress.[39]

Spiegel's report was a watershed development in the field not only because of *what he found* but because of *who he was*. He had all the right markings for the study to have a powerful impact. He was a Stanford professor, and beyond that he had—ideally from the point of view of maximizing the impact of the study—undertaken the study without any belief that psychological interventions had an effect on life extension with cancer. Moreover, he never conveyed to the group that he thought participation in the intervention would extend their lives. Spiegel's study offered the first solid scientific evidence in support of Cunningham's observation that the cross-study consistency of uncontrolled studies which show life extension might be "both true and important."

When the Spiegel study came out, one leading psychooncologist commented to me that perhaps it was the "social support" aspect of the intervention that was primarily responsible for the outcome. She was referring to the studies, described above, that show that people with strong social support networks live longer with cancer, and specifically to the study by J.R. Marshall and D.P. Funch (1983) that younger women with breast cancer who had higher levels of social support lived longer.[40] Other studies show that unmarried people with cancer have lower survival than married people.[41] And a number of important studies, most notably those of L.F. Berkman and S.L. Syme, have shown that people with more social support have lower mortality from a wide range of diseases than those with less social support.[42]

My colleague's point—that social support might be a critical explanation for the outcome of the Spiegel study—was well taken and likely true. But it also underscored the tenuousness of the distinction that psychooncology has drawn between "social support" and "psychological interventions." As I have mentioned before and want to reemphasize, in order to survive in their institutions, psychooncologists needed to minimize claims that what they did might extend the lives of cancer patients. They also needed to acknowledge the reality that strong social support often helps people live longer. Psychooncologists even took the professionally courageous position of welcoming support groups for cancer patients—on the grounds that these support groups helped improve quality of life—which many of the primary care physicians they worked with were deeply suspicious of. But they did not press the connection between enhancing social support by means of psychological intervention and extending life that the Spiegel study finally made inevitable.

As a result of the Spiegel study—but also because of trends in psychooncology and PNI that preceded its publication—it has now become professionally acceptable for top researchers to undertake studies that investigate the effects of psychological interventions on cancer survival. As I write, additional controlled randomized prospective trials by Spiegel and others examining the effect of psychological interventions on life extension are underway.

From the point of view of the cancer patient, the main problem with the new set of studies is that they often use psychological interventions that are far less intensive than the intervention some motivated cancer patients undertake for themselves. Nor do these studies address the question of whether or not there is a synergistic effect when cancer patients undertake intensive psychological interventions in combination with nutritional, physical, and other approaches to intensive health promotion. As you will remember, Spiegel found a "dose-effect" curve in his intervention group. The disturbing and important possibility exists that the "therapeutic dosage" of psychological and other health-promoting interventions in the prospective controlled clinical trials conducted to date is suboptimal in terms of extending survival, and that this remains true in the new generation of studies. In other words, exceptionally motivated patients who undertake integrated programs of intensive health promotion that include a strong psychological component may possibly be achieving results outside the curve that Spiegel and others reported. No current study that I am aware of tests this crucial hypothesis. On the other hand, the Spiegel study does show that an activity that is within the range of almost every patient—attending a weekly support group—was associated with a powerfully beneficial outcome.

Bernard H. Fox, Ph.D., Professor of Psychiatry at Boston University School of Medicine, one of the most respected, circumspect, and thorough of researchers in psychooncology, introduces a useful caution when he takes the view that if there is a contribution of psychological factors to survival in cancer, it is likely to be a very small one—a view that Holland cites as authoritative.[43]

More Support for the Life Extension Hypothesis: Fawzy I. Fawzy's Research on Malignant Melanoma

As this book was going to press, a second very important but far less widely reported study suggesting life extension as a result of a limited psychological intervention was published by Fawzy I. Fawzy, M.D., of the University of California at Los Angeles School of Medicine.

Like Spiegel, Fawzy had initiated a study some years before to assess the effects of psychological intervention of quality of life in cancer patients. He studied "changes over time in methods of coping and affective disturbance," and concluded in his earlier study that a brief psychiatirc intervention lowered depression, fatigue, and total mood disturbance and increased vigor in early stage melanoma patients.[44]

Six years later, Fawzy looked at the effects of the structured psychiatric intervention on survival and time to recurrence in his intervention group and the control group. He found that 10 of the original 34 patients in the control group with stage I disease had died, and 3 others had experienced local recurrences, while in the experimental group only 3 of the original 34 patients had died, and 4 had recurrences. The experimental group—those who participated in the psychiatric intervention—also achieved greater disease-free intervals than the control group.

Fawzy's intervention was strikingly minimal. It consisted of only six structured group sessions over a 6-week period, with each session lasting $1\frac{1}{2}$ hours. The group meetings offered (1) education on melanoma and basic nutritional advice; (2) stress management techniques; (3) enhancement of coping skills; and (4) psychological support form the staff and from other group members.

Like Spiegel, Fawzy emphasizes that his study was not originally designed to assess survival as an outcome, and says simply that, because of the small sample size and other methodological issues, the results warrant further research using a large number of properly stratified subjects.

He also found "to our surprise" that high levels of distress at the beginning of the study, rather than being a negative sign, were "a critical measure of awareness and behavioral motivation," and were associated with enhanced survival. The study also showed that "positive coping behavior can be learned or enhanced, and if implemented, improves health outcomes."[45]

The reader should bear these important findings in mind when reading elsewhere in this chapter about Lydia Temoshok's work with malignant melanoma, since the results of her research are so consistent with Fawzy's findings.

With all the qualifications that careful researchers introduce, Fawzy's research was a dramatic second positive finding regarding genuinely significant evidence of life extension with a very modest psychological interventions. But what if people go all out in a fight for life, with intensive and continuing psychological work, often in combination with other lifestyle interventions? This remains an unexplored frontier in mainstream psychological and behavioral research. But it brings us to the pioneering work of one of the great maverick psychologists in this field, Larry LeShan.

Psychotherapy and the Fight for Life: The Work of Lawrence LeShan

Perhaps the most remarkable claim for life extension with metastatic cancer comes from Lawrence LeShan, Ph.D., one of the pioneers of psychotherapeutic treatment for cancer. His reported success rate exceeds that of almost all other psychological investigators. LeShan writes:

> Ever since I learned how to use this approach some twenty years ago, approximately half of my "hopeless," "terminal" patients have gone into long term remission and are still alive. The lives of many others seemed longer than standard medical predictions would see as likely. Nearly all found that working in this new way improved the "color" and emotional tone of their lives and made the last period of their lives far more exciting and interesting than they had been before starting the therapeutic process.[46]

LeShan never published data in support of these claims, and other psychological investigators, including a number who share his psychotherapeutic philosophy and admire his contribution to the field, have never been able to replicate these results in their own experience with patients. But, while few psychotherapists would claim to have witnessed the frequency or extent of life extension that LeShan claims, many agree with him that life extension can be achieved using psychotherapeutic techniques similar to his. Because of the enormous influence that LeShan has had on psychotherapy and cancer, his work, recently summarized by him in *Cancer as a Turning Point,* is worth reviewing in some detail.

LeShan began researching the relationship of personality to cancer in 1947. "The first thing I found was that up to 1900 the relationship between cancer and psychological factors had been commonly accepted."[47] He cites Gendron, who in 1759 stressed the importance to cancer of "disasters in life, as occasion much trouble and grief."[48] He quotes Walter Hoyle Walshe, an authority on cancer in 1846:

> Much has been written on the influence of mental misery, sudden reverses in fortune, and habitual gloominess of temper on the deposition of carcinomatous

matter. If systematic writers can be credited, these constitute the most powerful cause of the disease. . . . I have myself met with cases in which the connection appeared so clear that I have decided questioning its reality would seem a struggle against reason.[49]

In 1885, Willard Parker in the United States summed up his half-century experience as a surgeon treating cancer: "It is a fact that grief is especially associated with the disease. If cancer patients as a rule were cheerful before the malignant development made its appearance, the psychological theory, no matter how logical, must fail: but it is otherwise. The fact substantiates what reason points out."[50]

After 1900, LeShan writes, the viewpoint that cancer had roots in the psyche disappeared from the literature as psychosomatic medicine went out of style. It lay dormant until LeShan and a few others began to revive it in the 1950s: "Since 1955 literally dozens of studies have shown conclusively that emotional life history often does play an important part in determining an individual's resistance to getting cancer and in how cancer develops after it appears. It is certainly not the only factor and does not play a part for every person with cancer by a long shot, but every cancer patient's emotional life should be considered."

In 1952, when LeShan began his clinical research into the question of whether or not psychotherapy could affect life expectancy with cancer, he applied for permission to conduct his studies at 15 New York hospitals. He was turned down by all 15 institutions—a reflection of the cultural status of this kind of research in medical centers at that time. He finally found "an excellent work relationship" at Trafalgar Hospital, the unconventional New York hospital then operated by Emanuel Revici, M.D., a leading unconventional cancer clinician and researcher (see chapter 23). He worked with patients at Revici's hospital for 12 years.

> The single thing that emerged most clearly during my work was the context in which the cancer developed. In a large majority of the people I saw (certainly not all), there had been, previous to the first noted signs of the cancer, a loss of hope of ever achieving a way of life that would give real and deep satisfaction . . . the kind of life that makes us look forward zestfully to each day . . .

Often, this lack of hope had been brought into being by the loss of the person's major way of expressing himself or herself and the inability to find a meaningful substitute.[51]

For years, LeShan struggled to treat these cancer patients with psychological support. For years, he reports, his cancer patients continued to die. His approach at the time was "very Freudian and psychoanalytic." He finally concluded that the psychological methods in which he had been trained were inadequate for the treatment of cancer.

Conventional psychotherapies, LeShan believes, ask three questions: (1) What is wrong with this person?, (2) How did he or she get that way?, and (3) What can be done about it? LeShan says: "Therapy based on these questions can be wonderful and effective for help with a wide variety of emotional or cognitive problems. It is, however, not effective with cancer patients. It simply does not mobilize the person's self-healing abilities and bring them to the aid of the medical program. We have now had enough experience in many different countries to state this as a fact."[52]

The therapeutic approach developed in his research work with cancer patients is based on entirely different questions:

> What is right with this person? What are his (or her) special and unique ways of being, relating, creating, that are his own and natural ways to live? What is his special music to beat out in life, his unique song to sing so that when he is singing it he is glad to get up in the morning . . .
>
> How can we work together to find these ways of being, relating and creating? What has blocked their perception and/or expression in the past? How can we work together so the person moves more and more in this direction until he is living such a full and zestful life that he has no more time or energy for psychotherapy?

LeShan found that this approach, in conjunction with medical therapy, seemed to help many of his patients extend their lives. Moreover, his patients taught him that there was more to a comprehensive approach to fighting for life than psychotherapy. He found that some patients "learned to work on all three levels of human life: the physical, the psychological and the spiritual. I began to realize that those patients who had gone beyond me, who were consciously working on all three levels, tended to do better than those who were not.

Over a period of time I learned about the holistic approach to illness and how to use it."[53]

LeShan's emphasis on the importance of the individuation process must be placed in the context that individuation has been the central goal of most of the humanistic and transpersonal psychologies that have developed out of the traditions of Jung, Maslow, Assagioli, and others. Jung wrote: "I have in fact seen cases where the carcinoma broke out . . . when a person comes to a halt at some essential point in his individuation or cannot get over an obstacle. Unhappily nobody can do it for him, and it cannot be forced. An inner process of growth must begin, and if this spontaneous activity is not performed by nature herself, the outcome can only be fatal."[54]

The Simonton Approach: Imagery and Cancer

Imagery is one of the most powerful tools in use with cancer. Though its potential for bringing about physical recovery remains an open question, it is practiced extensively by cancer patients and therapists who work with them.

What is imagery? Rachel Naomi Remen, M.D., often describes imagery as the language of the unconscious. It is the way in which all those parts of us that are not presently within our consciousness are able to speak to our conscious selves. If you are in France, she says, you need to learn to speak French in order to communicate. If you are undertaking an inner voyage of healing, it is useful to become acquainted with the inner language of imagery. Imagery is the language of dreams, poetry, the arts, religion, and myth.

O. Carl Simonton, M.D., and Stephanie Matthews Simonton were the pioneers who first used imagery with the goal of physically reversing the development of cancer. Their best-selling book, written with James Creighton, *Getting Well Again,* was a major, though controversial, contribution to this area when it was first published in 1978. It remains one of the most useful and comprehensive psychological self-help books for people with cancer. The Simontons recommended that a person first put himself into a deeply relaxed state. Then:

> Mentally picture the cancer in either realistic or symbolic terms. Think of the cancer as consisting of very weak, confused cells. Remember that our bodies

destroy cancerous cells thousands of times during a normal lifetime. As you picture your cancer, realize that your recovery requires that your body's own defenses return to a natural, healthy state.

If you are now receiving treatment, picture your treatment coming into your body in a way that you understand. If you are receiving radiation treatment, picture it as a beam of millions of bullets of energy hitting any cell in its path. The normal cells are able to repair the damage that is done, but the cancer cells cannot because they are weak. (This is one of the basic facts on which radiation therapy is built.) If you are receiving chemotherapy, picture that drug coming into your body and entering the bloodstream. Picture the drug acting like a poison. The normal cells are intelligent and strong and don't take up the poison so readily. But the cancer cell is a weak cell so it takes very little to kill it. It absorbs the poison, dies and is flushed out of your body.

Picture your body's own white cells coming into the area where the cancer is, recognizing the abnormal cells, and destroying them. There is a vast army of white blood cells. They are very strong and aggressive. They are also very smart. There is no contest between them and the cancer cells; they will win the battle.

Picture the cancer shrinking. See the dead cells being carried away by the white blood cells and being flushed from your body through the liver and kidneys and eliminated in the urine and stool.

Continue to see the cancer shrinking, until it is all gone.

See yourself having more energy and a better appetite and being able to feel comfortable and loved in your family as the cancer shrinks and finally disappears.

If you are experiencing pain anywhere in your body, picture the army of white blood cells flowing into that area and soothing the pain. Whatever the problem, give your body the command to heal itself. Visualize your body becoming well.

Imagine yourself well, free of disease, full of energy.

Picture yourself reaching your goals in life. See your purpose in life being fulfilled, the members of your family doing well, your relationships with people around you becoming more meaningful. Remember that having strong reasons for getting well will help you get well, so use this time to focus clearly on your priorities in life.

Give yourself a mental pat on the back for participating in your recovery. See yourself doing this mental imagery exercise three times a day, staying awake and alert as you do it.[55]

The Simontons stressed that it was not necessary to *see* the imagery if you could sense, think, or feel it. Among the benefits of relaxation and imagery that they listed were that it could: decrease fear; bring about attitudinal changes and enhance "will to live"; effect physical changes "enhancing the immune system and altering the course of a malignancy"; serve as a method for "evaluating current beliefs and altering those beliefs, if desired"; be used as a "a tool for communicating with the unconscious"; serve as a way of decreasing tension and stress; and help "to confront and alter the stance of hopelessness and helplessness. We have seen again and again how this under-lying depression is a significant factor in the development of cancer."[56]

In the Simontons' and some other imagery techniques, the immune system is considered to be the mechanism by which the body actively combats cancer. While we have cited the studies by Levy and Temoshok in support of this view, some researchers believe that other host resilience factors may contribute to life extension. The immune system may or may not turn out to be the most important system by which psychological practices modulate cancer survival.

The story of how the Simontons reached their conclusions about what was important to outcomes when patients used imagery is revealing: "We first began using mental imagery to motivate patients and provide them with a tool for influencing their immune systems, but we soon discovered that the activity revealed extremely important information about patients' belief systems." In brief, what they discovered was that the *content* of the imagery appeared as critical to positive outcomes as the regular practice of imagery. People with negative imagery in which the cancer appeared more powerful than the treatment or the response of their bodies often did not do well. Together with the assistance of Dr. Jeanne Achterberg, a research psychologist, they developed a list of criteria that can be used to evaluate the content of one's mental imagery:

> Representing cancer cells as ants, for instance, we have found is generally a negative symbol. Have you ever been able to get rid of ants at a picnic? Crabs, the traditional symbol for cancer, and other crustaceans are also negative symbols. These beasts are tenacious, they hang on. . . .
>
> Interpreting mental imagery is similar to interpreting dreams: It involves a highly personal, symbolic language. . . . The emotional meaning of a particular symbol may be very different for different individuals, so that a symbol that means

strength and power to you may mean anger and hostility to someone else. Thus, you should not automatically accept anyone else's interpretation of your symbols.[57]

But Achterberg and the Simontons believed there were certain *qualities* of successful imagery:

- The cancer cells are weakened and confused.
- The treatment is strong and powerful.
- The healthy cells have no difficulty repairing any slight damage the treatment might do.
- The army of white blood cells is vast and overwhelms the cancer cells.
- The white blood cells are aggressive, eager for battle, quick to seek out the cancer cells and destroy them.
- The dead cancer cells are flushed from the body normally and naturally.
- By the end of the imagery, you are healthy and free of cancer.
- You see yourself reaching your goals in life, fulfilling your life's purpose.[58]

Of all of these imagery processes, the Simontons regarded the imagery of the white blood cells as "aggressive, eager for battle, [and] quick to seek out the cancer cells and destroy them" as "the most crucial imagery process because it represents your beliefs about the body's natural defenses." They felt that critical elements in this imagery included the strength and number of white blood cells relative to cancer cells and the vividness of the imagery.[59]

The Simontons' and Achterberg's position that *aggressive* imagery—rather than gentle imagery—works better in support of physiological reversal of cancer remains the subject of an ongoing debate among clinicians who use imagery. One group of clinicians holds, with the Simontons, that aggressive imagery works better. Another group believes that, for some people, aggressive imagery is foreign to their personalities and to their sources of inner strength.

Rachel Naomi Remen uses the example of a client who tried to use aggressive imagery for his cancer but could not sustain the image of his white blood cells as sharks seeking out and destroying cancer cells. What came to him spontaneously, instead, was the image of a catfish, always awake, moving endlessly through the water and cleansing his blood of cancer cells. He also liked this image because he felt a great fondness for the catfish who he felt protected his blood—and he felt the catfish also loved and cared about him. To my knowledge, no research has yet been done that would offer any resolution to this debate.

A second debate in the imagery field centers on whether or not imagery that is anatomically accurate is more or less powerful than imagery that uses powerful symbolic representations. Should a cancer patient try to imagine as vividly and realistically as possible how the white blood cells and cancer cells look and how the white blood cells attack the cancer cells, or is he better off imagining his white blood cells as powerful forces of some kind overcoming the cancer cells? While not specifically addressing cancer, research studies are divided on this subject. Most clinicians are inclined to believe that symbolic representations can be just as powerful or more powerful for some patients than anatomically accurate ones.[60]

Martin Rossman: Self-Healing Through Imagery

Martin Rossman, M.D., has written one of the most accessible books on imagery: *Healing Yourself: A Step-by-Step Program for Better Health Through Imagery*. He also conducts one of the most respected imagery training programs for health professionals in the United States. While Rossman has not had a primary concern with cancer, he is widely admired by his colleagues for having articulated effectively one of the most comprehensive approaches to the use of imagery:

> Imagery is a flow of thoughts you can see, hear, feel, smell or taste. An image is an inner representation of your experience or your fantasies—a way your mind codes, stores and expresses information. Imagery is the currency of dreams and daydreams; memories and reminiscence; plans, projections and possibilities. It is the language of the arts, the emotions, and most important, the deep inner self.

> Imagery is a window on your inner world; a way of viewing your own ideas, feelings, and interpretations. But it is more than a mere window—it is a means of transformation and liberation from distortions in this realm that may unconsciously direct your life and shape your health.[61]

Rossman's imagery script for finding your own healing imagery starts with a standard "induction" that helps you reach complete relaxation. Then:

When you are ready, focus your attention on the symptom or problem that has been bothering you . . . simply put your attention on it while staying completely relaxed . . . allow an image to emerge for this symptom or problem . . . accept the image that comes, whether it makes sense or not . . . whether it is strange or familiar . . . whether you like it or not . . . just notice and accept the image that comes for now . . . let it become clear and more vivid, and take some time to observe it carefully . . .

In your imagination, you can explore this image from any angle, and from as close or as far away as you like . . . carefully observe it from different perspectives . . . don't try to change it . . . just notice what draws your attention . . .

What seems to be the matter in this image? . . . what is it that represents the problem? . . .

When you know this, let another image appear that represents the healing or resolution of this symptom or problem . . . again, simply allow it to raise spontaneously . . . allow it to become clearer and more vivid . . . carefully observe this image as well, from different perspectives . . . what is it about this image that represents the healing? . . .

Recall the first image and consider the two images together . . . how do they seem to relate to each other as you observe them? . . . Which is larger? . . . Which is more powerful? . . . If the image of the problem seems more powerful, notice whether you can change that . . . imagine the image of healing becoming stronger, more powerful, more vivid . . . imagine it to be much bigger and more powerful than the other . . .

Imagine the image of the problem or symptom turning into the image of healing . . . watch the transformation . . . how does it seem to happen? . . . Is it sudden, like changing channels on television, or is it a gradual process? . . . If it is a process, notice how it happens . . . notice if what happens seems to relate to anything in your life . . .

End your imagery session by focusing clearly and powerfully on this healing image . . . imagine it is taking place in your body at just the right place . . . notice whether you can feel or imagine any changing sensations as you imagine this healing taking place . . . let the sensations be sensations of healing . . . affirm to yourself that this is happening now, and that this healing continues in you whether you are waking or sleeping . . . imaging . . . or going about your daily activities . . .[62]

The session ends with instructions to return gradually to the external world.

Two other imagery strategies described by Rossman are "meeting your inner advisor" and "listening to your symptoms." The inner advisor, for Rossman, is a symbolic representation of our deepest inner wisdom who "may offer advice in areas as diverse as nutrition, posture, exercise, environment, attitudes, emotions, and faith. Your advisor can serve as a liaison figure to that part of your mind that thinks in images and symbols; as an ambassador between the silent and verbal brains, the unconscious and conscious minds."[63]

Another imagery approach that Rossman recommends, especially for those who feel uncomfortable with "inner advisor" imagery, is "listening to your symptoms." Citing the work of Edelstein and LeCron, Rossman suggests seven common unconscious reasons for the development of symptoms. They may be: (1) a symbolic representation of unexpressed feelings; (2) the result of unconscious acceptance of an idea or image of oneself from early life; (3) the result of past traumatic experience; (4) a way to resolve a current life problem; (5) the result of an unconscious identification with an important person in one's life; (6) a manifestation of an inner conflict; or (7) the result of an unconscious need for punishment. Using a script developed originally by Rachel Naomi Remen, Rossman takes the patient through a relaxation, suggests that the patient focus on the symptom, invites an image to appear that represents the symptom, suggests careful observation of the image, and then suggests:

> When you are sure about your feelings, tell the image how you feel about it—speak directly and honestly to it. . . . Then, in your imagination, give the image a voice, and allow it to answer you . . . listen carefully to what it says . . .
>
> Ask the image what it wants from you, and listen to its answer . . . ask why it wants that—what does it really need? . . . and let it respond . . . ask it also what it has to offer you, if you should meet its needs . . . again, allow the image to respond . . .[64]

Rossman goes on to suggest that the patient allow himself to *become* the image, to notice how he feels as the image and to look back at himself through the eyes of the image. Then the patient returns to himself, and may consult an "inner advisor" figure before coming to the end of the session.

Since Jeanne Achterberg's original collaboration with the Simontons, she and Frank Lawlis have over many years refined a theory and practice of imagery of great richness. Achterberg's insightful book, *Imagery in Healing*, traces the historical roots of modern imagery therapies. Her thesis is that imagery is a human potential deeply associated with the feminine aspect of humanity and with nature. The wisdom and consciousness of imagery has, she believes, been systematically suppressed in the modern era, just as women have been oppressed and the earth has been exploited. Drawing on two books written with Lawlis, *Image of Cancer* and *Bridges of the Bodymind*, Achterberg argues that the images that cancer patients develop of their immune systems and their cancers prove to be more predictive of outcome than any available medical tests.

They describe an imagery assessment technique that begins with a tape-recorded relaxation induction followed by a brief education on the disease process, how the treatment may be working to the patient's advantage, and the idea of host defense. Then the patient is advised to imagine these factors in operation in a guided, but not programmed, session that allows him considerable choice in imagery. The images are first drawn by the patient and then described in an interview, and both are scored on the basis of 14 dimensions, including: "vividness; activity and strength of cancer cells; relative comparison of size and number of cancer cells and white blood cells; vividness and effectiveness of medical treatment; the integration of the whole imagery process; the regularity with which they imaged a positive outcome; and a ventured clinical opinion on the prognosis, given the previous listed thirteen factors."

The total scores were found to predict with 100% certainty who would have either died or shown evidence of significant deterioration during the two-month period, and with 93% certainty who would be in remission [emphasis added]. Remember, the scores are just a numerical shape put on the imagination—it was the images themselves that so accurately predicted the future.

What the patients' imagination predicted were the dramatic changes that would occur within a short period of time. These results are often confusing to people who haven't witnessed the erratic course of cancer. Tumors can change as rapidly as nightblooming flowers, growing, shrinking, perhaps changing shape. People with Stage IV cancer can be living active lives with no pain, or they may be bedridden; and they can move from one of these conditions to the other, and back, within days.[65]

Achterberg and Lawlis's findings regarding the predictive power of imagery in cancer are startling. Their findings are so provocative and important that other research teams should replicate their studies.

Hypnosis and Cancer

Hypnotherapy for cancer is closely related to the use of imagery and relaxation, as both are part of the more general field—voluntary control of internal states of consciousness—that includes hypnosis, imagery, meditation, drug-induced alterations of consciousness, biofeedback, and traditional (preallopathic) systems of healing. Interest in these fields began to converge in the 1970s with annual conferences on the Voluntary Control of Inner States sponsored by Elmer and Alyce Green at the Menninger Foundation.[66]

What is hypnosis? Brown and Fromm describe it in *Hypnosis and Behavioral Medicine:*

> Hypnosis is a special state of consciousness in which certain normal human abilities are heightened while others fade more or less into the background. Roughly 90% of the population has the talent to go into a hypnotic state— some more talented than others. Hypnosis can be combined with any type of therapy. . . . Hypnosis itself is not a therapy, although the relaxation that accompanies it can be beneficial. . . . That hypnosis is an altered state of consciousness is now generally accepted. Ludwig (1966) coined the term "altered state of consciousness (ASC)," defining an altered state according to the subjective experience and altered psychological functioning.[67]

Numerous hypnotherapists have written of their experience using hypnotherapy for cancer patients. Brown and Fromm describe three basic strategies that hypnotherapists (and other psychotherapists) have used. They are *stress reduction, wellness enhancement,* and *direct immunotherapy.*

The stress reduction strategies of hypnotherapy and nonhypnotic therapies focus on identifying stressful situations in the patient's life and desensitizing the patient to them or teaching better communication skills, coping skills, deep relaxation, self-hypnosis, or meditation.

The wellness-enhancement strategies focus on enhancing well-being and mental health through humor, loving compassion, and a general focus on improving quality of life and quality of relationships: "The hypnotized patient visualizes his ego-ideal and merging into it, that is, becoming progressively more like the person he would like to be—healthy, competent and strong. He also imagines himself at various future times effectively living the kind of life he would most like to live.

Direct immunotherapy involves stimulating the immune system by imagery:

> The Simontons teach nonhypnotic relaxation combined with somatic imagery . . . Subsequent clinical studies suggest that routine application of such visualization is not in itself sufficient. Patricia Norris has her patients generate and experiment with a variety of images. She claims that certain spontaneous images (not always of immune functioning) have an experientially distinct "sense" about them and are highly specific, bodily felt images of one's natural healing forces. Their appearance increases the likelihood of a positive treatment response.[68]

The work of Bernauer Newton, Ph.D., presents a thoughtful exercise in the clinical use of hypnosis in cancer. Writing in a special issue devoted to cancer of the *American Journal of Clinical Hypnosis* in 1982–1983, Newton described 8 years of hypnotherapy at his center with more than 250 patients. Over this period, Newton and his colleagues began to emphasize quality of life rather than life extension per se:

> This shift does not reflect a lessening in our belief that a person can be successful in his fight against malignant disease, but rather a growing awareness that unless the quality of his life improves, he will not engage in an all-out fight. The patient frequently is in so much distress from symptoms and side-effects of medical treatment that he has lost all or most of his desire to live and the energy to go on. . . .

> Another change we have made is in the meaning we now attach to visualizations. We no longer pressure our patients to try for clearer visualizations. Many of our patients have done very well with weak and ephemeral images while others have gone down hill rapidly while visualizing vividly. We do believe that imaging assists some patients to strengthen their belief systems and certainly the results of biofeedback research point to its value. However this must be balanced against the possibility that urging the patient in this area . . . may result in his feeling that he is failing, experiencing guilt and depression, and raising his level of tension. . . .

Another change is really basic to nearly all that we do now. When we first began to work in this program, we were impressed with the need to help the patient make important psychological changes in what we feared might be a much shorter period of time than we usually had for non-cancer patients. This led us to be more confrontive and demanding. . . . As time went by, we were impressed by the progress some of our patients were making without this aggressive therapeutic interaction, and at the same time we were concerned about the rise in tension levels among those patients with whom we were being most "active." Then in 1976 we became aware of the work Ainslie Meares was doing in Australia. The patients, many of whom were in advanced stages, were having no other medical treatment. He was having most remarkable success by assisting them to achieve daily periods of the most complete inner calm induced by unique indirect and non-verbal techniques. This seemed to confirm what we were beginning to see and encouraged us to shift the emphasis we gave to various activities in our treatment program. We still have our patients engage in the visualizations and we carry out extensive and intensive hypnotically facilitated psychotherapy but we believe that *the cornerstone and absolutely indispensable part of our work is the patient's experiencing the most profound quiet on a regular daily basis* [emphasis added].[69]

Newton further reports clinical impressions of life extension based on a thorough review of patient records similar to, but more extensive than, that reported by the Simontons. Of the 283 patients seen over 8 years for at least one session, Newton decided that 105 would be considered "adequately treated" having had ten 1-hour sessions over a 3-month period. There were 57 "inadequately treated" patients seen three to nine times and 121 "unknown" patients seen fewer than three times. Almost all adequately treated patients experienced enhanced quality of life. There was no significant difference between adequately and inadequately treated patients with respect to diagnosis, stage of disease, age, or length of illness. But of 105 adequately treated patients, 54% were still alive at the time of the analysis, while of 57 inadequately treated patients, only 18% were still alive at the time of the analysis. And when he followed the Simontons' method of comparing length of life for his patients to national survival rates for advanced metastatic cancer of the breast, lung, and bowel, Newton reports: "The national figure for duration of life for breast cancer patients [with advanced metastatic illness] is 16 months while Simonton reported 35 months and the median for our patients was 42.5 months. The comparison for metastatic disease of the bowel and lung show equally favorable improvement in the duration of life, being twice, and in some cases, three times better than the national figures."[70]

Newton then goes on, responsibly, to emphasize that the data are "clinical impressions" and that there are numerous problems involving the small sample size, the selective nature of which patients stayed for "adequate" treatment, and other factors.

Newton disagrees with the Simontons and with Achterberg and Lawlis that clarity and power of images is an important predictor of survival. He has come to agree with Ainslie Meares, the late Australian psychiatrist, whose meditation technique places the patient in a very simple state of relaxation in which neither words nor images are used.

Meares, in fact, published one study in which he reported that a patient with advanced cancer went into remission while using intensive meditation but "a relapse occurred when she accompanied the meditation with vivid visualization of healthy cells eating cancer cells. The alertness caused by the visualization interfered with the state of regression needed for the therapeutic effect (activation of the immune system) to occur."[71] Yet, by contrast, a recent study comparing the effects on mood states of relaxation training compared with relaxation training plus imagery among 139 women with early-stage breast cancer found that both systems enhanced mood but that adding imagery further improved mood.[72] It is worth noting that Meares *believed and expected* that meditation without imagery was better for cancer patients than relaxation with imagery, while the authors of the breast cancer study believed and formally hypothesized the reverse.

These kinds of disagreements among clinicians and researchers should not surprise us. Some day answers may emerge as to whether or not aggressive imagery is preferable in cancer to nonaggressive imagery; whether vivid imagery is better than less vivid imagery or a nonimaging meditative state; and whether LeShan's individuation-oriented psychotherapy is decisively superior to other psychotherapies in cancer. But even if these answers emerge, they will almost certainly be generalizations about average responses. Most clinicians agree that there is tremendous individual variance. Brown and Fromm have noted a trend in behavioral medicine away from "uniform treatment packages" toward greater individualization, especially in the area of self-control strategies (i.e., muscle relaxation, imagery, hypnosis, biofeedback, and meditation). And with hypnosis and imagery, individuals respond differently to various types of suggestions and images.[73]

In reality, most clinicians in the field treat progressive muscle relaxation, hypnosis, biofeedback, imagery, and meditation as different techniques for reaching a common set of fields of altered states of consciousness in which certain forms of healing work are most effective. Here, for example, is the explanation Newton gives as to why he *presents* the work he does with cancer patients as hypnosis (as opposed to presenting it as meditation or relaxation):

> We have found that hypnosis has been most helpful in all phases of our program. We also believe that presenting it as hypnosis rather than as deep relaxation or meditation has a clear advantage. We have already acknowledged the importance to the patient's belief system; the probable placebo effect of what we do; the increase in the patient's sense that he has some control over what happens to him; and the value to the patient of achieving deeply altered states of consciousness. It is our strong belief that the use of the label "hypnosis"; the use of induction techniques rather than meditation; and having the patient experience hypnotic dissociative phenomena all have added impact and facilitate the treatment process. For this reason we use specific and rather mechanical and simplistic induction techniques rather than any more indirect and subtle ones. We want the patient to immediately begin to believe that something real and significant is happening and that he can make these important things happen for himself.[74]

From the beginning of human history, healers have developed their own strategies of putting their patients (and often themselves) in altered states of healing consciousness. The fundamental point here is that most of the disagreements are about how best to get into these altered states of healing consciousness and which are the best specific techniques to use once you get there. And as Fromm and Brown point out, and most clinicians would agree, the key variables are what works best for the individual patient *and* the individual clinician.

Is There a "Cancer-Prone Personality"?

Many cancer patients ask whether or not there is such a thing as a "cancer-prone personality"—a specific personality configuration, or certain personality traits, associated with a higher risk of developing cancer. Another question often asked is whether cancer may appear at a particular *site* in the body for psychological reasons.

Claus Bahne Bahnson, Ph.D., a professor of psychiatry at Jefferson Medical College in Philadelphia, has studied these questions extensively: "The relationship between stress and cancer has intrigued scientists for more than 2,000 years. Certain persons do appear to be at greater risk for developing cancer because of a personality makeup dominated by sadness, depression and unmet emotional needs."[75]

Bahnson reviews the historical literature and comes to the same conclusions that LeShan came to from his historical studies. Galen (c. 130–200 A.D.) saw breast cancer more often in "melancholic women"; Gendron (1759) saw more cancer in women prone to serious depression and high anxiety; Walshe (1846) found that "misery, sudden reverses of fortune, [and] habitual gloominess" cause cancer; Amussat (1854) found "the influence of grief appears to be . . . the most common cause of cancer."[76] Bahnson notes that between 1870 and 1890, a surge of "psychosomatic" statements concerning the influence of loss, bereavement, grief, and melancholy on the development of cancer appeared in the literature. Then, in 1926, E. Evans reported on 100 patients with cancer who had been evaluated through intensive psychotherapy. She found that her patients had lost, or had disrupted, a major emotional relationship prior to the development of the disease. Thus, Evans was, according to Bahnson, among the earliest investigators to express a dynamic formulation of cancer.

Bahnson found that psychology and psychoanalysis have developed two major theories about cancer. According to one, loss and depression are potential precursors. According to the second, "a particular personality configuration, characterized by denial and repression as well as by strong internalized control and commitment to social norms, increases the risk of cancer development." He cites numerous scientific studies that have lent support to the loss-depression hypothesis:

> Greene and associates and Schmale and Iker evaluated personality factors in patients with lymphomas and leukemias, and uterine cancer, respectively. These investigators found that severe loss or separation—with concomitant depression, helplessness, and hopelessness—is a characteristic antecedent to the development of these malignancies. With different collaborators, Greene has made carefully analyzed clinical studies and has consistently reported that separation from a significant person or the loss of a major goal, with ensuing depression, were the key psychological factors in the development of reticuloendothelial malignancies.

Bahnson also cites a study by Greene and Swisher showing that among monozygotic twins, the twin that developed leukemia was the one that suffered individual frustration or loss. Two separate investigators, Schmale and Spence, found that they could *predict* which women with higher-risk cervical cancer biopsies would actually develop cancer based either on a recent history of loss or on a computerized content analysis of words referring to depression and hopelessness in their speech.

> LeShan and associates, after working clinically with more than 500 cancer patients, reached a similar conclusion. LeShan emphasized that serious and incapacitating depletion and depression (or, as he calls it, "despair" in the sense of the Danish philosopher Kierkegaard) earmarked these patients who were experiencing insoluble life situations prior to the clinical onset of cancer. He also emphasized that cancer patients-to-be chronically have fragile or nonexistent affective object relations and a basic bleak hopelessness about ever achieving any real feeling or finding true meaning in life.[77]

Bahnson reports that LeShan and Worthington studied cancer patients and controls with a personal history test and found that cancer patients: (1) "had suffered the loss of an important relationship before the diagnosis," (2) "had no ability to express hostile feelings," and (3) "showed tension over the death of a parent, usually an event that had occurred many years previously."[78] Bahnson's own clinical experience led him to elaborate further a constellation of characteristics he found frequently among cancer patients:

- Childhood trauma, loss of close figures, lack of a protected and loving childhood, and parental deprivation and coldness.
- An encompassing underlying main affect of hopelessness that colors all experience—the certainty that everything must go wrong, coupled with simultaneous guilt feelings because of self-blame.
- A repetition compulsion of self-destructive drives, attitudes and acts, often manifested on anniversaries of other similar or related events.
- The development of a double life or double self within which realistic and adaptive ego operations unfold, separated from and independent of a parallel "shadow self" that feels isolated, unloved, hurt and deserted.[79]

Bahnson concluded that loss in adulthood is especially traumatic and crucial in the lives of cancer patients if they experienced a devastating childhood loss, particularly of parents, and above all if they had a conflicted and unsatisfying relationship with their mothers. The pattern of mistrust and hostility are transferred from the childhood experience into adult relationships, which are therefore precarious, and when the new relationships break down "the original despair and hopelessness of the deprived and longing child reemerge, throwing the individual back on his or her own resources in the face of a renewed insult from the environment. In essence, such persons are left with little hope that any warmth or solace can be obtained from others."[80]

Bahnson tested this theory by administering the Roe-Siegel Parent Child Relationship questionnaire to heart patients, cancer patients, and age-matched controls. "We found that cancer patients indeed remembered their parents as more neglecting and cold than do other patients or normal controls." As a child, according to Bahnson, the isolated cancer patient learned to inhibit the expression of feelings as a way of dealing with cold and conflicted parental relationships.[81]

C.B. Thomas reinforces Bahnson's view. In a prospective study of 1,337 medical students looking for predictors of later illness, Thomas and her associates found that "closeness to parents was a powerful factor among various groups. Tumor patients rated lowest on a closeness-to-parents scale, as did mental patients. However, mental patients rated highest, and cancer patients lowest, on matriarchal dominance. Thus of all the groups in this predictive study cancer patients were among the most emotionally deprived with regard to the mother."[82]

A prospective study of 2,500 participants in Sweden found that female cancer patients had a tendency toward depression that antedated their cancer. Another prospective study of 2,107 Western Electric employees found a significant correlation between their scores on the depression subscale of the Minnesota Multiphasic Personality Inventory and the later development of cancer.[83] Bahnson concluded: "There can be little doubt that a subtle relationship exists between loss and depression and the clinical onset or exacerbation of cancer."[84]

This hypothesis, however, does not hold up among other researchers. A recent study found no association between depression and the incidence of cancer, and led Bernard Fox to conclude that, if there was a relationship, it was only in a subset of cancer patients.[85] S. Greer and Peter M. Silberfarb, writing in

1982, emphasized the need to study patients with different kinds of cancer separately. They concluded that the "cancer personality" remains elusive:

> In ensuing investigations, it is essential to study separately patients with different kinds of neoplastic disease. Systematic controlled studies in this area . . . demonstrated that men with lung cancer differed systematically from controls with other pulmonary diseases in having restricted outlets for emotional discharge (Kissen, 1963). These results were confirmed in a replication study (Kissen et al., 1969). A subsequent investigation of men with lung cancer revealed that psychological differences between the cancer patients and the controls were most marked among younger men (Abse et al., 1974). This interesting and surprising result was also reported in a controlled study of women with breast cancer: suppression of anger was found to be correlated with the diagnosis of breast cancer, but the correlation reached statistical significance only in women aged under 50 (Greer and Morris, 1975). These authors found no significant association between breast cancer and either extraversion, depression during the preceding 5 years, or the loss of a loved person during their preceding 20 years. The hypothesis linking breast cancer with the previous loss of a major emotional relationship was also refuted in another controlled study by Muslin et al. (1966). . . . Is there a cancer-prone personality? The question has not been answered conclusively (Fox, 1978), and this remains a fruitful area for further inquiry. . . . Research workers would do well to heed the warning with which Fox (1978) concludes his comprehensive review of this whole field: "It is, truly, a most difficult type of research."[86]

Lydia Temoshok, who did the important studies with malignant melanoma described above, reviewed the literature on "personality, coping style, emotion and cancer" in the search for an "integrative model" of how these factors may affect one another. Her model is important in itself and also because Holland cited her study approvingly in the final section of her chapter, in her authoritative text.[87] Temoshok reviewed a large body of literature on the role of psychosocial factors in cancer initiation and progression.

> Given this heterogeneity [of the studies], we found it surprising that there were *any* consistencies in the literature. However, evidence from studies of various designs, using different cancer sites and different measures, converges for the most part on a constellation of factors that appear to predispose some individuals to develop cancer more readily or to progress more quickly though its stages. These factors include (a) personality traits of stoicism, niceness, industriousness, perfectionism, sociability, conventionality and more rigid defense controls, (b) difficulty expressing emotions and (c) an attitude or tendency toward helplessness/hopelessness.[88]

Temoshok developed the concept of a "Type C" behavior pattern which she conceived as "the opposite of Type A behavior shown to be predictive of the development of coronary heart disease": "Specifically, the Type C individual was hypothesized to be cooperative and appeasing, unassertive, patient, unexpressive of negative emotions (particularly anger), and compliant with external authorities, in contrast to the hostile, aggressive, tense and controlling Type A individual."[89] Temoshok described the hypothetical evolution of a Type C coping style through which—as a consequence of genetic dispositions or family interactions—a child learned to cope with the challenges of life by placing the needs of others in front of his own, suppressing negative emotions, and "being cooperative, unassertive, appeasing and accepting." This way of coping may be socially successful, but the chronic blockage of needs and feelings may exact a high psychobiological toll. "The Type C individual may be seen as *chronically* hopeless and helpless, even though this is not consciously recognized, in the sense that the person basically believes that it is useless to express one's needs: the needs cannot or will not be met by the environment."[90]

Why should this lead to the development of cancer? Temoshok developed an intriguing response. She proposed that there are basically two human ways of dealing with emotions: by externalizing them or internalizing them. People who internalize emotions would tend in general to develop physical rather than psychological problems under stress. She then suggested that an organism under stress generally seeks to respond to the stress at the highest level of mental organization available to it. If the problem overwhelms mental organization at that level, the organism responds at the next most primitive level. Both Type A and Type C people are prone to internalize emotional responses to stress and thus develop physical problems. But while Type A people prone to heart disease process stressful situations at the mental level of "motivation," which has as its biological basis the autonomic nervous system and endocrine system, Type C people process stressful situations at a lower level of organization—the mental level of "perception"—which has as its biological foundation immunomodulatory neuropeptides.[91]

Three things are particularly notable about Temoshok's model. First, while Temoshok posits a way of responding to stress learned or developed through genetic predisposition in childhood, she avoids the specific hypotheses about childhood loss and subsequent depression that entangled much of the research described previously. She does, it is true, describe the Type C personality as manifesting a learned or genetically predisposed helplessness/hopelessness, but does not posit a specific childhood loss behind it. Second, she writes as a researcher who conducts her work according to norms acceptable to the mainstream of psychooncology. As a result, her views on the role of Type C personality in cancer, while admittedly speculative, are accepted as a plausible way of integrating the wide and disparate body of research in this field. Third, and as a result of the preceding observations, her work has served as a vehicle by which hypotheses relating Type C behavior pattern to cancer incidence and progression—which closely parallel theories previously unacceptable to mainstream researchers—are sanitized, as it were, and enabled to enter the mainstream.

Does Personality Make a Difference in Recovery from Cancer?

It is one thing to wonder whether personality contributes to the incidence or progression of cancer. It is an additional step to consider whether, if personality does indeed appear to affect the progression of cancer, whether a cancer patient can do anything to alter this relationship between cancer and personality, coping style, and emotional expression. I will focus here on the research on whether or not any generalizations can be made about successful psychological responses to cancer. Greer and Silberfarb summarized the research in 1982. They found:

1. A flawed prospective study of different kinds of cancer by K.M. Stavraky revealed the most favorable outcomes in a group of patients who "differed strikingly from all others in its high proportion of individuals who had strong hostile drives without loss of emotional control." This personality profile, the authors point out, is the antithesis of the "hopeless" or "giving-up" reaction.
2. A study by A.D. Weisman and J.W. Worden that followed a series of patients at Massachusetts General Hospital with malignant melanoma, Hodgkin's disease, and lung, breast, and colon cancer: "They found that long survivors had closer personal relationships, were less emotionally distressed, regarded their physicians as more helpful, complained less and coped better with illness-related problems than was the case among short survivors."[92]

3. A contrasting study of metastatic breast cancer patients at Johns Hopkins Hospital, in which L.R. Derogatis found that long-term breast cancer survivors showed "more emotional distress (anxiety, depression, guilt, hostility), poorer adjustment to their illness and more negative attitudes toward their physicians."[93]

Greer conducted his own, now famous, study which prospectively followed women with early breast cancer treated by simple mastectomy with or without postoperative radiotherapy for 5 years. Their psychological response to breast cancer was analyzed 3 months after surgery by a structured interview:

> From an analysis of the patients' *verbatim* statements, it proved possible to group their psychological responses in 4 broad categories: denial, fighting spirit, stoic acceptance, and helplessness/hopelessness. Patients' psychological responses at 3 months were found to be related to outcome 5 years after operation: a favorable outcome (recurrence-free survival) was significantly more common among patients whose initial responses had been fighting spirit or denial than in patients who showed either stoic acceptance or a helpless/hopeless response.[94]

The finding that women showing "fighting spirit" or "denial" had better outcomes than "stoic" or "helpless" women was confirmed again at the 10-year follow-up. Using the same measurement tools, DiClemente and Temoshok found stoic acceptance in women and helplessness/hopelessness in men to be predictors of progression in melanoma 18 to 29 months after diagnosis. A half-dozen other studies cited by Temoshok found similar patterns in patients with cervical cancer, uterine or ovarian cancer, breast cancer, and (for men) the incidence of cancer in general.[95]

A public furor in this usually erudite research broke out in 1985 when Barrie R. Cassileth, Ph.D., of the University of Pennsylvania Cancer Center, published an article in the *New England Journal of Medicine* reporting that personality factors—and, indeed, all psychosocial factors—found to predict longevity in the general population did not affect survival in two groups of high-risk cancer patients. One group of 204 patients with advanced malignant disease was followed to determine length of survival. A second group of 155 patients with stage I or II melanoma or stage II breast cancer were followed to determine time to relapse. Cassileth measured psychosocial factors that included social ties, job satisfaction, drug use, life satisfaction, subjective view of adult health, hopelessness/helplessness, and perception of the adjustment needed to cope with the cancer diagnosis. She did not find that any of these factors affected length of survival or time to recurrence of the disease. "Our study of patients with advanced, high-risk malignant diseases," reports Cassileth, "suggests that the inherent biology of the disease alone determines the prognosis, overriding the potentially mitigating influence of psychosocial factors." Cassileth's study, by her own admission, did not "address the possibility that psychosocial factors or events might influence either the cause of disease or the outcomes for patients with more favorable cancer prognoses."[96]

The editor of the *New England Journal of Medicine* used Cassileth's article as a springboard to launch a broad attack against those who claimed that psychological factors might influence outcomes with cancer. This attack, in turn, was picked up by the press and widely disseminated as the *Journal's* swipe against all supporters of mind-body approaches to cancer and other life-threatening illnesses. Supporters of mind-body research responded with a barrage of letters to the *Journal,* most of them not published, criticizing the methodology of the Cassileth study or the inferences drawn in the editorial, for drawing, in Temoshok's words, "conclusions that were not based on evidence from a burgeoning literature in psychosocial oncology and psychoneuroimmunology."[97] Temoshok also pointed out that with the exception of some hotly debated studies by Grossarth-Matticek, there were not yet "[any] published studies . . . that have attempted to change emotional expression experimentally, and thereby beneficially alter the course of cancer (although a few such studies are underway)."[98]

Spontaneous Remissions

The new classic resource in this field is *Spontaneous Remission: An Annotated Bibliography*, by Brendan O'Regan and Caryle Hirshberg of the Institute of Noetic Sciences. At the start, the authors quote the renowned cancer researcher Lewis Thomas:

> The rare but spectacular phenomenon of spontaneous remission of cancer persists in the annals of medicine, totally inexplicable but real. . . . No one has the ghost of an idea how it happens. Some have suggested the sudden mobilization of immunological defense, others propose that an intervening infection by bacteria or viruses has done something to destroy the cancer cell,

but no one knows. It is a fascinating mystery, but at the same time a solid basis for hope in the future: If several hundred cancer patients have succeeded in doing this sort of thing, eliminating vast numbers of malignant cells on their own, the possibility that medicine can learn to accomplish the same thing at will is surely within the reach of imagining.[99]

Thomas spoke of "several hundred" cancer patients who had achieved spontaneous remissions, but in fact O'Regan and Hirshberg found more than 1000 articles in the world medical literature describing spontaneous remissions of cancer—often with reference to multiple cases. And, of course, these are only the published reports: conservatively, one would have to surmise that the people whose cases of spontaneous remission are not reported outnumber those reported by at least 10 to 1.

This master work by O'Regan and Hirshberg summarizes all the studies of spontaneous remission, categorizes the types of cancer for which remissions were reported, and describes the possible explanations for these remissions. Possible explanations on the list include fevers, infections, psychospiritual techniques, meditation, diet, Chinese herbs, and numerous other factors.

My inclination is to see spontaneous remissions of cancer not as an isolated phenomenon, but as the most dramatic endpoint of a continuum in many types of cancer in which a wide variety of mechanisms of self-repair may operate even as the malignancy works to turn the tide of battle the other way. I believe that the differential efficacy of these mechanisms of self-repair may help explain why, in so many cancers, there is such a wide variation in life expectancy. So I read the literature on spontaneous remissions not only with an interest in what may cause complete and lasting remissions but also for hints on what may cause partial remissions and life extension.

One article by Yujiro Ikemi and his associates at Kyushu University in Fukuoka, Japan, describes SRC (spontaneous regressions in advanced cancer). During a research trip to Japan, I visited Ikemi and spoke with him and his associates. They have published reports on five well-documented cases of SRC "among many possible SRC cases in the Fukuoka area." They have since collected numerous additional cases. Their cases make fascinating reading.

A 64-year-old man with a histologically confirmed cancer of the upper right jaw refused all medical treatment. A Shinto preacher, he felt that "this is God's will and I have no complaint about it. Whatever should happen will just happen." Ikemi reports:

> Ten days after the "sentence of cancer," he visited the president of the religious organization who said to him: "Remember that you are an invaluable asset for our church." This made him feel very happy and he shed tears of joy all the way back home. Since this moving experience, his hoarseness [a symptom of the cancer] began to improve. . . . Today Dr. F. says: "The cancer of this patient seems to be practically cured. When I looked into the vocal cord through the laryngoscope, the tumor was gone."

An 81-year-old church worker was diagnosed with a histologically confirmed tubular adenocarcinoma. Surgery was recommended but he declined:

> When he was told that he had cancer at the age of sixty-six and gastrectomy was suggested, he summoned a family council. He told his relatives that he wished to serve God as long as he lived, and that he would be satisfied if his life was taken away when God so wished, and that he did not want to undergo surgery but wanted to continue his usual life with his daily work and sake (a Japanese alcoholic beverage made from rice.) All the relatives approved of him. Since this time on, he complained less of symptoms of the stomach and worked as usual.

A 39-year-old housewife with extensive metastatic stomach cancer underwent a gastrectomy as a palliative operation but the metastases remained and the surgeon estimated her survival at 1 to 3 months. Nine years later, the woman was well at the time of Ikemi's report. The woman said:

> Frankly speaking, I was not afraid of cancer. That was because I had my religious faith. But without it, I would have given in to the fear of cancer. Now I am very grateful to my friend's mother who persuaded me to have this faith. . . . I suffered from cancer . . . before reaching what is called "the cancer age." Because of this, I was forced to an early mental awakening. I had been a stubborn person and I felt I had my corners rounded off by having cancer. Faith is to me not the attachment to life, just wishing to be saved, but it is the gratitude to God who saved my spirit. I have begun to live a real life since that time.

A 77-year-old man was diagnosed when he was 47 with a rectal cancer perforating the wall of the rectum. He declined surgery for economic reasons, and for 30 years has had no symptoms of rectal cancer: "When he was diagnosed," reports Ikemi, "he was not shocked, he says. . . . He learned that he had to pay 100,000 for surgery from his own pocket. He had no one to turn to to borrow that amount of money, so he decided that he would work hard as long as he could live even if it meant a year or two. He says that his Buddhist father served as a big support during those trying years. He has been unconcerned about worldly ambitions."

A 63-year-old farm wife was diagnosed at 58 with histologically confirmed extensive metastatic adenocarcinoma of the stomach. Palliative surgery was performed and she was given 1 to 3 months to live. The patient had worked extremely hard all her life on the farm. Reports Ikemi, "A drastic change took place in her pattern of life since she became ill. Before surgery she led a life of sacrifice for the family as mentioned above, while after surgery the attitude of the whole family has been very considerate and kind toward her. She was set free from many years of a self-sacrificing way of life, and was now protected by the love of the family."

The authors conclude that what their cases have in common is that these patients "suffered cancer under more or less severe existential crisis and seem to have overcome cancer by accepting the responsibility for resolving such a crisis for themselves." Second, "their psychological state at the time of 'a sentence of death' is the absence of anxious and depressive reactions. . . . All five of our patients completely committed themselves to the fate or the will of God." Third, "in all five cases, the dramatic change of an outlook on life has been observed, which resulted in the reconstruction of the patient's relationship with his human environment."[100]

One other study of spontaneous remissions was reported by Daan C. van Baalen and Marco J. de Vries of Erasmus University, Rotterdam. The authors identified seven SRC cases over a period of 19 months. Their success in finding these cases led them to believe "that SRC is a more common phenomenon than currently accepted." They then compared the behavioral characteristics of six of these patients with six patients suffering from advanced progressive cancer by comparing transcripts of in-depth interviews. Having identified what they regarded as key differences between the SRC cases and the progressive cancer cases, they gave the transcripts to six raters and asked them to score the transcripts independently for the eight characteristics that the authors believed differentiated the SRC cases from the progressive cancer cases.

Of all the patients, two (both SRC cases) had a tendency to deny that they had cancer. Said one: "I am a practical woman and I never want to know what I am suffering from." [You will recall that *denial,* along with a fighting attitude, was one of the predictors of longer survival among Greer's breast cancer patients.] In the behavioral sphere, the SRC patients were much more likely to make changes as a result of the cancer diagnosis, and the most common shift was in diet: five of the six SRC cases changed their diet by increasing food intake, paying more attention to the quality of food, or starting a specific diet, including diets prescribed by alternative medicine practitioners. By contrast, the progressive cancer patients were more likely to resist change.

In the sensory sphere, four patients reported altered perceptions of the world, and all four were part of the SRC group. Said one: "I could see the people around me so incredibly vividly . . . I heard what they said so much more clearly than in the past. Faces, expressions, everything was magnified in much more detail . . . like, gosh, how beautiful life can be."

One of the most significant differences was in the area of hopelessness and depression: "All SRC patients had profound fluctuations of mood around the time of tumor regression. They experienced periods of depression and hope-lessness alternating with shifts toward an attitude of hope. The PRC [pro-gressive cancer patients] showed less changes in mood."

In the sphere of autonomy, "all six SRC patients demonstrated a shift from dependence and helplessness towards autonomy or increased autonomy. . . . PRC patients had in general a greater tendency to comply with their doctors, partners and/or family than SRC patients."

In their cognitive lives, SRC patients had greater shifts in their concepts about cancer than PRC patients. Said one SRC patient: "Everybody knows that one dies of cancer, but I was not sure whether to apply this to myself. I considered this (common belief) as nonsense."

In the area of changes in existential perspectives on life, "all SRC patients indicated that they had experienced a more or less radical existential shift."

One, who had feared sharing a home with a man, and had thus experienced many broken relationships, dropped her studies and went to live with a man. Another previously well-behaved housewife began to curse her husband and swear obscenely at him. Said a third: "From the moment I got cancer I really began to live. I became much more gentle with other people. I did not judge people too soon. I enjoyed the time I had been given to turn into myself, attend to what I am essentially doing, what I am going to make of my life." Two of the six PRC patients also experienced important existential shifts.

In the area of social support, five of the six SRC patients experienced transformations in their support systems, while only two of the PRC patients did. In four of the five cases the relationships with spouses and family became more caring, and in three the SRC patients also became more demanding in a way that was ultimately accepted by the family. Only two of the six PRC cases experienced similar shifts.

The study has been criticized methodologically for obvious reasons, but I believe the criticism ignores the ingenuity of the approach and the potential significance of the findings. Acknowledging the limitations of this small retrospective study, the authors conclude that the results of their study suggest that there may be significant differences between the psychological history of patients who have a spontaneous regression of cancer and other cancer patients:

> The most significant correlates of SRC seem to be behavioral and sensory changes and shifts along the depression and autonomy axes. However, also belief and trust in medical procedures, among them alternative medicine, shifts in mental constructs about cancer and its treatment, existential shifts and improvement of social support and the quality of interpersonal relationships are significant. . . .
>
> The generally high scores of SRC patients [on depression] seem to suggest that allowing oneself to experience depression temporarily, rather than repressing such a state or staying in a depression, is associated with SRC. . . .
>
> Existential shifts may not be in a direction commonly regarded as "positive," such as an increased experience of meaning in life and so-called spiritual or religious conversions. This is demonstrated by two of our patients. Their existential shifts could easily be misinterpreted as "negative" in the sense of aggressiveness and being obnoxious.[101]

Conclusion

So after reviewing all this research and clinical work—much of it conflicting—what are the basic clues we are left with for cancer patients considering psychological work at present?

If I were to advise a friend, I would do so this way: "First and foremost," I would say, "because human healing systems are both complex and varied, each individual has his or her own unique personality and unique developmental history. As a result, the 'optimal' therapeutic strategy will vary from patient to patient and from therapist to therapist. Therefore, choose the therapies that seem to fit you best but do consider finding *some way* to enhance your psychobiological healing potential." With that fundamental thought in mind, I would make the following suggestions:

- Acute stress is known to enhance tumor growth in many animal experiments and probably does the same thing in some human cancers although we have evidence to the contrary as well. Nevertheless, I would recommend reviewing the major negative stress factors in your life and eliminating as many as you can. Look into stress reduction techniques—such as progressive muscle relaxation, meditation, hypnosis, and imagery—and see if they are helpful to you. Work psychologically to reach an inner state where you can carry the stresses of illness and life less heavily. These relaxation techniques are used both to enhance the quality of life and the possibility of life extension. Meares and Newton, for instance, believe the best outcomes are often associated with the capacity to enter into and practice a deep and simple meditative state. This is a teachable capacity.
- Social support also seems to be an enormously beneficial factor both for quality of life and perhaps for increasing longevity, as well. Consider strengthening your social support system, which may or may not include an organized cancer group. Be sure you choose supports that are personally meaningful to you.
- There are a wide range of behavioral or psychological techniques for reducing the side effects of cancer treatment and the discomfort of the disease itself, such as pain, weight loss, and sleeplessness. Make contact with a psychooncologist or other psychotherapist and see what he has to offer.

- Whether there is a "cancer personality" or behavior pattern—a personality that makes a person more likely to develop cancer or more likely to have it progress rapidly—remains debatable, but there is some consensus among researchers and clinicians that has led to credible hypothetical models. The implications from Temoshok's study are that learning to increase the capacity for emotional expression—especially anger—may mitigate the progress of cancer. Studies by Greer and Silberfarb and others suggest that interventions that reduce the sense of "helplessness/hopelessness" may also extend life. Individual or group psychotherapy can be of help here. If you feel you fall into some part of the hypothetical "cancer personality" or behavior pattern, look into what psychotherapeutic help may be available.
- The literature on spontaneous remissions from cancer offers an intriguing window on psychological attributes that may play a role in some recoveries from cancer.
- LeShan would say that a person with a personality that enables him to engage in the fight for life, to seek out and vigorously begin to engage with "finding your own song," would in general have a better prognosis than a person who could not fight for life or find a real reason to do so. Psychotherapy—either individual or group—is certainly a reasonable approach to the critical process of individuation.
- Achterberg and the Simontons have both associated better outcomes with a capacity for vivid visualization of a strong immune system overcoming a weaker cancer. This is usually a teachable capacity.

Research and clinical experience on psychological approaches to cancer make it clear that simplistic positions in this field are not tenable. We know that psychological practices can greatly enhance quality of life with cancer. We do not know whether, or to what degree, or in what cancers, or with what kinds of people, psychological practices extend life with cancer.

Skeptical scientists can still legitimately say that the evidence in support of the position that psychological interventions extend life with cancer is still not at all conclusive. But if you review the existing scientific, clinical, and popular literature, you can find ample support for a personal decision to fight for life using every psychological resource you have.

References

1   Robert Ader, David L. Felten, and Nicholas Cohen, eds., *Psychoneuroimmunology*, second edition (San Diego: Academic Press, 1991), xxv.

2   Bernie S. Siegel, M.D., *Love, Medicine, and Miracles: Lessons Learned About Self-Healing from a Surgeon's Experience with Exceptional Cancer Patients* (New York: Harper & Row, Publishers, 1988).

3   Lawrence LeShan, *Cancer as a Turning Point: A Handbook for People with Cancer, Their Families, and Health Professionals* (New York: E.P. Dutton, 1989). Copyright © 1989 by Lawrence LeShan, Ph.D. Used by permission of Dutton Signet, a division of Penguin Books USA Inc.

4   O. Carl Simonton, Stephanie Matthews-Simonton, and James Creighton, *Getting Well Again: A Step-by-Step Guide to Overcoming Cancer for Patients and Their Families* (New York: Bantam Books, 1978). Copyright © 1978 by O. Carl Simonton and Stephanie Matthews-Simonton. Used by permission of Bantam Books, a division of Bantam Doubleday Dell Publishing Group, Inc.

5   Joan Borysenko, Ph.D., *Minding the Body, Mending the Mind* (Reading, MA: Addison-Wesley Publishing Company, Inc., 1987).

6   Jimmie C. Holland, "Historical Overview" In Jimmie C. Holland and Julia H. Rowland, *Handbook of Psychooncology* (New York: Oxford, 1989), 11.

7   Julia H. Rowland, "Developmental Stage and Adaptation: Adult Model." In ibid., 25.

8   Ibid., 25–42.

9   Julia H. Rowland, "Intrapersonal Coping." In ibid., 44–5.

10 Julia H. Rowland, "Intrapersonal Resources: Social Support." In ibid., 59.

11 Ibid., 65.

12 Jimmie C. Holland, "Stresses on Mental Health Practitioners." In ibid., 680.

13 Rene Mastrovito, "Behavioral Techniques: Progressive Relaxation and Self-Regulatory Therapies." In ibid., 492.

14 William H. Redd, "Management of Anticipatory Nausea and Vomiting." In ibid., 423.

15 T.G. Burish, et al., "Behavioral Relaxation Techniques in Reducing Distress of Cancer Chemotherapy Patients," *Oncology Nursing Forum* 10:32–5 (1983). Abstract cited in Steven E. Locke, *Psychological and Behavioral Treatments Associated with the Immune System: An Annotated Bibliography* (New York: Institute for the Advancement of Health, 1986), 234.

16 Redd, in Holland and Rowland, *Handbook of Psychooncology*, 429–430.

17 D.F. Campbell et al., "Relaxation: Its Effect on the Nutritional Status and Performance of Clients with Cancer," *Journal of the American Dieticians Association* 4:201–4 (1984). Abstracted in Locke, *Psychological and Behavioral Treatments*, 235.

18 J. Cannici et al., "Treatment of Insomnia in Cancer Patients Using Muscle Relaxation," *Journal of Behavioral Therapy and Experimental Psychiatry* 14:251–6 (1983). Abstracted in Locke, *Psychological and Behavioral Treatments*, 235.

19 Mastrovito, in Holland and Rowland, *Handbook of Psychooncology*, 496–7.

20 Ibid., 498.

21   Daniel P. Brown and Erika Fromm, *Hypnosis and Behavioral Medicine* (New Jersey: Lawrence Erlbaum Associates Publishers, 1987), 135.

22   Yehuda Shavit, "Stress-Induced Immune Modulation in Animals: Opiates and Endogenous Opioid Peptides." In Ader, Felton, and Cohen, *Psychoneuroimmunology,* 789–90.

23   Janice K. Kiecolt-Glaser and Ronald Glaser, "Stress and Immune Function in Humans." In ibid., 854.

24   Shavit. In ibid., 791.

25   Ibid., 793.

26   Ibid., 795–6.

27   Kiecolt-Glaser and Glaser. In ibid., 850.

28   Ibid., 851.

29   Jimmie C. Holland, "Behavioral and Psychological Risk Factors in Cancer: Human Studies." In Holland and Rowland, *Handbook of Psychooncology,* 717.

30   Rowland, "Developmental Stage and Adaption: Adult Model." In ibid., 69.

31   Holland, "Behavioral and Psychological Risk Factors in Cancer: Human Studies." In ibid., 720–1.

32   Lydia Temoshok, "Biopsychosocial Studies on Cutaneous Malignant Melanoma: Psychosocial Factors Associated with Prognostic Indicators, Progression, Psychophysiology, and Tumor-Host Response," *Social Science and Medicine* 20(8):833–40 (1985).

33   A.J. Cunningham, "Psychotherapy for Cancer," *Advances* 1(4):8–14 (1984). Abstracted in Locke, *Psychological and Behavioral Treatments,* 223.

34   A. Meares, "What Can the Cancer Patient Expect from Intensive Meditation?" *Australian Family Physician* 9:322–5 (1980). Abstracted in Locke, *Psychological and Behavioral Treatments,* 228–9.

35   Ibid., 230.

36   O.C. Simonton, S. Matthews-Simonton, and T.F. Sparks, "Psychological Intervention in the Treatment of Cancer," *Psychosomatics* 21:226–33 (1980). Abstracted in Locke, *Psychological and Behavioral Treatments,* 232.

37   A.J. Cunningham, "From Neglect to Support to Coping." In C.L. Cooper, ed., *Stress and Breast Cancer* (New York: John Wiley & Sons, 1988), 148.

38   Janny Scott, "Study Says Cancer Survival Rises with Group Therapy," *Los Angeles Times,* 11 May 1989.

39   David Spiegel, "A Psychosocial Intervention and Survival Time of Patients with Metastatic Breast Cancer," *Advances* 7(3):10–19 (Summer 1991).

40   J.R. Marshall and D.P. Funch, "Social Environment and Breast Cancer: A Cohort Analysis of Breast Cancer," *Cancer* 52:1546–50 (1983). Cited in Holland and Rowland, *Psychooncology,* 713–4.

41   Ibid., 713.

42   L.F. Berkman and S.L. Syme. "Social Networks, Host Resistance, and Mortality: A Nine-year Follow-up Study of Alameda County Residents," *American Journal of Epidemiology* 109:186–204 (1979). Cited in ibid., 714.

43   Holland, "Behavioral and Psychological Risk Factors in Cancer: Human Studies." In Holland and Rowland, *Handbook of Psychooncology,* 723.

44 Fawzy I. Fawzy et al., "A Structured Psychiatric Intervention for Cancer Patients," *Archives of General Psychiatry* 47:720–35 (1990).

45 Fawzy I. Fawzy et al., "Malignant Melanoma: Effects of an Early Structured Psychiatric Intervention, Coping, and Affective State on Recurrence and Survival 6 Years Later," *Archives of General Psychiatry* 50:681–9 (1993).

46 LeShan, *Cancer as a Turning Point,* 21.

47 Ibid., 6–7.

48 Gendron (1759). Cited in ibid., 7–8.

49 Walter Hoyle Walshe (1846), *The Nature and Treatment of Cancer.* Cited in ibid., 8.

50 Willard Parker (1885). Cited in ibid., 9.

51 LeShan, ibid., 11–3.

52 Ibid., 22.

53 Ibid., 22–3.

54 C.J. Jung, quoted in Russell A. Lockhart, "Cancer in Myth and Dream." In James Hillman, ed., *An Annual of Archetypal Psychology and Jungian Thought* (Spring 1977), 2.

55 Matthews-Simonton, Simonton, and Creighton, *Getting Well Again,* 144–5.

56 Ibid., 148–9.

57 Ibid., 154.

58 Ibid., 155–6.

59 Ibid., 158–9.

60 Martin L. Rossman, *Healing Yourself: A Step-by-Step Program for Better Health Through Imagery* (New York: Walker and Co., 1987), 71.

61 Ibid., 14.

62 Ibid., 81–2.

63 Ibid., 88.

64 Ibid., 137–41.

65 Jeanne Achterberg, *Imagery in Healing: Shamanism and Modern Medicine* (Boston: New Science Library, Shambala, 1985), 188–9.

66 Brown and Fromm, *Hypnosis and Behavioral Medicine,* 2.

67 Ibid., 34.

68 Ibid., 140–3.

69 Bernauer W. Newton, "The Use of Hypnosis in the Treatment of Cancer Patients," *American Journal of Clinical Hypnosis* 25(2–3):105–7 (1982–3).

70 Ibid., 110–1.

71 Ainslie Meares, "A Vivid Visualization and Dim Visual Awareness in the Regression of Cancer in Meditation," *Journal of the American Society of Psychosomatic Dental Medicine* 25:85–8 (1978). Abstracted in Locke, *Psychological and Behavioral Treatments,* 227.

72 Linda R. Bridge et al., "Relaxation and Imagery for Breast Cancer Patients," *Advances* 6(2):28–30 (1989).

73 Brown and Fromm, *Hypnosis and Behavioral Medicine,* 32–3.

74 Newton, "The Use of Hypnosis," 108–9.

75 Claus Bahne Bahnson, "Stress and Cancer: The State of the Art," *Psychosomatics* 21(12):975 (1980).

76 Ibid.

77 Ibid., 976.

78   Ibid.

79   Ibid., 977–8.

80   Ibid., 978.

81   Ibid., 979.

82   C.B. Thomas, K.R. Duszynski, and J.W. Shaffer, "Closeness to Parents and the Family
     Constellation in a Prospective Study of Five Disease States: Suicide, Mental Illness, Ma-
     lignant Tumor, Hypertension, and Coronary Heart Disease," *Johns Hopkins Medical Jour-
     nal* 134:251–270 (1974). Cited in ibid., 979.

83   Ibid., 979–80.

84   Ibid., 980.

85   Bernard H. Fox, "Depressive Risk and Symptoms of Cancer," *Journal of the American
     Medical Association* 262(9):1231 (1989).

86   S. Greer and Peter M. Silberfarb, "Psychological Concommitants of Cancer: Current
     State of Research," *Psychological Medicine* 12:567–8 (1982).

87   Holland, "Behavioral and Psychological Risk Factors in Cancer: Human Studies." In Hol-
     land and Rowland, *Handbook of Psychooncology,* 722–3.

88   Lydia Temoshok, "Personality, Coping Style, Emotion and Cancer: Towards an Integra-
     tive Model," *Cancer Surveys* 6(3):545–67 (1987).

89   Ibid., 548.

90   Ibid., 559–60.

91   Ibid., 560.

92   Greer and Silberfarb, "Psychological Concommitants of Cancer," 568.

93   Ibid.

94   Ibid., 569.

95   Temoshok, "Personality, Coping Style, Emotion and Cancer," 547.

96   Barrie R. Cassileth et al., "Psychosocial Correlates of Survival in Advanced Malignant
     Disease," *New England Journal of Medicine* 312(24):1551–5 (1985).

97   Temoshok, "Personality, Coping Style, Emotion and Cancer," 546.

98   Ibid., 552.

99   Lewis F. Thomas, *The Youngest Science: Notes of a Medicine Watcher* (Viking Press,
     1982, 205) cited in Brendan O'Regan and Caryle Hirschberg, *Spontaneous Remission:
     An Annotated Bibliography* (Sausalito, Calif.: Institute of Noetic Sciences, 1993), 1.

100 Yujiro Ikemi et al., "Psychosomatic Consideration on Cancer Patients Who Have Made
     a Narrow Escape from Death," *Dynamische Psychiatrie* 8:77–93 (1975).

101 Daan C. van Baalen, Marco J. de Vries, and Marjolein T. Gondrie, "Psych-Social Corre-
     lates of 'Spontaneous' Regression in Cancer." Monograph, Department of General Pa-
     thology, Medical Faculty, Erasmus University, Rotterdam, The Netherlands, April, 1987.

PART FOUR

*Mainstream Nutritional Science and
the Unconventional Nutritional
Cancer Therapies*

eleven

What Science Says about Nutrition and Cancer: Macronutrients

Most physicians know little about the scientific literature on nutrition and cancer. Most patients who *think* they know about nutrition and cancer from popular health books actually know as little about the scientific nutrition literature as the physicians whose ignorance they decry.

When a cancer patient asks his doctor what he should do about diet, most oncologists simply advise that he "keep up his weight." If the patient asks whether there is any evidence that diet or nutritional supplements might affect the course of the cancer, most oncologists would answer with an emphatic no.

When someone asks a nutritionally oriented alternative cancer therapist what to do about diet, the therapist will usually prescribe a detailed and often rigorous nutritional program. If the patient asks whether there is any evidence that the diet might affect the course of the cancer, the therapist is likely to answer emphatically yes.

Interestingly enough, the oncologist and the alternative cancer therapist often have something in common: *neither has read the mainstream scientific literature on nutrition and cancer with any care*. If, for instance, the oncologist had read that literature, he might give the patient who asked a much different answer: "You know, this is a frontier area in medicine that, frankly, I was not trained in.

There are a lot of claims in the alternative therapies that I am cautious about, and I am convinced there are some dangers in some of the alternative therapies. But I have read enough in the literature to know that, at least in principle, diet and nutrition *can* affect the course of some cancers, either positively or negatively.

"If I were you, I would first try to eat a wholesome, nutritious diet, simply because you can use strength and energy to deal with both the cancer and the therapy. Take a few vitamin supplements—a multivitamin and perhaps some additional antioxidant vitamins C, E, and A—to ensure that your nutritional needs are met, especially as you go through hospitalization and treatment, which may cause nutrient deficiencies.

"As far as alternative nutritional therapies go, I have not studied them carefully but I would have to say to you that the evidence is mixed. Some patients apparently do well on those therapies, at least in terms of how they feel, but others do not. I would be particularly careful about any therapy if you begin to experience continuing weight loss and do not stabilize your weight at some reasonable level. Megavitamin therapy should only be done under expert supervision, since some nutrients may accelerate rather than retard the growth of a cancer. On the other hand, there is some positive evidence for the pharmacological uses of vitamins with cancer, both in support of radiation and chemotherapy and in cancer treatment. It will take some doing, but you and I should be able to look at the scientific studies or, even better, find a nutritionist familiar with this literature who can answer your questions."

That would, I believe, be a fair and balanced answer for an oncologist to give a cancer patient who inquired about diet and cancer or about alternative nutritional therapies. It is better than the standard answer that there is "no evidence" that diet affects the course of a cancer because the scientific litera- ture is *filled* with intriguing and often clearly important studies regarding not only cancer prevention but—far more important for the cancer patient—re- garding cancer treatment as well.

The problem for both the cancer patient and the oncologist trying to research this area is that, in the scientific nutrition texts, the most intriguing studies are usually presented with so much caution—and are surrounded by so many legitimately countervailing findings—that the probability of a cancer patient or even a physician sorting out these studies is low. In the unconventional therapies, on the other hand, claims are repeatedly made, and often stated as authoritative, that either flatly contradict the scientific literature or ignore key problems, especially by overinterpreting isolated studies. For the health practitioner or cancer patient who wants to begin to understand these issues, the starting point I would recommend is the authoritative textbook by Maurice Shils and Vernon Young (in former editions Goodhart and Shils), *Modern Nutrition in Health and Disease.*[1] The chapter by Shils on nutrition and cancer in this critical text is the place to start to see what the mainstream consensus is at this time.

In this and following chapters, I will walk in the no-man's-land between the scientific literature and the unconventional literature on nutrition and cancer. I will do so as responsibly as I know how, although the fact remains that, despite years of study, I am not an authority in this field. So the reader should take my use of data and my interpretations cautiously and, of course, talk with his physician and, if at all possible, with a qualified nutritional scientist before embarking on any drastic program of self-care.

My excursion into the nutritional approaches to cancer represents a rough mapping of a field that I believe neither scientific nutritional texts nor unconventional nutritional texts have done real justice to. The maps may need correction as time goes on, but I hope that I describe the general contours clearly. This chapter and the following one are necessarily two of the most technically difficult chapters in this book. Some readers may wish to skim the subheads or simply go directly to the conclusion, which describes the major findings.

Four Categories of Dietary and Nutritional Approaches to Cancer

Dietary and nutritional approaches to cancer can be divided into the following major categories:
1. Recommendations given by various governmental and nongovernmental agencies on dietary and nutritional approaches to lowering the risk of cancer.
2. Recommendations given by these same governmental and nongovernmental agencies on dietary and nutritional guidelines for cancer patients. This advice is given to the patient directly or to oncologists

and other professionals treating cancer. Interestingly enough, the first set of recommendations above for lowering cancer risk often directly contradict dietary recommendations given to cancer patients about how to maintain weight when diagnosed with cancer.

3. The epidemiological, experimental, and clinical *research literature* on nutrition and cancer, which very few oncologists or cancer patients are familiar with.

4. The claims and findings of a wide range of unconventional cancer therapists, researchers, and popularizers regarding dietary and nutritional approaches to cancer treatment.

The purpose of this chapter is to review the first two categories briefly and the third—the research literature on nutrition and cancer—in more detail. I have two reasons for this detailed treatment of the research literature on diet, nutrition, and cancer. First, *there is a tremendous wealth of scientific information on nutritional approaches which is buried deep in the literature that has direct application for cancer treatment, appropriate self-care, and for future research.* Second, only by carefully reviewing the scientific literature on nutrition can we be adequately prepared to review the claims of some of the major unconventional nutritional cancer therapies, which I will present in future chapters. This chapter considers macronutrients. The following chapter discusses micronutrients—vitamins and minerals.

Mainstream Recommendations for Cancer Prevention

Current views on nutrition and cancer prevention were shaped by the publication in 1982 of a report entitled *Diet, Nutrition and Cancer* by the National Academy of Sciences's National Research Council. The report was written at the direction of the National Research Council's Committee on Diet, Nutrition and Cancer, which was chaired by Clifford Grobstein, Professor of Biological Sciences and Public Policy at the University of California, San Diego. Based on its extensive review of the scientific literature, the committee issued a number of "interim dietary guidelines" to help Americans lower their risk of cancer. Among these were:

> 1. High fat consumption is linked to increased incidence of certain cancers (notably breast and colon cancer) and . . . low fat intake is associated with lower incidence of these cancers. The committee recommends that the con-

sumption of both saturated and unsaturated fats be reduced in the average U.S. diet. *An appropriate practical target is to reduce the intake of fat from its present level (approximately 40%) to 30% of total calories. The scientific data do not provide a strong basis for establishing fat intake at precisely 30% of total calories. Indeed, the data could be used to justify an even greater reduction* [emphasis added]. However, in the judgment of the committee, the suggested reduction (i.e., one quarter of the fat intake) is a moderate and practical target, and is likely to be beneficial.

2. The committee emphasizes the importance of including fruits, vegetables, and whole grain cereal products in the daily diet. In epidemiological studies, frequent consumption of these foods has been inversely correlated with the incidence of various cancers. Results of laboratory experiments have supported these findings in tests of . . . fruits (especially citrus fruits) and vegetables (especially carotene[3]-rich and cruciferous vegetables).

These recommendations apply only to foods as sources of nutrients—not to dietary supplements of individual nutrients. . . . There is very little information on the effects of various levels of individual nutrients on the risk of cancer in humans. *Therefore, the committee is unable to predict the health effects of high and potentially toxic doses of isolated nutrients consumed in the form of supplements* [emphasis added].

3. In some parts of the world, especially China, Japan and Iceland, populations that frequently consume salt-cured (including salt-pickled) or smoked foods have a greater incidence of cancers at some sites, especially the esophagus and stomach. . . . The committee recommends that the consumption of [these] food[s] . . . be minimized.

4. Intentional additives (direct and indirect) should continue to be evaluated for carcinogenic activity before they are approved for use in the food supply.

5. Excessive consumption of alcoholic beverages, particularly combined with cigarette smoking, has been associated with an increased risk of cancer of the upper gastrointestinal and respiratory tracts. . . . The committee recommends that if alcoholic beverages are consumed, it be done in moderation.[2]

In 1984, the American Cancer Society added to these recommendations: "eat more high fiber foods; include foods rich in vitamins A and C; include cruciferous vegetables; and avoid obesity."[4]

And in the most recent edition of *Cancer: Principles and Practice of Oncology,*[5] much of the same basic information appears as dietary guidelines from the National Cancer Institute:

1. Reduce fat to 30% of calories or less.
2. Increase fiber intake to 20 to 30 gm/day, with an upper limit of 35 gm/day.
3. Include a variety of vegetables and fruit in the daily diet.
4. Avoid obesity.
5. Consume alcoholic beverages in moderation, if at all.
6. Minimize consumption of salt-cured, salt-pickled, and smoked foods.

Why the Silence on General Nutritional Guidance for Cancer Patients?

Since weight loss can be a basic problem for some cancer patients, physicians usually advise that these patients eat whatever they feel is tasty and will help them maintain weight. Shils summarizes the advice in this way: "For the patient with mild to moderate anorexia and taste changes, careful evaluation of food likes and dislikes and properly timed provision of attractive solid and liquid foods can make the difference between weight maintenance and loss."[6] A large professional literature also exists on specialized nutritional support for patients with specific complications due to radiation, surgery, drug treatment, or the development of the cancer itself.[7]

However, the textbooks are remarkably silent on the subject of nutritional guidelines for people who do not have specific needs resulting from complications of treatment or the progress of cancer. DeVita's *Cancer: Principles and Practice of Oncology*, for example, devotes a large chapter to nutrition and cancer *prevention*, and a substantial section of a chapter to nutritional therapy for patients with disease or with treatment-related difficulties eating or digesting, but provides *no* general nutritional recommendations for the cancer patient who wants to eat a diet that will best support his general health, or support his resistance and recovery following cancer therapies.

On the face of it, this silence is curious, since a cancer patient might wonder whether he should try to follow the kind of healthy diet recommended for cancer *prevention* once he has cancer. The cancer patient might reasonably ask: If a specific diet, such as a low fat, high fiber whole-foods diet with an emphasis on fresh fruits and vegetables and whole grains lowers the incidence of some common cancers, might such a diet also slow or halt the development of one of these same existing cancers? And might a rigorous therapeutic diet along these same lines do even more to slow or reverse a cancer, or lower the chance of its recurrence, than a moderate diet that might be adequate for prevention?

None of these questions—the critical questions for cancer patients—were addressed in the National Academy of Sciences report on *Diet, Nutrition and Cancer,* nor, as I have said, are they addressed by the leading texts on oncology or nutrition. Nor have any of the other mainstream institutions that have issued guidelines for nutritional and dietary approaches to cancer *prevention* addressed these questions. Certainly, one of the reasons these critical questions of cancer patients are not addressed is because of the complexity of the scientific issues and the absence of adequate human clinical studies.

But there is also another reason for professional silence. In the sociology of American medicine, a mainstream nutritionist faces a great professional risk in studying the role of nutrition in the progress and treatment of cancer in areas that go beyond the current institutional consensus. The same dangers exist for an academic psychologist who chooses a career commitment to study the effects of psychological interventions on the progress of cancer. Therefore the mainstream nutritionist, like his psychologist colleague, risks powerful professional sanctions if he ventures into this field, even though the reasonable implications of nutritional research point inevitably to the question of whether or not the cancer patient, alone or with the aid of a physician or nutritionist, can do anything to slow or reverse the course of the cancer, or to protect himself from the side effects of treatment by altering his dietary and nutritional regimen.

Like his psychologist colleague, the nutritionist is sociologically marginal to the medical professions in charge of cancer treatment. Furthermore, like his psychologist colleague, he is often unable to get physicians to practice good nutritional interventions when there is *unimpeachable* scientific evidence of their efficacy. So why should the nutritionist venture into one of the most professionally forbidden zones in modern medicine, where the evidence is so complex and contradictory, when all of the professional sanctions are so high? From the nutritionist's perspective, working in these controversial fields will destroy his credibility as an advocate of nutritional treatment in areas that modern nutrition is sure of, but that mainstream medicine continues to neglect or ignore.

So, while the nutritionists and the oncologists are largely silent on the issue of therapeutic nutrition for reasonably healthy cancer patients, the *research literature* is filled with highly provocative studies that bear directly on the critical questions of diet and nutrition in cancer *treatment* as well as cancer *prevention*.

Again, a remarkable parallel exists between the studies that support nutritional approaches to cancer and the studies that support psychological approaches. As we will see in the next chapter, there is now significant evidence that nutritional support, like psychological support, can decrease the side effects of conventional therapies, and even in some instance *support* conventional therapies. There is also evidence that nutritional support can in some instances enhance chemotherapy and radiotherapy, while in other cases it can diminish their effectiveness. In addition, good evidence exists that diet and nutrition may enhance or reduce some measures of immunocompetence, whether or not enhanced immunocompetence effectively combats cancer. In animal and laboratory studies there is good evidence that diet and nutrition can also have a direct effect on cancer growth and regression, raising the question of whether or not this is also true for humans.

But controlled clinical trials of the radical therapeutic diets have simply not been done. And while it appears unlikely to me that any of the nutritional approaches represent anything approaching a definitive cure for cancer, the critical question is whether they may not contribute both to quality of life and life extension, especially when integrated with other health-promoting complementary therapies and the judicious use of conventional therapies.

Because these studies have not been done, mainstream statements that "there is no evidence that these therapies cure cancer" are doubly misleading: (1) the real issue is probably not cure but contribution to effective cancer management and treatment, and (2) the absence of evidence at this point represents an absence of scientific study, not a negative assessment based on extensive study.

"Underfeeding" and Caloric Restrictions

Nutritionists differentiate between "caloric restriction," which involves the restriction of a major contributor to calories in the diet, usually carbohydrates, and "underfeeding," in which all elements in the diet are restricted. Individual micronutrients, including vitamins and minerals, can also be selectively restricted.[8]

One of the most significant nutritional findings in cancer is the relationship between high caloric intake and the incidence of cancer. This is found in the epidemiological literature on the hormone-related cancers—breast, prostate, colon, and ovarian cancer. In *Diet, Nutrition and Cancer,* the National Academy of Sciences notes, "Berg (1975) pointed out that the international distribution of hormone-dependent cancers has generated suspicion that these cancers may be related to affluence. He suggested that diets typical of affluent populations, when ingested since childhood, could overstimulate the endocrine system, lead to aberrations in metabolic processes, and result in cancer."[9]

When Armstrong and Doll did a correlational study of cancer incidence and total caloric intake in 32 countries, they found significant correlations between the total calories ingested and the incidence of rectal cancer and leukemia in men, and mortality from breast cancer in women.[10]

The suspicion about the relationship of many common cancers to diets of affluence is well grounded in experimental research. Maurice Shils writes, "It is well established that experimental animals who have been deprived of food to the point of weight loss have a lower incidence of spontaneous tumors and a slower rate of growth of transplanted tumors." Not only does nutritional restriction slow the development of cancer and the rate of growth of transplanted tumors but: "Repletion with a complete diet of previously protein-deprived tumor-bearing rats also appreciably increases the ratio of tumor weight to host tissue weight."[11]

Lawrence Kushi, Ph.D., a knowledgeable nutritional epidemiologist who is presently an assistant professor in the Division of Human Development and Nutrition at the University of Minnesota School of Public Health, recasts the question of excessive nutrient intake and the potential benefits of nutrient restriction in the terms of appropriate balance:

> The key in this area is balance between physical activity and nutrient intake. The message from animal studies regarding underfeeding is not that caloric restriction may be a worthwhile approach for management of cancer. . . .

> Rather, I believe the interpretation is that an adequate physical activity and energy balance to maintain health may be an important part of the prevention of and recovery from many diseases, including cancer. . . . For humans living in our society, this may include reductions in the consumption of certain kinds of foods (e.g., meat) but perhaps an overall *increase* in food intake that is a *direct result* of increased physical activity in some cases.[12]

Research studies have shown that the extent of the inhibiting effect of "underfeeding" depends on the tumor type, the degree of diet restriction, and the presence of carcinogenic agents. According to Shils:

> When a commercial diet was compared to four purified diets varying in protein (casein), carbohydrate (sucrose) or in total calories in male rats, *total tumor risk was found to be directly and exponentially related to caloric intake. Within each dietary group, rats of heavier weight had greater tumor risk than lighter rats . . . Lowest incidence, greatest time in delay of occurrence, absence of malignant epithelial tumors and greatest life expectancy were observed when intakes of protein, carbohydrate and total calories were low.* [emphasis added].[13]

These findings would suggest, of course, that "underfeeding" (or the induction of macronutrient or micronutrient deficiencies) has potential therapeutic benefit for cancer patients. And as Shils notes:

> The rationale for attempting inhibition *or actual reversal of established neoplastic growth* by induction of nutritional deficiencies is based on the possibility that certain tumor cells may be more sensitive to such depletion than are normal tissues. An increased sensitivity may reside in the . . . differences in the requirements for certain nutrients so that depletion by dietary means . . . will adversely affect tumor cells to a greater degree than host cells.

> It has been concluded that *caloric intake can retard the establishment and growth of transplanted tumor cells only when the host weight diminishes.* Similarly, protein deprivation and other deficiencies are inhibitory only when associated with poor growth or weight loss [emphasis added].[14]

As we shall see, these scientific findings are of critical interest with respect to assessing the therapeutic claims of many of the alternative cancer therapies, which often restrict protein and total caloric intake, and which are often accompanied by significant patient weight loss. The question is, to the degree that alternative therapies employing these kinds of restrictions are beneficial for some patients, to what extent are the caloric and protein restrictions responsible for this effect?

Shils clearly states above—in a passage worth remembering—that the rationale for attempting to inhibit or reverse cancer nutritionally is that cancer cells *may be* more sensitive to nutritional "deficiencies" created by therapeutic diets than are healthy cells. The striking concept is that—as with chemotherapy—the diet will inhibit or reverse the cancer without too severely compromising the patient in terms of nutritional depletion. But it is important to add that, while Shils *describes* this rationale for such nutritional approaches, he does *not* endorse it.

If cancer cells may be more sensitive to nutritional restriction than normal cells, they also often have—in common with fetal growth tissue—a greater ability than normal cells to obtain their energy and nutrient needs in the face of nutritional deprivation. In other words, nutritional deprivation *does* inhibit the development of cancer in some experimental models at the point associated with weight loss. But does the cancer, in spite of this inhibition, still maintain a relative advantage over healthy cells in claiming whatever nutrients are available?

This is obviously a critical point for people with cancer. If a highly restrictive diet causes weight loss, with the result that the patient ends up stabilized at a healthy lower weight, and the cancer has been inhibited from further growth, that is a decisive clinical victory. If the patient temporarily stabilizes at a lower weight, but the tumor retains an advantage in nutrient uptake, it will grow—albeit more slowly because of nutrient restriction—and progressive weight loss will continue. If the patient fails to stabilize at a lower weight, it could either be because the diet is inadequate for that particular person to sustain healthy life or because the tumor has a great enough advantage in nutrient uptake that weight stabilization is unachievable. These are the hypothetical possibilities.

Researchers have also tried restricting intake of specific *micronutrients* (vitamins and trace minerals) as opposed to the *macronutrients* (fat, protein, and carbohydrate) we discussed above. For example, they have restricted different specific amino acids to see if it is possible to inhibit the development of cancers without excessive host weight loss. Phenylalanine and tyrosine restriction inhibited the growth of S91 melanoma in mice, for example.[15] As Shils points out, vitamins have also been restricted: "Deficiencies of folic acid, of pyridoxine, or of riboflavin have each been found to result in significant inhibition of the growth of certain tumors beyond the effect of vitamin deficiency per se."[16]

Immune status also has a complex relationship to restriction of diet or specific nutrients. While depressed immune function was initially believed to be a result of the cancer itself, numerous studies have now demonstrated that altered immune responses can result from malnutrition. According to Shils:

> Efforts can be made to improve immunity *either by improving nutritional status or, alternatively, by inducing certain deficiencies in an effort to slow tumor growth and enhance immune responses* [emphasis added]. In 1949 Stoerk and Emerson found that induction of riboflavin deficiency in C3H mice at 6 to 14 days after implantation of lymphosarcoma 6C3H-CD resulted in marked to complete regression of the tumor within 10 days and in a 30 to 37 per cent cure rate; tumor reinoculated into "cured" mice with or without riboflavin in the diet failed to "take." The authors believed that the [riboflavin] deficiency slowed tumor growth and permitted immune defenses to become effective.[17]

On the other hand, cellular immunity can also be *depressed* by protein restriction. And Shils, having set forth a provocative case for exploring "underfeeding" in cancer therapy, simply concludes:

> There is increasing clinical evidence that reestablishment of cellular immunity by nutritional means, together with control of infection, plays an important role in decreasing morbidity and mortality. A number of nutritional deficiencies can adversely affect the various parameters of immune mechanisms. The importance of optimum defenses against infection in the cancer patient emphasizes the need for providing adequate nutrition.[18]

The National Academy of Sciences report adds an additional caveat—that it is not clear in many caloric restriction studies whether reduction in total caloric intake is the key variable or whether the critical factor is the reduction in dietary fat.[19]

In a 1988 contribution to *Cancer,* Ludwik Gross, M.D., reviewed pertinent literature on the inhibition of tumors and leukemia in rats and mice with underfeeding. He found that by restricting food intake, tumor incidence in rats exposed to total body gamma radiation was reduced from 93% to 35% in females and from 59% to 7% in males. In a similar study with mice, radiation-induced leukemia dropped from 50% to 4% after food restriction:

> If the results of experiments carried out on rats and mice are extrapolated to humans, it would follow that all of us (particularly those who have had multiple cases of cancer or leukemia among family members) should aim at holding our weight below the limits considered normal for our age, sex and height. This appears particularly important for persons that have been exposed to large doses of ionizing radiation.[20]

And, as Gross points out, American Cancer Society data show that men and women who are overweight have an almost 50% higher incidence of cancer than those of similar sex and age who are not overweight.[21] His recommendation for restricting caloric intake seems particularly important for relatively young people with good survival potential who are undergoing radiotherapy for cancer and who have long lives ahead during which radiation-induced cancers might occur.

In summary, important research evidence exists on *both sides* of the critical question of whether total caloric restriction or restriction of specific macronutrients or micronutrients will enhance or diminish the patient's chances of recovery. Without question, populations with lower caloric intake have a lower incidence of some cancers. But whether dietary restriction will inhibit or reverse an established cancer—whether there is a significant nutritional margin at which human life and immunocompetence is sustained while the cancer is inhibited or reversed—has not yet been established scientifically.

Many alternative nutritional therapies—including the Gerson diet, the macrobiotic diet, the Hippocrates diet, and the Livingston-Wheeler diet, to name only a few—frequently result in weight loss. They restrict intake of some nutrients and increase intake of others. Many *healthy* people who try these diets *stabilize* at a lower weight, often their weight in high school or college. Some cancer patients, especially those with slow-growing cancers, also clearly stabilize on many of these diets. In experimental studies, this weight loss is the point at which cancer inhibition or reversal is also sometimes demonstrated. At the same time, ignorant or incautious use of alternative nutritional therapies has also been associated with continuing weight loss and with demonstrable diminished immunocompetence. Even more significant is the question of whether or not stabilizing at a lower weight on an alternative nutritional therapy is a net gain for the cancer patient, because of the possible competitive advantage in nutrient uptake of the tumor over the host and because of the high energy requirements of many cancers. On the one hand, the patient may have temporarily stabilized his weight, and even possibly slowed the growth of the tumor. On the other hand, he has lowered his body weight and energy reserves that are known to extend life with many cancers because of the energy uptake advantage that cancers often have. A study of small cell lung cancer patients, for example, found their level of energy expenditure was 37% above that of normal controls.[22]

Simplistic positions on both sides of this issue are simply not warranted. The question of whether dietary and nutritional therapies that restrict intake of some nutrients along the lines of many unconventional therapies are helpful or hurtful to people with some cancers remains unanswered scientifically. But, in my judgment, there is good reason to believe that both help and hurt are possible consequences of using these selectively nutrient-restricting therapies.

Dietary Fat, Proteins, and Carbohydrates

"Of all the dietary factors that have been associated epidemiologically with cancers of various sites, fat has probably been studied most thoroughly and produced the greatest frequency of direct associations," wrote the authors of the National Academy of Sciences Study, *Diet, Nutrition and Cancer*.[23] In epidemiological studies, correlations with high dietary fat have been reported for gastrointestinal cancers (especially of the large bowel) and endocrine cancers—breast, prostate, ovarian, and testicular cancers.[24]

Dietary fats are generally regarded as a promoter, rather than an initiator, of cancer. In experimental animal studies, increasing the level of dietary fat from 5% to 20% increases both the incidence and the rate of growth of chemically induced breast cancer. But the breast cancer levels increase *only* if the high fat diet is fed after, rather than before, the chemical initiation of the tumor.[25]

A study by Goodman et al. at the University of Hawaii, which compared the historical dietary fat and cholesterol intake of lung cancer patients with that of controls, showed that men in the highest quartile of cholesterol intake had a 2.2 times greater risk of lung cancer than those in the lowest quartile. The effect was not demonstrated for women, however, and was *restricted to heavy smokers*. Similar results were found for total fats, saturated fats, and, to some extent, unsaturated fats, but the high correlation between fat and cholesterol made it impossible to separate the effects of these nutrients.[26] This result could be interpreted as lending credence to the possible role of dietary fat as a promoter, rather than initiator, of lung cancer.

Finally, in a study of the relationship between dietary fat intake and disease progression and survival in breast cancer patients by Gregorio et al., at State University of New York, it was estimated that the risk of death at any time was increased 1.4-fold for each 1,000 gm in monthly fat intake, with the association strongest for patients with advanced disease.[27] This finding is consistent with that of P.I. Tartter and his associates at Mount Sinai who concluded that a lower preoperative serum cholesterol level (and lower weight) is associated with longer disease-free survival.[28]

Although the data are very strong, the mechanisms by which fat acts as a tumor promoter are not understood. But, says the National Academy of Sciences report:

> Of all the dietary components . . . studied, the combined epidemiological and experimental evidence is most suggestive for a causal relationship between fat intake and the occurrence of cancer . . . particularly [of] the breast and colon. Data from studies in animals suggest that when total fat intake is low, *polyunsaturated fats are more effective than saturated fats in enhancing tumorigenesis* [emphasis added], whereas the data on humans do not permit a clear distinction to be made between the different components of fat.[29]

This last point is surprising: in animal studies, polyunsaturated fats have a greater cancer-producing capacity than saturated fats when fat intake is low. On the other hand, in epidemiological studies, animal fats are correlated with *increased cancer incidence* when total fat consumption is *relatively high*.

Six years after the National Academy of Sciences report, Tim Byers reviewed progress on the fat-cancer question since the release of the report. He concluded: "There continues to be evidence, although it is inconsistent, that dietary fat may be an important factor in colon cancer. . . . However, the hypothesized relationship between dietary fat and breast cancer [has] been less consistently supported by new findings."[30] And Shils echoes Byers' caution: "A definite positive relationship remains to be demonstrated in view of mounting negative evidence."[31]

The research literature on dietary proteins and cancer is ambiguous. In a relatively short discussion, the National Academy of Sciences concluded: "Protein intake *may* be associated with an increased risk of cancer at some sites," but "because of the relative paucity of data on protein compared to fat, and the strong correlation between intakes of fat and protein in the Western diet, the committee is unable to arrive at a firm conclusion about protein."[32]

Similarly, the academy found data too sparse to reach any conclusions about the role of carbohydrates (with the possible exception of fiber) in cancer, except insofar as high carbohydrate intake contributes to high total caloric intake which, as we have seen, is associated with increased risk of cancer.[33]

Dietary Fiber

Dietary fiber includes indigestible carbohydrates and some carbohydrate-like elements. They provide bulk in food and are found in vegetables, fruits, and whole grains. Dietary fiber consumption often decreases with the consumption of a Western-style diet. Based on epidemiological studies, Burkitt and Trowell proposed in 1975 that the increased incidence of some cancers and other chronic illnesses may result from a low intake of dietary fiber.[34] Extensive research studies followed. The National Academy of Science report in 1982 stated that there was no conclusive evidence that dietary fiber protects against colorectal cancer, but that some specific components of fiber might have a protective effect.[35] The years that followed the publication of *Diet, Nutrition and Cancer* have borne out its prediction that some types of fiber have protective effects and that others do not, and still others may enhance tumor growth.

Lucien R. Jacobs of the University of California School of Medicine, Davis, reviewed the experimental literature and found that "most experiments with wheat bran and cellulose have shown evidence of a significant protective effect. In contrast, numerous other fiber supplements have been shown to enhance tumor development. These include pectin, corn bran, undegraded carrageenan, agar, Metamucil [a trademark for a preparation of psyllium hydrophilic mucilloid], and alfalfa."[36]

David M. Klurfeld and David Kritchevsky extensively reviewed the literature on human gastrointestinal cancer and fiber. They reported that the strongest correlations between dietary fiber consumption and gastrointestinal cancers are found in international studies "in which numerous environmental variables differ. Studies on smaller groups within a culture have not given strong support to the findings of international comparisons. Colon cancer rates within regions of the U.S. vary with sufficient magnitude that diet is unlikely to account for more than a minor proportion of risk. . . . It would be premature to suggest that a high fiber diet will confer protection against gastrointestinal cancer."[37] But investigators are divided, and the protective effects of fiber have been suggested for both breast and prostate cancer, as well as colon cancer.[38]

Conclusion

Epidemiological studies, laboratory research, and clinical research support the fundamental proposition that nutritional interventions hold great promise in cancer prevention, in reducing side effects of treatment, and in moderating or reversing the progress of some cancers.

What is shocking is that the same timidity characterizing psychological research on controlling cancer progression—which has not been aggressively pursued—is also characteristic of nutritional research. In laboratory studies, nutritional researchers are fairly bold in studying the effects of nutrients on cancer progression, and in protecting against the side effects of treatment or enhancing treatments. But, when it comes to testing these provocative animal and cell-line laboratory studies in humans, they are constrained by perceived professional sanctions, just as the psychological researchers have been constrained in studies designed to test whether psychological interventions extend life with cancer.

In recent years, the atmosphere at the National Cancer Institute (NCI) and American Cancer Society has changed somewhat with respect to nutritional therapies—almost to the same degree that it has changed with respect to psychological therapies. Yet the NCI clinical intervention trials currently under way focus primarily on preventing cancer—or at most preventing the recurrence of cancer—and they primarily test individual nutrients, or small combinations of nutrients.[39] The nutritional interventions that are actually examined are characteristically *puny* in comparison with the vigor of alternative nutritional interventions, where fundamental dietary change—sometimes in combination with multivitamin therapy (see next chapter)—is used with existing cancers as well as in prevention.

This failure to assess comprehensive nutritional interventions in existing cancers is all the more distressing because nutritional interventions, like psychological interventions, are characteristically nontoxic and generally enhance the quality of life, and researchers could readily find volunteers among cancer patients to participate in such clinical trials.

Neither the psychological studies nor the nutritional studies answer the real question of exceptional cancer patients, which is whether or not a combination of vigorous psychological, nutritional, and (often) other interventions can cascade into cancer inhibition or actual reversal. There is absolutely no scientific reason why these combined modalities—like combined chemotherapies or combined programs of radiation, chemotherapy, and other interventions—cannot and should not be assessed together.

Many researchers believe, for instance, that in early-stage metastatic breast cancer, *patients have little, if anything, to gain by early initiation of chemotherapy or radiotherapy.* This is also true for many non-small cell lung cancer patients, metastatic colon cancer patients, and metastatic prostate cancer patients. Hence we are in a position where all the major American cancers—colon, prostate, breast, and lung—do not, at certain important points in the illness, require immediate conventional interventions. Many of those patients—certainly a significant minority—would like nothing better than to be involved in vigorous clinical trials of less toxic or nontoxic therapies.

It is evident, therefore, that while both the nutritional and psychological literatures point to the potential benefits of vigorous interventions, the combined interventions that interest exceptional cancer patients most—and that most resemble the alternative therapies for which some successes are clinically reported—are simply not being tested in clinical trials. There is no legitimate scientific reason why evaluation of such combined therapies to determine whether or not they have a role in enhancing quality of life or extending life should not be a national research priority.

So what can we conclude from this somewhat complex and confusing data? Some practical guidelines:

1. For cancer prevention, dietary fat should be kept as low as possible —at least to 30% of total caloric intake, according to the National Academy of Sciences. This applies to *all* fats—including vegetable or polyunsaturated fats as well as animal fats. The controversy continues over the relationship of dietary fat to common cancers such as colon, prostate, and breast cancer, with the correlation clearest in international epidemiological studies (in which there may be confounding factors) and conflicted in studies within countries.

2. Ideally, weight should be kept within normal range—both for prevention and treatment. The unanswered question is whether or not caloric restriction (as well as the restriction of other nutrients) that is prescribed by some alternative nutritional therapies results in a state of health where the cancer is underfed and inhibited but the body retains adequate nutrition.

3. For cancer prevention, fresh fruits and vegetables should be eaten daily.

4. For cancer prevention, alcohol should be consumed in moderation, if at all. Smoking should be completely terminated.

5. Fiber—wheat bran and cellulose—have been shown in animal studies to have some protective effect against cancer, while corn, Metamucil, and alfalfa fiber may promote cancer.

In reviewing this nutritional literature, the most striking impression is that nutrition appears to hold considerable promise in cancer prevention, in reducing the side effects and augmenting the benefits of conventional treatment, in enhancing general health and quality of life, and in some instances in extending life with cancer. It is imperative that research in this area be accelerated.

Notes and References

1   Maurice E. Shils and Vernon R. Young, eds., *Modern Nutrition in Health and Disease* (Philadelphia: Lea & Febiger, 1988), especially M.E. Shils, "Nutrition and Diet in Cancer"; D.H. Hornig et al., "Ascorbic Acid"; and Q.N. Myrvik, "Nutrition and Immunology."

2   National Academy of Sciences, National Research Council, Committee on Diet, Nutrition and Cancer, *Diet, Nutrition and Cancer* (Washington, DC: National Academy Press, 1982), 1-15–1-16.

3   A precursor of vitamin A.

4   Marion Nestle, *Nutrition in Clinical Practice* (Greenbrae, CA: Jones Medical Publications, 1985), 183.

5   Vincent T. DeVita, Jr., ed., *Cancer: Principles and Practice of Oncology,* third edition (Philadelphia: J. B. Lippincott Company, 1989), 177.

6   Maurice E. Shils, "Nutrition and Diet in Cancer." In Shils and Young, eds., *Modern Nutrition in Health and Disease,* 1415.

7   Ibid.; see especially chart "Consequences of cancer treatment predisposing to nutrition problems," 1408.

8   Ibid., 1380–1.

9   National Academy of Sciences, *Diet, Nutrition and Cancer,* 4–1.

10   Ibid., 4–2.

11   Maurice E. Shils, "Nutrition and Neoplasia." In Robert S. Goodhart, and Maurice E. Shils, eds., *Modern Nutrition in Health and Disease* (Philadelphia: Lea & Febiger, 1980), 1187.

12   Lawrence Kushi, Ph.D., personal communication with the author, 25 January 1991.

13   Shils, "Nutrition and Neoplasia," 1153–4.

14   Ibid., 1159.

15   Ibid., 1160.

16   Ibid., 1160–1.

17   Ibid., 1161.

18   Ibid., 1162–3.

19   National Academy of Sciences, *Diet, Nutrition, and Cancer,* 4–4.

20   Ludwik Gross, "Inhibition of the Development of Tumors or Leukemia in Mice and Rats After Reduction of Food Intake: Possible Implications for Humans," *Cancer* 62:1463–5 (1988).

21   Ibid., 1464.

22   D. Russell et al., "Effects of Total Parenteral Nutrition and Chemotherapy on the Metabolic Derangements in Small Cell Lung Cancer," *Cancer Research* 44:1706 (1984). Cited in Moshe Shike and Murry F., Brennan, "Supportive Care of the Cancer Patient." In DeVita, ed., *Cancer: Principles and Practice of Oncology,* 2031.

23   National Academy of Sciences, *Diet, Nutrition and Cancer,* 5–1.

24   Ibid., 5–17.

25   Ibid., 5–19.

26 M.T. Goodman et al., "The Effect of Dietary Cholesterol and Fat on the Risk of Lung Cancer in Hawaii," *The American Journal of Epidemiology* 128(6):1241–55 (1988).

27 D.I. Gregorio, "Dietary Fat Consumption and Survival Among Women with Breast Cancer," *Journal of the National Cancer Institute* 75(1):37–41 (1986).

28 P.I. Tartter, "Cholesterol and Obesity as Prognostic Factors in Breast Cancer," *Cancer* 47(9):2222–7 (1981).

29 National Academy of Sciences, *Diet, Nutrition and Cancer,* 5-20–5-21.

30 Tim Byers, "Diet and Cancer: Any Progress in the Interim?" *Cancer* 62:1713–24 (1988).

31 Maurice Shils, "Nutrition and Diet in Cancer." In Shils and Young, *Modern Nutrition in Health and Disease,* 1396.

32 National Academy of Science, *Diet, Nutrition, and Cancer,* 6–11.

33 Ibid., 7–5.

34 Ibid, 8–1.

35 Ibid., 8–5.

36 Lucian R. Jacobs, "Modification of Experimental Colon Carcinogenesis by Dietary Fiber." In Lionel A. Poirier, Paul M. Newberne, and Michael W. Pariza, eds., *Essential Nutrients in Carcinogenesis* (New York: Plenum Press, 1986), 105–18.

37 David M. Klurfeld and David Kritchevsky, "Dietary Fiber and Human Cancer: Critique of the Literature." In Poirier et al., *Essential Nutrients in Carcinogenesis,* 119.

38 Melvyn R. Werbach, M.D., *Nutritional Influences on Illness* (Tarzana, CA: Third Line Press, 1987), 100.

39 Ralph W. Moss, *The Cancer Industry* (New York: Paragon House, 1989), 233.

twelve

Can Vitamins and Minerals Help?
The Scientific View: Micronutrients

There seems to be little question among scientists that vitamins and minerals can prevent, inhibit, and occasionally accelerate some forms of cancer. They may also play a role in reversal of some forms of cancer. Research has also shown in animal and clinical studies that vitamins may enhance the effect of anticancer treatments such as radiotherapy and chemotherapy, may protect against their side effects, and may possibly extend the life of cancer patients who are treated jointly with mainstream therapies and vitamins. I believe that careful review of these provocative scientific studies should be of real interest to both people with cancer and health professionals who are considering nutritional supplements or dietary manipulations as a form of treatment or self-care.

Vitamin A, Retinoids, and Carotenoids

By far the most extensive research on diet and cancer has been made for the retinoids. "Retinoids" refer to vitamin A (retinol) and its isomers, derivatives (retinal, retinoic acid), and synthetic analogues. According to Peter Greenwald, Director of the Division of Cancer Prevention and Control at the National Cancer Institute (NCI), retinoids have the capacity to modify the cancer cell, in some cases actually causing the differentiation, or return to a normal state, of cancer cells. "*Retinoids are of special interest for use in clinical prevention because they can exert their antineoplastic activity in cells that are already dedifferentiated or initiated into a malignant state* [emphasis added]."[1] In plain English, this means retinoids can sometimes stop the cellular process of loss of differentiation that characterizes the progression of cancer. This is of critical interest to people with cancer.

For example, researchers have found that vitamin A can suppress abnormal differentiation of prostate epithelial cells in laboratory tests *after* a potentially malignant state has been induced by chemical exposure or radiation. According to Greenwald, when the vitamin A was removed from the culture medium, "full expression of the malignant phenotype occurred."[2] And with human promyelocytic leukemia cells, retinoids returned malignant cells to full differentiation with the shape and biochemical characteristics of a healthy granulocyte.[3]

Other retinoids have "consistently arrested malignant progression in three different rodent bladder cancer systems" and have inhibited the development of cancer in chemically induced breast and skin cancer models. "Regression of chemically induced tumors and a delay in the appearance of transplanted tumors has been reported for several other synthetic retinoids."[4]

Greenwald goes on to say that beta-carotene, a dietary precursor of vitamin A, is particularly interesting for cancer patients because of its very low toxicity and because of the fact that blood levels are directly related to dietary intake, whereas the blood levels of retinoids are strictly controlled."[5] Says Greenwald:

> A direct chemopreventive role for beta-carotene has been suggested because of its very efficient ability to deactivate singlet oxygen and trap organic free radicals. . . . About 20 reports have evaluated cancer incidence and vitamin A or beta-carotene intake. In nine retrospective studies, a significant increase in cancer risk at various sites was associated with diminished vitamin A intake. Risks reported for groups with low vitamin A intake were about twice those for the high intake groups.[6]

The National Academy of Sciences *Diet, Nutrition and Cancer* report concluded: "Studies in animals indicate that an increased intake of this vitamin [A] has a protective effect against the induction of cancer by chemical carcinogens in most, but not all, instances."[7]

In epidemiological studies, low vitamin A intake has been associated with increased risk of colon, lung, cervical, larynx, bladder, esophageal, stomach, colon and rectal, prostate, and oral cancers. Three reports based on data from cohort studies have found a general inverse relationship between serum levels of vitamin A and cancer in general—although higher levels of serum vitamin A have not yet been decisively linked to higher levels of vitamin A intake.[8] For example, a study by Menkes and colleagues in the *New England Journal of Medicine* found a strong inverse correlation between serum beta-carotene levels and the risk of squamous cell carcinoma.[9] Similarly, a study of diet and lung cancer which compared the dietary histories of 332 lung cancer patients with 865 controls found a clear negative association between dietary beta-carotene intake and risk of lung cancer.[10] This finding is supported by a 1990 review of 12 studies by W.C. Willett at Harvard Medical School. In each study, high intake of fruits and vegetables containing carotenoids was associated with reduced risk of lung cancer, though this finding is also compatible with the possibility that some other factor in these foods is responsible for the result. At the same time, little relation was found between vitamin A intake and the risk of lung cancer.[11]

Vitamin A and retinoids have been demonstrated in clinical studies to reverse a variety of precancerous and cancerous conditions, primarily those related to epithelial tissue. In two clinical trials, the retinoid etretinate had a preventive effect on the recurrence of superficial bladder tumors and stimulated regression of bronchial metaplasias in smokers.[12] Similarly, in a randomized clinical trial of patients with oral leukoplakia, a premalignant lesion associated with oral cancer, 13-*cis*-retinoic acid was demonstrated to reduce the size of lesions in 67% of those treated (vs. 10% of controls) and reverse dysplasia in 54% of those treated (vs. 10% of controls).[13] This *reversal* of a premalignant lesion with a retinoid in humans is a dramatic finding.

As a result of the laboratory findings, the epidemiological studies, and the early clinical trials showing reversal of premalignant conditions and prevention of recurrence of some tumors, researchers have undertaken a broad range of intervention studies to test the efficacy of retinoids in the prevention and reversal of human cancers. In 1986, researchers at the NCI listed 19 "chemo-prevention intervention studies" in which retinoids were being evaluated for their capacity to "prevent precursor lesions, reverse precursor lesions, reduce the incidence of malignancy, reduce mortality due to malignancy, and reduce total malignancy."[14]

"Chemoprevention," in other words, has become the polite label under which the capacity of nutrients not only to prevent but actually to reverse cancers and precancers entered the world of mainstream cancer research. As nutritional researcher Lawrence Kushi points out, the approach of mainstream researchers to the question of nutrition in cancer as characterized by the term "chemoprevention" is essentially "the attempt to place a medical paradigm on what is essentially a behavioral/lifestyle intervention, that is, dietary change."[15]

One intriguing clinical study was reported by Frank L. Meyskens, Jr., then at the University of Arizona Cancer Center in Tucson:

> Extensive laboratory investigations have documented that Vitamin A and its natural and synthetic derivatives (the retinoids) can inhibit proliferation and stimulate differentiation and/or maturation in normal and many transformed [e.g., cancerous] cells. Epidemiological studies also support the general notion that vitamin A is a natural inhibitor of the development of human cancer. These observations have prompted us to examine the role of retinoids as anticancer agents. *We propose a general strategy which defines precancer and cancer as a continuum from normality to abnormality in which the modalities of prevention and treatment are blurred* [emphasis added].[16]

Based on the laboratory research showing that retinoids acted as a differentiating agent in mouse and human melanoma cells, in 1978 Meyskens started, in an adjuvant trial, comparing BCG (attenuated bovine tubercle bacillus) injections alone with BCG plus vitamin A for stage I (high risk) and stage II malignant melanoma. At the time of publication in 1984 (based on the first 120 patients) those treated with BCG plus vitamin A were experiencing a "favorable" trend in relapse-free survival compared to those receiving BCG alone.[17] A subsequent unpublished study by Meyskens failed to support his early findings. But the effort was sufficiently intriguing to merit this brief review (Frank L. Meyskens, Jr., personal communication, 1993).

Meyskens also reported "considerable antitumor activity" in a broad phase II clinical trial with several malignant and premalignant skin conditions using the retinoid 13-*cis*-retinoic acid. He found positive short-term responses in skin or subcutaneous cancers in patients with advanced metastatic head and neck cancers, and positive responses in 8 of 12 patients with T-cell lymphoma mycosis fungoides, "with four demonstrating nearly complete resolution of the disease."[18]

The positive results in both experimental research and in the early clinical trial of vitamin A with melanoma, which the later study did not support, are particularly interesting in view of the fact that melanoma is reported to be one of the cancers that has responded most frequently to the Gerson alternative nutritional cancer therapy. The Gerson raw foods diet, with frequent ingestion of fresh vegetable juices, provides a very high intake of beta-carotene. I have personally known several melanoma patients who did well for periods of years on the Gerson program. On the other hand, the course melanoma takes is highly variable, and there may be, as I reported in chapter 10, an important psychological component in improved outcomes with this disease.

The B Vitamins

The National Academy of Sciences *Diet, Nutrition and Cancer* report said that the literature on the relationship of dietary B vitamins to the occurrence of cancer was inadequate to draw any conclusions.[19] The committee wrote: "Because the B vitamins are essential components of any adequate diet and are necessary for the continued maintenance of cellular integrity and metabolic function, severe deficiencies in any of them will clearly reduce the growth rate of tumor cells and interfere with normal functioning of the organism."[20]

Tannenbaum's studies in the 1950s, which played a key role in establishing that "underfeeding" reduced the incidence and yield of tumors in animals, nonetheless found no significant differences in the frequency of tumors in animals fed high, medium, and low levels of B vitamins.[21]

As with other vitamins, the synergistic effects of specific B vitamins and other nutrients can be striking. In one study of mice with transplantable tumors, a combination of vitamins B_{12} and C inhibited the mitotic activity of the tumor cells and "produced a 100% survival rate, while neither vitamin alone at the same dosage had any effect." The effect was specific to ascites tumors.[22]

On the other hand, vitamin B_{12} can also serve as a powerful tumor *promoter*. One researcher fed rats carcinogenic DAB (3,3$'$ = diaminobenzidine) and then divided them into two groups, one of which received a vitamin B_{12} supplement while the other was on a diet that excluded the vitamin. The supplemented rats had a 78% incidence of liver tumors, while the unsupplemented rats had a 17% incidence. When methionine was added to the diets of both groups, the tumor incidence dropped to 33% and 11%, respectively. A control group that received vitamin B_{12} but was not exposed to the carcinogen developed no tumors. Several other researchers have confirmed these findings, which show how vitamin B_{12}—so effective with vitamin C against mouse tumors in the previous study, and innocent of carcinogenic effects on its own—powerfully promoted tumor growth in the presence of a carcinogen, but was modified in this tumor-enhancing effect by the addition of another nutrient.[23]

Vitamin B_6 is one of the most interesting B vitamins for cancer patients. Hans Ladner and Richard Salkeld, a team of German and Swiss researchers, reported an important controlled clinical trial in which 300 mg of pyridoxine (vitamin B_6) was given throughout a 7-week course of radiotherapy to half of a group of 210 patients aged 45 to 65 with endometrial cancer.[24] *They found a 15% improvement in 5-year survival compared to patients who did not receive the supplement, and found no side effects from the supplementation.* The theoretical basis for the study was animal experiments showing that healthy animals subjected to whole body radiation, or animals carrying tumors, developed tryptophan metabolism disorders that resembled those created by vitamin B_6 deficiency states. In humans, these metabolic disorders resembling vitamin B_6 deficiency states are found in Hodgkin's disease, and bladder and breast cancer. One study suggested that vitamin B_6 supplementation to correct the metabolic abnormality might prevent recurrence of bladder cancer.[24] Ladner and Salkeld also "confirmed the beneficial effects of pyridoxine administration on radiation-induced symptoms—nausea, vomiting, and diarrhea—in gynecological patients treated with high-energy radiation, and observed that impairment of the vitamin B_6 status was corrected by 300 mg pyridoxine daily."

Ladner and Salkeld then studied vitamin B_6 status in 6,300 gynecological cancer patients with cervical, uterine, endometrial, ovarian, and breast cancers. They found that before radiotherapy, in uterine, ovarian, and breast cancer, "the more the tumor had progressed, the more pronounced was the impairment of vitamin B_6, B_1 and B_2 status. During the course of irradiation, the vitamin B status became progressively more impaired." This led to their important findings that quality of life and survival were both improved with B_6 supplementation. They also found that chemotherapy—doxorubicin, cisplatin, and cyclophosphamide—generated "no definite worsening" of vitamin B_6 status in women with metastatic endometrial or breast cancer.[25] This study of the improved quality of life for women with gynecological and breast cancer who use vitamin B_6 supplements with radiotherapy is particularly provocative when we consider a similar report on vitamin C below.

Vitamin B_6 has also been reported to be particularly effective in inhibiting melanoma cancer cells. Based on this experimental evidence, one research team developed a topical pyridoxal cream that, "when applied to patients with recurrent malignant melanoma, produced a significant reduction in the size of subcutaneous nodules and complete regression of cutaneous papules." While the results were considered preliminary, "they are provocative and may lead to a more successful topical treatment of this highly lethal cancer."[26]

Linus Pauling and the Controversy over Vitamin C

A major public controversy over the role of vitamin C in cancer has been waged ever since the double Nobel Prize laureate, Linus Pauling, endorsed high-dosage use of the vitamin for both cancer and the common cold. In 1976, Pauling and his Scottish colleague Cameron reported in the *Proceedings of the National Academy of Sciences* that they had conducted a study in which "hopelessly ill" cancer patients had been given 10 gm of vitamin C a day in divided doses. They reported that survival for more than a year after the date of "untreatability" was found in 22% of their experimental group but in only 0.4% of historical controls (past patients with similar diagnoses who did not take vitamin C). They also reported that 370 nonrandomized contemporary controls showed the same survival statistics as the historical controls.

Thunderous criticism of the study arose in the scientific community. Melvyn Werbach, M.D., of the UCLA School of Medicine summarized the criticisms: (1) lack of a prospective random double-blind study; (2) lack of rigidly defined criteria for "untreatability"; (3) failure to match patients by histological identification of type and origin of cancer cells; and (4) failure to ensure that cases and controls adhered to their medication schedules.[27]

At the Mayo Clinic, researchers conducted two experimental double-blind studies to determine whether the survival advantage that Pauling and Cameron had demonstrated would show up under what they considered optimal scientific conditions. The first study by E.T. Creagan and his colleagues randomized 150 patients with advanced cancer into two groups:

Sixty "evaluable" patients received vitamin C and 63 similar, randomized patients received a lactose placebo, while 27 of the randomized patients elected not to participate. Neither vitamin C nor the placebo improved survival times which averaged 51 days; *however, those who withdrew survived only 25 days, raising the question of how the decision to withdraw may have influenced survival* [emphasis added]. The authors note that, in contrast to the earlier Pauling and Cameron study, a large proportion of patients in this study had received radiation and/or chemotherapy.[28]

In the second effort at the Mayo Clinic to replicate or disprove the Pauling-Cameron findings, Charles Moertel (who had been second author on the first study) and colleagues conducted a randomized controlled double-blind study of 100 advanced large-bowel cancer patients who had not received chemotherapy and who were given either the 10 gm of vitamin C that Pauling recommended or a placebo for 2½ months. There were no differences in survival between the two groups, *although none of the patients on vitamin C died while they were taking the vitamin.* Moertel et al. concluded: "On the basis of this and our previous randomized study, it can be concluded that high-dose vitamin C therapy is not effective against advanced malignant disease regardless of whether the patient has had any prior chemotherapy."[29]

Following publication of this study, its senior investigator Moertel went on network television to denounce vitamin C as "absolutely worthless." Pauling responded by accusing the Mayo Clinic of making "false and misleading" claims about the study and asked for a retraction, correction, and apology from the *New England Journal of Medicine*, which had published the study. The editor refused. The journal also refused to publish two letters from Pauling and at least two other letters critical of the study. Evelleen Richards in the highly respected British journal *New Scientist* reported:

> Pauling has never been content with unorthodox backing. He has consistently sought recognition of his claims from the establishment. Yet, in spite of his belief that the medical profession has never dealt with his claims in an unbiased and objective manner, his faith in the scientific method as the supreme arbiter of truth remains undiminished. Cameron, who describes his own professional background as "perfectly conventional, even conservative by some standards," shares Pauling's attitude. Cameron remains optimistic that once someone has demonstrated the "flaws" in the latest study from the Mayo Clinic, the National Cancer Institute will find a new trial. A fresh trial, he emphasizes, "must not be carried out by vitamin C enthusiasts nor by bigots, but by fair-minded

physicians, and conducted not in secrecy but in open cooperation using a mutually agreed protocol."

Therein lies the crunch. The idea of a cooperative approach embodying agreed criteria is not easily realized. Even if both sides to the dispute could agree about how to evaluate their respective claims about vitamin C, recent studies in the sociology of scientific knowledge suggest that impersonal rules of experimental procedure do not necessarily resolve disputes about "facts" and their interpretation. Such studies indicate that it is not always possible to dissociate the design of an experiment from the commitments of those who frame and evaluate the experiment. This latest chapter of the controversy over vitamin C tends to support this sociological contention. On the most superficial analysis, the Mayo Clinic's team is simply not talking the same language as Cameron and Pauling.

Throughout, Cameron and Pauling have emphasized that the massive doses of vitamin C that they recommend (10 grams or more daily) are essential to patients with cancer, who show an increased need for this vitamin. They say that, unlike conventional chemotherapy, vitamin C restrains rather than kills cancer cells, and that vitamin C plays a vital part in stimulating the immune system, improving the general health and well-being of the patient. Pauling and Cameron are not, therefore, offering a "cure" for cancer, although they have described some cases that seem to deserve this label. What they would expect, on the basis of their studies, is that, in patients given vitamin C, tumors would grow less quickly and some of the distressing symptoms of cancer would be alleviated. These patients would survive slightly, but significantly, longer and enjoy better quality of life. Cameron and Pauling also point out that vitamin C does not have the debilitating side effects of conventional chemotherapy, and that it is not expensive and does not need elaborate equipment.

Richards then reviewed Pauling and Cameron's critique of the methodological problems of the study of Moertel et al. First, urine tests for vitamin C levels were not routinely done, and those that were done indicated that at least one of the controls was found to be taking vitamin C independently. Second, in the Mayo Clinic study, vitamin C was stopped as soon as tumors started to grow again, which worked out to a median time of 10 weeks. In the Cameron-Pauling studies, vitamin C was continued indefinitely. "So the effect observed was related not only to the question of whether or not the tumor began to progress, but also to the subsequent rate at which the tumor grew under continued administration of vitamin C, and to any effect on the patient's general health that might contribute to his or her capacity to resist death from cancer."[30]

Third, and perhaps most important, Pauling and Cameron were concerned with the "rebound effect." Said Richards:

> If someone suddenly stops taking large doses of vitamin C, the level of vitamin C circulating in their body drops to well below normal. Doctors have known about this effect for about 12 years. Pauling and Cameron have repeatedly warned patients of its possible dangers. They believe the resultant temporary depression of the immune system may induce tumors to grow more quickly. The Mayo Clinic's team either ignored or was unaware of this possibility. The clinic's doctors abruptly discontinued vitamin C for those patients who showed signs that a tumor was progressing, thus inducing the rebound effect. According to Pauling and Cameron, this oversight invalidates the clinic's study; they say that the study does not refute their findings. They even suggest that the combination of the rebound effect and the subsequent highly toxic chemotherapy may have shortened the lives of patients participating in the Mayo Clinic's study.

> Irrespective of the cogency of Pauling and Cameron's criticisms, the clinic's study clearly demonstrates how vested interests intrude on the evaluation of treatments. At the beginning of the study, the team at the Mayo Clinic conceded that the powerful cytotoxic drug fluorouracil (either alone or in combination) was of no value in the treatment of colorectal cancer. Yet it fell back on this treatment for more than 50 per cent of patients in the study when it found vitamin C ineffective by the same criteria. The doctors' preference was for a treatment which is professionally controlled and administered and fits the established theoretical framework: yet this treatment is therapeutically useless and highly toxic. . . . In the face of the Mayo Clinic's own evaluation of this treatment, it is difficult to justify the decision, which Moertel subsequently defended on ethical grounds, to withdraw vitamin C or placebo and substitute chemotherapy for so many patients. . . .

> In spite of the orthodox medical profession's repeated emphasis on the need properly to evaluate Cameron and Pauling's research, most chemotherapies for cancer, including fluorouracil, have been widely applied in practice without previous evaluation by randomized controlled trials. Several studies have demonstrated that, once a therapy is professionally adopted and endorsed, there are significant financial, public and professional obstacles in the way of abandoning it, even if it is demonstrated to be ineffective and to harm patients.[31]

Adherents of Pauling's position have thus been able to argue, with some legitimacy, that neither of the two Mayo Clinic studies actually tested Pauling and Cameron's thesis—the first because patients were pretreated with chemotherapy and the second because (a) controls were not adequately tested for "out-of-study" use of vitamin C; (b) vitamin C was withdrawn as soon as tumors began to grow, thus possibly initiating a "rebound effect"; and (c) subsequent chemotherapy may have compromised survival.

While the mainstream scientific community has stuck close to the current consensus position that the Mayo Clinic studies "disproved" any positive role for vitamin C in cancer treatment, the most recent edition of the authoritative nutrition text edited by Maurice E. Shils and Vernon R. Young, *Modern Nutrition in Health and Disease,* gives two very different treatments to the vitamin C and cancer controversy, depending on which section you read. Shils, in his overview of nutritional approaches to cancer, dismisses the whole controversy in a paragraph without mentioning Pauling's work or the critique of the Mayo Clinic studies: "Ascorbic acid in the high dose of 10 g daily had no advantage over a placebo in 100 patients with advanced colorectal cancer who had no previous chemotherapy. The double blind study indicated no difference in the progression of measurable disease or survival. The same group had demonstrated earlier that this vitamin had no advantage over placebo when given in conjunction with chemotherapy."[32]

But, in the same book, Hornig and his co-workers in their chapter on vitamin C give Pauling's work a more subtle treatment. After describing Pauling's study and the two Mayo Clinic studies, they take note of the controversy with the use of understatement and strategic placement characteristic of many scientists: "An exchange of views about this controversy has been published." They *then* go on to describe a Japanese study showing increased survival with high-dose vitamin C. The Japanese study that they describe here, though flawed, lends weight to the Pauling position:

> Observation of terminal cancer patients in two hospitals who were receiving either a low-dose ascorbate (4 g daily or less) or high-dose ascorbate (5 g daily or more) showed a significantly higher median survival of 105 days in the high-dose group compared to 35 days in the low-dose group. The administration of ascorbic acid seemed to improve the well-being of many cancer patients, as measured by decreased requirement for pain-controlling drugs, improved appetite, and increased mental alertness. However, these studies were poorly controlled, and the classification of "low dose" and "high dose" was arbitrary. *Furthermore, the site of primary tumors seems to be important for the effectiveness of ascorbic acid; uterus and stomach are the most promising.* In vitro, an inhibitory effect of ascorbic acid on the growth of human melanoma cells was demonstrated. In 1 mmol ascorbate, no melanoma colonies were observed

and in 0.6 mmol ascorbate, the ability of melanoma cells to form colonies was 10 to 20 times less than for normal human amniotic cells. *Again, additional controlled studies are needed to eventually establish a role for vitamin C in cancer* [emphasis added].[33]

This gives you a taste of the public controversy over vitamin C. Note especially that some of the foremost authorities on vitamin C research are now more open to the potential for vitamin C in cancer treatment.

Cancer Prevention and Vitamin C

Epidemiological studies demonstrate an indirect association (indirect because they analyze foods known to contain high levels of vitamin C, not vitamin C itself) between high vitamin C intake and a lowered risk of cancer, particularly cancer of the esophagus and stomach. High consumption of fresh fruit specifically has been shown to protect against gastric cancer. A case-controlled study of vitamin C consumption and uterine cervical dysplasia, a premalignant condition, also showed a protective role for vitamin C; but a case-controlled study of colon cancer did not.[34] Note that in the Japanese study cited above, stomach and uterine cancer were considered the best responders to vitamin C therapy.

More recently, 33 of 46 epidemiological studies surveyed by Gladys Block, Ph.D., of the NCI showed significant protective effects of vitamin C. In aggregate, those in the top fourth of vitamin C intake had approximately half the cancer risk of the lowest fourth in terms of vitamin C consumption. Twenty-one of 29 studies assessing fruit intake demonstrated a protective effect, particularly for cancers of the esophagus, larynx, oral cavity, pancreas, stomach, rectum, and cervix. Block concluded that: "While it is likely that ascorbic acid, carotenoids, folate and other factors in fruit and vegetables act jointly, an increasingly important role for ascorbic acid in cancer prevention would appear to be emerging."[35]

A recent combined analysis of 12 case-controlled studies by Geoffrey Howe at the National Cancer Institute in Canada found that fruit and vegetable intake, and most notably vitamin C intake, provided a consistent protective effect for breast cancer. *Howe concluded that if North American women increased*

their fruit and vegetable intake to reach an average 380 mg/day of vitamin C fr
those sources, the breast cancer risk in the population would be decreased by 16%.

One aspect of the protective effect of vitamin C may lie in its ability to inhibit the oncogenic transformation of cells. Richard Schwarz of the University of California at Berkeley demonstrated that the presence of vitamin C in a culture of primary avian tendon cells and oncogenic Rous sarcoma virus "stabilizes the normal state [of the cells] by reducing virus production and promoting the synthesis of differentiated proteins."[37]

Experimental evidence demonstrates that vitamin C can also inhibit the formation of carcinogenic nitrosamines, which are found in tobacco smoke, marijuana, some cosmetics, corrosion inhibitors, rubber products, rubber nipples for baby bottles, and cured meats. Precursors of nitrosamines are found in many foods: they react with sodium nitrite, a food preservative, to form carcinogenic nitrosamines in the acidic environment of the human stomach.[38] Since vitamin C can inhibit the formation of nitrosamines in the stomach, this is widely assumed to be the basis for its protective effect against gastric cancers specifically.

This capacity of vitamin C to reduce nitrosamine levels in the stomach was demonstrated with esophageal cancer patients in a study performed in northern China's Lin-Xian province, an area where esophageal cancer is common. Researchers measured levels of nitrosamines in the stomach and lesions in the esophageal epithelium, and found a positive correlation: the higher the nitrosamine levels, the more lesions were found. They then gave experimental subjects 100-mg vitamin C supplements three times a day, an hour after meals. They found a marked decrease in urinary nitrosamine products, which became comparable to those in people in areas with low esophageal cancer risk.[39]

Another protective aspect of vitamin C is its antioxidant activity. This discussion of vitamin C is an appropriate place to describe briefly the broader question of how vitamin C, selenium, and other antioxidants, several of which we discuss below, protect the organism against the wonderfully named "free radicals."

Free radicals are potentially carcinogenic compounds created by both healthy and diseased cells in the course of cell respiration and intermediary metabolism. According to Carmia Borek of the departments of pathology and radiology at Columbia University College of Physicians and Surgeons:

> The cellular oxidant state is of the utmost importance also in cellular protection against the oncogenic potential of radiation and chemicals. . . . Inherent cellular factors comprised of enzymes, vitamins, micronutrients and low molecular weight substance are protectors. *These include superoxide dismutase and catalase, peroxidases and thiols, vitamin A, vitamin C, and vitamin E and the micronutrient selenium* [emphasis added]. These antioxidants serve to defend the cells against elevated levels of free radicals produced by radiation, chemical carcinogens and tumor promoters. The free radicals . . . to varying degrees damage the cell.[40]

Borek summarizes the field as follows:

> Free radicals are continuously produced by living cells. . . . Under optimal cellular metabolic conditions cellular antioxidants are sufficient to impart protection against oxidant stress. However, under conditions of exposure to carcinogens or to unfavorable metabolic stress which enhances free radical levels, inherent protection may prove to be inadequate leading eventually to neoplastic [cancerous] transformation. . . . Under stressful conditions cells require the external addition of antioxidants to enable them to cope with the excess load of free radicals and to minimize the oxidative damage and oncogenic transformation. Some nutrient antioxidants act directly, other agents such as selenium will impart their protection by inducing high levels of inherent protective enzyme systems which destroy peroxides. This enables the cell itself to increase its scavenging powers and to cope with the "overload" of free radicals and their toxic products thus preventing the onset and progression of malignant transformation.[41]

Two antioxidant enzymes, superoxide dismutase (SOD) and superoxide catalase, are also of interest in some alternative cancer therapies. These substances form part of the antioxidant cellular defense system against free radicals.

The role of vitamin C as one of the primary defenses against oxygen radicals is described by Etsuo Niki at the University of Tokyo: "Free radicals attack lipids, proteins, enzymes and DNA to eventually cause a variety of pathological events and cancer. . . . *When aqueous radicals were generated in the whole blood, ascorbic acid [vitamin C] scavenged them faster than any other antioxidants* [emphasis added] and protected lipids and proteins more effectively than bilirubin, uric acid or tocopherol (vitamin E)."[42]

Similarly, Balz Frei and Bruce Ames at the University of California at Berkeley investigated the effectiveness of selected antioxidants in human blood plasma. *Ascorbic acid proved to be the most effective of all the antioxidants they tested* and the only one which could prevent the initiation of lipid peroxidation, rather than simply lowering the rate at which the process occurs. They also found that the effect increased with the plasma concentration of ascorbic acid.[43]

Another pathway for the protective effects of vitamin C was proposed by Joachim Liehr at the University of Texas Medical Branch who found in animal studies that *vitamin C may also play a role in inhibiting estrogen-induced carcinogenesis by reducing concentrations of metabolic byproducts of estrogen.*[44] The potential effects of vitamin C are closely related to dietary iron. According to Swiss researcher Alfred Hanck:

> Iron deficiency is an aggravating factor in cancer patients. . . . Only ferrous iron is absorbed and ascorbic acid converts food ferric iron to bioavailable ferrous iron. . . . Vitamin C improves hemoglobin status and thus oxygen supply of tissue, with an increase in oxidative energy production. . . . The cytotoxic effect of ascorbic acid against malignant cells is significantly increased by chelation with ferrous iron. . . . This increased efficacy is attributed to the longer half-life of the ascorbate iron complex during cell contact compared to ascorbic acid.[45]

Vitamin C Inhibits Growth in Human Tumor Cell Lines

Vitamin C has also been shown to demonstrate an inhibitory effect on tumor growth. In an important 1989 study,[46] a group of Belgian researchers reported in *Cancer* that sodium ascorbate (vitamin C) and vitamin K_3 were administered separately and in combination to human breast, oral, and endometrial cancer cell lines. While both had an inhibiting effect on cancer cell growth at high concentrations, combined administration of both vitamins demonstrated a synergistic inhibition of cell growth at much lower concentrations where vitamins given separately are not toxic. The inhibitory effect was suppressed by the addition of catalase to the culture, which suggested that the observed effect on cancer cells was connected to the formation of hydrogen peroxide.[46] This study is obviously rich in possibilities for clinical trials of the combined vitamins. It has further interest because the presumed mechanism of the synergistic effect of these vitamins is hydrogen peroxide production. Hydrogen peroxide has long been a chemical of interest among some practitioners of alternative cancer therapies.

Other studies have demonstrated that stress linked to cancer lowers plasma levels of vitamin C in patients and in experimental animals. This has been demonstrated recently in patients with uterine, cervical, and ovarian cancer, and in leukemia and lymphoma patients.[47] If cancer stress lowers vitamin C levels, and below-normal vitamin C levels diminish immune function, this would appear to be an additional rationale for vitamin C supplementation in cancer.

Vitamin C Is Helpful with Radiation and Chemotherapies

Apart from the controversy over the Pauling-Cameron studies, the most important report I have seen on vitamin C is a trial showing the benefits of vitamin C when used in conjunction with radiotherapy. Hanck reviews the literature and describes the study:

> During radiotherapy, decrease of several vitamin levels [including] vitamins E, B_{12}, folic acid and C have been observed. A decrease of vitamin C plasma levels due to irradiation treatment has been reported by several investigators. *In addition, potentiation or augmentation of the lethal effect of radiation against tumor cells was demonstrated when ascorbic acid was co-administered* [emphasis added]. Recently the effects of radiation therapy with adjunct ascorbic acid treatment have been investigated in 50 cancer patients in a prospective clinical trial. The patients were divided into two groups by random allocation. [Patients had cancers of the tongue, tonsil, cervix, esophagus, neck, skin, lip, and cheek, and Ewing's sarcoma.] . . . Progressive disease was seen after one month in 5% of the control group and 3% of the study group. These values had increased to 20% of the control group after 4 months and 7% in the study group.

Based on 20 cases, Hanck found 45% of the control group surviving without disease and 50% with disease at 6 months; and 67% of the vitamin C group surviving without disease and 33% with disease at 6 months. He also found that, with the administration of vitamin C, patients suffered less anemia, less pain, less loss of appetite and weight. All the side effects of radiotherapy tended to be fewer. And since it is tolerated extremely well, he also urged further clinical investigations of the effects of high doses of vitamin C.[48]

In a related study, Paul Okunieff of Massachusetts General Hospital also found vitamin C to protect both the skin and bone marrow against the effects of radiation. It was not found to be toxic to the tumor itself, nor did it protect the tumor from radiation.[49]

Another potentially significant finding for cancer patients is the protective effect vitamin C has displayed against potential damage to the heart by Adriamicin (ADR, doxorubicin) in animal studies. According to Kan Shimpo and his colleagues at the Fujita Health University in Japan,

> One possible mechanism of ADR-induced toxicity is the induction of peroxidation in cardiac lipids. Ascorbic acid is a potent antioxidant. Thus, the lipid peroxidation and cardiac toxicity of ADR are expected to be reduced by prior treatment of the animals with ascorbic acid. . . . Ascorbic acid . . . significantly prolonged the life of mice and guinea pigs treated with ADR. . . . The results also suggest the clinical efficacy of the combined treatment of ADR and ascorbic acid or the derivatives.[50]

Experimental studies by Kedar N. Prasad of the University of Colorado Health Science Center have also demonstrated that two forms of vitamin C, sodium L-ascorbate and sodium D-ascorbate, enhanced the effectiveness of radiotherapy and the chemotherapeutic agents 5-fluorouracil (5-FU) and bleomycin when used on mouse neuroblastoma cells but *not* on rat glioma cells.[51] When one reads the experimental research literature on nutrients and cancer, it is replete with descriptions of studies where vitamins acted on one cell line but not on another, or even in opposite ways in different cell lines.

Vitamin C May Help or Harm with Leukemia

The complexity of the question of just how nutrients affect cancer cells is underscored by an experiment that suggests a significant potential hazard in using vitamin C for *some* people with leukemia—but a significant possible benefit for *others*. Vitamin C has an apparent paradoxical effect in cell cultures from cancer patients with acute nonlymphocytic leukemia and preleukemia, or myelodysplastic syndrome (MDS). A study by Chan H. Park at the University of Kansas found that L-ascorbic acid and glutathione (which potentiates the effects of L-ascorbic acid) *enhanced* leukemia cell growth in samples from one third of the patients, *suppressed* leukemia cell growth in one sixth of the patients, and had no effect on the rest. It is intriguing that the effect was replicable: in repeated trials, cell cultures from affected patients responded in the same way, either toward enhancement of growth or suppression of growth. The ascorbic acid compound used in the experiment also enhanced cell growth in 24% of the normal control cell cultures.[52] Park and Bruce F. Kimler also found that the reported effects of L-ascorbic acid had prognostic value for patients with MDS; patients sensitive to L-ascorbic acid have shorter survival times than patients who are not sensitive. The authors conclude that MDS is the ideal disease for in vivo trials to investigate the control of the disease process through L-ascorbic acid manipulation. Such trials are currently being planned.[53]

This suggests that leukemia patients considering experimenting with vitamin C therapy should do so only in careful collaboration with oncologists, preferably after ascertaining that their tissue culture was one of the minority that responds positively to vitamin C. The experiment, however, has the broader implication that *different patients with the same histological type of cancer may respond in different directions to the same nutrient.* The finding that vitamin C enhanced normal cell growth in 25% of the control cell cultures from healthy people is also intriguing. It is important to emphasize that a laboratory study of the effect of vitamin C on a cell culture does *not* predict how the vitamin will act on the cancer cells in a patient. But, for the many cancer patients who consider taking vitamins on their own—or on the advice of clinicians unfamiliar with the research literature—the potential hazard of vitamin C to patients with leukemia is worth noting. Above all, as Hippocrates said, never do harm to anyone.

In its summary of vitamin C research in 1982, the National Academy of Sciences report said that "the limited evidence suggests that vitamin C can inhibit the formation of some carcinogens and that the consumption of vitamin C–containing foods is associated with a lower risk of cancers of the stomach and esophagus."[54] Since then, the literature has continued to add intriguing and potentially significant pieces. The controversy over whether vitamin C extends life in cancer patients with advanced metastatic disease is scientifically unanswered due to the deficiencies of both the Cameron-Pauling studies and the replication studies. But the Japanese study, though flawed, again supports the Pauling hypothesis.

The Hanck study, although conducted with a mix of different tumor types, raises the real possibility that vitamin C may both extend survival and enhance the effects and diminish the side effects of radiotherapy. The Park laboratory experiment on human leukemia cell lines, on the other hand, emphasizes that in leukemia, at least, vitamin C may represent a hazard for some patients, while it may be helpful to others. And the study of vitamin C and vitamin K_3 administered synergistically in breast, oral, and endometrial cell cultures suggests that the yield of a chemotherapeutic use of these vitamins might be much higher if they were given together.

Vitamin E May Help with Cancer, Chemotherapies, and Radiation

The summary of the National Academy of Sciences *Diet, Nutrition and Cancer* report on vitamin E was brief: vitamin E (specifically alpha-tocopherol), like vitamin C, inhibits the formation of carcinogenic nitrosamines. But the committee found no reports indicating an effect of vitamin E on nitrosamine-induced cancers. Limited experimental evidence in several studies, however, showed that vitamin E inhibited tumor development.[55] But this short summary greatly understates the potential significance of vitamin E for cancer patients.

First, while both vitamin C and vitamin E (alpha-tocopherol) block the formation of carcinogenic nitrosamines and reduce levels of fecal mutagens, they work *better* in combination than they do independently to reduce fecal mutagen levels. Similarly, while vitamin E had no independent effect on chemically induced cancers in animals, it enhanced the preventive effects of selenium.[56] Second, some forms of vitamin E are effective in reducing growth and enhancing differentiation in mammalian cancer cells. Prasad, one of the leading authorities on vitamin E, has demonstrated that, among the several forms of vitamin E, vitamin E succinate appears to be the most effective in reducing growth and enhancing differentiation of mammalian cancer cell lines in laboratory experiments, perhaps because "tumor cells pick up this form of vitamin E more readily than they do other forms."[57] Third, high-dose alpha-tocopherol has reduced growth of human neuroblastoma cells in living cancer patients, and has reduced benign mastitis (inflammation) of the breast.[58] Fourth, and very important, vitamin E enhances the effectiveness of some chemotherapies, radiation, and hyperthermia on cancer cell lines. According to Prasad:

> Vitamin E enhances . . . the effect of ionizing radiation on tumor cells in culture without affecting the radiation response of normal tissues. Vitamin E also enhances the effects of hyperthermia on tumor cells in culture, and inhibits the production of prostaglandin E series which are known to suppress the host's immune system. Finally, vitamin E reduces the toxic effects of some chemotherapeutic agents. These studies suggest that vitamin E may be one of the important anticancer agents which could play a very significant role in the prevention and treatment of cancer.[59]

In animal studies, vitamin E has been shown to reduce cardiac and skin toxicity from doxorubicin, and lung fibrosis related to bleomycin—two very widely used chemotherapies.[60] In addition to protecting the heart against damage from doxorubicin in animal studies, vitamin E has been reported to have a possible protective effect in humans against hair loss from doxorubicin therapy. Werbach summarizes a study by Wood in the *New England Journal of Medicine:* "69% of patients on doxorubicin [Adriamicin] receiving 1600 IU *dl*-alpha-tocopherol acetate [vitamin E] daily did not develop alopecia [hair loss]. Those who did develop alopecia were believed to have received the vitamin E too late before chemotherapy, as it should be started 5–7 days prior to commencement."[61]

These vitamin E studies represent, in my judgment, stunning examples of the underutilization of scientific nutrition in cancer. Each year, hundreds of thousands of women around the world take doxorubicin at the same time that they undergo breast surgery. They not only undergo the personal loss of part or all of their breast, they also lose their hair. In addition, many end up with heart damage, a known side effect of doxorubicin in many situations. If vitamin E in an admittedly preliminary study was shown to *protect* against hair loss with doxorubicin, *why has this study not been replicated as a real priority in cancer research?* Further, since animal studies show that it may protect against heart damage, *why does this not add an even stronger argument for full replication?* I can see no good answer to these questions. If some oncologists maintain that we do not yet have enough evidence to recommend to patients undergoing doxorubicin treatment that they take vitamin E, then getting that evidence should be a national research priority. If others answer that there is already sufficient evidence to recommend taking vitamin E with doxorubicin, *that raises the equally troubling question of why most patients are not told they should take vitamin E when undergoing this therapy.* For the biomedical cancer researcher, protecting women against hair loss when fighting for their lives with breast cancer may seem trivial. But for the patient-centered medical practitioner, protecting women with breast cancer against hair loss is not at all trivial. Hair loss makes a profound difference in the *suffering* that women undergo. Therefore, if this is a preventable problem, it should be a vital matter to conduct the inexpensive and innocuous research that would settle the matter of hair loss and vitamin E and make the outcome a standard element in doxorubicin protocols. But even for the strictly biomedical researcher, unconcerned with hair loss, the issue of *preventing heart damage* with vitamin E should have some real salience. Again, the studies would be inexpensive and potentially lifesaving.

Finally, it is worth remembering that many of the salutary effects of the antioxidant vitamins A, C, and E on cancer, according to Prasad, are achieved best by their synergistic interactions.[62] Thus, studies of the individual nutrients may understate their potential for suppressing cancer cell growth, encouraging cell differentiation toward normality, enhancing immune function, potentiating the effects of existing anticancer therapies, and protecting the organism from the harmful side effects of some of these therapies.

Minerals and Cancer

Minerals play a role in both the enhancement and inhibition of human cancers. We will look at the evidence on selenium and zinc. Selenium is important because of its broad anticancer effects. Zinc is important because it is an antagonist to selenium and may in itself enhance or inhibit different tumors.

Selenium in minute quantities is essential to human health. According to Prasad, among the minerals, "only selenium has been shown to have a role in cancer prevention":

> Like vitamin E, selenium acts as an antioxidant and strengthens the body's immune defense system. Thus, many of the effects which are produced by vitamin E deficiency can be reversed or prevented by selenium. Some laboratory experiments have suggested that the combination of vitamin E and selenium is more effective in preventing cancer than either of them alone.

> Certain metals such as lead, cadmium, arsenic, mercury and silver block the action of selenium. . . . Recent laboratory experiments have shown that *high doses of zinc* block the action of selenium. Therefore, *one has to be careful about taking excessive amounts of zinc (over 20 milligrams per day from diet and supplements) while taking selenium* [emphasis added].

> Protein-rich and unsaturated fat–rich diets have been shown to increase the selenium requirements of the body. . . .
>
> Commercial preparations of selenium include inorganic selenium (sodium selenite) and various organic compounds of selenium. It has been reported that sodium selenite is not absorbed adequately, whereas organic selenium, including yeast-selenium, is absorbed very well. For this reason, yeast-selenium is considered best for human consumption. . . . It has been reported that selenium doses of about 250–300 micrograms a day (diet and supplements) would be helpful in preventing cancer. If an average person consumes 125 to 150 micrograms of selenium a day, an additional supplemental amount of 100 micrograms is unlikely to produce any major side effects.[63]

One of the foremost selenium investigators, Gerhard Schrauzer of the University of California at San Diego, says:

> Apart from its functions as an essential micronutrient, selenium also appears to have other physiological functions in which it acts as a physiological *resistance factor* [emphasis added]. Its cancer protecting effects fall into this category. In addition, selenium protects against free radicals, mutagens, toxic heavy metals and certain bacterial, fungal and viral pathogens. The selenium requirement increases under stress, just as the requirement for certain vitamins increases during infections.[64]

Selenium, according to Schrauzer, is most effective as a form of nutritional cancer prophylaxis. In animal research, its protective effect is greater the earlier in life it is given, and its shielding effect against virally induced cancer disappears if the nutrient is no longer fed to the animal. Nevertheless, selenium does have an effect on slowing the rate of growth of established spontaneous or transplanted breast tumors in animals, and in reversing the development of some malignant cell lines when used at pharmacological levels.[65] Further, selenium has shown a general capacity to stimulate the immune system in several animal models, which may add to its anticancer effects.[66]

It is of special relevance to cancer patients undergoing chemotherapy that selenium "has by now been shown to prevent or retard tumorigenesis induced by virtually all the major known carcinogens," probably, Schrauzer believes, "by modulating the rate of cell division."[67] For those undergoing radiotherapy, research by Carmia Borek is of interest: she found that pretreatment of a mouse cell line with nontoxic levels of sodium selenite "inhibits the induction of malignant transformation by x-rays" as a result of the ability of selenium "to induce high levels of free radical scavenging systems in the cells exposed to the oncogenic agents."[68] She writes:

> There is a close interrelationship between selenium and vitamin E in their antioxidant actions. However, the role of vitamin E as an anticancer agent varies with the model studied and probably depends on the tissue content of the vitamin. We found selenium to be a true protector. Its maximum effectiveness was imparted when cells were preincubated with the trace element. Thus, selenium can serve as a true radioprotective and chemoprotective agent.[69]

Zinc, like selenium, is widely taken as a supplement by many people interested in nutritional supplements. A mineral that is essential to life, it plays a key role in cell replication, tissue repair, and growth. Zinc-deficient children are frequently small in stature. Marginal zinc deficiency is suspected to be quite widespread in the United States. Pronounced zinc deficiency depresses immune function in both humans and animals.[70]

Zinc can both enhance and retard tumor growth. In epidemiological studies, the National Academy of Sciences report described a study in England and Wales where gastric cancer was higher in people whose gardens had high zinc levels in the soil. Schrauzer and his colleagues examined food intake in 27 countries and reported a direct correlation between higher zinc intake and a higher incidence of leukemia and cancers of the intestine, breast, prostate, and skin. They concluded that zinc increases cancer risk by its known antagonism to selenium. Schrauzer also found that high zinc in blood samples collected from healthy donors across the United States correlated directly with mortality rates from large bowel, breast, ovary, lung, bladder, and oral cancer in the different areas where the blood was collected. Zinc and selenium levels in the blood were inversely related. *On the other hand,* two studies of esophageal cancer found zinc levels to be lower in the diet of countries where that cancer is common and lower in the blood of patients with esophageal cancer than in normal controls. Clearly, in the latter studies, "the altered zinc levels may have followed, rather than preceded, the onset of cancer."[71]

The experimental evidence collected in the National Academy of Sciences report supports the epidemiological evidence, showing both the enhancing and retarding effects of zinc on tumor growth:

Zinc deficiency appears to retard the growth of transplanted tumors, whereas it enhances the incidence of some chemically induced cancers. In some experiments, dietary zinc exceeding nutritional requirements has been shown to suppress chemically induced tumors in rats and hamsters, but when given in drinking water it counteracts the protective effect of selenium in mice. These data are insufficient to explain the effects of zinc and of interactions between zinc and other minerals on tumorigenesis.[72]

While the evidence on the effect of zinc on tumor development is complex, it strongly suggests that, in general, one should be cautious about taking zinc supplements if one has cancer. And since selenium has a wide spectrum of demonstrable anticancer effects, cancer patients should be particularly cautious with zinc, since it is a selenium antagonist. I have seen many cancer patients taking moderately large amounts of zinc as part of a comprehensive megavitamin nutritional supplement program. In view of the available scientific evidence, this is another critical example of an area where uninformed nutritional supplementation may do harm.

Allergy, Food Sensitivities, and Cancer

Early in the twentieth century, mainstream medicine in America had a significant interest in food allergies and sensitivities. This interest diminished drastically as modern pharmaceutical research created the potential to control many allergic reactions with antihistamines, and the field of allergy research moved from the clinician's office into the laboratory. As the new focus on laboratory research on antigen-antibody interactions developed, a splinter group of allergists called "clinical ecologists" broke off from the mainstream and kept their focus on empirical relationships between foods and other allergens and clinical responses to them. Moreover, the clinical ecologists came into existence just as the petrochemical revolution after World War II was sweeping through the American economy, creating a whole new realm of chemical exposures for the American public that no medical specialty was addressing adequately. So the clinical ecologists added an empirical interest in chemical sensitivities to their interest in food allergies and other allergenic problems.

The clinical ecologists remain an "alternative" medical group, largely despised by their mainstream colleagues. As with many other splinter groups, the clinical ecologists attract many "true believers" who make excessive claims for the field. Yet in my judgment the clinical ecologists are pursuing an important line of inquiry concerning patterns of human reaction to foods, chemicals, and other substances.

In mainstream nutritional research, the relationship of allergies to cancer is a minor, yet potentially significant issue. *The central question raised is whether allergies may have a protective effect against development of cancer or predispose people to it.* A 1988 report by William McWhorter of the NCI summarizes the research from a series of studies over the last three decades: "Thirteen [studies] reported allergy to be protective, three found no association, and two found allergy to be a risk factor. The hypothesis often given to explain a protective effect is that individuals with allergies may have hyperstimulated immune systems, which are better able to detect and eliminate incipient malignancies."

McWhorter reported a prospective study of 6,108 adults surveyed during 1971–75 in the First National Health and Nutrition Examination Survey.[73] His objective was to focus on the relationship between a history of allergy and the subsequent risk of developing cancer. The group with allergies—those who had been told by a physician that they had asthma, hay fever, hives, food allergy, or any other allergy—constituted 30.1% of the sample, or 26.3% if the category was restricted to those who had allergic histories of more than 5 years. He found that allergy sufferers—controlling for race, sex, age, and smoking history—had a "highly significant positive association between history of any allergy and development of any cancer." A family history of allergy was also a risk factor for subsequent cancer.

Breaking down the allergies into specific subgroups, and the cancers into specific diagnoses, McWhorter found that *the strongest cancer association was with hives and "lymphatic and hematopoietic malignancies, which included leukemias, lymphomas, and myelomas* [emphasis added]. . . . The adjusted risk factor of developing a lymphatic-hematopoietic malignancy for persons with hives was particularly strong."[73]

This study is, the author notes, the first prospective study that controls for age, sex, smoking, and race, and the first based on a population derived from a national probability sample. The limitations of the study included the small numbers of people with specific allergies and specific cancer types, and the very real possibility that allergic symptoms were underreported by people with higher cancer risk—nonwhites, smokers, males, and older people.[74]

In *Modern Nutrition in Health and Disease,* Maurice Shils supports McWhorter's findings in one significant area: he reports on a series of studies which document an increased risk of intestinal lymphomas among patients with celiac syndrome. Celiac syndrome is an allergy or hypersensitivity to the gliadin fraction of grain protein gluten. Three separate studies reviewed by Shils found a very high incidence of intestinal lymphomas in a series of celiac patients: 10% in one study, 6.2% in a second, and 6.9% in a third: "Because of this relationship, lymphoma should be suspected with the onset of celiac syndrome in middle age especially, but also in young people particularly with certain racial backgrounds. *Males above 40 years of age with long-standing celiac syndrome who are not eating a gluten-free diet are a major risk group* [emphasis added].[75]

To this, I would add some personal and clinical notes. I have a special interest in this subject because my father developed an intestinal non-Hodgkin's lymphoma and my brother was born a celiac syndrome child. I developed a celiac condition when I was 40, accompanied, when uncontrolled, by hives, and my son has also been diagnosed with a wheat allergy which may well reflect broader celiac sensitivity. I have strong reason to suspect an undiagnosed celiac condition in my father, based on a lifelong history of skin rashes similar to those my brother and I experience when we do not follow a celiac diet. To my knowledge, lymphoma patients (including Hodgkin's disease patients) are rarely, if ever, informed of the high incidence of celiac syndrome preceding lymphoma. I wonder—as I do with other nutritionally related cancer research—whether a diet that may well prevent the development of lymphomas might play some adjunctive role in controlling an established lymphoma, particularly when there is a history of celiac disease.

I would hypothesize further that allergy may play a protective role against some cancers—especially in certain phases of an allergic life history—but that it might play a contributing role at other times or for other cancers. Borrowing from Hans Selye's stress studies, some allergists believe that allergies may stimulate the immune system for a considerable period of time, but that sustained stress over long periods (including allergic stress) may result ultimately in depleted resilience. Thus, the allergy might be protective in an earlier period of life, but if allergies and other stresses exhaust immunocompetence in later life, it might become a risk factor. One finding in the McWhorter study is intriguing in this regard: the one age period in which allergy appeared to have a protective effect was in the youngest adults surveyed—the 25- to 34-year-olds—where the risk odds ratio of having allergies and developing cancer was less than one—0.7.[76]

Immune function in cancer patients is sometimes tested by seeing whether they are *capable* of generating an allergic response. Both mainstream and some alternative medicines (notably the Gerson program) recognize the return of capacity for allergic response as evidence of a recovering immune system. Many alternative nutritional cancer therapies are widely reported to diminish allergic responses in healthy people, and for good reason: they often eliminate or greatly diminish exposure to common food allergens such as wheat, dairy products, caffeine, refined carbohydrates, chocolate, and eggs. That raises the question of whether or not there may be a benefit in reducing exposure to nutritional, chemical, or other allergic or hypersensitivity stresses in cancer. The hypothesis would be that relieving the significant immune stress of the allergy or hypersensitivity might support the recovery of immune potential to combat the cancer. I know of no research on this significant point.

Conclusion

So what can we conclude from the vitamin and mineral research? Certainly as much as this:

1. Vitamins A (with the retinoids and carotenoids), C, and E and several of the B vitamins have shown significant anticancer effects in experimental, epidemiological, and clinical studies. The most significant vitamins for general anticancer effect are the antioxidant vitamins A, C, and E. The use of these vitamins should be considered in both prevention and treatment.

2. Vitamin C has been the subject of a great controversy: it is not yet clear whether, in pharmacological doses, it enhances survival, as Cameron and Pauling claim. But more recent studies do indicate that it may have a protective effect against cancer, some antitumor

effects, and the capacity to diminish side effects of radiotherapy and chemotherapy and improve outcomes. A few recent studies support Pauling and Cameron's hypothesis that vitamin C may help slow tumor progression and extend life. Interesting cell line research proposes that vitamin C may be powerfully potentiated when administered in combination with vitamin K_3.

3. *Patients with leukemia should be cautious in taking vitamin C.* One study shows that it enhanced leukemia development in some human leukemia cell lines and inhibited leukemia development in other cell lines. This raises the more important proposition that nutrients, in general, may act to enhance or inhibit cancer. This can be true not only in different cell lines or animal models, or in different human cancers, but the same nutrient may enhance or inhibit histologically identical cancers in different patients. However, this capacity of some nutrients to affect the same cancer in different directions is probably relatively rare, in comparison with the ability of specific nutrients to inhibit or enhance cancer unidirectionally.

4. Vitamin E has a wide range of positive effects in cancer—particularly vitamin E succinate. It enhances the effects of selenium, and enhances some chemotherapies, radiotherapy, and hyperthermia. It also may help prevent hair loss, and it protects the heart (in animal studies) from cardiac toxicity from doxorubicin.

5. B vitamin supplementation should be approached with care. Vitamin B_{12} can act both as a tumor promoter and a tumor-inhibitor; its tumor-enhancing activities are partially controlled by methionine. Vitamin B_6 (pyridoxine) is deficient in many cancer patients and has been used to enhance the outcome of radiotherapy in a controlled prospective trial.

6. Among the minerals, selenium has broad immunopotentiating and anticancer effects, whereas zinc is a selenium antagonist. While zinc is an essential nutrient for life, great care should be taken in using zinc supplements with cancer.

References

1   Peter Greenwald, "Principles of Cancer Prevention: Diet and Nutrition." In Vincent T. DeVita, Jr., ed., *Cancer: Principles and Practice of Oncology* (Philadelphia: J.B. Lippincott Company,1989), 169.

2   Ibid.

3   Ibid.

4   Ibid.

5   Ibid.

6   Ibid.

7   National Academy of Sciences, National Research Council, Committee on Diet, Nutrition and Cancer, *Diet, Nutrition and Cancer* (Washington, DC: National Academy Press, 1982), 9–5.

8   Greenwald, "Principles of Cancer Prevention: Diet and Nutrition." In DeVita, ed., *Cancer: Principles and Practice of Oncology,* 170. See also Melvyn R. Werbach, *Nutritional Influences on Illness* (Tarzana, CA: Third Line Press, 1987), 103–4 and National Academy of Sciences, *Diet, Nutrition and Cancer,* 9-2–9-3.

9   M.S. Menkes et al., "Serum Beta-Carotene, Vitamins A and E, Selenium and the Risk of Lung Cancer," *New England Journal of Medicine* 315:1250 (1986). Abstracted in Werbach, *Nutritional Influences on Illness,* 104.

10   L. LeMarchand, et al., "Vegetable Consumption and Lung Cancer Risk: A Population-Based Case-Control Study in Hawaii," *Journal of the National Cancer Institute* 81(15):1158–64 (1989).

11   W.C. Willett, "Vitamin A and Lung Cancer," *Nutrition Review* 48(5):201–11 (1990).

12   W. Bollag, "Vitamin A and the Retinoids: From Nutrition to Pharmacotherapy in Dermatology and Oncology," *Lancet* 8329(1):860–3 (1983).

13   Waun Ki Hong et al., "13-*Cis*-Retinoic Acid in the Treatment of Oral Leukoplakia," *New England Journal of Medicine* 315:1501–5 (1986).

14   William D. DeWys et al., "The Chemoprevention Program of the National Cancer Institute." In Frank L. Meyskens, Jr. and Kedar N. Prasad, *Vitamins and Cancer: Human Cancer Prevention by Vitamins and Micronutrients* (Clifton, NJ: Humana, 1986), 301–10.

15   Lawrence Kushi, personal communication with the author, July 1990.

16   Frank L. Meyskens, Jr., "Prevention and Treatment of Cancer with Vitamin A and the Retinoids." In K.N. Prasad, ed., *Vitamins, Nutrition and Cancer* (Basel: Karger, 1984), 266.

17   Ibid., 270.

18   Ibid., 271.

19   National Academy of Sciences, *Diet, Nutrition and Cancer,* 9–15.

20   Ibid., 9–12.

21   Ibid., 9–13.

22   M.E. Poydock et al., "Inhibiting Effect of Vitamins C and B12 on the Mitotic Activity of Ascites Tumors," *Experimental Cell Biology* 47(3):210–7 (1979). Abstracted in Werbach, *Nutritional Influences on Illness,* 109.

23   Isao Eto and Carlos L. Krumdieck, "Role of Vitamin B12 and Folate Deficiencies in Carcinogenesis." In Lionel A. Poirier et al., eds., *Essential Nutrients in Carcinogenesis* (New York: Plenum Press, 1986), 313–30.

24   Hans A. Ladner and Richard M. Salkeld, "Vitamin B_6 Status in Cancer Patients: Effect of Tumor Site, Irradiation, Hormones and Chemotherapy." In George Tryfiates and Kedar N. Prasad, eds., *Nutrition, Growth and Cancer* (New York: Alan R. Liss, 1988), 273–81.

25   Ibid., 278.

26   Robert D. Reynolds, "Vitamin B_6 Deficiency and Carcinogenesis." In Poirier, et al., eds., *Essential Nutrients in Carcinogenesis,* 339–45.

27   E. Cameron and L. Pauling, "Supplemental Ascorbate in the Supportive Treatment of Cancer: Prolongation of Survival Times in Terminal Human Cancer," *Proceedings of the National Academy of Sciences USA,* 73:3685–9 (1976). See also "Supplemental Ascorbate in the Supportive Treatment of Cancer: Reevaluation of Prolongation of Survival Times in Terminal Human Cancer," *Proceedings of the National Academy of Sciences USA* 75:4538–42 (1978). Both abstracts cited in Werbach, *Nutritional Influences on Illness,* 107–8.

28   E.T. Creagan et al., "Failure of High-Dose Vitamin C (Ascorbic Acid) Therapy to Benefit Patients with Advanced Cancer: A Controlled Trial," *New England Journal of Medicine* 301:687–90 (1979). Ibid., 107.

29   C.G. Moertel et al., "High Dose Vitamin C versus Placebo in the Treatment of Patients with Advanced Cancer Who Have Had No Prior Chemotherapy: A Randomized Double-Blind Comparison," *New England Journal of Medicine* 312:137–41 (1985). Ibid., 107.

30   Evelleen Richards, "Vitamin C Suffers a Dose of Politics," *New Scientist,* 27 February 1986, 46–9.

31   Ibid., 48–9.

32   Maurice E. Shils, M.D., "Nutrition and Diet in Cancer." In Maurice E. Shils and Vernon R. Young, eds., *Modern Nutrition in Health and Disease* (Philadelphia: Lea & Febiger, 1988), 1414.

33   Dietrich H. Hornig et al., "Ascorbic Acid." In Shils and Young, *Modern Nutrition in Health and Disease,* 425. The citation of the Japanese hospital study was to A. Murata, F. Morishige, and H. Yamaguchi, "Prolongation of Survival Times of Terminal Cancer Patients by Administration of Large Doses of Ascorbate." In A. Hanck, ed., *Vitamin C: New Clinical Applications in Immunology, Lipid Metabolism and Cancer* (Berne: Huber Verlag, 1982), 103–14.

34   National Academy of Sciences, *Diet, Nutrition and Cancer,* 9–8.

35   Gladys Block, "Epidemiologic Data on the Role of Ascorbic Acid in Cancer Prevention." Meeting abstract, "Ascorbic Acid: Biological Functions and Relation to Cancer," National Institutes of Health, Bethesda, MD, 10–2 September 1990.

36   Geoffrey Howe, "Dietary Factors and Risk of Breast Cancer: Combined Analysis of 12 Case-Controlled Studies," *Journal of the American Medical Association* 82(7)561–9 (1990).

37   Richard I. Schwarz, "Ascorbate Stabilizes the Differentiated State and Reduces the Ability of Rous Sarcoma Virus to Replicate and to Uniformly Transform Cell Cultures."

Meeting abstract, "Ascorbic Acid: Biological Functions and Relation to Cancer," National Institutes of Health, Bethesda, MD, 10–2 September 1990.

38   Alfred B. Hanck, "Vitamin C and Cancer." In Tryfiates and Prasad, eds., *Nutrition, Growth and Cancer,* 307–20.

39   Ibid., 309.

40   Carmina Borek, "Free Radicals, Dietary Antioxidants and Mechanisms in Cancer Prevention: In Vitro Studies." In Meyskens and Prasad, eds., *Vitamins and Cancer,* 68.

41   Ibid., 75.

42   Etsuo Niki, "Action of Ascorbic Acid as a Scavenger of Active and Stable Oxygen Radicals." Meeting abstract, "Ascorbic Acid: Biological Functions and Relation to Cancer," National Institutes of Health, Bethesda, MD, 10–2 September 1990.

43   Balz Frei and Bruce N. Ames, "Ascorbic Acid Protects Plasma Lipids Against Oxidative States." Meeting abstract, "Ascorbic Acid: Biological Functions and Relation to Cancer," National Institutes of Health, Bethesda, MD, 10–2 September 1990.

44   Joachim G. Liehr, "Inhibition by Vitamin C of Incidence and Severity of Renal Tumors Induced by Estradiol or Diethylstilbestrol." Meeting abstract, "Ascorbic Acid: Biological Functions and Relation to Cancer," National Institutes of Health, Bethesda, MD, 10–2 September 1990.

45   Hanck, "Vitamin C and Cancer." In Tryfiates and Prasad, eds., *Nutrition, Growth and Cancer,* 310.

46   Vincenzo Noto et al., "Effects of Sodium Ascorbate (Vitamin C) and 2-Methyl-1,4-Naphthoquinone (Vitamin K_3) Treatment on Human Tumor Cell Growth in Vitro," *Cancer* 63:901–6 (1989).

47   Hanck, "Vitamin C and Cancer." In Tryfiates and Prasad, eds., *Nutrition, Growth and Cancer,* 312.

48   Ibid., 312–4.

49   Paul Okunieff, "Interactions Between Ascorbic Acid, Radiation Therapy, and Misonidazole." Meeting abstract, Ascorbic Acid: Biological Functions and Relation to Cancer," National Institutes of Health, Bethesda, MD, 10–2 September 1990.

50   Kan Shimpo et al. "Ascorbic Acid and Adriamycin Toxicity." Meeting abstract, "Ascorbic Acid: Biological Functions and Relation to Cancer," National Institutes of Health, Bethesda, MD, 10–2 September 1990.

51   K.N. Prasad et al., "Sodium Ascorbate Potentiates the Growth Inhibitory Effect of Certain Agents on Neuroblastoma Cells in Culture," *Proceedings of the National Academy of Sciences USA* 76(2):29–32 (1979). See also K.N. Prasad, "Modulation of the Effects of Tumor Therapeutic Agents by Vitamin C," *Life Sciences* 21(2):275–80 (1980). Abstracts cited in Werbach, *Nutritional Influences on Illness,* 108.

52   Chan H. Park, "Vitamin C in Leukemia and Preleukemia Cell Growth." In Tryfiates and Prasad, eds., *Nutrition, Growth and Cancer,* 321–30.

53   Chan H. Park and Bruce F. Kimler, "Growth Modulation of Human Leukemic and Preleukemic Progenitor Cells by L-Ascorbic Acid." Meeting abstract, "Ascorbic Acid: Biological Functions and Relation to Cancer," National Institutes of Health, Bethesda, MD, 10–2 September 1990.

54   National Academy of Sciences, *Diet, Nutrition and Cancer,* 9–10.

55   Ibid.

56   Kedar N. Prasad, "Summary and Overview." In Poirier et al., eds., *Essential Nutrients in Carcinogenesis,* 543–7.

57   K.N. Prasad, "Mechanisms of Action of Vitamin E on Mammalian Tumor Cells in Culture." In Tryfiates and Prasad, eds., *Nutrition, Growth and Cancer,* 363–75.

58   Ibid., 364.

59   K.N. Prasad, "Modification of the Effect of Pharmacological Agents, Ionizing Radiation and Hyperthermia on Tumor Cells by Vitamin E." In Prasad, ed., *Vitamins, Nutrition and Cancer,* 76–104.

60   K.N. Prasad et al., "Vitamin E Enhances the Growth Inhibitory and Differentiating Effects of Tumor Therapeutic Agents on Neuroblastoma and Glioma Cells in Culture," *Proceeds of the Society for Experimental Biological Medicine* 164(2):158–63 (1980). Abstracted in Werbach, *Nutritional Influences on Illness,* 109–10.

61   L. Wood, "Possible Prevention of Adriamiacin-Induced Alopecia by Tocopherol," *New England Journal of Medicine* 312:1060 (1985). Abstract cited in Werbach, ibid.

62   K.N. Prasad, *Vitamins Against Cancer: Fact and Fiction* (Denver: Nutrition Publishing House, 1984), 91.

63   Ibid., 65–7.

64   Gerhard N. Schrauzer, "Selenium in Nutritional Cancer Prophylaxis." In K.N. Prasad, ed., *Vitamins, Nutrition and Cancer,* 240–50.

65   Ibid., 243.

66   Ibid., 244.

67   Ibid., 243.

68   Carmia Borek, "Free Radicals, Dietary Antioxidants and Mechanisms in Cancer Prevention: In Vitro Studies." In Meyskens and Prasad, eds., *Vitamins and Cancer,* 65–92.

69   Ibid., 73.

70   National Academy of Sciences, *Diet, Nutrition and Cancer,* 10–8.

71   Ibid., 10–8–9.

72   Ibid., 10–10–11.

73   William P. McWhorter, "Allergy and Risk of Cancer: A Prospective Study Using NHANESI [First National Health and Nutrition Examination Survey] Followup Data," *Cancer* 62:451–5 (1988).

74   Ibid., 454.

75   Maurice E. Shils, "Nutrition and Neoplasia." In Robert S. Goodhart, M.D., and Maurice E. Shils, M.D., eds., *Modern Nutrition in Health and Disease* (Philadelphia: Lea & Febiger, 1980), 1177.

76   McWhorter, "Allergy and Risk of Cancer," 453.

thirteen

Unconventional Nutritional Approaches to Cancer—An Overview

In any discussion of the unconventional nutritional approaches to cancer, it is useful to develop a typology that clarifies the basic differences between these various approaches. For example:

- Most unconventional nutritional cancer therapies are vegetarian, but some are not.
- Some nutritional cancer therapies involve primarily raw foods (such as the Gerson diet and the Hippocrates wheat-grass therapy), while others (such as macrobiotics) involve primarily cooked foods.
- Many nutritional cancer therapies use nutritional supplements as well as diet (such as the Livingston program), but others (such as macrobiotics) do not use supplements.
- Some nutritional cancer therapies place major emphasis on the inclusion of specific foods known in scientific studies to have anticancer effects (such as Keith Block's nutritional program), while others do not.
- Some therapies place emphasis on different foods believed in traditional medicines to have anticancer effects, but these recommendations—as in macrobiotic and Ayurvedic cancer diets—may often be directly contradictory.

- Some therapies (such as the Gerson diet) place a major emphasis on low sodium, high potassium foods, while others (such as macrobiotics) do not.
- Some therapies (such as the Gerson diet) place a stringent emphasis on organic foods, while others do not.
- Some therapies are protein-restrictive, while others are not.
- Some therapies include detoxification measures (such as the Gerson and Hippocrates program enemas), while others do not.
- Some therapies are purely nutritional, while others integrate nutritional, psychological, spiritual, immunosupportive, and other forms of treatment.

From the great variety of unconventional nutritional approaches, certain commonalities emerge. Most of the alternative nutritional approaches to cancer involve fresh, whole foods eaten in nutritionally balanced combinations with a strong emphasis on a primarily vegetarian diet. Fundamentally, they shift the diet in directions known from epidemiological studies to be helpful in lowering the incidence of many of the common cancers. If they sometimes recommend drastic dietary changes, it is because reversing an established cancer is obviously a much more difficult proposition than preventing the development of cancer.

A critical distinction for cancer patients exists between nutritional programs *known* to be nutritionally adequate and other programs which apparently work, when they do, by the cancer-inhibiting effects of selective nutrient restriction (see chapter 11). These latter approaches, like chemotherapies, involve a real element of danger: they assume that the cancer is more vulnerable than the host organism to nutrient restriction, and that the cancer will be controlled before the patient loses too much weight.

In reality, different patients respond very differently to all nutritional cancer therapies, including both those known to be nutritionally adequate for most people and those that are severely nutrient-restrictive. A specific cancer patient may find even the nutritionally adequate diet personally inadequate for him, as shown by continuing weight loss without stabilization at some healthy level. Yet another person with cancer may stabilize at an adequate, if low, weight on a quite restrictive diet. But the restrictive diets clearly involve additional risk.

These are excellent reasons why *intensive* nutritional therapies for cancer should, in the ideal world, be medically supervised by broad-minded, nutritionally trained oncologists who are aware of how to modulate a nutritional program according to the individual patient's responses and nutritional needs. One of the unfortunate realities is that such broad-minded nutritionally trained oncologists are extraordinarily rare. So the patient is usually left to his own devices, or to supervision by a physician with at best broad practical nutritional experience. The tragic cases are when self-supervision, or supervision by an untrained practitioner, leads to progressive weight loss, decisive weakening of the patient, and death.

The Problem of Weight Loss in Nutritional Cancer Therapies

I want to tell the story of Luis, a wonderful South American man with metastatic prostate cancer who came as a participant to the Commonweal Cancer Help Program. He had done extremely well with the support of a gifted mainstream doctor using a hormonal therapy and a macrobiotic program. His cancer was in remission for several years. One day I had a call from the macrobiotic practitioner who had taught Luis the macrobiotic diet. He described how, with a recurrence of his cancer, Luis had gone to a Mexican clinic where he had been put on a highly restrictive raw foods diet. He grew progressively weaker, but his symptoms of physiological decline were interpreted to him by the staff at the clinic as "healing crises." He finally grew so weak from the diet that he died. The macrobiotic practitioner was distraught. It was, he said, a profound lesson to him about the dangers of some nutritional therapies. While he believed that "healing crises" (in holistic health theory, the temporary augmentation of some symptoms as the body detoxifies and begins to recover) are a reality in many holistic treatments, he saw how destructively the term had been used at the Mexican clinic where Luis had gone: how in fact this nutritional program had cost Luis his life.

The experience of Luis is not a common one. But it is not, unfortunately, entirely uncommon. I also knew the wife of a senior American scientist, who described to me how her husband, with a liver cancer, had gone on the Hippocrates wheat-grass program. There are many people with cancer who believe that the Hippocrates program has been a benefit to them, particularly as a short-term detoxification program. But this man followed the highly restrictive raw foods diet rigorously despite the fact that with his particular physiology and condition he experienced progressive weight loss without any sign of stabilization. His wife had supported him wholeheartedly in undertaking the program, given that conventional medicine had nothing to offer him. But as he became progressively more emaciated, she became more and more concerned. She was convinced, she told me, the diet was a significant contributor to his death.

In still another case with which I am familiar, a man with prostate cancer and his woman partner undertook a macrobiotic diet together. The man did very well on the macrobiotic program, but his partner, seeking in solidarity to eat exactly what he ate, progressively lost weight until friends became very concerned for her. The friends convinced her that *she* simply was not physiologically the same as her mate and that she needed to broaden her diet. She did so, while remaining primarily macrobiotic, and stabilized at a healthy weight.

My point is that nutritional approaches to cancer, while characteristically nontoxic and generally health-promoting, *can be dangerous* if not appropriately supervised or if not undertaken with self-awareness and common sense. The razor's edge with nutritional therapies, as I said in chapter 11, is with those nutrient-restrictive therapies which—like chemotherapies—require finding the margin where life is sustained but the cancer is, in theory, inhibited. This usually requires a carefully supervised course of treatment. The critical question appears to be whether or not an individual's weight *stabilizes*—often at his college or high-school weight—after a few months on the program. If there is no stabilization, and weight loss is progressive, the patient is almost certainly on a diet that is nutritionally inadequate.

On the other hand, it is important to point out the fact that moderate weight loss is what many cancer patients need, especially in breast cancer and other cancers in which obesity is a known risk factor. Chapter 11 reviewed in some detail the reasons why caloric restriction may be helpful both in primary prevention and in preventing recurrence in some cancers. Nor should we be surprised that a given nutritional therapy can produce positive results for one person and negative results for another. Just as different people with the same cancer have different responses to a specific chemotherapy, the same is true with nutritional approaches. Because few clinical trials of these therapies have been conducted, both the physician and the patient should carefully watch for any changes brought about by the diet.

Ian Gawler's Approach to Anticancer Diets

Ian Gawler, an Australian veterinarian, has developed a good example of a reasoned integral approach to cancer that utilizes diet, meditation, and some of the other therapies that we have already discussed. Following the amputation of his leg and the development of inoperable and highly visible chest wall tumors extruding from his chest, Gawler recovered from an advanced metastatic osteosarcoma. He worked with the late Ainslie Meares, an Australian psychiatrist, who wrote up his recovery as an example of the effects of intensive meditation. Subsequently, Gawler became one of the leading exponents in Australia of holistic approaches to cancer. Although his nutritional perspective is not well-known in the United States, he serves as an example of someone who developed a highly intensive holistic nutritional-psychological program based on sane principles and inferences from the nutritional and psychological literature.

To begin with, Gawler makes a sensible overview of the main dietary options. There are, he suggests, basically four alternatives:

First, you may not wish to make any changes in your diet. This, as Gawler emphasizes, is fine for some people. And it is true that exceptional recoveries from cancer do take place without any dietary change. At the same time, as Daan C. Baalen and Marco J. de Vries of Erasmus University found in their study of remissions from cancer in the Netherlands, dietary change is one of the most frequent concomitants of spontaneous regression of cancer.[1]

Second, you may adopt a maintenance diet that is basically a healthy, wholefoods diet that avoids foods and substances known to be injurious to health. This is a beneficial step and, as Gawler points out, a major one for some people who have eaten poor diets in the past. Simply starting to eat a healthy whole-foods diet—such as that recommended by the National Academy of Sciences—can make a major contribution to health.

Third, you may develop an individualized nutritional program of any level of vigor and intensity. This is what Gawler himself finally did, based on experience he developed after following the Gerson diet for 3 months. The sensitivities he developed to foods that helped or hurt him on the Gerson diet led to an awareness of how to individualize his own nutrition optimally.

Fourth, you can commit yourself to one of the intensive programs, such as the Gerson diet, macrobiotics, or the Bristol diet program, preferably seeking professional help to undertake it.[2]

From his years of dietary experimentation, Gawler proposed four basic principles for nutritional cancer therapy: (1) the body should be detoxified; (2) any vitamin and mineral imbalances need to be corrected; (3) digestion should be restored and the diet made up of only fresh, vital, pure, and suitably prepared food; and (4) the patient needs to develop and maintain a positive attitude, both in general and toward his diet in particular.[3] Let us discuss each of these briefly.

Detoxification

It is fascinating that the concept of detoxification—the removal of existing toxins from the system—and the avoidance of introducing new toxins—have virtually no credibility in mainstream nutrition *despite the fact that the carcinogenic impact of toxic substances in human biology is well known*. Yet detoxification is a fundamental practice in many forms of traditional medicine, especially naturopathic medicine. Writes Gawler:

> It makes good sense to remove any toxins in the system and then avoid introducing any new sources of toxic material. The latter is easier than the former, and can be done by avoiding those things incriminated as having an increased risk of cancer.

> Removing toxins from the body is not such a simple business in theory or practice. It is certainly more open to medical debate. Again, these principles do work, and I suggest they can be validated. . . . What is not so reasonable is the emphasis some patients put on detoxifying [e.g., through excessive emphasis on enemas]. Perhaps this is because of feelings of uncleanliness that sometimes accompany disease, but it disappoints me to see some people seeming to delight in detoxifying through cleansing and purging in a rather violent way. Detoxifying is not just cleansing the bowels with gusto! It is a *thorough* spring cleaning for the *whole body* and can be done gently.[4]

Gawler recommends "eating a lot of fresh, vital foods [to] get the process in motion." He agrees with Gerson on the use of freshly prepared vegetable and fruit juices, but does not agree that these juices are always needed hourly 12 times a day. He also accepts Gerson's concept that raw organic liver juice may help build the blood. He also found Gerson's coffee enemas effective as a liver stimulant—a point to which I will return in my discussion of Gerson.

Nutritional Supplementation in Vitamin and Mineral Imbalances

As I mentioned in chapter 11, there is good evidence that modern American diets are often nutritionally unbalanced, that cancer patients specifically often demonstrate nutritional imbalances both prior to and after development of cancer, and that, in laboratory and animal experiments, specific nutrients can slow, stop, or reverse the progress of some cancers. This research raises the issue of whether cancer patients should use nutritional supplements. This, Gawler correctly concludes, is one of the most difficult nutritional areas in which to say anything definitive. His view is that the Gerson diet and some other intensive regimens provide very high levels of needed nutrients in natural forms and balances.

But many cancer patients on intensive programs still use supplements despite the fact that the proponents of the therapies often, in principle, recommend against them. Gawler tried megavitamin therapy but found it did not help him, although "at specific times I have felt the need for specific supplements and benefitted from them . . . supplements are a difficult question, the one I find the hardest to be clear about and I make no definite recommendations."[5]

Digestion and Fresh Food

With regard to restoring the digestion and switching the diet to fresh, vital, pure, and suitably prepared food, there is good evidence for the higher nutrient values of such foods. At the same time, one rarely finds mainstream physicians or nutritionists speaking in these essentially holistic terms about the quality of food patients should eat. Gawler observes:

Here again the idea of supplementing the digestive functions is medically questionable. I find this easier to put forward [than recommendations for nutritional supplements] as there is little doubt that most cancer patients initially do have an impaired digestion. Gerson recommended supplementing stomach acid and pancreatic enzymes. There have been several claims that pancreatic enzymes can actually attack cancer cells and digest them. I find the evidence for this to be sketchy. It is hard to imagine such supplements doing harm, however, and there is a body of circumstantial evidence which suggests that they might do good. I took them while I was on Gerson's therapy but they were one of the first things I discontinued.[6]

Positive Attitude toward Food

The idea that it is important to develop and maintain a positive attitude in general and toward a healthy diet in particular is virtually never discussed in mainstream nutrition but is one that Gawler emphasizes:

> This whole area of diet is full of excitement, controversy and the definite prospect of being helpful. It is essential to be clear in your own mind as to the relevance it has for you. You should feel good about your choices. It is very necessary to think about the whole area and come to definite conclusions. In the final analysis, food should be a happy thing. You should be able to sit down before it, give thanks for what you have to eat, know that it is appropriate for your situation, and eat with a smile on your lips and a song in your heart![7]

In short, the four basic nutritional-psychological concepts that Gawler discusses—which are broadly representative of many alternative cancer therapies—are not inconsistent with any scientific evidence but do go beyond science in proposing that such a diet and attitude may assist in recovery from cancer.

What is particularly valuable about Gawler's contribution to the field of holistic nutritional-psychological approaches to cancer is that his position is not doctrinaire. He personally has experienced a documented recovery from an advanced cancer from which he was expected to die. He achieved his recovery while using intensive nutritional and psychological measures. And yet he did not come out of this recovery experience—as many understandably do—a true believer and zealot for a specific nutritional program as *the answer* for everyone with cancer. Rather, he takes a balanced and at the same time very vigorous perspective on nutrition as a key for some people to cancer recovery. He carefully notes that detoxification is not discussed in the contemporary mainstream medical literature, and that nutritional supplementation represents a problematic area. He allows everyone room to choose his own type and level of nutritional intervention. He personally undertook one of the most rigorous nutritional programs—the Gerson diet—and then continuously modified it until he reached an individualized program.

Keeping in mind Gawler's example of a flexible and reasoned approach to nutrition in cancer, in the next four chapters we look at some of the major nutritional therapies.

References

1   Daan C. van Baalen, Marco J. de Vries, and Marjolein T. Gondrie, "Psycho-Social Correlates of 'Spontaneous' Regression in Cancer." Monograph, Department of General Pathology, Medical Faculty, Erasmus University, Rotterdam, the Netherlands, April 1987, 6.
2   Ian Gawler, *You Can Conquer Cancer* (Melbourne: Hill of Content, 1986), 99.
3   Ibid., 90–1.
4   Ibid., 91.
5   Ibid., 97.
6   Ibid., 97.
7   Ibid., 9.

fourteen

The Gerson Diet—A Radical Anticancer Therapy

"I see in Max Gerson one of the most eminent geniuses in medical history."

Albert Schweitzer

Until the advent of the macrobiotic diet, the Gerson therapy was, for many years, the best-known nutritional therapy for cancer in the United States. Today, thousands of cancer patients still practice the Gerson diet and diets based on Gerson's regimen. The Gerson Institute in Bonita, California, directed by Charlotte Gerson, Max Gerson's daughter, and the Gerson Clinic in Tijuana, Mexico, continue his work. Derived from a combination of scientific research and the European folk medical tradition by German physician Max B. Gerson, the therapy requires a patient to eat a raw vegetarian diet for a prolonged period. Cooked foods and some animal products may be added later. A patient drinks specific freshly prepared vegetable and fruit juices every hour, takes four types of enemas, including coffee enemas, and also consumes two to three glasses of fresh calf's liver juice each day.[1]

The Gerson regimen as currently offered in Mexico is a radical anticancer therapy in that it involves a *tremendous* level of personal commitment. When fully undertaken, it requires a full-time effort by a reasonably mobile and energetic person who does not have to work and who has access to the requisite fresh organic produce year-round. It works best when undertaken jointly by a cancer patient and a spouse or friend, and even then it is close to a full-time project for both people. The psychological consequences of making and sustaining such a full-time commitment to physical recovery are potentially a significant element in recoveries associated with the Gerson program.

Patricia Spain Ward, Ph.D., a medical historian at the University of Illinois at Chicago, has outlined the history of the Gerson therapy for the Office of Technology Assessment:[2]

> It is one of the least edifying facts of recent American medical history that the profession's leadership so long rejected as quackish the idea that nutrition affects health. Ignoring both the empirical dietary wisdom that pervaded western medicine from the pre-Christian Hippocratic era until the late nineteenth century and a persuasive body of modern research in nutritional biochemistry, the politically-minded spokesmen of organized medicine in the U.S. remained long committed to surgery and radiation as the sole acceptable treatments of cancer. . . .

> The historical record shows that progress lagged especially in cancer immunotherapy—including nutrition and hyperthermia—because power over professional affiliation and publication (and hence over practice and research) rested with men who were neither scholars nor practitioners nor researchers themselves, and who were often unequipped to grasp the rapidly evolving complexities of the sciences underlying mid-twentieth-century medicine.

> Nowhere is this maladaptation of professional structure to medicine's changing scientific content more tragically illustrated than in the American experience of Max B. Gerson (1881–1959), founder of the best-known nutritional treatment for cancer of the pre-macrobiotic era. A scholar's scholar and a superlative observer of clinical phenomena, Gerson was a product of the German medical education which Americans in the late 19th and early 20th centuries considered so superior to our own that all who could afford it went to Germany to perfect their training.[3]

Gerson's Biography

Gerson graduated from the University of Freiburg in 1909, having studied with leading specialists in internal medicine, physiological chemistry, and neurology. By 1919 he had set up a practice and had devised an effective dietary treatment for migraine, from which he himself suffered. "In 1920," Ward reports, "while treating migraine patients by this salt-free diet, he discovered that it was also effective in lupus vulgaris (tuberculosis of the skin, then considered incurable) and, later, in arthritis as well."[4]

His success with tuberculosis of the skin brought Gerson renown and an opportunity to test the diet with larger numbers of lupus patients at a special Bavarian government–sponsored clinic. The diet was then extended to cases of pulmonary tuberculosis as well. He served as a member of the State Board of Health in Prussia, and also as a consultant to the Prussian Ministry of Health on how to restore depleted soils for agriculture. Ward says: "When he learned that modern farming methods often rob plants of their natural mineral and vitamin riches, while increasing their sodium content, he began to think of the earth's well-being as our own. Eventually, he began to refer to the soil, which nourishes the food we eat, as our "external metabolism."[5]

Gerson first used his diet for cancer in 1928, when a woman with bile duct cancer that had metastasized to the liver insisted he put her on the diet, despite his reluctance to do so. The patient introduced him to a special soup which, according to German folk medical lore, Hippocrates had used for cancer, and which Gerson later adopted for his own therapy. "Having taken up this challenge against his will, with no hope of success," reports Ward, "Gerson was astounded when his patient seemed fully recovered within six months. In quick succession he had the same good results with two patients with inoperable stomach cancer."[6]

After the rise of Hitler, Gerson moved to Vienna where he reported the diet failed with six cancer patients, in his view as a result of poor dietary supervision at the institution where he worked. He then moved to Paris, where he reported the diet produced good results in three of seven cases. He emigrated to the United States in 1938 and in 1939 passed the state medical boards in New York, where he continued to perfect his diet.[7] Ward continues:

> Despite the fact that he had no in-patient facility until 1946, when he opened a clinic in Nanuet, New York, Gerson managed, through his thriving Park Avenue practice and an affiliation at Gotham Hospital, to amass enough data to publish a preliminary report in 1945. He presented his rather remarkable cases modestly, concluding that he did not yet have enough evidence to say whether diet could either influence the origin of the cancer or alter the

course of an established tumor. He claimed only that the diet, which he described in considerable detail, could favorably affect the patient's general condition, staving off the consequences of malignancy and making further treatment possible.[8]

The AMA did not openly attack Gerson until November, 1946, a few months after he testified in support of a Senate bill to appropriate $100 million to bring together the world's outstanding cancer experts in order to coordinate a search for the prevention and cure of cancer.[9]

In many respects, the Senate hearing was hostile to conventional approaches to cancer therapy, and it would have been naive for anyone not to anticipate a possible reaction from the American Medical Association. Gerson presented patients of his who had failed on conventional therapies; he received a strong testimony of support from the medical director of Gotham Hospital, who also reported the results of a study which found that patients who received no treatment for cancer lived longer than conventionally treated patients; and another witness called Gerson's successes "miracles" and, as Ward reports, urged the Senators to secure their future cancer commission against control by any existing medical organization.[10]

Historically, this was a period in which the AMA had recently established its hegemony over American medicine. It was headed by Morris Fishbein, a pugnacious physician who was to make himself infamous in the eyes of many advocates of unconventional cancer therapies for his attacks on Gerson, Hoxsey, and other pioneers of unconventional therapies. It is no surprise to me that Fishbein, faced with congressional hearings inimical to conventional cancer treatment and AMA hegemony, went on the attack. The details of the process by which the AMA destroyed Gerson's professional reputation have been described by Ward and others. Gerson lost his hospital affiliation and was denied malpractice insurance:

According to a 1981 publication of the Gerson Institute, headed by his daughter, Charlotte Gerson, a manuscript for a book he was writing about his therapy disappeared from his files in 1956. At the age of 75, isolated from medical colleagues and unable to find assistants, Gerson undertook the work of rewriting the entire manuscript in order to show "that there is an effective treatment of cancer, even in advanced cases." It was published in 1958 as *A Cancer Therapy: Results of Fifty Cases*. Gerson died of pneumonia the following year.[11]

Interpreting the AMA Attack on Gerson

In evaluating this history, I come down somewhere between the interpretation offered by advocates of the Gerson therapy and that offered by the mainstream critics of Gerson. Many medical historians would agree with Ward that the rejection of nutritional approaches to health in general, and cancer in particular, is among the "least edifying facts" of recent American history. As time passes and scientific evidence supportive of the Gerson and other nutritional approaches to cancer gradually grows, Fishbein's and the AMA's attack on Gerson appears in a less and less favorable light.

On the other hand, a close reading of Ward's recounting of the history of what happened to Gerson shows that the AMA attack on Gerson was scarcely an unpredictable event. An immigrant refugee physician from Germany appears in New York and, in a few short years, opens a thriving Park Avenue practice using an unconventional cancer therapy, opines loudly regarding the health dangers of tobacco (Philip Morris was then the *Journal of the American Medical Association*'s main source of advertising),[12] and on top of that has the temerity to testify before Congress, showing off his recovered patients who had failed on conventional therapies. At the same hearing, others propose that $100 million be spent to investigate apparently allied innovative approaches to cancer; Gerson's hospital chief offers testimony that no treatment at all is better than conventional treatment for cancer; and another witness warns the legislators not to let "any existing medical organizations" (a clear reference to the AMA) control their search.

Regardless of the merits of the Gerson therapy, mainstream medical opinion at that time firmly held the view that nutritional therapies had nothing to offer for cancer treatment, and to this day the evidence for decisive, positive results from Gerson therapy remains highly questionable. In contemporary studies, the Gerson program emerges as a potentially useful *complement* to conventional therapies. But even if, as Ward emphasizes, Gerson was modest in his testimony regarding his claims for his therapy, he allowed himself to be part of a very public critique of the medical establishment of his time, and he did not disassociate himself from testimony by others that his cases were "miracles." He and his colleagues should certainly have been aware of the enormous political risk they were taking. Nor did the AMA attack Gerson before he participated in this hearing before Congress. Prior to that time, he was allowed to develop a thriving medical practice using an alternative therapy for cancer and was affiliated with a New York hospital. The point simply is that the mythological view of some Gerson advocates that Gerson discovered a "cure" for cancer and was, as a result, made the innocent victim of an unprovoked witch-hunt by the AMA, does not stand up to scrutiny, any more than does the view of Gerson critics that he was simply a "quack" who deserved the professional assault he received.

In my view, the question of Gerson's motivations for participating in the congressional hearings could benefit from further historical inquiry. As a recent immigrant, Gerson was either naive about the politics of American medicine, or very poorly advised, or he felt that he had a great mission to accomplish to alert the American public to the potential benefit of nutritional approaches to cancer, and therefore went forward with the hearings despite full knowledge of the dangers. It is not uncommon, among some of the best-known practitioners of unconventional cancer therapies, that they have, rightly or wrongly, a sense of mission that is sometimes accompanied by a sense of personal invincibility and self-confidence that can at times appear grandiose. Nor are charismatic leaders in mainstream medicine any more exempt from these particular characteristics.

For whatever reasons, Gerson, in participating in the congressional hearings, undertook a course of action that appears, at least in retrospect, professionally suicidal. History cannot tell us what would have happened if he had quietly continued his practice, strengthened his contacts with the medical profession, and continued to publish a stream of professional reports in which he made it clear that his nutritional therapy for cancer was not a cure but deserved further evaluation as a useful adjunctive cancer treatment. Instead, he died as another martyr in the cause of alternative cancer therapies.

The Gerson Therapy

According to Gerson, in order to heal,

> "The body must by detoxified—activated with ionized minerals, natural food so that the essential organs can function. For healing the body brings about a kind of inflammation. That is a tremendous transformative reaction. This renders

the body hypersensitive or allergic to the highest degree against abnormal or strange substances (including bacilli, cancer cells, scars, etc.). Consequently the more malignant the cells, the more effective the treatment."[13]

The critical elements in the Gerson therapy are[14]:

1. Salt and water management through sodium restriction and potassium supplementation.
2. High doses of micronutrients through frequent administration of raw fruit and vegetable juices.
3. Extreme fat restriction.
4. Temporary protein restriction through a basic vegetarian diet.
5. Thyroid administration.
6. Frequent coffee enemas.

Raw calf's liver juice, an iodine solution, thyroid extract, extra potassium, pancreatin, and vitamin C were later added to the regimen.[15]

A scholarly man, Gerson continuously explored the medical literature of his day for explanations of why, in his experience, this empirically derived nutritional treatment appeared to work to the degree that some patients achieved cures and many others had positive responses. He came to regard cancer as one of a family of degenerative illnesses in which impaired metabolism underlay the degenerative process. He believed that a number of metabolic functions were deficient in cancer patients, including the metabolism of fats, proteins, carbohydrates, vitamins, and minerals. He also believed that oxygen-supplying enzymes had been inactivated and that the vitality of intestinal bacteria had been impaired.[16]

Gerson believed that his therapy reversed these elements of impaired metabolism. But he also believed that, if the diet and other medications were given without active detoxification, the patient could often die from a liver overburdened by the toxins being released from the body. He placed a central significance on the health of the liver, and sought to stimulate the detoxification of the liver by prescribing coffee enemas as frequently as every 3 or 4 hours, which he believed stimulated the release of bile and aided in the release of toxins.[17] In 1978, the editors of *Physiological Chemistry and Physics* stated that "caffeine enemas cause dilation of the bile ducts, which facilitates excretion of toxic cancer breakdown products by the liver and dialysis of toxic products from blood across the colonic wall."[18] Coffee enemas, long a respected entry in the *Merck Manual*, represented to him a logical component of the detoxification process. He emphasized restoring the oxidative enzymes in the diet, since he believed cancer cells grow in the absence of oxygen and can be inhibited or destroyed by replenishing cellular oxygen supplies. He sought to supply this oxygen using fresh organic fruit and vegetable juices prepared with a stainless steel grinder and press.[19]

The third central element in Gerson's effort to restore healthy metabolism was balancing potassium and sodium in the body. He believed that high-sodium, low-potassium diets contributed to tumor growth, and that high-potassium, low-sodium diets and potassium supplementation could help reverse the unhealthy balance.[20]

Scientific Support for the Gerson Therapy

Because of the attack by the AMA, Gerson's therapy was, for decades, considered one of the prototypical "quack" cancer therapies. But in recent years—as the nutritional research literature on cancer quietly mounted behind doors closed by professional prejudice against nutritional elements in cancer therapy—an increasing number of physicians and researchers have been asking whether Gerson may have had something to contribute after all.

In 1980, writing in the same *Journal of the American Medical Association* that had attacked Gerson, William Regelson, M.D., suggested that "we may shortly have to ask if Gerson's low-sodium diet, with its bizarre coffee enemas and thyroid supplementation, was an approach that altered the mitotic regulating effect of intracellular sodium for occasional clinical validity in those patients with the stamina to survive it."[21]

Similar suggestions, that a more favorable sodium-potassium ratio (such as that created by the Gerson therapy) might affect malignant mitogenesis, had been offered 9 years earlier by Clarence D. Cone, Jr., writing in the *Journal of Theoretical Biology*.[22] In a series of studies, Cone found evidence that the level of electrical polarization found in the membranes of healthy cells was significantly higher than that found in the membranes in proliferating cancer cells.

This "electrical transmembrane potential" can affect, among other things, the capacity of the cell to keep sodium and potassium levels in healthy relationships inside and outside the cell membranes.[22] Basically, the healthy cells had a high potassium and low sodium content and high electrical polarization of their cell walls, while the cancer cells had higher sodium, lower potassium, and lower electrical polarization.

In 1983, a molecular biologist named G.N. Ling wrote an article[23] exploring the clinical implications of this emerging work and its possible theoretical substructure. In it, he explained:

> The recognition of cells as the basic unit of life implies that living matter is not a continuous mass but consists of separate units. This discontinuity between the cell and its aqueous environment is selective in a subtle manner. Thus from the earliest days of biology, it was recognized that water can move in and out of the cells with relative ease. . . . It [later] became clear that the living cell membrane is not just permeable to water but is also permeable to a host of other solutes dissolved in water. The most surprising of this new revelation concerns the permeability of sugar, free amino acids, and salt, which at high strength cause sustained cell shrinkage. . . .

> If the cell membrane is permeable to a particular solute, one expects that over a long period of time, this solute would reach and be maintained in the cell wall at the same concentration as that in the external medium. Yet old cells as well as young cells share the striking characteristic of maintaining the same high level of potassium and the same low level of sodium in the cell water while the aqueous environment in which these cells are bathed contains as a rule a low level of potassium and a high level of sodium.[23]

Ling went on to propose a highly technical explanation of how the relationship was maintained. This line of research was seized on by F.W. Cope, M.D., in an article entitled "A Medical Application of the Ling Association-Induction Hypothesis: The High Potassium, Low-Sodium Diet of the Gerson Cancer Therapy."[24] Cope wrote:

> This paper shows how modern work on cation association [i.e., the behavior of ions in a solution] and water structuring in cells supports and makes more precise some of the deductions Gerson made from his medical experiments with cancer patients. An essential component of Gerson's cancer therapy was the use of a low sodium, high potassium diet. Indeed, he found experimentally

that cancers regressed faster if large quantities of inorganic solutions of potassium were given in addition to a diet which was already high in potassium.

Gerson attempted to understand the biochemical and biophysical reasons for the observed success of low sodium and high potassium diets in the cure of cancer. He recognized the significance of this question and devoted much space in his book to correlations with known experimental facts. He observed that cancer patients always had marked degeneration of other tissues. . . . Gerson made the general deduction that a major part of the reason for the observed success of the low sodium, high potassium diets in the treatment of cancer was that they forced a correction of the generalized tissue damage . . .[24]

Tissue damage, from any cause and in any tissues, produces a similar set of changes in tissue salt and water, which Cope called "the tissue damage syndrome."

The most easily observed components of the tissue damage syndrome . . . are decreased cell potassium, increased cell sodium, and increased cell water (cell swelling or tissue edema). . . .

The high potassium, low sodium diet of the Gerson cancer therapy is a logical strategy for improving the health of the body tissues, of which probably all, and certainly the liver, are suffering from the tissue damage syndrome. . . .

In the damaged or partly damaged cell, the cell proteins lose all or part of the preference of their sites for associating with potassium rather than sodium. Therefore if in the environment around the cell the concentration of potassium is increased compared to sodium, the association sites are forced to accept more potassium and less sodium. . . . This tends to restore the normal configuration of the proteins. Therefore treatment with the Gerson diet to increase tissue potassium concentration and to decrease tissue sodium concentration is a logical therapy for the tissue damage syndrome in the cancer patient.[24]

Up to this point, I have reported primarily on hypotheses concerning the molecular biology and chemistry of the Gerson diet. There is evidence from clinical research as well.

In a 1983 study published in *Cancer Research,* a Hungarian team led by Zs.-Nagy performed x-ray microanalyses of intraoperative biopsy material from human thyroid cancers, and compared these cells with normal human epithelial cells. They then compared the levels of sodium and potassium in the malignant and normal cells, and found that increasing levels of sodium in relation to potassium were associated with increasing malignancy in the human thyroid, thereby supporting Cone's theories concerning the relationship of cell membrane depolarization and rate of cell division.[25]

Two years later, two researchers from the University of Texas M.D. Anderson Cancer Center in Houston reported that high concentrations of potassium altered the shape and the ability to grow of rat kidney cells infected with a sarcoma virus. High concentrations of potassium returned 100% of the cells to their normal structure. They also noted that other researchers were reporting positive effects of high potassium concentrations on cellular differentiation.[26]

A Partially Controlled Clinical Trial of a Modified Gerson Diet

The ultimate evaluation of the Gerson program must come from controlled clinical trials. Recently, an enterprising surgeon in Austria and his colleagues conducted what they admitted was a flawed controlled clinical trial using patients from their own practice who were willing to go on a modified Gerson diet.[27]

Dr. Peter Lechner and his colleagues of the Second Surgical Department of the Landeskrankenhaus in Graz have used a modified Gerson treatment for 4 years. They exclude the liver juice, and, except in hypothyroidism, the routine thyroid supplementation. They also exclude niacin "for fear of severe bleeding complications—especially in patients with a derangement of hemostasis caused by liver metastases."

> Our patients do not take more than two coffee enemas a day, one in the morning and the other one in the afternoon not later than 5 P.M. to avoid disturbances of sleep. *Four enemas a day led to colitis in three patients in the very beginning of the therapy* [emphasis added].

> We use the Gerson therapy not as an alternative but as an additive treatment, e.g. often combined with chemo- and/or radiation-therapies, and without exception in patients who had operations before. So diagnosis is verified at least by tissue biopsy in every single case.[27]

The 60 patients were male and female, 23 to 74 years of age, with many types of cancer and many kinds of prior treatment. The Gerson program was given on an outpatient basis, so the level of compliance could not be carefully assessed. And Lechner warns that they have used the therapy for only 4 years: "It is commonly accepted that oncological treatments demand a period of observation, documentation and evaluation of at least five or, better, ten years before final conclusions can be drawn." He continues:

> There is a very personal aspect, too: All our doctors are general surgeons, thus being conservatively or even skeptically minded, and none of us is an enthusiast as far as so-called alternative methods are concerned. We do watch our patients very carefully and from a rather critical point of view. For the same reason, we try to learn more about how and why the therapy might work, and we also do fundamental research work with special regard to the coffee enemas in cooperation with leading physiologists and biologists. Experiments performed in rats convinced us that two constituents of the coffee enemas lead to an enhanced production of bile. Applied rectally, these substances are absorbed into the portal venous blood and accelerate the excretion of phenacetin and some free radicals into the bile. Further data shall be published in the near future.[27]

Lechner found that only a small percentage of their patients were willing to follow the modified but still restrictive Gerson program. Among the refusers, they sought patients whose cases were similar to the Gerson patients so they could form "pairs" for the sake of comparison. There are, as we will see, methodological problems with this procedure. They surveyed 19 pairs of women with breast cancer who had radical mastectomies, with type and stage of malignancy verified in all cases. Of six pairs of premenopausal women, all belonging to a high-risk group, one Gerson patient (GP) developed a metastasis while three non-Gerson patients (NGP) developed metastases. Of seven pairs of premenopausal women, two NGPs had local recurrence and two NGPs had metastases to the spine. Of six pairs of postmenopausal women, none have shown further signs of disease so far.

The GPs also showed markedly better tolerance for radiotherapy, and especially chemotherapy. They did not show alterations in liver or kidney function or depressions of red or white blood cell count. Chemotherapy had to be interrupted with two NGP women because of severe depression in the blood count. Clinical side effects such as nausea, vomiting, loss of appetite and weight, and loss of hair were seen three times more frequently in the NGP group.

Among patients with liver metastases, GPs again showed "significantly increased tolerance" for chemotherapy. Lechner said this about the three pairs of patients with liver metastases: "Five of the six women are dead by now—only one, a GP, is still alive, her disease having been in a 'no change' state for fourteen months. Her partner died more than eight months ago. *In no case did the Gerson Therapy lead to a complete remission, but the two GPs survived their partners for at least twice the time* [emphasis added]. This might be an effect of the coffee enemas."

Among four patients with metastases to the lungs, a condition that usually causes pleural effusion of fluids and a need for puncture and drainage, "the two NGPs had their hydrothorax punctured twice as frequently as the GPs. The much slower recurrence of the effusion in GPs might be a result of the strict avoidance of dietary sodium."

Two patients had brain metastases:

> The GP "recovered" for a period of three months, and most of the symptoms disappeared. CT-scan showed that peritumorous edema was reduced by more than 30%. The underlying mechanism might be the same as it is in pleural effusions. Both patients died, the GP four months later than the NGP.

> Metastases to the bone are very frequently seen, and so we had 12 pairs of patients who belong to this subtype. *This kind of tumor, usually treated with chemotherapy, responds only poorly to the Gerson therapy* [emphasis added]. There is no significant difference between the NGP and the GP group as far as tumor size and survival are concerned. Only the quality of life seems to be better in the GP group, probably for two reasons: (1) The coffee enemas, taken twice a day, give some pain relief so that most of the GPs only need low doses of non-steroidal antirheumatics (aspirin or other similar analgesics). They usually do not take alkaloids, so that they can lead quite an active life in spite of their disease. (2) Hypercalcemia, which can alter kidney function, does not occur in GPs, maybe as a result of the intake of more than two litres of juices per day.[27]

Among patients with colorectal carcinoma, Lechner found no significant difference between the two groups regarding local recurrences or distant secondary metastases. "After the operation, GPs usually recover better than NGPs and seem to gain weight more easily." This observation of improved *weight gain* in Gerson patients is intriguing, given the concerns I have previously expressed regarding the potential for *weight loss* in the radical nutritional therapies.

"Patients with metastases in the liver seem to be the best responders to the Gerson therapy," Lechner found. After radical surgical resection, Lechner's patients are no longer given intravenous or intraarterial chemotherapy, "the results having been rather poor in the past." For most patients—except those opting for liver transplants—"the Gerson therapy remains the only treatment. . . . We have already surveyed eight pairs by now, ten men and six women between 32 and 74 years of age. The laboratory findings of all of them show significant differences between the GP and NGP groups." Lechner continues:

> The hepatic enzyme profiles, in four patients more than four times beyond the normal range at the beginning of treatment, became completely normal in the two GPs within four months and remained so for more than one year. One of the two women had her gallbladder removed and . . . died of liver failure. The other is still leading an active life. Ultrasound and CT-scan show no growth of the metastases.

> In another four pairs success was not so evident; the enzyme profiles remained high and the disease was apparently progressing. Although all these patients died within two years after operation, lifespan of the GPs was in all cases more than double the NGPs. As described in breast cancer patients, the GPs usually needed less analgesic drugs than the NGPs and, as a result of the regularly applied enemas, none of them developed a bowel obstruction although two of them suffered from far advanced peritoneal carcinosis. Among the last four patients of this subtype there is one of the GPs who came into a complete remission and remained in this state for about half a year. . . . Among all our patients this is the only one where the Gerson therapy might have had a tumoricide effect, but we tend to interpret this as a "spontaneous remission" rather than as the result of the dietary treatment.[27]

Lechner's account is worthy of careful consideration. There are methodological problems with selecting the "pair" for each Gerson patient from the patient who turned down Gerson treatment. Among the GPs there may simply have been a higher motivation to live. On the other hand, Lechner has at least provided an invaluable rough estimate of the effects of a modified Gerson therapy over 4 years with 30 pairs of patients.

From his experience, Lechner found significant advantages for Gerson patients. Some lived longer. Others were healthier, had better responses to conventional therapies and fewer side effects, less pain, and better quality of life. Some of these advantages seemed directly related to the Gerson regimen. But the psychological and physical characteristics that enabled these people to undertake the regimen undoubtedly played a part in the superior results in many categories.

These findings, while significant, are a far cry from the dramatic results claimed by Gerson or claimed in his name by colleagues and admirers while he was alive and leaders of the Gerson Institute after his death. At the same time, Robert Houston has properly pointed out that Lechner did use a reduced therapy and also combined it with chemotherapy and radiation, both of which are immunosuppressive. Any immune enhancement brought about by the Gerson program itself may therefore have been compromised by its use as complementary therapy.[28]

Claims for the Gerson Diet

The question of what Gerson claimed and what others claimed in his name is confusing. Gerson himself said different things in different places as his experience with the treatment evolved. In an early report, published in 1949, he said: "The difficulty of evaluating any therapy, especially in a disease so protean in character as cancer, is fully appreciated by us. It is too early to make any definitive statement as to the value of the Gerson Dietary Regime at this time, but we hope to be able to report a sufficient number of cases later to allow statistical analysis."[29]

By the time he was rewriting *A Cancer Therapy* near the end of his life, Gerson wrote: "This book has been written to indicate that there is an effective treatment for cancer, even in advanced cases." What does that mean? If we look at Lechner's results in Austria, it might be fair to call the Gerson therapy an "effective treatment," just as a chemotherapy that enhances outcomes significantly over other chemotherapies may be described as an "effective treatment." But Gerson writes those words in the context of presenting 50 cases of advanced cancer patients whom he regarded as individually "cured" by treatment. And a lecture given in 1956 was entitled, "The Cure of Advanced Cancer by Diet Therapy." In it Gerson said: "I should like to tell you what we do to prove that this treatment really does work for cancer. Number one, the results. I think I can claim that I have, even in these far advanced cases, 50% results. The real problem arises when we cannot restore the liver."[30]

What does Gerson mean by "50% results" in far-advanced cases? Gerson explains: "The number of terminal cases among my patients increased to more than 90 per cent of the total, having come to me after the applied treatments had failed. . . . About 50 per cent of these cases could be improved and saved; the percentage could be higher if there were better cooperation from the family physician, the patient himself, and less resistance from the family against such a strict regime."[31] Gerson believed that he had accomplished a rate of *cure* of 50% for advanced cancers after mainstream treatments had failed. I find this claim very difficult to believe.

There is the further question of just how strong the evidence was in the 50 cases that Gerson presented in *A Cancer Therapy* as among his best cases. Mark F. McCarty, of the McNaughton Foundation, offered the following comment:

> Dr. Gerson published 50 cases which he believed best documented the success of his methods. A survey of these cases shows that many of them offer less than adequate evidence of response to the diet: recent prior treatment with standard modalities occurs in some cases; lumps or radiological findings appearing after surgical extirpation of the primary tumor are often assumed to indicate recurrence without proof; a few cases were never biopsied; and several were of tumor types that occasionally remit spontaneously. Nevertheless, barring outright deception on Gerson's part (and it was generally admitted by his opponents that Gerson was sincere), it is my impression that at least some of these cases indicate objective tumor regression in response to the Gerson methods. At a Senate Select Committee hearing on cancer research in 1945, five independent M.D.s who had personal experience with patients treated by Gerson submitted letters indicating that they had been surprised and encouraged by the results they had seen, and urged a widespread trial of the method. One of these doctors claimed that relief of severe pain was achieved in about 90% of cases. No controlled trial of Gerson's methods was ever undertaken.[32]

Gar Hildenbrand, the scholarly current director of the Gerson Institute, believes that the results the Gerson Institute is getting today are analogous to those Gerson achieved. But neither he nor other long-time observers of the Gerson program suggest that they achieve anything approaching cure in 50% of advanced cancer patients.

Scientific Evaluations of the Gerson Program

In 1987, Gar Hildenbrand undertook an important and ambitious "best-case" review of patients on the Gerson program. The review was intended to focus on patients who had either had no previous conventional treatment or who had not been helped by previous conventional treatment.[33] The study was a heroic undertaking, and doubly important because it represented one of the most important efforts so far *by a proponent of an alternative cancer therapy* to design, fund, and carry out a major assessment of the objective benefits of the therapy. Unfortunately, the study turned out to be impossible to complete because the Gerson practitioners were relying on blind recall as to who had done well on the program, the number of "pure" cases in which neither allopathic intervention nor the natural history of the disease could possibly account for the favorable outcome was very small, complete records for patients seen over many years are very difficult and extremely expensive to get, and necessary reassessment is even more difficult and expensive. The study demonstrated the difficulties inherent in the full-scale best-case review as a prelude to controlled clinical trials or other formal evaluations.

In 1989, an objective and qualified British research team headed by Karol Sikora, Professor of Clinical Oncology at the Royal Postgraduate Medical School, University of London, visited the Gerson Clinic on behalf of a British insurance company. They observed clinic operations freely and were offered information from the files on what were considered by the clinic staff to be the best cases of the Gerson treatment. In addition to their best-case study, the researchers conducted a psychological assessment of patients currently at the clinic:

> During our assessment we had free access to all the inpatients and their notes, and also a sample of notes gathered as examples of best responses. Out of a total of 3000 patients treated since 1974, 149 case histories were examined, having been selected by the Gerson Institute on the basis of replies to a postal questionnaire sent to patients over the past two years. The commonest tumours were melanoma (24), breast carcinoma (29), colorectal cancer (21), prostate cancer (11), and lung cancer (15). . . . Of the patients responding, 27 had independent documentation of their disease status from their "conventional" physicians and thus were assessable according to standard oncological criteria [see table 14.1].[34]

Table 14.1

Patients with Assessable Disease

Tumor	No.	Response	Clinical course
Melanoma	9	N/A	Within natural history
Prostate, microinvasive	2	N/A	Within natural history, no evidence of spread at 9 and 13 yr
Prostate, metastatic	1	CR	Elevated acid phosphatase (23 units / L, 1984) returned to normal (0–6 units / L, 1986)
Breast	2	N/A	Residual masses post biopsy persisted; 1 patient also took hormones
Low-grade non-Hodgkin's lymphoma	3	1 CR 2 N/A	2 were unassessable because of concurrent conventional therapy, 1 had 4 × 4 cm mass (biopsy confirmed), which regressed
Endometrium	3	1 CR 1 N/A 1 PD	1 in situ carcinoma became invasive, 1 biopsy-proven Ca subsequently showed no disease at hysterectomy
Cervix	1	N/A	Stage 1A Ca completely excised at cone biopsy
Astrocytoma	1	PD	Slowly progressive disease after initial response
Pancreatic gastrinoma	1	PD	Node and liver metastases at operation; slowly progressive disease
Pancreas	2	2 N/A	1 unbiopsied tumor regressed, 1 no information after positive biopsy
Hard-palate adenocarcinoma	1	SD	Positive biopsies in 1975, 1977, 1984; no progression
Bladder	1	N/A	Stage 2B (1966), poorly differentiated, excision biopsy only; declined chemoradiotherapy and cystectomy

From Reed et al., *Lancet* 336:676–7 (September 15, 1990).
CR, complete response; PD, progressive disease; SD, stable disease; N/A, not assessable; Ca, carcinoma.

In their psychological study, the researchers found a very marked enhancement of quality of life and of pain control without the need for opiates, even in advanced cancer:

> Psychological information was obtained from the patients present at the centre. . . . [A] striking feature was the high degree of control the patients felt they had over their health and, perhaps as a consequence, their high ratings for mood and confidence. Particularly intriguing were the low pain scores and analgesic requirements for all the patients, despite the presence of extensive metastatic disease in many and the fact that several had been on opioid medication previously.[34]

In terms of tumor response to the therapy, the researchers concluded:

> We could find little objective evidence of an antitumour effect from the Gerson therapy, although most patients were not assessable because of concomitant conventional therapy. However, in a few patients definite tumour regression was documented. In view of the poor prognosis of most of the patients, perhaps it is more important that there was a subjective benefit both to them and to their families. There is evidence that a "fighting spirit" response is associated with a better prognosis, and Spiegel and co-workers have shown that patients with metastatic breast carcinoma treated with psychotherapy in addition to conventional chemotherapy had a significantly improved survival. Judged in this context, the improvement in the Gerson patients' sense of wellbeing may take on a greater importance.[34]

The researchers pointed out that the example of the Gerson therapy did demonstrate a "way forward" for oncology practice: "The nature of the therapy requires a positive contribution to be made by the patient to his or her health and meets a need not satisfied by conventional therapy, in which the role of the patient is essentially passive. These approaches may suggest ways forward for oncologists in the management of desperate cancer patients and their families."[34]

Conclusion

I undertook this extended review of the Gerson therapy for several reasons. First, the Gerson therapy is the oldest and best known of the modern Western alternative nutritional therapies for cancer, and there is more scientific information available on it than for most other nutritional treatments. Second, the complexities of evaluating the therapy, the historical and scientific issues, are similar to those raised by many other nutritional therapies. Third, in my judgment, the evaluation suggests the general range in which we might expect outcomes to be achieved with other intensive nutritional therapies.

What conclusions can we reach? I suggest that the most reasonable conclusion based on the currently available evidence, which is suggestive, but not definitive, is that the Gerson therapy sometimes enhances outcomes for patients with some types of cancer who have the stamina and the willingness to undertake it. Also, we can conclude that the Gerson therapy does not approach being a *decisive cure* for any type of cancer.

If adequate controlled clinical trials of the Gerson therapy are undertaken by open-minded and reasonably sympathetic researchers who have carefully studied the cancers in which Gerson therapy seems to yield the best results, I predict that the therapy will prove to be a significant adjunct to the judicious use of conventional therapies for those cancers. Further, it may also improve outcomes for some cancers where conventional treatment would bring few—if any—results. And I believe it would prove a legitimate option in some cancers where standard modalities have demonstrated only limited efficacy—in, say, 10% to 25% of cases—but the costs in toxicity and quality of life are very high. I also predict that in controlled clinical trials, there would be a small but significantly increased number of *cures,* along with a wide range of increases in life expectancy and improved quality of life.

Gar Hildenbrand, current executive director of the Gerson Institute, has expressed his view that the Gerson therapy is a *necessary adjunct* to standard modalities. This move away from the original claims of cure is an important move toward a scientific middle ground. One day, the Gerson therapy may be recognized as being of supreme historical importance in the recovery of the nutritional component in cancer management. However, I believe it will prove to be only one version of a necessary adjunctive nutritional treatment. There are and will be other adjunctive nutritional treatments, and some may ultimately prove to be better approaches than Gerson's. I believe Max Gerson, the great pioneer of nutritional cancer therapies, the scholar's scholar, and the supreme empiricist who believed that results at the bedside were decisive, would be content to be remembered that way.

Albert Schweitzer said: "I see in Dr. Max Gerson one of the most eminent geniuses in medical history."[35] If one immerses oneself in Gerson's writings, the writings about him, and the scientific mystery story we have set out to unravel here, it is not difficult to see why he has inspired such admiration. He was a profoundly ethical man who helped recover for our time the great healing potential of a nutritional medicine based on the conventional scientific understanding of his time and on his own empirical experience. He sought to modernize and understand nutritional therapy in the context of a commitment to science and to his patients with cancer.

Notes and References

1 In October 1989, the Gerson Institute issued instructions to all patients to substitute carrot juice for calf's liver juice obtained from growers in the United States. This decision was based on multiple outbreaks of bacterial infections at the Hospital de Baja California where liver juice was part of the therapy. Liver juice was added to the therapy by Gerson in 1950 in the belief that the nutritional quality of fruits and vegetables was declining due to modern farming practices. According to the Gerson Institute, the rise of modern organic farming holds out the promise of higher-quality fruits and vegetables than were available during Gerson's lifetime.

2 Patricia Spain Ward, "History of Gerson Therapy," contract report for the U.S. Congress Office of Technology Assessment (OTA), revised June 1988. This report created a storm of controversy at OTA when a staff member commented in writing that the paper seemed unduly favorable to Gerson, and proponents of alternative therapies vigorously protested the comment as evidence of bias against Gerson and against alternative therapies more generally. Rosemary Stevens, Ph.D., chair of the OTA Advisory Panel on the Unconventional Cancer Therapies Report subsequently commented at an open review session that Ward's paper was a professionally competent review of the subject.

3 Ibid., 1–2.

4 Ibid., 2.

5 Ibid., 4.

6 Ibid.

7 Ibid., 5.

8 Ibid., 11.

9 Ibid., 12.

10 Ibid.

11 Ibid., 15.

12 Ibid., 12.

13 Max Gerson, *A Cancer Therapy: Results of Fifty Cases* (Del Mar, CA: Totality Books, 1977), 7–10.

14 Gar Hildebrand, "Let's Set the Record Straight, Part 5—Bread, Propaganda and Circuses," *The Healing Newsletter,* The Gerson Institute, March-June 1987.

15 Max Gerson, "Effects of a Combined Dietary Regime on Patients with Malignant Tumors," *Experimental Medicine and Surgery* 7(4):299–317 (1949). Cited in U.S. Congress Office of Technology Assessment, *Unconventional Cancer Treatments* (Washington, D.C.: Government Printing Office, September 1990), 45.

16 Max Gerson, "Cancer, A Problem of Metabolism," translated from *Medizinische Klinik* 49(26):1028–32 (1954). Cited in Office of Technology Assessment, *Unconventional Cancer Treatments,* 45.

17 Max Gerson, "The Cure of Advanced Cancer by Diet Therapy: A Summary of 30 Years of Clinical Experimentation," *Physiological Chemistry and Physics* 10:449–64 (1978). Cited in Office of Technology Assessment, *Unconventional Cancer Treatments,* 45–6.

18 Freeman W. Cope, "A Medical Application of the Ling Association-Induction Hypothesis: The High Potassium, Low Sodium Diet of the Gerson Cancer Therapy," *Physiological Chemistry and Physics* 10:465–68 (1978).

19 Gerson, "The Cure of Advanced Cancer by Diet Therapy," 46.

20 Ibid., 45–6.

21 William Regelson, "The 'Grand Conspiracy' Against the Cancer Cure," *Journal of the American Medical Association* 243(4):337–9 (1980).

22 Clarence D. Cone, Jr., "The Role of the Surface Electrical Transmembrane Potential in Normal and Malignant Mitogenesis," *Annals of the New York Academy of Sciences* 420–32 (1971).

23 G.N. Ling, "The Association-Induction Hypothesis: A Theoretical Foundation Provided for the Possible Beneficial Effects of a Low Sodium, High Potassium Diet and other Similar Regimens in the Treatment of Patients Suffering from Debilitating Illnesses," *Agressologie* 24(7):293–302 (1983).

24 Cope, "A Medical Application of the Ling Association-Induction Hypothesis: The High Potassium, Low Sodium Diet of the Gerson Cancer Therapy," *Physiological Chemistry and Physics,* 465.

25 Imre Zs.-Nagy et al., "Correlation of Malignancy with Intracellular Na-K Ratio in Human Thyroid Tumors," *Cancer Research* 43:5395–7 (1983).

26 Chiu-Nan Lai and Frederick F. Becker, "Potassium-Induced Reverse Transformation of Cells Infected with a Temperature-Sensitive Transformation Mutant Virus," *Journal of Cellular Physiology* 125: 259–62 (1985).

27 P. Lechner, "The Role of a Modified Gerson Therapy in the Treatment of Cancer." Typescript, Second Department of Surgery, Landeskrankenhaus, Graz, Austria, 1987.

28 Robert Houston, personal correspondence with the author, 4 May 1991.

29 Max Gerson, "Effects of a Combined Dietary Regimen," *Experimental Medicine and Surgery,* 299–315 (1949).

30 Max Gerson, "The Cure of Advanced Cancer by Diet Therapy: A Summary of 30 Years of Clinical Experimentation," *Physiological Chemistry and Physics* 10:449–63 (1978).

31 Gerson, *A Cancer Therapy*, 33.

32 Mark F. McCarty, "Aldosterone and the Gerson Diet—A Speculation," *Medical Hypotheses* 7:591–7 (1981).

33 Office of Technology Assessment, *Unconventional Cancer Treatments*, 50.

34 Alison Reed, Nicholas James, and Karol Sikora, "Mexico: Juices, Coffee Enemas, and Cancer," letter to the Editor, *Lancet* 336:676–7 (September 15, 1990).

35 Gerson, *A Cancer Therapy*, cover.

fifteen

Macrobiotics—A Diet and a Way of Life

Today, macrobiotics is the most widely used unconventional nutritional approach to cancer in the United States. Best known for its primarily vegetarian, high complex carbohydrate, low fat diet, macrobiotics also offers a spiritual philosophy of life that is embraced to varying degrees by many thousands of practitioners around the world. Michio Kushi, the focus of this chapter, is the most influential macrobiotic teacher today. Kushi's approach to macrobiotics is by no means the only one in the macrobiotic "movement," but because he is the best-known macrobiotic teacher and made the choice to make significant claims for success with cancer, he is the proper focus for this analysis.

As the preeminent teacher in a very widespread movement, Kushi necessarily generates a wide range of responses—some critical, some laudatory—both from within and outside macrobiotic circles. But what is unquestionably true is that he is a philosophical thinker in the great tradition of what Aldous Huxley called the perennial philosophy—the philosophy that appears at the core of all the great spiritual traditions of the world. He is a contemplative observer of both the microcosm of human health and the macrocosm of planetary history and evolution. In this he is reminiscent of Rudolf Steiner, founder of anthroposophy, and Edgar Cayce, the American seer: all three provide their followers with a spiritual perspective based on the perennial philosophy, with prescriptions for healthy and balanced living, and with detailed recommendations for the treatment of disease, including cancer.

The word "macrobiotics" comes from the Greek *macro,* meaning "great" or "large," and *bios,* "life." In its current manifestation, macrobiotics originated in the late nineteenth and early twentieth centuries with an educator named Yukikazu Sakurazawa and a physician named Sagen Ishisuka. They reportedly cured themselves of serious illnesses by changing from the modern refined diet then sweeping Japan to a simple diet of brown rice, miso soup, sea vegetables, and other traditional Japanese foods. After restoring their health, they went on to integrate traditional Oriental medicine and philosophy with Vedanta (a Hindu spiritual tradition), original Christian and Jewish teachings, and holistic perspectives in modern science and medicine.[1] (Some critics have asserted that Sakurazawa and Ishisuka never intended this theological base, and that later proponents of macrobiotics, particularly Michio Kushi, were responsible for the religious element.) When Sakurazawa came to Paris in the 1920s, he adopted George Ohsawa as his pen name and called his teachings macrobiotics.

Kushi's Biography

Michio Kushi was born in 1926 in Japan. Kushi studied political science and law at Tokyo University, the premier university of Japan, during World War II. According to a biography of Kushi published by the Kushi Institute:

> The atomic bombing of Hiroshima and Nagasaki made a deep impression on him, and he decided to devote his life to world peace. After the war, he continued graduate studies in Tokyo in international law. With the support of Norman Cousins, editor of the *Saturday Review,* Professor Shigeru Nanbara, chancellor of Tokyo University, and Rev. Toyohiko Kagawa, the Christian evangelist, he came to the United States in 1949 to pursue his studies of world order.[2]

Kushi continued graduate studies at Columbia University. He began to question the possibility of bringing about social change through political means and went to see Albert Einstein, Thomas Mann, Upton Sinclair, Robert M. Hutchins, Harold Urey, Pitrim Sorokin, and other prominent scientists, authors, and statesmen. They all offered encouragement with his search but told him they knew of no lasting solution to make humanity peaceful.[3]

Before leaving Japan, Kushi had studied briefly with George Ohsawa at the Student World Government Association. It was Ohsawa's belief that food was the key to health and that health was the key to peace. By returning to a traditional diet of whole, natural foods, he believed that humanity could regain its physical and mental balance and therefore become more peaceful. While living in New York, Kushi experienced positive changes in his own health and consciousness after changing his own diet. Over the next 10 years, with the support of his wife Aveline, he began to study traditional and modern approaches to diet and health and to teach macrobiotics.[4]

In the 1960s, Kushi moved to Boston and founded Erewhon (one of the early natural foods distributors) to make available the foods necessary for a macrobiotic lifestyle. In 1971, his followers founded *East-West Journal,* and the following year the East-West Foundation was started to support macrobiotic education and research. In 1978, Michio and Aveline Kushi founded the Kushi Institute for One Peaceful World, with affiliate organizations throughout Europe. Kushi has met many national and international leaders, lectured to thousands of health professionals, and been profiled in dozens of leading newspapers and magazines.[5]

Today, Kushi describes macrobiotics as

> a unique synthesis of Eastern and Western influences. It is the way of life according to the largest possible view, the infinite order of the universe. The practice of macrobiotics involves the understanding and practical application of this order to our lifestyle, including the selection, preparation and manner of eating our daily food, as well as the orientation of consciousness. Macrobiotics does not offer a single diet for everyone, but a dietary principle that takes into account differing climactic and geographical considerations, varying ages, sexes and levels of activity, and ever changing personal needs.[6]

Twenty years ago, Kushi made an interesting, critical, and intriguing decision. He decided to present macrobiotics to the world with a major emphasis on its role in the prevention and alleviation of cancer. His son, Lawrence Kushi, Ph.D., a respected nutrition researcher, commented in a discussion I had with him, "Twenty years ago, macrobiotics was generally seen in its role as a philosophy of life focused on the order of the universe. Later it became most widely known for the cancer prevention diet. Michio Kushi moved in that direction. Some would ask whether that was the right decision, or whether cancer was necessarily the right disease."[7]

The question is a fair one because Michio Kushi is not a careless man, but one who teaches and practices taking "the large view." Granting that Kushi's life purpose was to support a movement toward world peace through health, pure food, and right living, still there was no clear imperative for him to give a primary emphasis to the role of macrobiotics in preventing or "relieving" cancer. Moreover, a macrobiotic diet has not yet been scientifically demonstrated to be effective with cancer in the way it appears to have been with heart disease. In heart disease, the work of Dean Ornish, M.D., and others has suggested that a very low fat vegetarian diet in combination with yoga-based stretching and group support can not only decisively ameliorate the symptoms of angina[8] but may slowly reverse arterial blockage.[9] Similarly, Frank M. Sacks, M.D., of Harvard Medical School and his colleagues found that macrobiotic populations had much lower blood pressure and serum cholesterol levels than were found in the general population.[10] Macrobiotics, like other nondairy vegetarian diets, is an effective preventive strategy for heart disease and hypertension and, very likely, if the studies by Ornish are confirmed by others, an effective approach to symptom control and reversal of arteriosclerotic blockage as well. Because of the more limited evidence for macrobiotics in the "relief" of cancer, the question remains whether or not cancer was the right disease for Kushi to choose as a focus.

With cancer, macrobiotics and similar vegetarian diets are arguably preventive for those cancers most closely associated with a high fat Western diet, although, again, this relationship is not nearly as clear as the relationship between high fat diets and heart disease. These diets may also some day prove to be effective for patients with some types of cancer, in the inhibition or reversal of tumor progression as well as in the extension of disease-free and overall survival after surgical or medical treatment. However, well-designed scientific research will be necessary to determine whether, and in what ways, macrobiotics is helpful with cancer, and the results of these studies will not be in for at least another decade.

The Cancer Prevention Diet: Michio Kushi's Blueprint for the Relief and Prevention of Disease,[6] written with Alex Jack, is Kushi's major treatise on the macrobiotic approach to cancer. The book, worthy of close study by any serious student of alternative cancer therapies, has three parts.

Part I, "Preventing Cancer Naturally," discusses cancer, diet, and macrobiotics in the context of modern civilization. It argues persuasively that our increasingly unnatural lifestyles, out of touch with nature and the order of the universe, predispose us to a wide range of degenerative disorders, including cancer. There is little doubt that this is true.

Part II applies the general theory of macrobiotics to 14 of the most common types of cancer.

Part III is entitled "Recipes and Menus" and also has a very important discussion of "home remedies based on traditional macrobiotic Oriental medicine and folk medicine, modified and adjusted for practical use in modern society."[11] The most intriguing "home remedy" is a clay-cabbage compress said to be capable of drawing a tumor up through the skin without surgery. I will discuss this remedy in some detail later in the chapter.

Though the title of Kushi's book presents the program as primarily a dietary program, the text introduces the reader to the whole philosophical-spiritual and lifestyle system that macrobiotics encompasses. And while the title of the book emphasizes *prevention,* the text focuses primarily on the use of the program for "relief" of the disease. The text also often makes clear Kushi's disapproval of many forms of conventional treatment. In fact, to a large degree this is a book about modalities that, from a commonsense perspective, could be described as adjunctive or complementary *treatments.* I raise these points neither as criticisms nor endorsements, only as observations.

Kushi, cautiously, does not choose to present macrobiotics as an adjunctive treatment system. He has stated emphatically in a letter to the Office of Technology Assessment that "macrobiotics is neither a treatment nor a therapy, but a commonsense approach to living."[12] But some of the specific recommendations he makes for cancer go beyond a simple "commonsense approach to living."

Breast Cancer as an Example

Kushi's chapter on breast cancer in *The Cancer Prevention Diet* is one of the best examples of Kushi's approach to cancer, and I will report on it in detail because so many women with breast cancer consider adopting a macrobiotic diet. The chapter starts with a discussion of survival rates for patients with breast cancer who follow conventional treatment:

> About 65 percent of women with breast cancer survive five years or more. In 1973 researchers at Italy's National Cancer Institute in Milan reported that studies showed no difference in survival or recurrence rates between women who had complete mastectomies and those who had partial ones. In 1977 Dr. Jan Sytgersward, a Swiss cancer researcher, reported that breast cancer patients who received no radiation therapy survived 10 percent longer than those who received radiation treatment. On March 15, 1980, *The Lancet,* a British medical journal, noted: "The overall survival of patients with primary breast cancer has not improved in the last ten years, despite increasing use of multiple drug chemotherapy for the treatment of metastases. Furthermore, there has been no improvement in survival from first metastasis, and survival may even have been shortened in some patients given chemotherapy."[13]

Two problems with Kushi's book are that the medical references are not footnoted for the articles cited, and that references are often incomplete or selected in a biased manner. In this instance, Kushi's first statement regarding the equivalence of partial and complete mastectomies for survival is generally regarded as correct. The second statement regarding the survival *dis*advantage of radiation treatment is too broad a statement to assess and would generally be regarded as incorrect. The third statement regarding the absence of progress in life expectancy in primary breast cancer is widely debated. The fourth statement regarding the lack of progress in life extension after first metastasis is widely regarded as correct. The general point I wish to make here is that, in his book and elsewhere, the citation of scientific studies is very loose, and the real scientific issues are not always fairly stated.

Kushi then discusses his views of the causes of breast cancer. While there is scientific support for his views on the role of a high animal fat, low fiber diet in the development of breast cancer (although the subject is still debated), his view of the mechanisms by which breast cancer develops are at most only partially shared by scientists. If we eat poorly over a long time, Kushi says, we lose our ability to discharge excess wastes and toxins. Thus far, he would find agreement. But his statement of the mechanism of tumor formation goes beyond currently accepted scientific theories of tumorigenesis:

> This can be serious, if an underlying layer of fat has developed under the skin, which prevents discharge toward the surface of the body. Repeated overconsumption of milk, cheese, and other dairy products, eggs, meat, poultry, and other fatty, oily, or greasy foods brings about this stage. When it has been reached, internal deposits of mucus or fat begin to form, initially in areas with some direct access to the outside such as the sinuses, the inner ear, the lungs, the kidneys, the reproductive organs, and the breasts.[14]

According to Kushi, this deposit of mucus or fat in the breast can become a cyst, and the process is accelerated by ingesting ice cream, milk, soft drinks, fruit juice, and other foods with a "cooling or freezing effect." Breast-feeding is protective against formation of cysts or tumors in mothers, Kushi says, and cow's milk is unsuited for human consumption because of the differences between it and human milk: "The abuse of dairy food in the modern diet and its degenerating artificial quality are major factors in the rise of breast cancer, heart disease, and other serious illnesses. The quality of our food determines the quality of our blood. The quality of blood, in turn, determines the quality of mother's milk and the biological strength of the next generation."[15]

Many scientists would agree with Kushi's comments on the role of excessive nutrient intake and the possible role of toxins in the etiology of breast cancer, as well as with his comments on the protective value of breast-feeding. However, the rest of the theory is unsubstantiated from a general mainstream perspective.

In a following section entitled "Medical Evidence," Kushi cites a number of intriguing findings from the history of medicine and more contemporary science. The bulk of the evidence that Kushi reports supports his views that a grain-based diet can relieve cancer and permit the patient to live a long time; that artificial infant feeding is associated with an increased incidence of breast cancer among mothers; that caloric restriction results in a lower incidence of breast cancer in animals; and that a vegetarian diet prevents breast cancer.[16]

A section entitled "Diagnosis" first discusses conventional methods of diagnosis, and then diagnosis from a macrobiotic or Oriental medical perspective:

In addition to self-examination of the breasts, Oriental medicine looks for signs of developing mammary disorders in the condition and complexion of the cheeks. As a result of parallel embryonic development, the cheeks reflect underlying changes in the chest region, including the lungs and breasts, and in the reproductive region.

Cheeks with well-developed firm flesh and a clean, clear skin color show sound respiratory and digestive functions, especially if there are no wrinkles or pimples in the area. Red or pink cheeks, except during vigorous exercise or when out in the cold weather, show abnormal expansion of the blood capillaries, caused by heart and circulatory disorders due to the overconsumption of yin foods and drinks, including fruits, juices, sugar and drugs. Milky-white cheeks are caused by the overconsumption of dairy products such as milk, cheese, cream and yogurt. A pinkish shade mixed with the white indicates excessive intake of flour products and fruits. Both these colors indicate accumulation of fat and mucus in various regions of the body including the breasts, lungs, intestines, and reproductive organs.

Fatty spots that are dark, red, or white in color on the cheeks are a sign of fat accumulation in either the lungs or breast and often accompany the beginning of a cyst or tumor formation. Coffee or other stimulant, aromatic beverages may contribute to the appearance of this color in the cheeks. . . . Certain colors and marks appearing on the white of the eye also indicate abnormal conditions in corresponding areas of the body. . . . Green vessels appearing along the Heart Governor meridian or Lung meridian from the wrist toward the elbow on the inside softer side of the arm also show the development of cancerous conditions in the breast or lung region. [The references to "meredians" are to energy channels postulated in acupuncture.] [17]

All of this is, of course, outside the ken of mainstream medicine.

The next major section of the chapter on breast cancer discusses "Dietary Recommendations" and begins with what should be avoided:

For breast cancer, all dairy food and all fatty, oily food including meat, poultry, eggs and other animal products are to be eliminated. Sugar, honey, and other sweeteners as well as soft drinks and other foods and beverages treated with sugar are also to be avoided. Tropical fruits, fruit juices, and vegetables such as potato, yam, sweet potato, asparagus, tomato and eggplant should not be consumed. Because they are excessively mucus-producing, all flour products are to be avoided except for occasional consumption of nonyeasted unleavened whole-wheat or rye bread. Chemicalized and artificially produced and treated foods and beverages are to be completely eliminated. Even unsaturated vege-table oil is to be completely avoided or minimized in cooking for a one- or two-month period. All ice-cold foods and drinks including ice-cream should be avoided. Although they are not the cause of breast cancer, all stimulants, spices, coffee, alcohol, and aromatic, fragrant beverages and drugs should be avoided because they enhance tumor development.[18]

Kushi then discusses the recommended diet for breast cancer, which involves relatively small modifications of his basic cancer prevention diet[19]:

- Fifty to sixty percent of daily consumption, by volume, should be whole-cereal grains. The most preferred are pressure-cooked medium or small-grain brown rice and, frequently, millet or barley.
- Five to ten percent soup, consisting of two bowls per day of miso soup or tamari soy sauce broth cooked with kombu, wakame, or other sea vegetables and various land vegetables such as onions and carrots.
- Twenty to thirty percent vegetables, cooked in a variety of forms.
- Five percent small beans, such as azuki or lentils, may be used daily, cooked together with sea vegetables such as kombu or with onions and carrots.
- Five percent or less sea vegetable dishes.

Kushi then goes on to specify condiments (sesame salt, kelp, or wakame powder). "Finely chopped scallions mixed and heated with an equal volume of miso and a small portion of grated ginger are helpful to soften hardening of tissues and tumor."[19]

Mainstream medicine would find the diet nutritionally balanced but many of the specific recommendations nonsensical.

Kushi's Recommended "Home Cares"

The following section, "Home Cares," is one of the most intriguing and important. In it Kushi discusses home remedies that reportedly enable the tumor to be drawn out through the surface of the skin and purged through the application of clay-cabbage compresses:

For breast tumors, a towel soaked in hot water and squeezed out can be applied over the affected area for about three to five minutes to stimulate circulation. Afterwards, a compress containing about 50 percent green clay and 50 percent cabbage leaves or other natural plant leaves may be applied over the area to help facilitate the discharge of accumulated toxic matter. . . . This clay-cabbage compress may be left in place for about four hours or overnight, and it may be applied daily for up to one month, preferably under the supervision of an experienced macrobiotic counselor. *This compress will gradually help draw the excess mucus and fat from the inner parts of the mammary tissues toward the surface of the skin. Eventually, the fatty mucus, sticky substances, and unclean blood that make up the tumor will drain out* [emphasis added].

In cases where a breast has already been surgically removed and the surrounding lymph nodes, neck and in some cases arm have become swollen, a buckwheat plaster can be applied following a brief ginger compress.[20]

This section is intriguing because Kushi makes a specific claim that there is an alternative to surgery for the removal of some breast tumors. This claim is necessarily either true and important—in which case it should be scientifically validated—or untrue and potentially dangerous, because women would, in trying this method, avoid early removal of a breast tumor and wait until the tumor had progressed. The use of compresses must be approached with some caution, however. Keith Block, M.D., an Evanston, Illinois, internist-oncologist who serves on the faculty of the University of Illinois, reports observing some women who have been referred to him following prolonged use of compresses. In his experience, initial examination of some of these patients demonstrated tumors having grown so large that they broke through the skin and were draining fluids and blood; what might have been a simple resection earlier on now left these patients with limited options for recovery.[21]

A section entitled "Other Considerations" advises daily scrubbing of the whole body with a towel that has been immersed in hot gingerroot water as well as avoiding wool and synthetic fibers and metallic jewelry ("It is fine, though, to wear a wedding ring").

Kushi also cautions against long periods in front of a television or other source of electromagnetic energy: "Radiation weakens the chest area." Psychologically, he advises, "Breast-cancer patients are subject to depression and should do everything possible to maintain a cheerful and calm attitude. Smile, be optimistic, dance, sing, and enjoy each day for itself."[22]

The last section in the breast cancer chapter is the case history of Phyllis Crabtree: "In October, 1972 . . . a fifty-year-old homemaker, nursery school teacher, and grandmother from Philadelphia, had an operation for cancer in which her uterus, ovaries, and Fallopian tubes were removed. By January, 1973, the tumor metastasized, and she had a modified radical mastectomy of the right breast." Kushi then tells how her son Phillip, who had studied macrobiotics, brought her macrobiotic food in the hospital and how she gradually began to implement the macrobiotic diet. She then consulted Kushi, who recommended a stricter healing diet.

> The next summer Mrs. Crabtree returned, and I told her that she was 60 percent healed and to continue eating carefully. By autumn of 1978, Phyllis had completed the five-year "cure" period for her original illness and outlived 85 percent of women who had had similar operations on the uterus and breast.
>
> "I'm grateful to macrobiotics for more than a cancer 'cure', she stated. "For myself there has been an improvement in my aching back (caused by osteoporosis) and a urinary infection (both ailments of thirty years' duration). The migraine headaches are fewer in number and less in intensity and duration. Even my motion sickness has lessened.
>
> "My husband has benefitted from the diet through weight control. Michio's lectures in Los Angeles many years ago were instrumental in returning Phil to us from his 'hippy' world. My daughter adopted a baby girl because she was unable to conceive. She now has three daughters, two of them 'macrobiotically brewed'."[23]

Analyzing Kushi's Breast Cancer Program

In analyzing Kushi's recommendations for breast cancer, five major points can be made:

1. As I have noted, the use of medical literature is profuse but sketchy and sometimes unbalanced. Often the implied criticisms of mainstream treatment are fair and would be acknowledged as such by objective oncologists, but these fair criticisms are placed side by side with poorly substantiated claims, and all are given equal weight.
2. Kushi's theory of the *causation* of breast cancer combines the mainstream position that a high fat diet may contribute to breast cancer

(which he does not acknowledge as debated) with the macrobiotic theory (of the formation of mucus into cysts and tumors), which is poetic, intriguing, and unproven.

3. Kushi's discussion of the *diagnostic* system of macrobiotics incorporates a skeptical review of mainstream diagnosis with his own interpretation of Oriental medical diagnosis, which is unproven by conventional medicine.

4. Kushi's *dietary recommendations* provide for a healthy and nutritionally balanced diet, but are based on a complex macrobiotic dietary theory that also has no foundation in scientific medicine. Moreover, the specific foods that are included and excluded by macrobiotics for breast cancer differ from those recommended by many other systems of diet coming from other traditional medicines of equally noble lineage. Ayurvedic medicine from India, for example, gives dietary recommendations for breast cancer that are quite different from, and often contradict, macrobiotic recommendations. So it is true not only that macrobiotics has a dietary theory that is "unproven" from a mainstream perspective but also that its system, in many respects, contradicts other traditional dietary regimens, such as naturopathic or Ayurvedic dietary programs. These other traditional dietary systems, incidentally, also contradict one another. However, Kushi would point out legitimately that although the dietary therapies of the great systems of traditional medicine differ in their details, they are generally united in their recommendation of fresh whole foods with a primary emphasis on grains. Kushi's recommendation of sea vegetables is supported by suggestive scientific evidence, as we shall see later.

5. Perhaps most interesting is the astounding assertion (from the mainstream perspective) that a clay-cabbage compress applied regularly to a breast with a malignant tumor can draw the tumor up through the skin and out of the body. This assertion cries out for objective scientific evaluation. Can the success of this clay-cabbage compress be documented based on past case records, as Kushi states? Can this success be replicated by independent scientific observers? What is the further course of the disease in patients who have treated their tumors in this way as opposed to having them surgically removed? What is the comparative rate of metastasis? Are there medical complications with the compress method, and

how do they compare with complications of surgery and radiation therapy? What are the comparative experiences with quality of life and life expectancy? What are the dangers in the procedure when the tumor enlarges or ruptures?

Given the observations of cases mentioned above, these are very serious issues indeed. The concept of using compresses to remove fat and mucus, thereby eliminating tumors, does not square well with current medical observation of the contents of breast tumors. And the dangers of delaying medical, radiological, or surgical treatment of breast cancer would be, from the physician's point of view, grave indeed. On the one hand, if success with this treatment were documented, it could well represent an important advance in the treatment of breast cancer—potentially rivaling in importance the adjunctive role of diet as a supportive treatment. On the other hand, if the treatment does *not* work, it could be dangerously misleading or simply dangerous. It is a mark of the absence of careful studies of macrobiotics by researchers that this question, to my knowledge, has never been addressed.

Kushi's assertion that this procedure works *at all* would create incredulity—if not shock—in many mainstream physicians. But my suspicion that there may be something here worth studying was raised by my having met a cancer patient early in my research (before I realized the importance of documenting this assertion) who told me firsthand that her tumor had been drawn out through the skin using similar compresses. John Fink of the International Association of Cancer Victors and Friends in Santa Barbara also reported a case to me of a woman who had treated her cancer in this way. These reports add to my sense that this is an important area for objective assessment.

The lifestyle recommendations regarding maintenance of a positive attitude, avoiding wool, synthetic fibers, metallic jewelry, and electromagnetic fields from televisions and other apparatuses are harder to assess. Many psychotherapists would disagree with Kushi's recommendation that women "do everything possible to maintain a cheerful and calm attitude," and would instead encourage women to be aware of their inner states, including fear, anger, and so forth. Kushi's recommendations are, nonetheless, consistent with many of the attitudinal recommendations of other Eastern traditions, which often teach that *replacement* of "negative" emotions with "positive" emotions is generally superior to the modern Western tradition that emphasizes *expression* of emotions so that one can "move through" them, rather than being caught in them.

The experience of Mrs. Crabtree with "metastatic breast cancer" is very problematic. Based on the available information, it does not sound as if Mrs. Crabtree had metastatic breast cancer at all. Rather, it sounds as though she had uterine or ovarian cancer which subsequently metastasized to the breast. This is very different from metastatic breast cancer. On the other hand, the recovery story is balanced; the point is made that at least 15% of women with similar cancers live as long as Mrs. Crabtree, and the story of the numerous health improvements experienced by Mrs. Crabtree and her family ring true to anyone familiar with the benefits of a program like macrobiotics.

Kushi's Cancer Program in General

Kushi states that the cancers that respond best to the macrobiotic approach are cancers of the breast, cervix, colon, pancreas, liver, bone, and skin. Cancer of the lung, he says, is "more difficult to change," and "cancers caused by eating eggs are among the most difficult, particularly when they appear deep within the body such as in the ovaries or testicles."[24]

When Kushi moves from specific recommendations to a broader overview of cancer, he moves toward safer—though obviously still contested—ground. He believes that modern science has overlooked the root cause of cancer, which he suggests is the comprehensive biological decline brought about by modern civilization and modern diet.[25] He believes that to respond to cancer we must enlarge our perspective and create a new civilization which is not primarily competitive and materialistic. He also believes we must overcome dualism in thinking about cancer, and understand the beneficial nature of disease. In his view: "cancer is only the final stage in a sequence of events in an illness through which individuals in the modern world tend to pass because we fail to appreciate the beneficial nature of disease symptoms."[26]

A healthy organism, he believes, can discharge through normal channels of elimination a limited excess of nutrients and toxins, but if overconsumption continues, the body reverts to "more serious" measures of discharge such as fever, skin disease, and other superficial symptoms. If we suppress or ignore these symptoms, the body seeks to localize deposits of impurities in the form of fat deposits, chronic mucus, vaginal discharges, cysts, benign tumors, and other similar conditions. If we still persist in unhealthy living, a "critical mass" is reached where these accumulations may become malignant:

As long as we continue to take in excessive nutrients, chemicals and other factors that serve no useful purpose in the body, they must continue to accumulate somewhere in order to continue our normal living functions. If we don't allow them to accumulate in limited areas and form tumors, they will spread throughout the body, resulting in a total collapse of our vital functions and death by toxemia. Cancer is only the terminal stage in a long process. . . . Cancer is the body's last drastic effort to prolong life, even a few more months or years.[26]

In this line of reasoning, although not in all details, Kushi shares the company of many other practitioners of Eastern and Western nature-based healing systems.

Kushi's Use of Yin and Yang in Individual Diet

The modification of the Cancer Prevention Diet to the type of cancer that the individual has is based on a fundamental division that macrobiotics posits of virtually all phenomena in the universe—as manifestations of the interplay of "yin" and "yang" forces.

Yin and yang are two ancient philosophical concepts from China said to represent the "universal laws of harmony and relativity." Kushi traces them back to Confucius and Lao-tzu.[27] Yin, the feminine principle, represents the outward, centrifugal, movement of matter or energy. It is expansive. Yang, the masculine principle, represents an inward, centripetal, movement of matter or energy. It is contractive. Virtually everything can be classified in terms of yin and yang, including foods and cancers. Kushi provides a classification table of yin and yang foods (see table 15.1).

One intriguing question is whether macrobiotics means the same thing by the terms yin and yang that traditional Chinese medicine means. A number of very knowledgeable persons, including Keith Block, Lawrence Kushi, and Gordon Saxe, have suggested that the meaning, or at least the application, of these concepts is significantly different in macrobiotics from the usage in traditional Chinese medicine. One respondent suggested that one of the reasons that some practitioners ultimately abandon macrobiotics or go on to study traditional Chinese medicine in more depth is because of their dissatisfaction with the ambiguities involved in the application of these terms in macrobiotics.

Table 15.1

Yin and Yang Foods

Strong Yang Foods	Balanced Foods	Strong Yin Foods
Refined salt	Whole-cereal grains	Temperate-climate fruit
Eggs	Seeds	White rice, white flour
Meat	Beans and bean products	Tropical fruits and vegetables
Cheese	Nuts	Milk, cream, yogurt
Poultry	Sea vegetables	Oils
Fish	Root, round, and leafy vegetables	Spices (pepper, curry, nutmeg, etc.)
Seafood	Spring or well water	Aromatic and stimulant beverages (coffee, black tea, mint tea, etc.)
	Nonaromatic, nonstimulant teas	Honey, sugar, refined sweeteners
	Natural sea salt	Alcohol
		Foods containing chemicals, preservatives, dyes, pesticides
		Drugs (marijuana, cocaine, etc.)
		Medications (tranquilizers, antidepressants, etc.)

From Kushi and Jack, *The Cancer Prevention Diet*, (New York: St. Martin's Press, 1983), 118.

Another felt that Ohsawa believed that Westerners would have difficulty comprehending the kinetic nature of yin and yang and so he used the terms based on a structure rather than dynamic interrelationships. Therefore the usage of the terms *yin* and *yang* in macrobiotics is often opposite to the usage in traditional Chinese medicine. Alex Jack, co-author with Michio Kushi of *The Cancer Prevention Diet*, takes a constructive view of the relationship between yin and yang in macrobiotics and traditional Chinese medicine: "As for the differences between the way yin and yang are used in traditional Chinese medicine and macrobiotics, modern macrobiotics approaches the subject with a dynamic understanding of structure and energy flow that is based on the traditional Oriental view. Contemporary Chinese medicine sometimes takes a more static perspective. However, these views are more complementary than antagonistic."[28]

The debate underlines the broader point that macrobiotics is very much Michio Kushi's own interpretation of certain underlying principles in traditional Chinese medicine viewed through the lens of his personal interest in health-promoting therapies.

"Medically Terminal or Macrobiotically Hopeful"

Kushi's broader recommendations for "preventing cancer naturally" are very much a part of the great perennial teachings found in all the great healing and spiritual traditions. In his version, these teachings include[29]:

- Self-reflection to develop a more natural, harmonious, contemplative, appreciative, and contributory perspective on life.
- Respect for the natural environment, so that we do not continue to degrade the earth for which we depend on life.
- A naturally balanced diet, in harmony with evolutionary order, universal dietary traditions, the ecological order, the changing seasons, and individual differences.
- An active daily life.

In a discussion of whether cancer patients are "medically terminal or macrobiotically hopeful," Kushi addresses the truly difficult and delicate problem of the relationship of the macrobiotic regimen to conventional therapies:

> The recovery of patients who have received medical intervention may be complicated and more difficult as a result of the side effects of treatment and the general weakening produced by chemotherapy, radiation, or other methods. With macrobiotics, we try to change the quality of the blood and cells through living a natural daily life and strengthening the body's natural system of immunity . . .
>
> A medically terminal case is one for which present treatments offer no hope of recovery. In some cases, an exploratory operation is performed and the patient is told that no treatment will be applied. Persons in this situation often

have a better possibility of recovery on the Cancer Prevention Diet than those who were considered hopeful by modern medicine and who received conventional treatment.[30]

This is, again, a very concrete statement, and it would be interesting indeed to evaluate it scientifically. I would be very surprised if Kushi's assertion turned out to be correct.

Kushi then lists factors that may interfere with the process of recovery. These include:

- Lack of gratitude: A spirit of thankfulness is essential to the healing process. The person needs to see that his or her way of eating and living created the cancer and that he is fortunate to have the opportunity to change his diet and lifestyle. However, many cancer patients . . . constantly complain when the new diet is introduced. . . . Such persons think that cancer happened to them by accident and that they have done nothing to deserve it. . . . This type of person has no understanding of himself, nature, or God, and is incapable of self-reflection. . . . For such people, macrobiotics is just another pill to be taken and discarded when their symptoms disappear. They may survive for a while, but will never fundamentally heal themselves or be happy. The death certificate will say cancer, heart attack, or the flu, but the real cause is arrogance.
- Inaccurate dietary practices: . . . Another mistake is to confuse the macrobiotic approach with other dietary or nutritional approaches to cancer and "to be on the safe side" try to combine them all.
- Lack of will: In some cases persons who have no desire to live are introduced to the Cancer Prevention Diet, often by some well-intentioned family member or friend. Such persons, who frequently ignore the advice they are given, have a very slight chance of recovery. We can extend to them our love, sympathy and prayers, but ultimately we must respect a person's decision to die.
- Lack of family support: Among the many patients whom I have counselled were a number of middle-aged men who, although they were married, visited us by themselves. When asked why their wives had not come, they often replied that their wives did not agree with their desire to begin macrobiotics. . . . I have also met many women who did not have the support of their husbands or children whose parents were not sympathetic. I sympathize very much with these people because in a real sense they are alone. Their families lack the understanding, love and care that are essential for their recovery. . . . Despite their courage, the chances of succeeding are low. Among all the cancer patients I have met, those who recovered were

primarily single and cooked for themselves or had the full support of their families, even to the extent that other family members also started the diet and learned to cook macrobiotically. Therefore, the cancer patient in this situation should investigate the possibility of another living situation until his or her condition improves.[31]

Kushi points to spiritual awareness, the experience of deep suffering leading to a desire to embrace the macrobiotic program, will and determination, and the love and care of family and friends as powerfully supportive of recovery.[31]

In his list of impediments to healing, the combination of perennial wisdom and the controversial application of particulars that characterizes so much of macrobiotic philosophy is vividly apparent. Kushi's strong position on the patient's need to accept that his way of life caused the cancer, and his rigorous condemnation of those who complain about the diet or who are not grateful for the opportunity cancer has given them to change their diet and lifestyle, are profoundly controversial among many progressive psychotherapists who share a more positive orientation toward nutritional and psychospiritual approaches to cancer.

Nor is Kushi's strong position in this area universally shared among macrobiotic teachers. Those who take issue with his approach feel that it is irresponsible to insist that the patient "caused" his cancer, and that his denunciation of people who object to a macrobiotic diet, or who do not feel "grateful" for the opportunities cancer has afforded them, are prime examples of serious "guilt-tripping" and "blaming the patient," which can be found in a number of New Age theories of cancer. But, in his defense, one anonymous Kushi advocate said:

> The motivation behind this view is to provide the perspective that "if I caused the illness, then I can get rid of it." This . . . has the potential of bringing the patient to see that he or she has the responsibility and means to take charge of his or her treatment/recovery. Thus, it can be an enlightening source of empowerment. . . .
>
> I also point out that this idea that one has caused one's cancer is *directly* substantiated by the growing evidence that one's lifestyle (diet, smoking, exercise, etc.) strongly influences the risk of developing disease.

Kushi's position that the macrobiotic diet should not be modified would also not meet with agreement among many clinicians who utilize a modified macrobiotic regimen. But his belief in the importance of the "will to live" and "family support" would certainly meet with deeper agreement.

Kushi's Strategy

Strategically, Kushi made some adept decisions in choosing to present macrobiotics as "a commonsense approach to living" and as an educational program. In contrast to the proponents of many alternative nutritional approaches, his book does not call his approach a *cancer cure*. While he gives examples of patients who reportedly recovered from metastatic or otherwise life-threatening cancers using macrobiotics, the cases often include explicit evidence that misdiagnosis might have been involved or that the case was not entirely hopeless from a mainstream perspective.

He also developed an educational model for delivering the program, as well as a systematic program for training many others in how to use it. He himself has written ten books and helped others write and publish books and articles on the use of the macrobiotic diet. For all of these reasons, macrobiotics was strategically placed at a comparative advantage over most of the medically based alternative nutritional programs that represented their approaches as cancer *cures,* thereby engendering a far more virulent opposition from the medical community.

One of the few other groups of practitioners who have exhibited similar strategic skill in avoiding serious conflict with mainstream medicine is, not coincidentally, the practitioners of traditional Chinese medicine; they have often (not always) been even more cautious than Kushi. They make no special claims about cancer; many practitioners even refuse to treat cancer; and those who do treat it emphasize the purely adjunctive nature of their treatment. As a result, tens of thousands of American cancer patients are able to avail themselves of the supportive treatment of traditional Chinese medicine. Strategic placement of treatments outside the medical mainstream are the skills of people from Oriental cultures, accustomed to taking the long view in strategy, and to achieving goals by indirect means when direct assaults on governmental authorities would be counterproductive or dangerous.

Case histories, physician reports, and scientific studies that relate to the use of macrobiotics in cancer are sketchy. But nonetheless they are suggestive that macrobiotics may have, at least, some positive impact for some people with cancer.

One of the most credible independent witnesses for a macrobiotic approach to cancer was Anthony Sattilaro, M.D., whose book, *Recalled by Life,*[32] published in 1982, describes his recovery from prostatic cancer, which had metastasized to his skull, shoulder, spine, sternum, and ribs. He underwent conventional therapy, but his physician told him that he had at best only a few years to live. Then he turned to macrobiotics, experienced a spiritual awakening, and subsequently recovered. The story of his recovery did for macrobiotics something akin to what the story of *New York Times* columnist James Reston's experience with acupuncture did for that approach: it brought a heretofore very foreign-sounding therapy to public attention through a single person's account. The key point here is that both authors had credibility. Reston was a respected reporter and columnist. Sattilaro was chief executive of Methodist Hospital in Philadelphia, having previously served as chairman of the anesthesiology department. Some mainstream critics questioned whether Sattilaro's cancer was *truly* as life-threatening as he portrayed it. (Sattilaro subsequently laid this debate to rest by dying of a recurrence of his cancer in 1989.)

After his initial recovery using macrobiotics, Sattilaro distanced himself from the macrobiotic movement, especially from its more particularistic components and its belief systems. But his belief in the importance of his own spiritual awakening and the whole-foods vegetarian diet remained.

A second important independent witness for the benefits of some of the nutritional building components of the macrobiotic approach is Keith Block, M.D., whose treatment program I discuss in chapter 17. Block is an especially credible observer because he clearly distinguishes between the particularistic and ideological components of macrobiotics and its fundamentals. Once a believer in macrobiotic nutrition, Block gradually moved away from macrobiotics and developed his own system:

I found problems within the macrobiotic system, but also a great deal that was significant and valuable in concert with certain other regimens whose principal emphasis has been on complex carbohydrates, high fiber, low fat and moderate protein intake.

Do I believe that food cures cancer? Certainly not in and of itself. Do I believe food can cause cancer or militate against its control? I absolutely do. Do I believe that appropriate nutrition has a series of unacknowledged and complex consequences which affect other biochemical systems in the struggle to retard tumor growth and elaboration? I absolutely do.[33]

Block has collected a number of well-documented cases in which he believes his individualized and modified macrobiotic-based nutritional system played a significant role in controlling or reversing cancer. He has presented his cases to professional audiences and welcomes open evaluation of his results.[33]

While the scientific literature contains no published studies on macrobiotics and cancer treatment, there are three unpublished studies, each of them flawed but nonetheless intriguing both for what they show and what they do not show. Vivien Newbold, M.D., a charismatic young emergency-room physician, tells the following story:

In December, 1983, a close friend was found to have inoperable colon cancer that had spread to the liver. He was given just four to six months to live. Since there was then and, at this writing, still is no known treatment for this disease once it has spread beyond the intestines, and since chemotherapy could, at best, offer only a possibility of temporary prolongation of life, he chose not to receive any medical treatment, but instead to try macrobiotics. He and his family followed the macrobiotic diet one hundred per cent, without any deviations, and became totally involved in the macrobiotic way of life. Almost every night his wife and son gave him *shiatsu* massage. Within three months of being on the macrobiotic diet, he began running, and by September of 1984 he ran half a marathon. In November, 1985, a CT scan could find no sign of cancer and his present health is excellent. This is truly astounding in view of the fact that there is only one recorded case of spontaneous regression of metastatic colon cancer.[34]

Following this experience, Newbold set out to document the results of cancer of patients who (1) used macrobiotics with or without chemotherapy; (2) used macrobiotics for pancreatic or brain cancers in particular; (3) used macrobiotics for other serious illnesses; and (4) were documented cases of medically advanced, incurable, biopsy-proven cancer who had followed macrobiotics and recovered completely.[35] Just as Gar Hildenbrand discovered in his effort to find "pure" Gerson recoveries for a best-case analysis of the Gerson therapy, Newbold found the task extremely difficult. After a very extensive search, she ultimately found six cases of complete remission from advanced malignant disease using both conventional therapies and macrobiotic diet. Newbold had the cases reviewed independently, and the diagnoses confirmed by pathologists and radiologists, and offers copies of clinical records to other researchers for confirmation.

Newbold offered her paper to three major medical journals, the *New England Journal of Medicine, Lancet,* and the *Journal of the American Medical Association.* She says, "On every occasion it was turned down for publication on the grounds of insufficient interest to their readership or similar reasons. On no occasion was any attempt made to review the evidence supporting the paper in depth."[36]

In summarizing her study in another publication, Newbold wrote: "The number of patients in this . . . group is small, and although it does not prove that macrobiotics can bring about recovery from cancer, it indicates that for the patient who cannot be offered hope medically, it is certainly worth a try."[37]

Efforts to Study Macrobiotics and Cancer Scientifically

James Carter, Chairman of the Department of Nutrition at the Tulane School of Public Health, and Gordon Saxe, M.P.H., a Ph.D. candidate in Epidemiologic Science at the University of Michigan, and their colleagues conducted two retrospective studies on the effects of the macrobiotic diet. The first study examined primary cancers of the pancreas to determine if patients following a macrobiotic diet survived longer than pancreatic cancer patients from the National Cancer Institute's SEER (Surveillance Epidemiology and End Results—a national cancer registry) data from the same period. Pancreatic cancer was chosen because it has a very poor prognosis, is rapidly fatal (therefore a relatively short period of follow-up is required to see evidence of life extension), and is a cancer for which macrobiotics claims positive results.

Carter and Saxe studied pancreatic cancer patients treated from 1980 to mid-1984 by macrobiotic counselors and who reported following macrobiotic diets for at least 3 months. (Of 109 patients who had been counseled, 36 were reached and 23 met the study criteria.) Carter and Saxe compared mean and median length of survival, as well as the proportion of patients surviving at various time points (e.g., 1 year after diagnosis), for these 23 patients with that of all SEER patients who had pancreatic cancer diagnosed during the same period. The mean and median survival for the macrobiotic patients was 17.3 and 13.3 months, respectively, compared to 6.0 and 3.4 months for the SEER group. The 1-year survival rate was 52.2% for the macrobiotic group compared with 9.7% for the SEER subjects. Carter and Saxe observed that the macrobiotic patients lived significantly longer than the nonmacrobiotic population, but that this difference may have resulted from selection or other biases. They concluded that these results did not prove that dietary modification was the reason for the longer survival. However, they noted that these findings, taken together with several medically documented reports of remission in macrobiotic pancreatic cancer patients, was suggestive of a possible dietary effect.[38]

The important question is whether it was the practice of macrobiotics per se, or rather some type of selection or other bias, which accounted for the dramatic difference between the survival of macrobiotic patients and those in the SEER sample. The answer is uncertain. A related question is what happened to the 67% of macrobiotic patients that Carter and Saxe could not locate. If, hypothetically, Carter and Saxe's 23 participants represented some of the top survivors among all the macrobiotic patients originally identified, and if all the other macrobiotic patients made the same marked dietary changes but had the same survival curve as the SEER patients (a very conservative assumption), then Carter and Saxe calculate the macrobiotic patients would have had a 1-year survival rate of about 20%, compared to the 9.7% reported for the SEER patients. If the group Carter and Saxe contacted were the longest-lived survivors among the macrobiotic patients, then the survival rate for the macrobiotic patients was only about 12% compared to 9.7% for the SEER group—virtually no difference at all in a sample this size.[39]

In a subsequent analysis, Saxe found that when the survival comparisons were restricted to those SEER patients alive at least 4 months after diagnosis, the difference shrank but was still statistically significant (and could, of course, still be accounted for by other biases). For example, after 1 year, the difference narrowed from 52.2% vs. 9.7% to 52.2% vs. 37.7%. On the other hand, he noted that few of the macrobiotic patients received adequate follow-up counseling, cooking instruction, dietary monitoring, or social support. As a result, dietary compliance may have been overestimated and the therapeutic potential of dietary modification underestimated.[40]

In my estimate, these studies suggests the possibility of a significant survival advantage for the patients who undertook the macrobiotic diet. The range of improvement reported is in keeping, incidentally, with the doubling of survival reported by David Spiegel in his study of psychological group support for women with metastatic breast cancer and, as we saw in chapter 10, similar reports from several other studies of psychological interventions that matched participants against historical controls or other partial controls. It appears to be an outcome in the same range that Lechner's Austrian group found in its poorly controlled study of participation in the Gerson diet (see chapter 14).

In a second study, Carter and colleagues examined 11 cases of prostate cancer. The 11 men, all of whom were receiving conventional treatment and following a macrobiotic diet, were matched with controls receiving conventional treatment only, and also were compared with similar-stage cancer patients reported in the literature. The median survival of the macrobiotic group was 81 months, compared to 45 months for the nonmacrobiotic population. In describing the study, the Office of Technology report *Unconventional Cancer Treatments* concluded that the same methodological difficulties that were present in the first study also made it impossible to interpret the results of the second.[41]

Barry R. Goldin of the New England Medical Center Hospital in Boston and his colleagues compared the excretion of estrogens in healthy pre- and post-menopausal macrobiotic and omnivorous women. They found that "vegetarian" (macrobiotic) women excrete two to three times more estrogens in feces than do omnivores and that omnivores have about 50% higher mean plasma levels of estrogen products than do vegetarians. "[The] data suggest that in vegetarians a greater amount of the biliary estrogens escape reabsorption [in the intestines] and are excreted with the feces. *The differences in estrogen metabolism may explain the lower incidence of breast cancer in vegetarian women*" [emphasis added].[42]

Evidence also exists that a macrobiotic diet might influence important prognostic factors in breast cancer. L.E. Holm and his colleagues at the Karolinska Hospital in Stockholm studied women who had had surgery for breast cancer and found that tumor size at the time of surgery was inversely related to fiber intake, and that patients having estrogen receptor–rich tumors received proportionately more calories from carbohydrates and foods containing retinol. They concluded that "these results suggest that the dietary patterns of the western world (e.g., high fat intake and low intake of carbohydrates and fiber) affect certain prognostic factors in breast cancer, such as tumor size and ER [estrogen receptor] content of the tumor."[43] Similarly, in a preliminary analysis of a recent study involving 225 breast cancer patients at the University of Michigan Hospital, Saxe found that overweight patients were almost three times as likely as lean patients to be diagnosed with an advanced-stage malignancy.[44]

Takeshi Hirayama of the National Cancer Center Research Institute in Japan reported in 1981 that daily intake of soybean paste (miso) soup correlated with dramatically reduced gastric cancer rates in a large-scale prospective study of over 260,000 Japanese men and women. The standardized mortality rates for men who drank miso soup daily was 171.9 per 100,000 compared to a rate of 255.9 for men who never drank miso soup, with intermediate values for men who drank miso soup occasionally or rarely. The rates for women were 77.8 for daily miso soup drinkers and 113.6 for women who never drank miso soup. Hirayama noted that the results could result from beneficial compounds such as protease inhibitors or other nutritious factors in the soybean paste, or that it could reflect other beneficial foods that frequently accompany soybean soup consumption, such as intake of green and yellow vegetables.[45]

Another study by Goro Chihara and his colleagues at the same institute in Japan found that two polysaccharide preparations from *Lentinus edodes,* a mushroom eaten frequently in the macrobiotic diet, had strong antitumor effect in the growth of sarcoma 180 implanted in mice.[46]

Two studies on seaweeds used in macrobiotics are of interest. Jane Teas of the Harvard School of Public Health and colleagues, noting that breast cancer is three times lower in premenopausal Japanese women than in premenopausal American women, decided to look at the possibility that brown seaweed (kelp), which is widely consumed by Japanese women, might be a factor. "Several studies have shown that seaweed extracts can prevent the growth of tumors transplanted to laboratory animals. We were interested in whether the regular intake of dietary seaweed could be prophylactic for carcinogen-induced mammary tumors in rats."[47]

The Sprague-Dawley rats treated with the carcinogen DMBA (7,12-dimethyl-benz[a]anthracene) were considered a good model because the breast cancers in rats arise, as in humans, in the ductal system of the mammary gland. The tumors are hormone-dependent and are thus analogous to estrogen receptor–positive breast cancer in women. Experimental rats fed kelp took almost twice as long to develop tumors as the control rats and had a 13% reduction in the number of adenocarcinomas that developed.[47]

The second seaweed study, by Y. Tanaka and his colleagues at McGill University in Montreal, looked at the role of polysaccharides from brown seaweed (kelp) in inhibiting the intestinal absorption of radioactive strontium:

> Polysaccharides prepared from brown seaweeds are unique agents from the practical as well as the theoretical point of view because they selectively bind strontium. . . . We became interested [in them] because of their importance as a source of material that can prevent the intestinal absorption of radioactive products from atomic fission, and in their possible use as natural decontaminators because of their ability to concentrate metal ions from seawater.[48]

Whether this ability of kelp to prevent the absorption of radioactive products is of value to patients undergoing radiation therapy is a question of some interest.

A small cluster of epidemiological studies also lends credence to the value of assessing the role of macrobiotic diet as a preventive measure for breast cancer. Ernst Wynder of the American Health Foundation in New York and his colleagues describe research showing a marked increase in the incidence of breast and prostatic cancer among Japanese migrants to Hawaii.[49] This increase is best explained by the adoption of American diets by these migrants and by their offspring, whose cancer incidence rates approach the rates for Hawaiian whites. Similarly, the gradual increase in breast and prostatic cancer rates in

Japan since the 1950s can be correlated with the increase in dietary fat intake in that country. Wynder et al. conclude that a threshold exists between 20% and 30% of caloric intake in the form of fat where the stimulatory effect of fat on breast carcinogenesis manifests itself. The researchers therefore recommend a diet for the population at large, and particularly for high-risk women, that limits fat intake to 25% of total calories.

Analyzing breast cancer survival rates, Wynder et al. cited studies indicating that these rates are higher for women in Japan than in the United States and that the major survival difference is found among postmenopausal women. These findings are compatible with case-controlled studies showing that breast cancer patients on high fat diets have poorer survival times than those on low fat diets. Wynder et al. conclude, "We are surprised that most physicians pay so little attention to the likelihood that metabolic overloads in terms of nutritional intake could have a deleterious effect, aside from obvious obesity, on many bodily functions. Therefore, nutritional adjustments are very likely to be an effective pharmacologic intervention, particularly when used early in a disease process; in fact, 'we are what we eat'."[49]

The macrobiotic diet, then, might well be a good model for individuals interested in implementing a diet based upon the above recommendations, since it is to a large degree derived from the traditional Japanese diet. But the data on breast cancer cited by Wynder et al. can be interpreted in several ways. It may suggest that a Japanese-style diet might have its greater effect on older American women, who are less likely today to be attracted to it, and is much less likely to help younger American women, who are more likely to belong to the subcultures that more readily accept such diets. Following this interpretation, a key issue is the level of cultural stress involved for older women in adapting to such a diet. Acute stress, I pointed out in chapter 10, is often a proven enhancer of tumor development in animal studies, and is also believed to be a tumor promoter for humans. If adopting a radically different diet is experienced by some older women as a major life stress, the stress effect could very plausibly offset any potential benefit of the low fat diet.

A second interpretation of the Wynder et al. data suggests that at the time the authors did their study, older Japanese women were more likely to be eating a traditional, low fat diet than younger women, who had westernized their diets. Therefore, this—rather than biological or hormonal factors—may account for the fact that younger Japanese women had nearly the same survival as younger American women. If this were the case, a Japanese or macrobiotic diet might be useful to premenopausal women with breast cancer as well as to older women.

Conclusion

In summary, the scientific evidence, case reports, and clinical assessments by physicians lead us to much the same conclusions about the macrobiotic diet that we reached about the Gerson diet. The macrobiotic program is clearly not any kind of definitive "cure" for any cancer. If it were, the researchers who worked hard to gather "best cases" for analysis would have found many more striking recovery stories.

On the other hand, there are a considerable number of well-documented, unexpected recoveries, including recoveries from metastatic cancers. The available data suggest, as the Gerson data suggest, that the kind of person who chooses the rigors of the macrobiotic program may be likely, for psychological reasons, to have a somewhat more optimistic outlook regarding his quality of life and life extension, in addition to possible positive effects of the diet. To venture a grossly rough guess on the magnitude of the effect of macrobiotic diet in the instances when it appears helpful, it might be in the range of doubling the length of survival, which is the same rate reported by a number of the psychological interventions and, with some cancers, for the Gerson regimen.

But is this hypothetical enhancement of survival to be credited to the diet? Lawrence Kushi, Michio Kushi's son, believes that, although it is not the macrobiotic diet per se that has an anticancer effect, but probably any healthy vegetarian diet (that does not contain substantial amounts of dairy food), still the macrobiotic *philosophy* "helps to provide a framework by which to evaluate potential dietary approaches to cancer therapy. . . . Certain principles of application are likely to have some benefit; however, how these are applied may not resemble (superficially, at least) a 'macrobiotic' diet as most people consider it."[50] Certainly, if similar effects are found for some patients with vegetarian diets as diverse as the Gerson diet and macrobiotics, it is not a *single* vegetarian diet that achieves these effects.

I believe, as Michio Kushi clearly believes, that the will to live, a healthy attitude toward life, and the macrobiotic diet work together to produce whatever outcomes are possible. I must also say that for myself, a 10-year vegetarian, a broad and somewhat flexible macrobiotic diet generally makes me feel better than any other vegetarian diet. I feel grounded, stronger, and experience fewer addictive food cravings than when I eat a wholly flexible vegetarian diet. Once old cravings from an earlier diet have been overcome, I believe that how one feels is often an excellent guide to what diet really works for oneself. Therefore, *for me,* I suspect that a macrobiotic-oriented diet is more than a bizarre, restricted variation of a healthy vegetarian diet, but has some real wisdom to it. I suspect that a large portion of my benefits result from the proportions of different recommended food types, the food preparation methods, the sea vegetables, and the miso soup. Before moving gradually toward a broadly macrobiotic diet, I had for years eaten too many salads and raw vegetables, which left me feeling weaker and with a craving for oils and dairy products. Increasing grains to 50% of my intake played a major role in changing that. So my guess is that a very broadly based macrobiotic diet is, at least for some vegetarians, including myself, healthier than other vegetarian diets.

It is striking, however, that a community as large, intelligent, and generally well situated as the macrobiotic community has produced so little in the way of definitive research on the effects of macrobiotics on cancer. The available evidence is certainly suggestive that macrobiotics may be of at least modest help in some types of cancer, but it is no more than suggestive. I think it is incumbent on the macrobiotic physicians and their colleagues in the medical research community to move beyond suggestive studies, case histories, and the clinical-philosophical treatises of Michio Kushi and other macrobiotic teachers and to do some serious studies. The studies should evaluate both the diet and some of the more striking "home remedies"—most notably the clay-cabbage compresses said by supporters to be capable of drawing tumors out through the skin and by critics to be potentially dangerous. For a community that defines itself as taking the long view, the time has come to do some small but well-designed case-control, prospective, or randomized clinical trials with cancer. Given the resources that the Kushi Institute and other macrobiotic programs generate nationally, and the willingness of well-qualified macrobiotic researchers to stretch dollars and work inexpensively, there should be no need to wait for federal research support. The money should be raised within the macrobiotic community and the prospective clinical trials undertaken.

As this book was going to press, Alex Jack, co-author with Kushi of *The Cancer Prevention Diet*, wrote to me regarding the extensively revised and expanded edition that was published in 1993:

> The new edition incorporates ten years' of refinement and evolution in Michio's understanding and approach, including some new dietary recommendations, new home cares, and new recipes and menus. On the surface, these may not appear to be significant to the general reader, but to the experienced macrobiotic teacher or health care professional they represent an important development.
>
> Overall, I think the last ten years have seen a detente or rapprochement between holistic health and conventional medicine, including macrobiotics. I think macrobiotic teachers are more appreciative of the usual medical doctors and therapies and willing to integrate them or refer others in that direction if necessary. Similarly, the medical profession is more tolerant of macrobiotics and a good number of doctors are very supportive and encouraging. This coexistence, I believe, is reflected in the new edition of *The Cancer Prevention Diet* and many of the sections critical of modern medicine have been deleted. In fact, Michio added a section on adjusting dietary recommendations for those undergoing radiation, chemo[therapy], or other conventional therapy.[51]

Notes and References

1 *Biography of Michio Kushi*, Kushi Institute, undated, 2.
2 Ibid.
3 Ibid.
4 Ibid.
5 Ibid., 3.
6 Michio Kushi with Alex Jack, *The Cancer Prevention Diet: Michio Kushi's Nutritional Blueprint for the Relief and Prevention of Disease*, (New York: St. Martin's Press, 1983), 17.
7 Lawrence Kushi, telephone conversation with author, July 1990.
8 Dean Omish et al., "Effects of Stress Management Training and Dietary Changes in Ischemic Heart Disease," *Journal of the American Medical Association* 249(1):54–9 (1983).
9 *New York Times*, "Health Section," 16 November 1989.
10 Frank M. Sacks et al., "Blood Pressure in Vegetarians," *American Journal of Epidemiology* 100(5):390–8.

11 Kushi, *The Cancer Prevention Diet,* v–vi.

12 Michio Kushi, letter. Cited in U.S. Congress Office of Technology Assessment, *Unconventional Cancer Treatments,* (Washington, D.C.: Government Printing Office, September 1990), 59.

13 Kushi, *The Cancer Prevention Diet,* 146.

14 Ibid., 147.

15 Ibid., 149.

16 Ibid., 150–5.

17 Ibid., 156–7.

18 Ibid., 157.

19 Ibid., 159.

20 Ibid., 160–1.

21 Keith Block, M.D., letter to the author, 27 November 1991.

22 Kushi, *The Cancer Prevention Diet,* 161.

23 Ibid., 162–3.

24 Ibid., 76–7.

25 Ibid., 19.

26 Ibid., 24.

27 Ibid., 58.

28 Alex Jack, personal communication with the author, 16 April 1991.

29 *Cancer Prevention Diet*, 26–34.

30 Ibid., 90.

31 Ibid., 90–7.

32 Anthony Sattilaro, *Recalled by Life* (New York: Avon Books, 1982).

33 Block presented some of his cases where diet and psychosocial factors may have played a significant role in controlling or reversing cancer at the Symington Foundation Conference on New Directions in Cancer Care at Commonweal in February 1989 to an international audience of oncologists, psychotherapists, and other professionals concerned with cancer.

34 Vivien Newbold, "Macrobiotics: An Approach to the Achievement of Health, Happiness and Harmony." In Edward Esko, ed., *Doctors Look at Macrobiotics* (New York: Japan Publications, 1988), 45.

35 Ibid.

36 Vivien Newbold, letter to Helen E. Sheehan, Director of Professional Education Programs, American Cancer Society, 4 March 1988.

37 Newbold in Esko, ed., *Doctors Look at Macrobiotics,* 46.

38 James Carter et al., "Cancers with Suspected Nutritional Links: Dietary Management?" Typescript, Nutrition Section, Tulane University School of Public Health and Tropical Medicine, New Orleans, LA, February 1990. Cited in Office of Technology Assessment, *Unconventional Cancer Treatments,* 64–5.

39 Gordon Saxe, telephone conversation with author, July 1990.

40 Gordon Saxe, personal communication with the author, 31 January, 1991.

41 Carter et al., "Cancers with Suspected Nutritional Links." Cited in Office of Technology Assessment, *Unconventional Cancer Treatments,* 65.

42   Barry R. Goldin et al., "Effect of Diet on Excretion of Estrogen in Pre- and Post-menopausal Women," *Cancer Research* 41:3771–3 (1981).

43   L.E. Holm, "Dietary Habits and Prognostic Factors in Breast Cancer," *Journal of the National Cancer Institute* 81(16):1218–23 (1989).

44   Gordon Saxe, personal conversation with the author, 21 August 1991.

45   Takeshi Hirayama, "Relationship of Soybean Paste Soup Intake to Gastric Cancer," *Nutrition and Cancer* 3:223–33 (1982).

46   Goro Chihara et al., "Fractionation and Purification of the Polysachharides with Marked Antitumor Activity, Especially Lentinan, from *Lentinus edodes* (Berk.) Sing. (An Edible Mushroom)," *Cancer Research* 30:2776 (1970).

47   Jane Teas et al., "Dietary Seaweed (Laminaria) and Mammary Carcinogenesis in Rats," *Cancer Research* 44:2758–61 (1984).

48   Y. Tanaka, "Studies on Inhibition of Intestinal Absorption of Radioactive Strontium," *Canadian Medical Association Journal* 99:169–75 (1968).

49   Ernst L. Wynder et al., "Diet and Breast Cancer in Causation and Therapy," *Cancer* 58:1805–11 (1986).

50   Lawrence Kushi, personal communication with author, 24 January 1991.

51   Alex Jack, letter to the author, 29 September 1993.

sixteen

Virginia C. Livingston—Integrating Diet, Nutritional Supplements, and Immunotherapy

The story of Virginia C. Livingston, a physician who died in her late eighties in 1990, is at once dramatic and prototypical of those who venture off the path of mainstream cancer medicine. After undertaking some exacting research, she claimed that she had discovered a microbe that caused cancer and then developed a vaccine that she claimed would help control that microbe. Whether or not her claim has any validity has not yet been fully evaluated, although it has been categorically dismissed by mainstream medicine.

In addition to her vaccine, Livingston also developed a multifaceted nutritional, medical, and immunosupportive program, which can be traced back in part to the German naturopathic tradition of Max Gerson and Josef Issels. She can therefore be considered a "second-generation" nutritional cancer therapist, especially since fully half of her program is nutritional in content. Livingston's treatment is still being offered at the Livingston Clinic in San Diego.[1]

Livingston's Biography

Virginia Livingston started her medical career as one of the pioneering women physicians of her time. Her great-uncle and father were both physicians, and her father was one of the early members of the American College of Physicians. She was one of only four women to receive her M.D. from New York

University in 1936 and was appointed the first woman resident physician at a New York hospital—the prison hospital for venereally infected prostitutes.[2]

While at the prison hospital, she became interested in tuberculosis and leprosy, which were being treated in nearby infectious disease units. As a school physician a few years later, she became interested in scleroderma, a degenerative disease of the skin and tissue that Livingston came to see as related etiologically to tuberculosis, leprosy, and cancer. Livingston found that a red dye staining technique revealed numerous "acid-fast" organisms (organisms that stained when exposed to the diagnostic dye) in scleroderma. These organisms, she believed, were similar to those found in leprosy and tuberculosis. Because she saw scleroderma as similar to cancer, she began to wonder whether she might not find similar organisms in cancer tissue. "At this point," she writes, "I reasoned that perhaps scleroderma was a kind of slow cancer. I decided to begin examining cancer tissues with the same method. . . . Upon examining all kinds of cancerous tissues . . . I found that a similar microorganism was present in all of them."[3]

Livingston then made contact with Eleanor Alexander-Jackson, M.D., of Cornell University, who had found that the tubercle bacillus undergoes many changes in shape, and hence is "pleomorphic" (able to change shape and size.) At that time, cancer was thought to be caused by a virus, and the technique for differentiating a virus from a bacillus was to see whether it passed through a special filter; viruses are much smaller than bacilli and could pass through the filter. Her association with Alexander-Jackson led Livingston to conceive of the acid-fast organisms she saw in scleroderma, leprosy, tuberculosis, and cancer as a family of pleomorphic organisms that sometimes assumed very small forms similar to viruses and at other times had large forms similar to bacilli.[4]

Against considerable odds, Livingston was able to develop a research program to explore this world-class research hypothesis: a family of microbes—able to change dramatically in size and shape—were responsible for the development of cancer, tuberculosis, leprosy, and scleroderma. At a time when women physicians were scarcely welcome in leading roles in cancer research—much less as champions of major breakthrough concepts—she created the Rutgers-Presbyterian Hospital Laboratory for the Study of Proliferative Diseases associated with the Bureau of Biological Research of Rutgers University. She received funds from the American Cancer Society and an impressive group of foundations and medical laboratories. "The next few years at Rutgers," Livingston writes, "were to be the most significant period of my work in cancer research. Our research team was enthusiastic that our work would prove once and for all that the *Progenitor cryptocides* [or PC, the name she would later give the organism she believed she had discovered] microbe was the cause of cancer and that a vaccine could be made to defend against it."[5]

Alexander-Jackson left Cornell to work with Livingston at the new laboratory, and they built a small research team. In 1950, she and Alexander-Jackson published a paper in the *American Journal of Medical Sciences*, which was co-authored by four others including James Hillier, developer of the electron microscope and head of electron microscopy at RCA Victor Laboratories in Princeton, and John Anderson, head of the department of bacteriology at Rutgers and a noted histologist and pathologist. In this paper, they described how Koch's postulates ("the accepted foolproof method of proving the cause of a disease") could be satisfied in the case of *P. cryptocides*. Pure *P. cryptocides* cultures were obtained from both human and animal cancers and injected into animals capable of being infected. Disease areas then developed resembling those from which cultures were taken. Pure cultures were then reisolated from the infected animals. "Koch's postulates," Livingston writes, "were fulfilled to the satisfaction of our entire group and to that of our biology superiors at Rutgers."[6]

Livingston had thus demonstrated to her own satisfaction, and to that of some colleagues, that she had isolated a microorganism that caused cancer in both animals and humans. Needless to say, for Livingston and anyone who credited her discovery, this was a historic accomplishment. "The next step," she says,

> was to prove that the cancerous growth was not the whole disease. For more than one hundred years people like Rudolf Virchow thought that cancer cells themselves were parasites within the body. He did not understand that the small coccuslike granules he saw dividing in the cancers were not the development of daughter cells within mother cells, but instead they represented the true intracellular parasite that was the causative agent. . . . The whole truth may be that the parasite within the cancer cell transforms the normal cell into a sick cell that cannot mature by normal cell growth processes. In other words, the tumor is *not* the disease.[7]

Her claims did not, however, find approval in the medical community. In 1953, a spokesman for the New York Academy of Medicine, Dr. Iago Gladston, discounted her claims, echoing the attitude of most of the medical community. "This is an old story," he said, "and it has not stood up under investigation. Microorganisms found in malignant tumors have been found to be secondary invaders and not the primary cause of malignancy."[8]

That Livingston's bold thesis did not find approval in the medical community is not surprising, but the strong opposition to allowing her to continue her efforts to develop and defend her thesis was scientifically unconscionable. As a result, Livingston's laboratory in New Jersey was forced to close in 1953 due, according to her, to the efforts of leading researchers at Memorial Sloan-Kettering Cancer Center in New York opposed to her research.[9] Deeply disappointed, Livingston moved to California to live near her family. But in Europe, and within a small faction of the microbiology research community in the United States, interest in theories similar to hers continued to develop.

Livingston became an Associate Professor of Microbiology at the University of California in San Diego to continue her research. In 1969, she and Alexander-Jackson and their colleagues presented a group of papers at a New York Academy of Sciences meeting on "microorganisms associated with malignancy." Some of the articles were published in the *Annals of the New York Academy of Sciences.*[10]

Livingston viewed *P. cryptocides* as what she called an "obligate symbiont": an organism necessarily present in all human cells, in fact one that plays a vital role in all reproductive life, including fertilization and pregnancy and the development of the cancer cell.[11] But this obligate symbiont is susceptible to a malignant transformation and proliferation in disease states, especially those that depress normal immune function. She saw cancer as an immunodeficiency condition caused by environmental toxins and inadequate diet.[12]

In other words, in the classic dispute between researchers who give primary importance to the infectious agent in a disease and researchers who believe that the infectious agent only takes hold in an organism weakened by poor nutrition, toxins, or other stressors, Livingston came down in the middle. The agent did, she believed, play a critical role: it could be isolated and a vaccine effective for the prevention of cancer and modulation of existing cancer could be developed. But the weakened terrain of the organism was also critical, for it provided the depleted environment in which the infectious agent took on pathological shape and multiplied out of control.

In 1990, the Office of Technology Assessment summarized the prevailing attitude about Livingston's work within the research establishment:

> [Dr. Livingston has] little support, outside of a few researchers, for her belief that the different microbes observed in the tissue and blood of cancer patients are actually different forms of the same microbe. At present, no independent evidence exists to corroborate her contention that the microbial forms are related to each other as different forms of a single, pleomorphic organism. Evidence does show that the bacterial culture Livingston isolated is not a new and unique species as claimed: *P. cryptocides* supplied by Livingston were identified as different species of the genus *Staphylococcus* and *Streptococcus*. The issue of isolating bacteria of any kind from tumor tissue and urine of cancer patients, however, is generally not disputed, since many groups of researchers have reported isolating various species and strains of bacteria from such sources. Some of these bacteria have also been showed to undergo morphogenic alterations characteristic of cell wall deficient (or pleomorphic) bacteria.[13]

The Livingston Cancer Treatment Program

In 1965, a friend convinced Livingston to try to help her husband, a physician with a malignant lymphoma of the thymus gland. She "treated him with an autogenous vaccine [a vaccine cultured from his own blood] as a nonspecific immune stimulation, mild antibiotics, and diet. He died only recently, of a heart attack, after living almost twenty additional years."[14]

In 1968 she founded what was to become the Livingston-Wheeler Medical Clinic. Over the 22 years from 1968 until Dr. Livingston's death in 1990, the Livingston-Wheeler Clinic became one of the landmark alternative therapy clinics in the United States and one of the treatment centers of choice for many cancer patients seeking other options. It is still in operation, essentially providing the same treatment originally designed by Livingston. The program is complex and sophisticated. It includes:

- A primarily vegetarian whole-foods diet, with a major emphasis on elimination of poultry products and a prohibition on smoking, alcohol, coffee, refined sugars, and processed foods. "Microbes *love* sugar, iron and copper. Iron deficiency in a cancer patient is a defense mechanism and a sign that something else is wrong, not a disease in itself."[15]

- Fresh, whole-blood transfusions from a young, healthy person—preferably a family member—and gamma globulin (often of placental origin) as a source of antibodies.

- Splenic extract to "increase the white blood count [and] enhance immunogenic systems."

- A variety of vaccines, including an autogenous vaccine prepared from the patient's own blood, BCG vaccine (an attenuated bovine tuberculosis bacillus vaccine that Livingston describes as "a close relative of *Progenitor cryptocides*") to stimulate immune function, and other nonspecific vaccines.

- A supplement program that includes vitamins B_6, B_{12}, liver, multiple vitamins, and sometimes intravenous vitamin C. "We believe that vitamins A, C, and E are effective anti-cancer agents."[16] Trace minerals, especially organic iodine (such as that found in kelp), are prescribed, since "iodine is essential to the metabolism of thyroid, the oxidative hormone. Additional thyroid is also given whenever tolerated."[17] [Note the research evidence cited in chapter 12 that vitamin B_{12} can sometimes *promote* tumor growth.]

- Antibiotics, which Livingston reports can sometimes shrink tumors but which more generally reduce the number of *P. cryptocides* (the cancer microbe) organisms circulating in the blood.

- A program to acidify the blood, "since an imbalance toward the alkaline side is known to exist in tumor patients. Hydrochloric acid in various forms can be given."[18]

- Attention to dental hygiene with a view to eliminating dental, tonsillar, and sinus infections that may diminish immune function (an emphasis she shared with the German cancer therapist Josef Issels).[19]

- A program of frequent baths in a hot tub with one cup of white vinegar to help "eliminate toxins through the skin," along with "purging and enemas," which Livingston believed reduced the *P. cryptocides* population and contributed to detoxification.[20]

- Enemas, including coffee enemas, and sometimes high colonics, for detoxification.[21]

- A selective approach to conventional therapies. To affect the course of the disease, Livingston postulated, "two courses of action are possible: One is to destroy the cancer cells in any way possible and the other is to build immunity in the host to resist the inroads of the infecting agent, the PC. The well known destructive route is to employ surgery, radiation and chemotherapy. The first, surgery, is probably the most useful of the three methods because it removes physically as many cancer cells as possible so that the immunological drain on the patient is lessened."

Livingston believed that radiation destroyed immunity but had limited usefulness for localized bone lesions. She thought radiation was also useful in early treatment of some solitary cancers, in some minute metastatic lesions, and in some early lymphomas. The role of chemotherapy, she maintained, was difficult to evaluate, but generally ran counter to the immunological treatment of the disease. She cited acute leukemia, premenopausal breast cancer, lymphoma, multiple myeloma, Wilms's tumor in children, and chorioepithelioma as cancers in which chemotherapy had a role, though often a restricted one. "Even when chemotherapy is used," she said, "immunization should also be instituted at the same time or at intervals between short courses of chemotherapy. However, it must clearly be understood that the patient will eventually survive only because of the stimulation of a potentially intact immune system. Everything else is of secondary importance."[22]

The Diet

Livingston subtitled her book, *The Conquest of Cancer,* with the words *Vaccines and Diet*. Diet played a critical role in her therapy as a way of supporting the renewal of the compromised immune system. She devised three diets for her patients: one for acutely ill patients, one for recuperating patients, and one for patients on a maintenance program.

The strict diet (for acutely ill patients) included at least 50% raw foods (some patients were given completely raw foods diets for up to a year) and included up to a quart of fresh carrot juice a day, other fresh vegetable juices, whole-grain breads, whole-grain cereals, fresh fruits, nuts, baked or boiled potatoes, salads, homemade soups, and raw or freshly cooked vegetables.[23] The diet was based around the fresh juices, which, in addition to pure carrot juice, included carrot juice mixed with apple juice, spinach juice, cabbage juice, cucumber juice, beet juice, or tomato juice.[24] To a large degree, the Livingston diet is strikingly similar to Gerson's diet, but considerably more permissive.

Vitamin Therapy

Livingston summarizes her view of megavitamin therapy in her *Physician's Handbook*.[25]

> We use megavitamins in our program because it is not feasible to attempt to determine what individual deficiencies may exist. We find from experience that high dosage gets the best results. . . . We use only natural oils for vitamin A. Many mucous membrane and skin lesions respond to high dose vitamin A. We advocate megadoses of vitamin C and relatively high doses of vitamin E. In general, these dosages are well tolerated, but if an idiosyncrasy develops to any one of them, the dose can be lowered or a substitution made. . . . *The dosage should be individually adjusted by the physician* [emphasis added]. We often give vitamins by injection, particularly in the paraneoplastic syndrome and after chemotherapy when there is pain along nerve roots and peripheral nerves. B_{12}, liver, and B complex without folic acid can relieve pain in many cases. Abscisic acid, an analog of vitamin A, appears to have an inhibitory effect on tumor growth. Unfortunately, it is very expensive and in short supply so we recommend foodstuffs which contain it in large amounts such as the nuts, seeds and root vegetables as well as mature leaves and vegetables, but definitely avoid green sprouts and green juices which contain growth factors for tumor.[26]

We should note again the research cited in chapter 12 that vitamin B_{12}, which Livingston recommends, may promote tumor growth.

Livingston's Shortcomings

One of Livingston's striking defects as a cancer researcher was the poor job she did in documenting the effects of her treatment on cancer patients, as opposed to her apparently rigorous work in the laboratory.

In *The Conquest of Cancer*, Livingston presented some data on 100 cases that, she said, were selected at random from the clinic files. After excluding noncancer patients, those who did not follow the program, and recent arrivals, the researcher was left with 62 charts, of which 17 were of patients officially diagnosed as terminal. The 62 cases included 21 breast cancer patients of various types, 5 lung cancer patients, 3 uterine cancer, 3 ovarian cancer, 6 colon cancer, 6 melanoma, 2 basal cell skin cancer, 3 prostate cancer, 2 kidney cancer, 1 pancreatic cancer, 1 pelvic cancer, 1 esophageal cancer, 1 larynx cancer, and 6 Hodgkin's disease patients. In summarizing these cases, Livingston claimed, "an examination of the sixty-two random cases shows that our success rate has been 82%. Considering the patients we called inconclusive but for whom we were able to be of *some* help, it is over 90%." She concluded by saying,

> With the approval of the patient, we will provide access to photocopies of any patient's chart to any licensed physician or qualified researcher. Also with patient approval, we will put such qualified investigators in touch with the patient for personal interviews. The clinic is open for inspection or educational visit to any physician, prospective patient, or representative of an accredited institution. As always, we invite any member of the American Cancer Society or the National Cancer Institute to make a careful investigation of our clinic, our program and our results with cancer patients.[27]

For a scientist, Livingston's cursory description of her "success rate" as being "82%" is stunningly imprecise. A great deal of positive anecdotal evidence does come from patients who have been helped at the Livingston Clinic. I have had some well-informed friends who went there and who saw patients with serious prognoses who have done well. Others, of course, were not visibly helped.

In the meantime, two independent researchers in Virginia have developed preliminary data that is supportive of some of Dr. Livingston's claims. Vincent Speckhart, M.D., is Assistant Clinical Professor of Medicine at the Medical College of Hampton Roads, East Virginia Medical School, and Alva Johnson, Ph.D., is Professor of Microbiology at the same institution. According to Dr. Speckhart, they have isolated a pleomorphic organism that fits Livingston's description in some regards. In work with 40 patients, Speckhart has found that the autogenous vaccine made according to Livingston's instructions is useful in reversing immunosuppression in cancer patients.[28]

Speckhart reports a complete response in three patients with minimal disease who used the vaccine—a chronic lymphocytic leukemia patient, a malignant lymphoma patient, and a breast cancer patient. He also reports a partial response in a malignant melanoma patient.[29] Speckhart and Johnson are currently using the autogenous vaccine in a prospective clinical trial.[30] Anthony Strelkauskas, M.D., of the University of South Carolina, is presently studying the immune response of breast cancer patients to the autogenous vaccine.[31]

Livingston's vaccine also bears a strong resemblance to the Maruyama vaccine from Japan, which is perhaps the most widely used Japanese alternative cancer therapy. The Maruyama vaccine is like BCG but is derived from human tuberculosis rather than bovine tuberculosis. I know of no one who has published a study of the relationship between the Maruyama vaccine and Livingston's autogenous vaccine based on *P. cryptocides*. Nor are there, unfortunately, any controlled clinical trials of the Maruyama vaccine in Japan, which might give us some baseline for comparative assessment of the Livingston vaccine.

Cassileth's Case-Control Study of Livingston's Therapy

One of the most credible researchers among mainstream observers of unconventional cancer therapies has ventured the opinion that Livingston probably did "about as well as the oncologists do" in the treatment of advanced metastatic cancer. The first systematic evaluation of this proposition was a study by Barrie Cassileth and colleagues of the University of Pennsylvania that appeared in the April 25, 1991 *New England Journal of Medicine*.[32] The study of Cassileth et al. found that there was no difference in survival between a group of patients with metastatic cancer and poor prognoses who were treated at the Livingston Clinic and a similar group treated with conventional therapy at the University of Pennsylvania Cancer Center. But, interestingly (and ambiguously), the study found quality of life to be *lower* for those at the Livingston-Wheeler Clinic than for those at the University of Pennsylvania from enrollment on. The patients studied were people with Dukes' stage D or recurrent unresectable colon or rectal cancer, metastatic non-small-cell lung cancer, disseminated melanoma, and unresectable adenocarcinoma of the pancreas.

Barrie Cassileth is, in my judgment, a conservative but fair researcher assessing unconventional cancer therapies, although some proponents of these therapies regard her as seriously prejudiced against them. The rhetoric at the beginning of the study sets up the authors' position as inclined to be unfavorable to unconventional treatments. But the study is a fascinating political as well as scientific document. Take the essential conclusion: "For this sample of patients with extensive disease and for this particular unorthodox treatment regimen, conventional and unorthodox treatments produced similar results." That is actually a very striking finding. "We hypothesized that survival time would not differ between the two groups on the basis of the assumption that the unproved remedy would be no more effective with end-stage disease than conventional care, *itself largely ineffective*" [emphasis added].[32]

One way to read this finding is that patients should not waste their time and money on this alternative treatment. Another way to read the finding is that conventional treatments are equally dubious: "Our findings suggest that conventional therapy for the kinds of diseases studied here should be measured against a no-treatment alternative involving only palliative care."

A third possibility, not mentioned in the study, is that both the conventional and alternative therapies studied here were somewhat beneficial for these groups, either for their placebo value or because they were both modestly biologically effective. This could only be assessed if both types of therapy were measured against a no-treatment, palliative care group. Thus, in terms of life extension, if any, this study suggests that, with selected serious metastatic cancers, cancer patients can do just as well at the Livingston Clinic as they can with ongoing chemotherapy and radiation. "The conventional and unproved treatments studied were similar in efficacy." Cassileth et al. continue: "This study explored only one unorthodox therapy, the regimen of the Livingston-Wheeler Clinic, and it involved only patients with diagnoses and stages of disease for which there is no effective conventional treatment. Therefore, the results cannot be generalized to patients with less advanced stages of disease or to other treatment regimens."

The second research hypothesis in the study was that quality of life would be better in patients at the Livingston-Wheeler Clinic. "This hypothesis was based on the benefits that patients are thought to receive from the various aspects of unorthodox therapy, especially its self-care components, and on the absence of the toxicity often associated with chemotherapy." Popular media reports have suggested that the surprise in the study was that quality of life was worse for Livingston's patients. In fact, a close reading shows that the study explicitly found that quality of life was better for University of Pennsylvania patients "at all times including enrollment," and that "quality of life deteriorated at an equal rate in the two patient groups."

The fact that quality of life was significantly better *from the start* for patients on conventional treatments raises the question of whether the Livingston patients were in fact *significantly sicker from the start,* despite the best efforts of the researchers to obtain fair matches for all patients. If a reanalysis of the data in this study were to find that the difference in quality of life reflected the fact that the Livingston patients were in fact significantly sicker from the start—purely a hypothetical possibility—then the fact that they lived as long as the University of Pennsylvania patients would suggest that the Livingston regimen was slightly more efficacious than conventional therapy for patients with these diagnoses and stages of disease.

On the other hand, the Livingston study adds another small but significant piece of evidence to the increasingly numerous studies that suggest no dramatic benefit from the nutritionally based unconventional cancer treatments for patients with advanced metastatic disease—at least no benefit unless one focuses (as the studies have not) on patients who pursue the therapies vigorously and consistently.

What all of this suggests is that, in nutritional (as well as psychological) studies of adjunctive therapies, there seems to be little alternative to controlled clinical trials to assess the efficacy of these therapies. We will not know until someone conducts a controlled clinical trial what the effects of nutritional interventions on cancer are, nor will we know whether the combined effects of psychological and nutritional interventions are greater (or lesser) than the sum of the parts. But we do know that clear-cut "cures" do not show up frequently in the available case studies of nutritional cancer therapies and that the case-control studies—for all their methodological difficulties—certainly do not show dramatic survival benefits for everyone who undertakes the nutritional therapies. Whether a study of those who intensively follow the nutritional programs would show better outcomes we do not know.

Conclusion

In evaluating Livingston's work, we should ask the following questions:

- Does her autogenous vaccine based on *P. cryptocides* work empirically?
- If it does, does it work for the reasons she believed, or for other reasons?
- Has she identified a microbe that causes cancer and, if so, is she correct in describing it as pleomorphic and as functioning as she claimed?
- How many other components of her therapy contribute to her clinical outcomes? Did the diet, vitamins, enemas, and selective use of conventional therapies play a major role, either separately or in combination?
- Did she, in fact, achieve the levels of clinical success that she reports?

I remain agnostic about Livingston's claim that she found a cancer microbe. It is an interesting hypothesis which should be scientifically evaluated. As I mentioned, a small but identifiable international coterie of physicians and researchers is currently investigating pleomorphic organisms and cell wall–deficient bacteria, so the ideas are unlikely to go away. Whether or not someone will do a rigorous, independent evaluation to test Livingston's claims remains unclear.

While her claims in regard to her "cancer microbe" and her vaccine are an unresolved issue of high science, it is easy to overlook the comprehensive nature of the immunosupportive and nutritional program she designed around her vaccine. Livingston was both a brilliant researcher (whether or not she was correct) and an inspired pragmatic clinician who took ideas that made sense to her where she found them and wove them into her treatment program. Livingston was a careful observer of the methods of others, including the Gerson program and other nutritional-metabolic programs in the San Diego-Tijuana area, which is one of the hotbeds of alternative cancer therapies in North America. She often attended conferences at which practitioners from these clinics spoke. She was also a good friend of Josef Issels, a pioneering nutritional-metabolic practitioner from Germany, and drew on his work. So her nutritional-metabolic program is an example of a coherent program that can readily be replicated by others with a genuine research interest in her results.

But Livingston's claimed 82% success rate is entirely noncredible to me, similar in its exaggeration to Max Gerson's claim of a 50% success rate with advanced cancers and the claims made by many of the other alternative cancer clinics in the San Diego-Tijuana area. These grossly overstated claims of success are, it is true, endemic among alternative cancer therapists. These claims greatly diminish their credibility. Livingston, as a physician and research scientist, should have known better than to publish these claims. Her poor judgement helps account for her marginalization in the scientific and medical communities.

Yet Livingston is certainly one of the best examples of an ethical, credentialed, research-oriented practitioner who made her rationale for treating cancer and her treatment protocols explicit, and who welcomed outside evaluation. If she erred in failing to do careful clinical research on her work, it is a common failing among clinicians. The possibility that her work may, in retrospect, appear historically significant—either as a result of her microbiology research and her vaccine or as a result of her nutritional and immunosupportive treatment protocol—is still open.

Notes and References

1   Virginia Livingston was also known for many years as Virginia Livingston-Wheeler, and her clinic was known as the Livingston-Wheeler Clinic. I have used her unhyphenated name at her family's request.
2   Virginia Livingston-Wheeler, *The Conquest of Cancer: Vaccines and Diet* (New York: Franklin Watts, 1984), 55–6.
3   Ibid., 57.
4   Ibid., 57–8.
5   Ibid., 59.
6   Ibid., 63.
7   Ibid.
8   Ibid., 87.
9   Ibid., 88.
10 Ibid., 98–9.
11 Ibid., 129.

12   U.S. Congress Office of Technology Assessment, *Unconventional Cancer Treatments* (Washington, D.C.: Government Printing Office, September 1990), 109.

13   Ibid., 108.

14   Ibid., 97.

15   Livingston-Wheeler, *The Conquest of Cancer,* 24.

16   Ibid., 127.

17   Ibid., 128.

18   Ibid., 125–30.

19   Virginia Livingston-Wheeler, *Physician's Handbook: The Livingston-Wheeler Medical Clinic* (San Diego: Livingston-Wheeler Clinic, 1980), 5.

20   Ibid., 5.

21   Office of Technology Assessment, *Unconventional Cancer Treatments,* 110.

22   Livingston-Wheeler, *Physician's Handbook,* 3–4.

23   Livingston-Wheeler, *Conquest of Cancer,* 153–4.

24   Ibid., 162.

25   The *Physician's Handbook* is no longer in print and some aspects of the therapy it describes are no longer in use. However, it does describe the megavitamin therapy that Livingston employed.

26   Livingston-Wheeler, *The Microbiology of Cancer: Physician's Handbook* (San Diego: Livingston-Wheeler Medical Clinic) 14.

27   Ibid., 15–38.

28   As measured by reversing antigenic response to skin tests from negative to positive.

29   Vincent Speckhart, M.D., personal communication with author, 1990.

30   Office of Technology Assessment, *Unconventional Cancer Treatments,* 111.

31   Ibid.

32   Barrie R. Cassileth et al., "Survival and Quality of Life Among Patients Receiving Unproven as Compared with Conventional Cancer Therapy," *New England Journal of Medicine* 325:1180–5 (1991).

seventeen

Keith Block—Integrating Diet, Fitness, and Psychological Support into an Oncology Practice

Keith Block, M.D., is one of the significant figures in the emerging "middle ground" approach to integrated management of cancer. Although he has received considerable publicity in the Midwest, he is not highly visible either in conventional cancer therapy or in alternative cancer therapy. Rather, like many of the best individual therapists I have met, he is known to a network of people around the country who respect his work.

Block is an example of the kind of physician we are going to need more of in the future: a clinical internist who has conducted postgraduate research in nutritional and behavioral oncology and who is dedicated to the judicious and effective use of conventional cancer treatments. At the same time, he places a strong emphasis on the use of appropriate complementary therapies as adjunctive treatments. Although little objective evidence exists as yet on the efficacy of Block's approach, it is nevertheless a model that could fit easily into the future mainstream practice of hematology-oncology.

Block's Biography

Soon after entering medical school, Keith Block developed an illness that conventional medicine was unable to remedy. After attempting a number of different therapies, he found clinical relief with a macrobiotic diet. He emerged from medical school as a practicing physician publicly committed to investigating the macrobiotic approach to health. Early in his involvement, however, he recognized what he thought were numerous weaknesses in the macrobiotic system and gradually became aware that he had some significant differences with the way macrobiotics approached cancer and other health problems. He separated himself from macrobiotics and began to develop his own adjunctive treatment program.

Currently, Block has a private practice in Evanston, Illinois, and has developed a unique and multifaceted cancer care program which includes an inpatient ward at Edgewater Medical Center (EMC) in Chicago, an affiliate hospital of the University of Illinois School of Medicine. He is medical director of the cancer treatment program at EMC and, additionally, is vice president of a Chicago chapter of the American Cancer Society. A large proportion of the people who come to see him—both locally and from across the country—are cancer patients.

I came to know Block well when he joined a community of other progressive practitioners and researchers concerned with new approaches to cancer at Commonweal's annual Lloyd Symington Foundation Conference on New Directions in Cancer Care. We also worked together on the advisory board of the Office of Technology Assessment Report on Unconventional Cancer Therapies for the U.S. Congress.

Medical Caritas

Block describes his program as being based on *medical caritas* (Latin *caritas*, charity), meaning "compassionate caring for others." He says: "At the heart of the model is a carefully developed, very special doctor-patient relationship. . . . The primary care physician seeks not only to understand and treat the patient's ailments but also to identify the patient's psychological, biomechanical, nutritional and physiological resources. In addition, the physician functions as a . . . coordinator of medical care for patients."[1]

Block's treatment model consists of six components: biomedical, biopsychosocial, biochemical, biomechanical, medical gradualism, and the use of innovative diagnostic and therapeutic tools which are minimally invasive. The last two components exemplify Block's philosophy and "caritas" approach. By "gradualism" he means using the most effective, least invasive procedures first, before adopting more invasive procedures as and if they become necessary. He also uses innovative diagnostic and therapeutic tools which are noninvasive or only modestly invasive. These include sensitive laboratory evaluations which assess the activity and aggressiveness of malignancies; antagonists to side effects from conventional therapy (SEAs); and therapeutic agonists (TEAs), which consist of treatments or pharmacologic agents aimed at enhancing the effectiveness of conventional cancer therapies. SEAs and TEAs include a variety of food components that may enhance immune response. Where necessary, Block uses a modified version of enteral (via the small intestine) and parenteral (by injection) feeding intended to nourish the patient rather than the tumor. He is currently researching psychological interventions aimed at disrupting adverse conditioned responses to chemotherapy, and plants that have interesting immune system activities.[2]

One of Block's fundamental premises, echoing one of the great themes in medical history, is the need for compassionate caring that focuses not only on the diagnosis of a physical disease, such as cancer, but also on understanding *what kind of person has this disease*. This concept receives lip service in conventional medicine, but Block focuses fully on its importance and on how to implement it systematically:

> This clinical model can be used to develop treatment modalities that are based not simply on a diagnosis of a patient's condition but on a deep understanding of that patient's total psychosocial-cultural gestalt. Without a clear recognition of what is deeply important to the patient—e.g., prestige, libido, safety needs, control issues—the physician may propose a treatment that the patient cannot psychologically, culturally, or socially accept. As many physicians have found to their dismay, treatment urged on a frightened or unwilling patient often compounds the problem rather than alleviating it. Unfortunately, rather than examine their own clinical approach, many physicians may blame the patient or even the procedure for the failure. What is required is not an adjustment in technical procedures, but a change in the clinical model itself.[3]

The significance of this statement cannot be overemphasized. Block is going beyond the common contribution of many alternative and adjunctive therapies which propose the addition, or substitution, of complementary therapies for conventional therapies. Rather, he is saying that *the entire package of both conventional and complementary therapies needs to be designed around the specific persona of the individual patient, and that this design process is the focus of a special and profound relationship between the patient and the physician.* What Block is saying is not new—it is as old as the oldest shamanic tradition—but he is adept at reminding us of it and practicing it.

The key points from the other four components of Block's *medical caritas* model are:

The biomedical profiles: Block does a full workup on each patient, including etiologic review, physical examination, laboratory work, diagnostic testing, and review of pathology specimens. His innovations fall primarily in the technical use he makes of a panel of biomedical tests for nutritional and immune assessment.[4]

The psychosocial profiles: In a careful interview with each patient, Block develops four key psychosocial profiles of the patient: a patient-needs profile, an attitudinal profile, a stress level profile, and a learning profile. He also investigates the patient's support systems and lifestyle. From the results of these profiles—together with the biomedical evaluation—he designs an individualized treatment regimen.

Based in part on Abraham Maslow's well-known "hierarchy of needs," the patient-needs profile explores what the patient feels is basic to his survival as a person. "To develop this profile," says Block,

> I try to determine whether a patient is driven most strongly by the degree of safety needs (the need to be physically, biologically, psychologically secure), membership needs (the need for warm, mutually satisfying relationships), self-esteem needs (meeting one's own self-imposed criteria and standards of performance), or status-prestige needs (to receive acknowledgement, recognition, or approval from others). This knowledge . . . enables me to relate to the patient in an informed way and to establish the kind of relationship that provides me with the most significant feedback I need to accomplish our diagnostic and therapeutic goals.[5]

For example, a patient with high safety needs usually responds well to support and reassurance. "On the other hand," says Block, "a patient with high self-esteem needs can be challenged to perform (e.g., meet treatment goals), and, if safety needs are low, provided with information and counseled in a direct manner that a person with high safety needs could find paralyzing."[6]

The attitudinal profile is based on Steven Greer's work with breast cancer patients at Kings College in England. Greer divided breast cancer patients into four groups: hopeless-fatalistic, stoic-suppressor, denier, and feisty fighter. He found that the "feisty fighters" and, surprisingly, the "deniers" had the longest survival, while the "stoics" and the "hopeless-fatalistic" patients did less well. Says Block:

> This particular profile must be correlated with the Patient-Needs Profile. It serves no purpose to identify someone as belonging to the stoic-suppressor group if one does not recognize that this is a manifestation of high self-esteem needs . . . To the clinician, this is a signal that forcing "reality" on some people can break through a defense that is critical for their survival. Such qualifications on "truth-telling" are critical for clinicians to understand if they are to serve their patients' best interests. This particular area of communication requires great skill and tact to maintain an honest response while affirming a patient's emotional integrity.[7]

The stress level profile uses the well-known Hohme Stress Rating Scale and other instruments to assess the stress that patients have been under during the previous year. Says Block, "Stressful events in themselves do not always precipitate a health crisis. Rather, it is how the patient *perceives* those stressful events—how the events affect the patient's social needs and coping capacity—that can result in a major health problem."[8]

The learning profile focuses on the learning pathways through which a particular person processes information about himself and the rest of the world. Some techniques involve assessing whether the patient is more auditory, visual, or kinesthetic in information processing. Others address the level of the patient's hypnotizability or "suggestibility quotient." Still others look at how the patient can manage stress or learn progressive deep relaxation.

> [These] can provide the physician with additional insight into what degree of influence they may have on the patient, the patient may have on himself, and what particular techniques best suit the patient—i.e., biofeedback, hypnosis, repetitive work techniques—and whether they should use primarily verbal, visual or kinesthetic methods. . . . Developing and implementing this profile is

[essential] since it is in this area that patients are frequently able to experience the most control in taking charge of their medical care and their ability to heal.[9]

While Block addresses a professional audience in discussing these issues, we can (and Block does) readily adapt these issues to self-care. Block is in effect suggesting that each of us seeking healing in the face of serious illness should ask:

- What are my needs? What matters to me fundamentally as a person? Who am I, at the deepest level I can reach, and what matters to me most at that level?
- How do I face a serious challenge in my life? What is my style in meeting such a problem, and what does that say about the kinds of interactions and information that are most helpful to me?
- What are the stresses in my life, and how do I experience those stresses? How have they affected my deepest experience of myself over the past year?
- How do I learn? How do I process information about myself and the world? What are the approaches to cognitive and affective information that work best for me? What do I find most relaxing and healing?

In short: *what we need, how we respond to challenges, what we experience as stress,* and *how we learn* are the four psychological areas Block suggests we need to address, either with a physician or for ourselves.

The biochemical profile: "Since I use diet as an important part of my clinical methodology," says Block, "I need to know a patient's eating habits and attitudes toward food. Trying to change someone's diet without understanding what food means to him can simply add another level of stress to a patient's life."[10] To assess eating habits, Block uses a food/social profile which helps him distinguish between the biological and the social needs for food and thereby develop a realistic nutritional program for each patient.

The biomechanical profile: Block does better work in the area of physical conditioning than most other practitioners involved with complementary approaches to cancer, who typically focus on spiritual, psychological, nutritional, or immunosupportive approaches, but rarely on biomechanical or physical approaches. He uses "the body composition analysis along with the patient's exercise history, past and present, and his current cardiovascular, respiratory, and muscle-skeletal needs. These factors help me determine what type of exercise regimen is best suited for his condition, keeping in mind not only what he is capable of but *willing* to do." His approach is cardiovascular, aerobic, isometric, structural, and neurokinesthetic (using movements that reinforce a "cross-crawl" patterning). The movements are patterned after specific components modified from Western and Eastern systems of exercise.[11]

Block describes three objectives for his physical conditioning protocol:

> 1. Produce maximum possible efficiency in terms of *all* life support systems—cardiovascular, pulmonary, skeleto-muscular, neurologic, metabolic, immunologic, and total organic functioning. *Programs that produce results in only one organo-physiologic system are severely deficient* [emphasis added].

> 2. Maintain in the individual the capacity to work hard and to function at the level of peak performance possible to each. . . .

> 3. Produce a heightened sense of well-being, vitality, and emotional resilience. It seems pointless to achieve great physical results if the patient is emotionally depleted most of the time. An appropriate program must be able to help the patient overcome the impact of psychological stress—regardless of whether the stress comes from internal or external pressures.[12]

Block's basic physical conditioning program often starts with 30 minutes of vigorous walking 5 days a week for patients who are able to do so. Others may start with isometric, flexibility, or minimal aerobic exercise. All patients then gradually work into a more comprehensive program.

Applying the Findings to Diagnosis, Treatment, and Patient Training

In presenting the diagnosis, Block discusses at length the high art of finding an approach "that immediately begins marshalling the patient's own inner resources in the fight against his disease."[13]

In treatment planning, he distinguishes between the biomedical therapy and the complementary adjunctive program. Block's approach to biomedical therapy is based firmly on the Hippocratic doctrine of "doing no harm." The complementary adjunctive program consists of individualized programs that "help patients break out of negative thinking patterns and adopt life-affirming patterns."

> The adjunctive program is designed to enhance and support the biomedical therapy. One of the primary benefits is that the patient always has something constructive and positive to do on behalf of his own care. He is not simply a passive recipient of medical treatment. . . . Even in what may prove to be a terminal case, these combined activities can help a patient come to terms with his life, optimize what time remains, achieve resolution of many issues before the finality of his death, and be able to bid farewell to family and friends who have shared so much of his life.[14]

Block has designed a $3\frac{1}{2}$ day training program that includes practicing the biochemical, biopsychosocial, and biomechanical protocols developed for each patient. It includes nutritional instruction, physical conditioning counseling, and stress-reduction programs. "The objective of the Intensive Health Training sessions," Block says, "is to create a sense of control and competence on the part of the patient, an ingredient I believe is deeply missing in the treatment of disease of all types. Giving the patient personal responsibility and a sense of personal power regarding his care is as important as prescribing the right medication." Minimizing negative physical or psychological factors and en-hancing emotional vitality "*builds a foundation upon which invasive techniques, when needed, can work most effectively. There isn't a physician or surgeon practicing today who wouldn't prefer to have a patient attain maximum condition prior to dealing with the compromises inherent in any invasive procedure* [emphasis added]."

The Block Nutritional Program

Block developed his nutritional program from macrobiotics. But, while mac-robiotics generally makes fewer excessive claims than many of the other alternative nutritional approaches to cancer, Block is even more cautious, and takes what I regard as the most reasonable stance. Says Block,

> Although the nutrition and diet part of my clinical program has received the widest attention, it is neither more nor less important than the other compo-nents. I am not a nutritionist or dietitian, nor do I claim that the diet has miraculous or curative powers. I believe strongly that diet is a critical factor in health—that what we eat makes a significant difference in our body's ability

to resist disease and maintain health. I believe that diet can act therapeutically as well as adjunctively in treatment.[15]

The Block diet is based on traditional diets that have historically been considered to support good health in countries around the world. Its principle components are whole cereal grains, vegetables, legumes, fruits, nuts and seeds, and optional use of animal products. (When desired, Block permits limited use of certain fish and free-range poultry.) The Block diet is also remarkably similar to the diets that the American Cancer Society, the National Cancer Institute, the American Academy of Sciences, and the American Heart Association have endorsed as having some *preventive* value in protection against cancer and coronary disease.[16] As part of an ongoing scientific literature review of the latest nutritional findings, Block and his staff continue to modify and individualize regimens based on the patient's disease, his physical condition, and his food needs and therapeutic adjustments.

> For most physicians, nutrition is the least understood and most poorly used tool in the treatment arsenal against cancer. Most physicians received little or no training in nutrition during their medical school years. As a result, they remain unaware of the potential of diet and nutrition, either as an adjunct to conventional therapy or as a therapeutic tool . . . to maintain patient morale and well-being before, during and after treatment. While many physicians support the National Cancer Institute and American Cancer Society nutritional guidelines for a "cancer prevention diet," few are versed in the rationale behind these guidelines or what makes it a "prevention" diet.
>
> Unfortunately, *once their patients develop cancer, the prevention diet is abandoned and nutritional support for the patient, if it is considered at all, becomes a matter of trial and error. Or worse, it is either completely discarded or switched to a regimen that is comparable to a diet identified as cancer promoting. Thus, it is not surprising that one of the leading causes of mortality among cancer patients is death from severe malnutrition* [emphasis added].[17]

The importance of this point is difficult to overemphasize. What, we may reasonably ask, is the scientific basis for encouraging people who develop cancer to abandon a diet known to offer some protection against the development of cancer in favor of a diet identified as cancer-promoting? There is, actually, an answer, which goes like this: There is no reason to assume that the diet that prevents cancer also slows its development once it is established. And, precisely because malnutrition is a major threat with many cancers, the patient should be encouraged to eat a diet as high in caloric intake as possible. But while this is a reasonable argument, can we in any way say that it represents a more "scientific" position than the one Block has taken?

Nutrition researcher Lawrence Kushi points out that

> If we believe that dietary factors act as *promoters* of carcinogenesis, then the influence of diet on tumor growth and spread should not necessarily be much different before or after clinical expression of the tumor. . . . Specifically, one can make a strong case that the time of clinical presentation of cancer is fairly arbitrary. This is particularly so when one considers the evolving technology and acceptance of screening procedures. Of course, there will be cases where caloric support is paramount, but for the otherwise healthy cancer patient . . . the same dietary approach for prevention, broadly speaking, could be used for treatment as well.[18]

In his 12 years of clinical experience, Block reports that the diet he uses provides four major benefits:

> (1) Patients manage their disease and treatment better. The dietary regimen gives patients both a continual reinforcement that they are doing something for themselves by being involved in their treatment and a strong sense of control in dealing with their fight against cancer. (2) Patients experience fewer side effects as they undergo conventional treatments. They report a reduction or cessation of pain, nausea, vomiting, skin irritations, and other side effects commonly produced by cancer treatments. . . . (3) Some patients appear to experience slower rates of tumor growth, fewer tumors at cancer sites, reversals of early stages of tumor development, and increases in survival time. This appears to occur even among patients with advanced disease. (4) Terminal patients are often more comfortable in the final stages of their disease, suffering less pain, requiring less medication, and experiencing diminished mental and emotional difficulties. There have been a stream of responses from patients' families regarding patients' unusual levels of activity, alertness, and ability to interact and engage with loved ones during the last days.[19]

Block specifically addresses the ongoing research debate, which I described in chapter 11, over whether a low calorie diet retards tumor growth without a dangerous level of weight loss or whether a high fat, high calorie diet is the only reasonable one for cancer patients with weight problems. His position is that *appetite* rather than *weight* is the critical factor: "As long as appetite is maintained and patients stabilize without continued loss [of weight], a limited initial drop in weight [as is often found with primarily vegetarian therapeutic diets] should not be a cause for concern."[20]

The Block Diet

The Block diet provides 50% to 60% of nutrients in complex carbohydrates and a range of fat intake from 12% to 25%, as required, primarily from vegetable sources, with the remainder of calories coming from protein. Using that framework, the diet is tailored to the taste of the individual patient using extensive exchange lists.[21] The exchange groups are: (1) grain, pasta, and bread, (2) legumes, (3) soy foods, (4) vegetables, (5) nuts, seeds, and oils, (6) fish, poultry, and dairy, and (7) fruits. Foods are grouped in each list by shared levels of nutrient and caloric value. Thus Block has made it easy for patients to "trade" different foods or drinks from the same list. Each patient is given an individualized menu based on his physical condition, cultural background and tastes, climate and geographical location, activity level, and physical needs.

Block works with three levels of dietary change: transitional, maintenance, and therapeutic. Transitional diets are for patients who are just beginning to make changes in their eating patterns. Maintenance diets are for healthy persons who follow all of the guidelines set out in Block's programs. Therapeutic diets are for patients who have more or less active diseases that require intensive dietary management, and who are willing and able to follow the dietary program conscientiously. Seven different exchange lists were originally developed during Block's research on the program; each one was based on a different protein type, since different protein sources vary widely in fat content. In clinical work, however, a single "averaged" exchange list has been found to be most practical for daily use by patients.[22]

The diet includes not only commonly eaten foods but also a variety of lesser-known foods that provide variety or special nutritive values: cereal grains such as quinoa, teff, and amaranth; soy products such as tempeh, tofu, and miso; shiitake mushrooms and a wider variety of leafy greens than most people are familiar with; and sea vegetables such as kombu, dulce, hijiki, arame, and wakame. Vegetables from above and below ground, including burdock root, daikon, and lotus root, also make their appearance on the diet.[23] Many of these foods were initially popularized by macrobiotics.

Restricted or eliminated are most dairy products, eggs, red meat, refined sugar, caffeinated or alcoholic drinks, processed foods, some less healthy oils, and some vegetables in the nightshade family such as eggplant and green peppers.[24]

Scientific Rationale of the Block Nutrition Program

Block provides a very lengthy scientific rationale for each of the components of his nutritional program, discussing clinical, epidemiological, and laboratory evidence supportive of the choices he has made. A review of the literature is beyond the scope of this book, but Block's theory of how the diet may work can be summarized:

1. The amounts and types of fat in the diet may affect tumor promotion and growth, especially in cancers of the reproductive and digestive systems. Rapidly growing cancer cells need large amounts of lipids, a critical component of cell membranes. Restricting fat intake may deny tumor cells this important nutrient. It is interesting to note that postmenopausal Japanese women with breast cancer following peasant diets have been observed to have much longer survival periods than postmenopausal American breast cancer patients following Western diets.[25] There are also some preliminary investigations indicating that lower fat diets may increase natural killer cell activity in humans,[26] which can be critical in destroying tumor cells in the body. The types of fat consumed may also influence tumor growth. Fats high in linoleic acid appear to promote tumor growth: Block emphasizes the use of low linoleic fats such as olive oil and canola oil for cancer patients.
2. Compounds in shiitake mushrooms (*Lentinus edodes*) and *Laminaria* sea vegetables (kombu, kelp) have been shown to have potent anti-cancer properties, even at relatively low levels of dietary intake. Some of these compounds act in a manner similar to interferon or boost the activity of interferon-like protein polysaccharides, which attack and destroy cells. They also interfere with the initiation and promotion stages of carcinogenesis.
3. A vegetarian diet contains a variety of plant foods whose protective-compounds act as prohibitive, blocking, and suppressing

agents. These agents, which include phenols, indoles, aromatic isothiocyanates, methylated flavones, coumarins, plant sterols, selenium salts, protease inhibitors, ascorbic acid, tocophereols, retinols, and carotenes, interrupt cancer initiation and promotion stages. Foods that contain these substances include vegetables in the cabbage family, onions and related vegetables, winter squashes, carrots, and a number of other plant foods. These compounds act on many stages of cancer development to detoxify carcinogenic substances, trap free radicals, combine with heavy metals to form inert products, repair damage to DNA and RNA, and suppress the formation of tumors. Protease inhibitors, such as those found in soybean products, also increase excretion of bile products and excess protein and protect cells from transformation due to ionizing radiation, including x-rays used in cancer therapy.

4. Dietary fibers play a protective role, particularly fiber rich in phytates, compounds which may be important inhibitors of colon cancer formation owing to their ability to lower production of certain types of oxygen free radicals (harmful chemical species that contain an unpaired electron, which makes them highly reactive). Phytates are found primarily in cereal grains. Fiber can increase fecal bulk, speed up transport of potentially carcinogenic substances through the bowel, and act as a prohibitive or blocking agent in the presence of carcinogens.

5. Though he deemphasizes the use of supplements in megadose quantities, Block uses both nutritional and botanical supplementation in cases where there is clinical evidence that such interventions are likely to be of value. Various nutrients, such as the fat-soluble vitamins A and E, and trace minerals, including selenium, working in combination, can boost both cell-mediated and antibody-mediated immune functions and increase the antigenicity of tumor cells. This has value not only as a protective measure against cancer but also as a therapeutic measure for cancer patients whose immune functions have been impaired through malnutrition, conventional treatment, or the effects of the disease itself.

Improved immune functions also can speed healing and reduce the risk of secondary or opportunistic infections, as well as aid in the fight against tumors. A vigilant, strong immune system may help to prevent a recurrence of cancer by destroying remaining cancer cells before they have an opportunity to proliferate.

Botanical supplements include such agents as *Echinacea* and garlic; their use is chiefly aimed at boosting immune function and counteracting side effects of cancer treatments. In the course of his clinical work, Block feels that he has consistently found that precise use of selected nutritional or botanical agents does indeed aid in diminishing side effects and enhancing effects of treatment.

6. The diet may be effective in helping patients remain in remission and help prevent the recurrence of neoplastic disease. Some researchers have suggested that the recurrence of some tumors may be due to the survival of "micrometastases" that escape conventional therapy. Components in the diet that block or suppress carcinogenesis may prevent these cells from establishing new colonies or may even destroy them.[27]

Conclusion

In my judgment, the Block program is clinically, scientifically, and historically significant for a number of reasons:

First, Block is not an alternative practitioner but a mainstream internist practicing within the paradigm of mainstream medicine and medical director of a multifaceted cancer care program which includes an inpatient ward in a Chicago medical center.

Second, I believe he has placed his nutritional program in precisely the right *practice framework*. It is a critical but coequal component of his program, whose six points include biomedical, biopsychosocial, biochemical-nutritional, and biomechanical-fitness components, as well as medical gradualism and therapy-mediating tools. I believe that is exactly as it should be.

Third, Block does not make excessive claims for the efficacy of good nutrition in cancer and at the same time he does not underplay its potential contribution. He has gathered the scientific evidence, made his clinical observations, and proposed a theory for how the scientific and clinical observations fit together, which I have outlined above. Block states clearly that while good nutrition is no panacea or cure for cancer, it appears clinically to enhance quality of life, to enhance resilience and response to conventional therapies, and possibly to slow tumor development, reduce the size and number of tumors that do occur, and reduce or delay recurrence in some patients.

In deemphasizing the standard use of supplements in megadose quantities, Block shares common terrain with macrobiotics and (to a large degree) the Gerson program, but not with Livingston and the majority of nutritional support programs for cancer. Whether or not a program that relies on diet alone for nutritional support in cancer is generally superior to a program that uses megavitamins is an important research issue that urgently requires further investigation.

Summary

From reviewing both the conventional and unconventional nutritional approaches to cancer discussed in the preceding chapters, I have reached the following conclusions:

The preponderance of the scientific and clinical evidence supports the hypothesis that there may be some beneficial effect for many cancer patients from a nutritional component in cancer treatment and care. This conclusion is not yet supported by controlled clinical trials, but I believe that the dominant mainstream position—that there is "no evidence" that nutrition makes any difference in cancer—is also not supported by the evidence. We should more properly say that the available laboratory and animal evidence, and the fragmentary evidence from human studies, suggests the possibility of some positive effects in some people with some cancers from nutritional treatment, and that controlled clinical trials are warranted and urgently needed.

We do not yet know how much difference nutrition makes in cancer in general, how much difference it makes in specific cancers at different stages, or how much difference it makes in different kinds of people with different cultural backgrounds, different biochemistries, and different attitudes about using nutrition in their fight for survival. But for some significant proportion of these people facing cancer, I predict that adjunctive nutritional support will ultimately be shown to make at least a modest difference in cancer survival.

It is equally clear that nutritional support will not prove to be any kind of panacea. From the extensive efforts that have been made to find people who have done well on the Gerson, macrobiotic, and Livingston programs, it is apparent that while some individuals have achieved *individual* "cures" or lasting remissions on nutritional programs, nutrition does not approach being a cure for cancer for most people who use these therapies. At best, it shifts the survival curve up in the way an effective chemotherapy does. If this is true, there will be more people who achieve lasting remissions at one extreme end of the curve for very serious cancers (which we find in the well documented case reports of survival), and more people who live longer all along the curve. There would, most important, be more people who do not have recurrences of cancer. We have no idea whether nutritional therapies will function this way across the broad range of cancers or, more likely, to very different degrees for different cancers. There is also the strong probability that some nutritional therapies may prove genuinely counterproductive for some specific cancers.

I believe that what the available evidence supports is a middle ground between the typical claims of most alternative cancer therapists and the typical critiques of the "Quack Busters." Many, if not most, supporters of nutritional therapies for cancer have made excessive claims for the efficacy of these therapies. Some have touted their therapies as suppressed "cures" for cancers. Others have given excessive publicity to cancer patients who have apparently done well on these therapies, while failing to provide prospective patients with adequate information on what the *general experience* of cancer patients is with a particular nutritional therapy. Quack Busters, by contrast, dismiss nutritional therapies as quackery, with equally dubious justification.

We are only at the beginning of objective scientific evaluation of nutritional approaches to cancer treatment. But the information that we do have shows that, for some cancers, nutrition does make a significant difference in prevention and may make a difference in treatment. The magnitude of that difference in treatment, the degree of individual variation, the responses of specific cancers to nutritional regimens, and the effectiveness of specific nutritional programs remains, for now, unknown.

References

1   Keith I. Block, "Part 1—Block Nutrition Program." In *New Clinical Care Model: Applications to Cancer Patient Care,* November 1989, 1–2. Prepared for Office of Technology Assessment. Reference updated by personal communication from Keith Block to author, 14 September 1990.

2   Ibid.

3   Ibid., 3.

4   Ibid., 4–5.

5   Ibid., 7.

6   Ibid., 7–8.

7   Ibid., 8–9.

8   Ibid., 9–10.

9   Ibid., 12.

10 Ibid.

11 Ibid., 15.

12 Ibid., 15–16.

13 Ibid., 18.

14 Ibid., 20.

15 Ibid., 25.

16 Ibid., 25–6.

17 Ibid., 27–8.

18 Lawrence Kushi, personal communication with author, 24 January 1991.

19 Block, "Part 1—Block Nutrition Program." In *New Clinical Care Model,* 29–30.

20 Ibid., 33.

21 Ibid., 45.

22 Ibid., 48.

23 Ibid., 53.

24 Ibid.

25 G. Sakamoto, H. Sugano, and W.H. Hartmann, "Comparative Clinicopathology Study of Breast Cancer Among Japanese and American Females," *Japanese Journal of Clinical Oncology* 25:161–70 (1979). Cited by Keith Block in personal communication with the author, 14 September 1990.

26 J. Barone, J.R. Herbert, and M.M. Reddy, "Dietary Fat and Natural Killer Cells Activity," *American Journal of Clinical Nutrition* 50:851–67 (1989). Cited by Keith Block in personal communication with author, 14 September 1990.

27 Block, "Part 1—Block Nutrition Program." In *New Clinical Care Model,* 52–6.

PART FIVE

Physical, Traditional, and Pharmacological Therapies

Physical and Energetic Approaches—Exercise, Massage, Therapeutic Touch, and Chiropractic

I have described spiritual, psychological, nutritional, and physical approaches to healing with cancer as a special "quartet" of therapies that are intrinsically health-promoting. It is noteworthy that the physical approaches to cancer are given less emphasis in the American cultures of complementary cancer therapies than the other three components of the "quartet." This deemphasis of physical approaches to cancer is not characteristic of all countries. In China, as we shall see in the next chapter, qi gong—a Chinese psychophysiological discipline—has many adherents who believe it is useful as an adjunctive cancer treatment.

But while physical approaches to cancer are rarely given primary emphasis in the United States, they are frequently assigned a leading supportive role. A great variety of physical approaches to health and energy-centered treatments are recommended by practitioners and used by patients seeking to recover from cancer. The physical approaches include exercise, massage and other forms of bodywork, chiropractic, movement therapies, and dance. Energetic therapies, closely related to physical therapies, include the laying on of hands, acupuncture, acupressure, bioenergetics, Therapeutic Touch, and other forms of energy manipulation and balancing techniques. Much of energy medicine has early antecedents in traditional Chinese medicine and its theory of qi (vital energy) which moves along meridians in the body and controls the health of the blood, nerves, and vital organs. I describe qi and the practice of acupuncture further in chapter 19, "Traditional Chinese Medicine." In this chapter I discuss exercise, massage, Therapeutic Touch, and chiropractic.

Exercise

Exercise is one of the most common supplements to complementary cancer therapies. Josef Issels, one of the great pioneering German alternative cancer therapists, regularly instructed the patients who came to his clinic in the Bavarian Alps to "go climb a mountain." In fact, that was the title of a well-known BBC television documentary about Issels. Similarly, internist-oncologist Keith Block, whose work is described in chapter 17, recommends a comprehensive fitness training program for his patients.

A man with a rare documented recovery from metastatic colon cancer from Memorial Sloan-Kettering Hospital in New York told me that he attributed his recovery to his iron determination to keep playing tennis even when chemo-therapy made him feel he could not take another step. Indeed, many cancer patients I have met intuitively made some regular form of exercise part of their recovery effort. And yet, as with every other major component of intensive health promotion, the available research data indicate that the benefits of exercise in recovering from cancer are not entirely straightforward.

Max Gerson, the pioneering German nutritional cancer therapist whose work is described in chapter 14, strongly opposed exercise for his cancer patients. He believed they needed deep rest and that exercise was counterproductive. Practitioners of yoga and meditation do not oppose exercise in health and healing but believe that aerobic activity brings the "heat" to the surface of the body, while yoga and meditation bring heat to the internal organs which, they believe, is more important for healing than is aerobic activity.

Animal studies of the effects of exercise on experimental cancers show that in some cases exercise does retard the development of the cancer, but that in other cases it accelerates it. R.A. Yedinak, D.K. Layman, and J.K. Milner, researchers at the University of Illinois, reported an exciting study in 1987 designed to determine whether the "tumorigenic effects of dietary fat could be modified by routine exercise." They assigned female Sprague-Dawley rats to four groups: low fat diet and sedentary life; high fat diet and sedentary life; low fat diet and exercise; and high fat diet and exercise. The rats then received a dose of the carcinogen DMBA (7,12-dimethylbenz[a]anthracene) after 2 weeks on the program. They found that the high fat diet doubled the number of tumors in both sedentary and exercised rats. Exercise *lowered* the incidence of tumors 25% in the low fat diet rats. By contrast, exercise *stimulated* tumor development in the rats on a high fat diet.[1]

However, in a telephone interview, Layman told me that he had found to his frustration that he was not able to replicate the study. One problem with the exercise studies on animals, he pointed out, was that virtually all of them *force* the animals to exercise, and that may cause the exercise to be a stress on the organism rather than a source of health promotion. One researcher, he said, has tried allowing experimental animals to exercise voluntarily and found some protective effect against cancer in animals that choose to exercise a lot, but this raises the question whether the protective effect is from the exercise itself or from factors that predispose the animal to high levels of exercise.[2]

In human studies, some of the most important work has been done by Rose E. Frisch of Harvard. Frisch and colleagues surveyed 5,398 women ages 21 to 82.[3] According to a summary in *Oncology Times,* they found that "in every age group, the non-athletes had a higher life-time occurrence of cancers of the reproductive system, which covered cancers of the uterus, ovary, cervix, and vagina. The non-athletes had 2.5 times the risk of the athletes."[4]

The risk of breast cancer for nonathletes was approximately twice the risk that athletes faced. The study was carefully controlled for confounding variables including family history of cancer, age at menarche, number of pregnancies, age at first pregnancy, use of oral contraceptives, use of estrogen during menopause, leanness, smoking history, and current diet. Frisch also found that exercise during the college years was far more protective against cancer than exercise initiated by nonathletes in later life, although exercise initiated later did have some effect. Of nonathletes who exercised later in life, 50% had a reduced risk of cancer. *Oncology Times* reported:

> Dr. Frisch . . . postulates reasons for the lower risk in former athletes. First, the athletes may have made less estrogen because they were leaner and had less adipose tissue, which converts androgen to estrogen. A decrease in estrogen, which causes breast and reproductive tissue to divide, would result in less tumor cell division. Secondly, the estrogen athletes made may have been less potent. It has been previously shown that the leaner one is, the more one's estrogen

metabolism produces a less potent estrogen, which does not let uterine and breast cells divide.[5]

That vigorous exercise reduces body levels of the highly active form of estrogen was confirmed in a study by Rachel Snow, a graduate student working with Frisch, who measured body fluids of athletes and nonathletes. She found that girls and women with anorexia and an irregular menstrual cycle develop an excess of the inactive form of estrogen. An Olympic gold medal figure skater, Tenley Albright, later became a specialist in female disorders and took part in Frisch and Snow's research. Albright reported that in view of recent findings, an athlete's irregular menstrual cycle should be considered an "appropriate response" by the body that would disappear when a less active life was resumed.[6]

Frisch also found that hard exercise is often associated with the delay of the onset of menstruation. She believes this may be protective against breast and reproductive system cancers. In fact, she postulates that the higher the total number of ovulatory periods in a woman's lifetime, the greater her susceptibility to cancer may be. She noted that 100 years ago menarche typically took place at $15\frac{1}{2}$ years of age. It is now, in general, 3 years earlier, but remains $15\frac{1}{2}$ for girls who exercise hard. "I don't think there is anything great about menarche at twelve-and-one-half," she said.[7]

In another study, Frisch found that cancers of the digestive system, thyroid, lung, and other sites, as well as the hematopoietic cancers (lymphoma, leukemia, myeloma, and Hodgkin's disease), were also lower for the college athletes. Interestingly, the prevalence rates of malignant melanomas and skin cancers did not differ significantly between the two groups.[8]

Further evidence of the protective benefits of exercise in later life was found by Lawrence Garfinkel and Steven D. Stellman of the Department of Epidemiology and Statistics of the American Cancer Society. In a study published in 1988, they reported that "exercise is inversely related to mortality in males and females in both smokers and non-smokers." But the detailed findings were more intriguing: while people who did not exercise had markedly higher cancer mortality levels—and the drop in mortality was substantial for those who described their exercise pattern as "slight" or "moderate"— there was an increase in cancer among male and female smokers who described their exercise as "heavy." In addition, female nonsmokers who exercised "moderately" enjoyed no gain in cancer protection compared with women who exercised "slightly," whereas those who exercised "heavily" did show an increase in cancer risk. Male nonsmokers, by contrast, had some additional gain in cancer protection as they moved from slight to moderate exercise, and a very small amount more as they moved to heavy exercise. These correlations, while fascinating, were *too small to achieve significance* statistically. The elevated risk for cancer associated with intense exercise referred specifically to lung, colorectal, and pancreatic cancers—not, interestingly, to breast or reproductive system cancers.[9]

But the evidence does not all point in the same direction. Ralph S. Paffenbarger of Stanford University Medical School found in another extensive retrospective review of the effects of physical activity (participation in college sports) on students that the active male students, while considerably *less* likely than inactive students to develop rectal cancer, were considerably *more* likely than inactive classmates to develop prostate cancer. He also did *not* find in his sample the protective effects of athletics for breast cancer that Frisch had reported—in fact he found none of the protective effects for women's cancers that Frisch had reported in her sample.[10]

Thus we find that the picture is complex when we link exercise and cancer. It is striking that the greatest protective effect of exercise against cancer may be associated with *concomitant protective factors*. Exercise helps men and women—smokers and nonsmokers—but it helps the nonsmokers more and it helps most if done in moderation.

So exercise may work by many complex and varied pathways in either lowering or increasing cancer risk. Its association with leanness, which is protective against cancer, has been noted, as has its effect on estrogen, ovulation, and other factors related to female breast and reproductive cancers. Another protective pathway by which exercise may modulate the development of cancer is through its effect on depression. In a number of studies, exercise has been shown to have an antidepressive effect, and depression is a common precursor and concomitant factor in cancer. Moderate exercise can have a powerful protective effect against depression, which in turn may work through complex mind-body pathways to help prevent or modulate the development of a cancer.

Some researchers have hypothesized that at high exercise levels the body may experience an increase in free radicals and peroxide production in the body, which might account for the increase in cancer in some animal studies and the increase (albeit statistically nonsignificant in the previously cited study) in humans, particularly in smokers.

Still another interesting perspective on cancer and physical activity comes from Ron E. LaPorte, Associate Professor of Epidemiology at the School of Public Health at the University of Pittsburgh. LaPorte believes *physical activity* rather than *exercise* may be the important protective factor against cancer. As *Oncology Times* reported, LaPorte believes "there is . . . some evidence . . . that increased physical activity alters bowel transit time. Decreased transit time might be related to reduced colon cancer risk, said Dr. LaPorte, because there is less time for carcinogens to be produced. He also cited evidence for decreased cancer risk related to physical activity via increased thermal effects, and increased concentrations of vitamin A."[11]

One very striking gap in the literature on exercise and cancer is that there are no studies that I have been able to find assessing the effect of exercise on an existing cancer—only cancer prevention. Indirect evidence, however, shows the benefits of physical activity for people with cancer. The line of reasoning is that enhanced functional status or performance status is a predictor of better outcomes in some cancers, and "functional status" is a synonym for capacity to be physically active. Similarly, most oncologists regard a person who is in good physical shape as potentially more resilient to treatment.

The absence of studies of the effects of exercise on survival in people with cancer is as striking as the paucity of psychological and nutritional cancer survival studies. It reflects the same astounding medical assumption that what we eat, think, feel, and do while we have cancer can have no possible effects on the outcome of established disease, and therefore that the subject is not worth studying.

Massage

In the weeklong retreats we offer for cancer patients through the Commonweal Cancer Help Program, we have found that the three hourlong massages each participant receives are among the most treasured forms of nurturance and relaxation that the program provides. We try to schedule the most anxious participants for the first massage appointments because the effect is often transformative. Participants whose skin color when they arrive is almost gray from chemotherapy often get pinker skin after one or two massage appointments. Areas of chronic pain and tension are often eased or fully relieved.

For many participants, the massage at Commonweal is the first they have ever had. And for many, the only touch they have experienced from health professionals during their illness has been associated with painful or, at best, neutral diagnostic or treatment procedures. Many participants have not shown their bodies and scars to anyone since they began cancer treatment. The experience of having a scarred body treated with love and compassion by a truly caring masseuse can be a profound one. (We select women as massage therapists, incidentally, because the large majority of participants are women.)

The sparse clinical literature on massage for cancer is mixed, but largely positive. The occasional concern, which is a legitimate one, is that massage might possibly help the cancer spread because it increases circulation. Based on this concern, some massage clinics have a policy of not providing massage for cancer patients, and a few texts recommend against massage for people with cancer on this basis. On the other hand, increased circulation and deep relaxation could well have protective benefits. The primary nursing literature supports massage for cancer patients.

Our own rule of thumb at Commonweal is to use gentle massage techniques and especially to avoid any form of deep massage in areas of known cancer activity. We also avoid pressure around bone metastases, and we avoid any form of massage that stimulates lymphatic movement in cancers that are in the lymph system. We also avoid pressure massage in leukemias because of the special characteristics of leukemic cells.

In the literature on massage for cancer patients, a number of nursing studies show that slow-stroke back massage enhances relaxation or the feeling of general well-being. For example, an article by K. Warren in *Nursing Times* recommends slow-stroke back massage, along with distraction, guided imagery, progressive muscle relaxation, systemic desensitization, hypnosis, and dietary adjustments, to help patients with chemotherapy-induced nausea and vomiting.[12] In the same journal, S. Sims reports a pilot study with six breast cancer patients undergoing radiotherapy for whom back massage resulted in

fewer symptoms, more tranquility and vitality, and less tension and tiredness.[13]
L.A. Barbour, in a descriptive study in *Oncology Nursing Forum*, found that
patients use an array of nonanalgesic methods to control pain that include heat,
deep breathing, massage, and exercise.[14] B.Z. Dobbs in *Nursing Mirror* reports
that reflexology was helpful to advanced cancer patients both in comforting
them and controlling pain.[15] Reflexology involves massage of the hands and
feet based on the theory that pressure points there correspond to different
parts of the body, including the internal organs.

In physical therapy, massage is frequently a necessary part of the management
of lymphedema, in which the protein-rich fluids of the lymph system accumulate in tissue after breast surgery or radiotherapy. One key to the treatment
of lymphedema is to spot it and treat it early, since prolonged presence of
lymphedema in the tissue can break down the structure of the tissue so that
it loses the elasticity necessary to squeeze out lymphatic accumulations. At Sir
Michael Sobell House in London, which specializes in the treatment of
lymphedema, diuretics are no longer used (they reduced edema at the expense
of dehydration). Instead, massage combined with a variety of sleeves and
stockings is used to control the movement of lymphatic swelling.[16]

Therapeutic Touch

*The implications of Therapeutic Touch for medicine and science are—if the scientific
studies of its efficacy are valid—truly awesome. Something is happening in these studies,
if they are correct, that medicine should attend to and science cannot yet account for.*

Therapeutic Touch is a modern version of the ancient practice of laying on of
hands. Many of our ancestors—in antiquity and throughout the Middle Ages—
believed that touch had a magical quality for healing, particularly if it were
administered by a holy man or healer. Today, the laying on of hands is being
revived in much of its original method in many churches. Therapeutic Touch,
however, is a new and systematic protocol for healing with the hands, originated by Dora Kunz, a famous healer, and Dolores Krieger, Professor of
Nursing at New York University. According to Krieger, although it had its
historical origins in the laying on of hands, Therapeutic Touch takes its
theoretical basis both from modern physics (which "posits that energy fields
are the basic units of all matter . . . that the human being extends beyond
what we perceive as a physical boundary and is, through energy, intercon-

nected with everything in the environment") and from the Eastern theories of qi and prana, the Chinese and Indian concepts of the life energy. Says Krieger

> Eastern literature states that a healthy person has an overabundance of "Prana" or "Qi" . . . and that an ill person has a deficit. Indeed, having a deficit of Prana is the Eastern definition of illness. Prana or Qi can be transferred from a healthy person to an ill one *if*—and this is very important—the healer has the conscious intent to do so. This transfer of energy will help the ill person to buttress his own energy system in the service of self-healing.[17]

Krieger believes that anyone can learn therapeutic touch: "It's a natural potential in all human beings and this potential can be developed."[17]

There are three major phases in the procedure: the first is *centering*—a short period in which the therapist enters a meditative state of awareness so that she washes away all the "busy-ness" of her own thoughts and becomes acutely open to any input from her client. Second, the therapist then "listens passively" with her hands as she scans the client's body a few inches *above* the skin, and "tunes in" to any disturbances in the energy field around the body. She is searching for temperature changes or other energy differences as clues to underlying energy imbalances. This is called *assessing*. In the third phase, with her hands still above the client's skin, the therapist "unruffles" or smoothes out the energy field surrounding the body and begins to concentrate on areas where she has sensed accumulated tension. She helps redirect the energy flow so that it is no longer congested and begins to move smoothly through the body. This is known as *rebalancing*.

Normally, the whole process takes no longer than 15 to 20 minutes and should not be drawn out, lest the client (in the vocabulary of Therapeutic Touch) receive too much energy and become irritable. "The basis of Therapeutic Touch," says Krieger, "lies in intelligently directing healing energy through the healer to the healee."[18]

Therapeutic Touch is now widely used by nurses in many major medical centers, hospices, and in home care throughout this country and abroad, albeit not without resistance from conservative physicians. Scientific studies of its effectiveness have been made by Krieger and many others, including Janet F. Quinn, R.N., Ph.D., Associate Professor at the Center for Human Caring at the University of Colorado School of Nursing, and Theresa Connell Meehan,

R.N., Ph.D., Associate Director of Nursing for Research at New York University Medical Center. To date, research has shown that Therapeutic Touch is effective in reducing acute pain in postoperative patients; in relieving pain in general; in helping the body's basic metabolism (by increasing hemoglobin values); in decreasing anxiety in hospitalized cardiovascular patients; in reducing behavioral stress in premature infants; and in decreasing headache pain in adults. In several other studies, by contrast, Therapeutic Touch produced no significant effects.[19]

In an innovative and well-designed study by Daniel Wirth, M.S., J.D., president of Healing Sciences International in Orinda, California, small experimental wounds were administered to the arms of college students, who then placed their arms through a special armhole in a wall and were randomized into a group that received Therapeutic Touch and a group that did not. The group receiving Therapeutic Touch experienced significantly faster wound healing.[20] Wirth and his colleagues obtained similar results in a subsequent replication of the original study.[21]

Obviously, Therapeutic Touch makes assumptions about the nature of reality that are not universally shared in our culture. But these assumptions have a history that goes back far beyond the beginnings of the great traditions of medicine. Every year, millions of Americans use laying on of hands in religious healing services. What is different about Therapeutic Touch is that it is employed systematically by nurses and researchers in a nonsectarian manner and that a strong effort has been made to develop systematic research on its effectiveness. Whatever the merits of its theory, Therapeutic Touch has been demonstrated in careful research to have efficacy in physical and psychological healing. Says Krieger, "Like acupuncture, the workings of Therapeutic Touch have not yet been adequately explained within the postulates of Western science. We know acupuncture works—and therein lies its value. But we have yet to understand just *how* it works from the Western scientific view. We have begun the scientific study but we still need more research."[22]

There is a very small literature on Therapeutic Touch in regard to cancer. M.L. Raucheisen at the Veterans Administration Medical Center in Washington, D.C., describes the use of Therapeutic Touch for relief of a "multitude of symptoms," including nausea and pain. She also describes its effectiveness in enhancing relaxation and quality and duration of sleep.[23] Cathleen Fanslow, R.N., M.A., a hospice nurse in New York and teacher of Therapeutic Touch, uses it extensively to relieve pain in cancer patients and to give dying patients the relaxation and reassurance to let go and die.

Using Therapeutic Touch or the simple laying on of hands with participants in the Commonweal Cancer Help Program, we have the participants work *with each other,* so that each participant has the opportunity to give a healing experience to someone, as well as to receive it. For the vast majority of participants, the experience of both giving and receiving some form of simple touch with intent to heal is a profoundly positive one. It often induces deep feelings of mental, emotional, and spiritual healing, and sometimes has significant effects on physical symptoms as well. Many participants say that they enjoy the giving of Therapeutic Touch more than receiving it. This is perhaps not surprising, given that Cancer Help Program participants consist in large part of women with breast cancer who often say that excessive giving and difficulty in receiving have been issues all their lives.

Chiropractic

Chiropractors are much more likely than physicians to be interested in unconventional health-promoting approaches to cancer. They are often familiar with a range of nutritional and physical supportive treatments for cancer, some possibly beneficial and some possibly harmful. The greatest harm that can take place with a chiropractor occasionally occurs when a cancer patient goes to the chiropractor with back or neck pain caused by an undiagnosed spinal metastasis. In such a case, a physical manipulation of the neck or spine could cause further damage or a break in the compromised vertebrae. Sophisticated chiropractors are well aware of this danger. W.D. Defoyd, a chiropractor, writes:

> Metastatic disease of the lumbar spine is a relatively common but catastrophic cause of low back pain. Because of an increasing role as primary care providers for back pain patients, it is essential that chiropractors keep this possibility in mind. Careful consideration of the patient's history, physical and laboratory findings, and the use of imaging procedures are helpful in establishing a correct diagnosis in those cases where metastasis is suspected.[24]

Historically, physicians have been hostile to chiropractors—and many still are today—since they often see patients who have done poorly with chiropractors, just as chiropractors often see patients who have done poorly with physicians. A typical warning comes from P. Shvartzman and A. Abelson at Ben Gurion Hospital in Israel:

> Back pain often causes patients great despair, and they expect the primary care physician or orthopedic surgeon to provide a quick, simple solution. Rest and analgesia are the most commonly prescribed treatments, and muscle relaxants, heat, traction, and physiotherapy are also used. If these treatments do not help, the patient may search for relief through faith healing, acupuncture, chiropractic treatment, or other nonconventional forms of treatment. Although chiropractic treatment is a popular alternative, its long-term effect is questionable and the medical literature contains numerous reports of patients whose condition has worsened as a result of it. Physicians should be aware of the dangers of chiropractic treatment, particularly in patients with severe spondylitic [inflammation of the vertebrae] changes, osteoporosis, fractures, [and] tumors.[25]

While the dangers to patients suffering from cancer who visit poorly informed chiropractors are real, physicians historically have grossly underestimated the relief and help that many patients experience from chiropractors, osteopaths, and other physical manipulators skilled in structural work.

As an example of the constructive use of chiropractic, imagine a woman with a primary breast cancer and no metastases who also has a history of spinal problems. She goes through conventional therapy but wants to take whatever measures she can to enhance her general health in order to lower the risk of recurrence. She visits a chiropractor who points out that the region of the spine connected by nerves to the breast is out of alignment, and also that other misalignments in her spine keep her from breathing deeply and effectively, lowering her capacity to oxygenate her blood fully. He recommends a short course of chiropractic adjustment (she has been warned against chiropractors who believe you should come back for an endless and expensive series of treatments, and is fortunate enough to find a like-minded practitioner). He also recommends gentle yoga and moderate exercise as ways to reinforce correct spinal alignment. Finally, he suggests a low fat diet and basic nutritional supplementation. She finds that the manipulations do, indeed, correct long-standing areas of pain in her back; that she is able to stand more erect and with less fatigue; and that her breathing is improved. This consultation certainly improved her basic health and quality of life. It may have been helpful to her in reducing the risk of recurrence of the cancer.

An example of successful collaboration between a chiropractor and an oncologist is recounted by S.E. Downs, who provided chiropractic treatment for a woman with bronchogenic carcinoma who was experiencing muscle spasms and pain in the neck, axilla, and ribs. His x-ray film showed a lesion in the lung and he referred the woman for conventional treatment of her cancer. While she was being treated for the cancer, Downs says, "a significant reduction in the pain experienced by the patient was achieved with spinal manipulative therapy."[26]

In summary, chiropractors, like physicians and, indeed, like all health care practitioners, are a mixed lot. There are excellent ones and there are poorly trained or negligent ones. But many cancer patients find that chiropractors represent one group of licensed health professionals with a broad general interest in supportive health promotion for people facing chronic or degenerative illnesses such as cancer. It is not insignificant, moreover, that many forms of health insurance reimburse for chiropractic treatment.

References

1   R.A. Yedinak, D.K. Layman, and J.A. Milner, "Influences of Dietary Fat and Exercise on DMBA-Induced Mammary Tumors." Meeting abstract, Federation Proceedings, 46(3):436 (1987).

2   D.K. Layman, personal communication with the author, 1991.

3   Rose E. Frisch et al., "Lower Prevalence of Breast Cancer and Cancers of the Reproductive System Among Former College Athletes Compared to Non-Athletes," British Journal of Cancer 52(6):885–91 (1985).

4   Sarah Tilyou, "Exercise May Reduce Risk of Certain Cancers," Oncology Times, 15 August 1987.

5   Ibid.

6   The New York Times, 16 February 1988.

7   Ibid.

8   R.E. Frisch et al., "Lower Prevalence of Non-Reproductive System Cancers Among Former College Athletes," Medicine and Science in Sports and Exercise 21(3):250–3 (1989).

9   Lawrence Garfinkel and Steven D. Stellman, "Mortality by Relative Weight and Exercise," Cancer 62:1844–50 (1988).

10   Robert S. Paffenbarger, "Physical Activity and Incidence of Cancer in Diverse Populations: A Preliminary Report," American Journal of Clinical Nutrition 45:312–7 (1987).

11   Tilyou, Oncology Times.

12   K. Warren, "Will I Be Sick, Nurse?" Nursing Times 84(12):53–4 (1988).

13   S. Sims, "Slow Stroke Back Massage for Cancer Patients," Nursing Times 82(47):47–50 (1986).

14   L.A. Barbour, "Nonanalgesic Methods of Pain Control Used by Cancer Patients," *Oncology Nursing Forum* 13(6):56–60 (1986).

15   B.Z. Dobbs, "Oncology Nursing 6: Alternative Health Approaches," *Nursing Mirror* 160(9):41–2 (1985).

16   C. Badger, "The Swollen Limb," *Nursing Times* 82(31):40–1 (1986).

17   *Therapeutic Touch—A New Skill From an Ancient Practice,* a half-hour videotape produced by Harriet Harvey for the Hospital Satellite Network and the American Journal of Nursing Company, 1985.

18   Ibid.

19   Ibid. See also, Janet F. Quinn, "Building a Body of Knowledge: Research on Therapeutic Touch 1974–88," monograph, table 1. Prepared for publication in *Journal of Holistic Nursing* Spring, 1988.

20   Daniel P. Wirth, "The Effect of Non-Contact Therapeutic Touch on Healing Rate of Full Thickness Dermal Wounds," *Subtle Energies* 1(1), Winter 1990.

21   Daniel P. Wirth, Joseph T. Richardson, and William R. Eidelman, "Full Thickness Dermal Wounds Treated with Noncontact Therapeutic Touch." Unpublished manuscript, 1991.

22   *Therapeutic Touch—A New Skill From an Ancient Practice,* videotape produced by Harriet Harvey.

23   M.L. Raucheisen, "Symptom Relief with the Use of Non-Invasive Techniques," *Oncology Nursing Forum* 12(2 Supplement):94 (1985).

24   W.D. Defoyd, "The Use of Imaging Procedures in the Diagnosis of Metastatic Disease of the Lumbar Spine," *Journal of Manipulative and Physiological Therapeutics* 13(3):161–4 (1990).

25   P. Shvartzman and A. Abelson, "Complications of Chiropractic Treatment for Back Pain," *Postgraduate Medicine* 83(7):57–8, 61 (1988).

26   S.E. Downs, "Bronchogenic Carcinoma Presenting as Neuromusculoskeletal Pain," *Journal of Manipulative and Physiological Therapeutics* 13(4):221–4 (1990).

nineteen

Traditional Chinese Medicine—A Favored Adjunctive Therapy for American Cancer Patients

In May of 1991, thirty-five alumni of the Commonweal Cancer Help Program gathered at Commonweal for one of our regular reunions. We sat together in a large circle for introductions. Each person gave his name, hometown, type of cancer, and a short list of resources that had proved particularly helpful. Participants described compassionate surgeons and oncologists, high-quality cancer support groups, and helpful psychotherapists. But the most commonly mentioned additional resource that the alumni talked about were practitioners of traditional Chinese medicine. One participant after another described how beneficial the acupuncture and herbal treatments were. They stressed particularly the value of Chinese medicine in coping with the side effects of chemotherapy and radiation.

I have suggested previously that spiritual, psychological, nutritional, and physical approaches to cancer represent a quartet of intrinsically open and ethical approaches to intensive health promotion in the face of cancer. Now I would like to add a fifth key approach to cancer. It differs from the quartet only in that it often contains elements that are not obviously intrinsically health-promoting. This fifth approach is found in the traditional medicines of the world.

When practiced with integrity by experienced practitioners, the traditional medicines of the world have often achieved highly significant benefits for patients. The World Health Organization recognizes these traditional medical systems as the primary providers of health care for much of the world. Although there are many different systems of traditional medicine around the world that have been developed over thousands of years of practice, I am choosing to describe traditional Chinese medicine because it is the traditional medicine best known in the West and the most widely used by Western cancer patients.

The Contrast Between Traditional Chinese Medicine and Mexican Alternative Cancer Therapies

Nowhere is the contrast in complementary cancer therapies greater than in the difference between how practitioners of traditional Chinese medicine have approached cancer and how some of the cancer clinics in the Tijuana area of Mexico—and others in the United States with similar medical cultures—have approached cancer.

Many of the Tijuana clinics make forceful claims that they can "cure" or otherwise effectively treat cancer in a high proportion of cases. They often denigrate conventional therapies as ineffective and harmful. They conduct little, if any, meaningful scientific research on their therapies.

Most practitioners of traditional Chinese medicine, by contrast, make modest claims for the efficacy of their cancer therapy. They often support the use of conventional cancer therapies. They offer treatments that are compatible with conventional therapies or that counteract the side effects of chemotherapy and radiation. Moreover, researchers in China, Japan, Hong Kong, and elsewhere conduct extensive research on virtually every aspect of traditional Chinese therapies—although not always to the standards that Western scientific medicine accepts.

If anything, most practitioners (there certainly are exceptions) of traditional Chinese medicine can—on the basis of the research literature—be criticized for *understating* the promise of their treatments for cancer. In fact, the practitioners of traditional Chinese medicine I have met in the United States and Japan usually go out of their way to minimize the potential of their therapies for cancer, *except* with respect to quality of life and alleviating side effects of treatment.

It was only when I began to undertake computer searches on the constituent parts of Chinese medicine that I began to discover the true magnitude of its clinical and research literature on cancer. I am not an expert on traditional Chinese medicine and the abstracts that are translated into English represent only a fragment of the total research effort, so I can offer only a preliminary sketch of this extraordinary literature.

Oriental medicine, of which traditional Chinese medicine is a part, constitutes a large and diverse field of practice, theory, and research. For example, the use of acupuncture and herbal therapies in Japan differs significantly from their use in China. There are also many different schools of traditional Chinese medicine within China, Hong Kong, and Taiwan. At the same time, a deep coherence of theory and practice exists even among the different schools. For the sake of simplicity, I focus primarily on traditional Chinese medicine as it is practiced in China, even though many of the studies I cite come out of Japan and do not strictly represent this school of practice.

English-Language Authorities on Traditional Chinese Medicine

Michael Broffman is an American acupuncturist who studied traditional Chinese medicine extensively in Taiwan. He works at the Pine Street Medical Clinic in San Anselmo—a town near Commonweal—and is one of the more sought-after traditional Chinese medicine practitioners in our area. Both a scholar and a practitioner, Broffman has many devoted cancer patients.

Among the English language authorities on traditional Chinese medicine that Broffman trusts the most are Paul Unschuld, author of *Medical Ethics in China* and *Medicine in China: A History of Ideas;* Nathan Sivin, author of *Traditional Medicine in Contemporary China;* and Ted Kaptchuk, author of *The Web That Has No Weaver,* one of the most accessible and beloved resources for Westerners who wish to understand traditional Chinese medicine, which is discussed below.

While practitioners like Broffman are using traditional Chinese medicine with cancer patients as an adjunct to mainstream treatments in communities across the United States, one academic medical researcher and physician is having a significant impact on the development of mainstream research in traditional Chinese medicine. David Eisenberg, M.D., of Beth Israel Hospital and Harvard

Medical School in Boston, was the first U.S. medical exchange student to study in the People's Republic of China. He made a series of trips between 1979 and 1985 and wrote, with Thomas Lee Wright, one of the best and most fascinating introductory books on traditional Chinese medicine, *Encounters with Qi*; it reads like a novel.[1] He is responsible for Harvard Medical School exchange programs with the Chinese Academy of Medical Sciences, and is actively encouraging the development of collaborative research programs on various aspects of traditional Chinese medicine involving Chinese and American scholars. He more recently updated his findings in a talk published in the *Noetic Sciences Review* called "Energy Medicine in China: Defining a Research Strategy Which Embraces the Criticism of Skeptical Colleagues."[2]

Integrating Eisenberg's observations of traditional Chinese medicine with other studies, the following is an overview of its four major treatment approaches, each of which has applications to cancer:[3]

1. *Acupuncture,* which is known primarily in the West as a system of pain control, is regarded in Oriental medicine as a way of "restoring energy balance." Its practitioners, Eisenberg notes, speak of "putting energy through the needles" or "taking energy out of the body." Acupuncture posits a system of "meridians" which run like energy pipelines through the body. The acupuncture "points" where needles are placed are like valves on these energy pipelines where the energy can be adjusted.

2. *Acupressure* is a system of massage in which finger pressure on the acupuncture points is used in place of needles, both in diagnosis and in treatment. According to Eisenberg:

   Claims of energy transfer were used by my mentors in describing what they were doing in diagnosing and treating patients on the massage table. I was impressed clinically by the extent to which patients with acute musculoskeletal pain and/or pain in association with chronic neurological or musculoskeletal problems found relief through massage therapy. More importantly, in many instances patients' relief was not short-lived, but rather lasted for days, weeks or months in a fashion I could not explain. These were among my most humbling observations."[4]

3. *Herbal medicine,* says Eisenberg, is "the principal mode of Chinese intervention." Most Westerners think of acupuncture as the primary system of traditional Chinese medicine. But over the past two mil-

lennia the Chinese have developed a vast pharmacopoeia of plant, animal, and mineral substances based on empirical and clinical experience.

4. *Qi gong*—energy medicine—is one of the most fascinating elements in traditional Chinese medicine. The physical movements of qi gong, which Eisenberg describes as "a martial art, are circular, symmetrical, and slow, and are similar to those movements used in other martial arts (such as Tai Chi Chuan and Kung Fu). However, in addition to the physical movements, the Qi Gong practitioner is instructed in the art of centering, of achieving a particular state of physical balance, and, simultaneously, to meditate."[5] Some qi gong practitioners make intriguing claims about the capacities of qi gong practice to help people overcome cancer, as we shall see.

Cross-cutting these four major fields, Eisenberg offers a summary of five major (though unproven) assertions regarding the "energy medicine" aspects of the system:

1. Qi (vital energy) exists as a physical entity. The Chinese claim qi can be measured and controlled and has biological and clinical significance.
2. "Qi meridians" (energy fields) exist as physical entities. The Chinese claim that meridians are measurable, and necessary for pulse, tongue, and energy diagnosis. The meridians can predictably be influenced by acupuncture stimulation, herbal therapies, massage, qi gong, or other cognitive interventions.
3. Tongue, pulse, and energy diagnoses are reliable and may help to elucidate important physiologic relationships. The Chinese claim that subtle variations noted on the radial artery, the tongue, and along acupuncture meridians can reveal the location and severity of internal organ abnormalities.
4. Internal or external manipulation of qi can alter the course of illness. The Chinese specifically assert that qi gong therapy can alter illness patterns in malignant cancers, chronic diseases (e.g., renal failure, chronic obstructive pulmonary disease, arthritis, etc.), psychiatric disorders (such as anxiety, depression, and schizophrenia), and immunodeficiency (e.g., AIDS).
5. Paranormal (i.e., psychic) abilities are "qi-related" phenomena. A long-held Chinese claim states that persons who practice and be-

come masterful at manipulating internal or external qi are capable of unique paranormal skills.[6]

The concept of qi, Eisenberg notes, is not unique to China. "It is found within the medical systems of Tibet, India, ancient Greece, branches of the Catholic Church, and also has similarities to more recent theories such as that of 'animal magnetism' proposed by Mesmer in the eighteenth century."[7] In yoga, qi is referred to as *prana*, a vital life force that is preserved and enhanced by yoga practices. The *Yoga Sutras* also note that yoga practitioners may develop paranormal capacities, but sternly warn against pursuing these powers, which may distract the student from the real end of self-realization.

Like yoga, Oriental medicine systems primarily emphasize prevention as superior to intervention. Says Eisenberg: "It also emphasized that one's life-style, including diet, exercise, thoughts and emotions, plays a critical role in the natural course of illness and one's ability to maintain health."[8]

Eisenberg's account of traditional Chinese medicine has the advantage that it comes from a physician-researcher at Harvard who combines knowledge of traditional Chinese medicine with a rigorous commitment to Western research methods and standards.

A second major resource, mentioned above, for those who want to understand traditional Chinese medicine in more detail is Ted Kaptchuk's *The Web That Has No Weaver: Understanding Chinese Medicine*. In reading Kaptchuk's more extensive account after I had read Eisenberg's book, I found that it deepened my understanding of the fundamental concepts of traditional Chinese medicine. Kaptchuk has little to say about cancer per se, and does not discuss qi gong at length. He focuses on explicating traditional Chinese medicine in its own terms. Kaptchuk shows how fundamentally different are the Eastern and Western ways of seeing and thinking about life in general, and about medicine in particular:

> The two different logical structures have pointed the two medicines in different directions. Western medicine is concerned mainly with isolable disease categories or agents of disease, which it zeroes in on, isolates, and tries to change, control or destroy. The Western physician starts with a symptom, then searches for the underlying mechanism—a precise cause for a specific disease. . . .

> The Chinese physician, in contrast, directs his or her attention to the complete physiological and psychological individual. All relevant information, including the symptom as well as the patient's other general characteristics, is gathered and woven together until it forms what Chinese medicine calls a "pattern of disharmony.". . . The question of cause and effect is always secondary to the overall pattern.[9]

Kaptchuk proceeds to discuss every major element of traditional Chinese medicine in depth. For cancer patients who want to understand exactly what a practitioner of traditional Chinese medicine is doing when you consult him, Kaptchuk makes this unfamiliar world comprehensible in detail.

Controlling Chemotherapy-Related Nausea

Before I begin to summarize pertinent parts of the research literature on traditional Chinese medicine, I would like to emphasize that I have access only to translated studies, have worked largely from abstracts of articles in the computer databases, and so cannot vouch for the design of many of the studies cited. Research design for traditional Chinese medicine studies in China is often sadly deficient by Western scientific standards.

The research on the uses of acupuncture and moxibustion (the application of heat to acupuncture points) strongly suggests that these treatments can be effective in controlling or alleviating vomiting and nausea related to chemotherapy; controlling or alleviating certain kinds of pain; alleviating side effects of radiation treatment, most notably edema; and *possibly* (the evidence is only from animal studies) in contributing to life extension. At the empirical level, as you read in my description of the Commonweal reunion, many patients report obtaining relief from chemotherapy and radiation side effects with traditional Chinese medicine.

A controlled clinical trial was reported by J. W. Dundee in Belfast in the *Ulster Medical Journal* in which either manual or electrical acupuncture stimulation of the P6 (neiguan) point prevented nausea and vomiting. Control over nausea could also be obtained by acupressure, but not as effectively as by acupuncture. The author concluded that "acupuncture is a useful adjuvant in reducing sickness after cancer chemotherapy. This effect can be prolonged for 24 hours by acupressure."[10]

A similar study of the effectiveness of elasticized wrist acupressure bands to control chemotherapy-related nausea was reported by Stannard in *Nursing Times*. The study compared periods when the 18 patients undergoing chemotherapy wore the wristbands with periods when they did not wear them or had them incorrectly positioned. "When acupressure bands were used correctly, nausea remained but, in most cases, it was greatly reduced. Vomiting was reduced both in number of times and amount of emesis; some patients did not vomit at all. Antiemetic drugs were still needed, but the amount of drugs used was greatly reduced." The authors recommended a randomized controlled clinical trial, since the study was exploratory in nature.[11]

Not insignificantly, sailors who are inclined to get seasick now frequently use these wristbands. They are on sale at almost every marine store—and sailors swear by them.

Controlling Pain

Acupuncture has the capacity, in the right hands, for controlling cancer-related or treatment-related pain. Many American cancer patients testify to the pain relief they have obtained with acupuncture. Eisenberg describes watching major brain surgery being done with acupuncture as the anesthetic. In spite of his initial reluctance, Lu, a 58-year-old Beijing University professor with pituitary cancer, agreed to have acupuncture analgesia during his surgery after he was assured that 90% of all head and neck surgeries at the Neurological Institute were performed successfully under acupuncture analgesia with fewer side effects than with other forms of analgesia.

Eisenberg then describes how Lu was first given a mild sedative by the staff anesthesiologist, who had 10 years of Western anesthesiology training before she ever learned acupuncture. The anesthesiologist selected six key points on the basis of the collective experience of the team of doctors in hundreds of similar operations. The points included two in the region of the eyebrows, two near the right temple, and two in the region of the left shin and ankle. The needles were connected to low-voltage electronic stimulating machines, often used in acupuncture, that sent electrical current through the needles at regular intervals. The anesthesiologist then waited 20 minutes for the acupuncture analgesic to take full effect.

Lu's head was held in a special metal frame to immobilize it for the surgery. A sterile sheet separated the surgeons and the operating field from Lu's field of vision: he could see only Eisenberg and the anesthesiologist:

> The anesthesiologist gave the go-ahead to begin, and the surgeons took up their scalpels. They made an incision along three sides of the rectangle outlined by the marking pen, and proceeded to lift a three-sided flap of full-thickness skin from Lu's skull. At the moment of incision, Lu failed to wince, grimace or give any hint of pain. He remarked he was aware of the surgeons applying pressure to his skin but that he experienced no discomfort. His pulse and blood pressure remained at the preoperative levels.
>
> Using high-speed bone drills with surgical bits, the surgeons bored holes through the four corners of the rectangular piece of bone. They threaded a wire saw between two adjacent holes and pulled it back and forth until the bone was sawed through. They repeated this procedure on all four sides of the rectangle until they could remove the large piece of bone. The manipulation of bony surfaces is usually extremely painful.
>
> Throughout the entire procedure, which continued for more than four hours, Lu remained conscious, and his vital signs remained stable. We conversed the whole time he was on the operating table.
>
> After the completion of the surgery, *Lu sat up from the operating table, shook the hand of his surgeon, thanked him profusely, shook hands with the anesthesiologist and me, then walked out of the operating room unassisted. The large tumor had been removed, and it subsequently proved to be benign* [emphasis added].[12]

Later, Eisenberg participated in two thyroid operations:

> In certain respects these neck operations were even more impressive than Professor Lu's brain surgery. A thyroidectomy (surgical removal of the thyroid gland) requires an extensive dissection of the neck and is almost always performed with the patient under general anesthesia. In the thyroid operations using acupuncture analgesia, no drugs whatsoever were administered. The analgesia consisted of two needles in the hand and nothing else.[13]

Eisenberg and Wright point out that although acupuncture is 3,000 years old, its application to surgery is very recent, since surgery played a very minor role in traditional Chinese medicine. It began to be applied to surgery when Chairman Mao called for the union of Chinese and Western medicine. Research showed that while acupuncture provided successful analgesia for 90% to 95% of head and neck surgeries, it was "only" successful in 70% to 80% of abdominal, gynecological, and chest surgeries. It could not relax the abdominal muscles in abdominal surgery or block pain related to the movement of internal organs. By the 1980s, Eisenberg reports, Chinese anesthesiologists were using acupuncture primarily for head and neck surgeries as a result of these findings.[14]

Kondo, in Nagoya, Japan, points out another aspect of the significant potential of acupuncture analgesia in cancers of the head and neck:

> Deterioration in the patient's general condition in cancer of the head and neck is slow in comparison to the extent of local disease. Counter-measures against pain, therefore, become very important in treating these patients. Cancerous pain may be divided into three stages, i.e., the early, middle and terminal stages. . . . Acupuncture is effective for early and middle stage pain and has a pain-relieving effect which is different in type from the relief gained by other analgesics.[15]

A review article from the former Soviet Union on the treatment of advanced cancer pain considered analgesic drugs, radiotherapy, nerve blocks, surgery, and acupuncture as pain relief methods. "Acupuncture has been found to have certain advantages over nerve block," the authors concluded.[16] A case report from Leningrad described three women with metastatic breast cancer confined to bed with severe pelvic pain. They were given acupuncture "which resulted in complete alleviation of pain and restoration of mobility."[17]

There are many more Chinese, Japanese, and Russian references to the use of acupuncture analgesia than there are American references. While some American studies clearly describe the efficacy of acupuncture in pain control, acupuncture analgesia is more typically discussed under "unproven methods" or "unusual methods" in discussions of the management of cancer pain.

No one knows precisely how acupuncture analgesia works. Eisenberg reports one of the leading hypotheses:

> Over the past few years scientists have discovered that acupuncture stimulates the production of certain morphine-like substances in the brain. These substances diminish pain perception. The newly discovered compounds are called

endorphins or enkephalins. They are small chains of amino acids that serve as neuromodulators, that is, regulators of neurological activity. There is evidence that acupuncture influences the production and distribution of a great many neuromodulators and neurotransmitters and that this in turn alters the perception of pain.[18]

Controlling Radiation-Induced Injuries

Edema caused by radiation treatment is one of the most vexing ongoing problems for many cancer patients, particularly those with breast cancer. A considerable number of studies, mostly from Russia, report on the value of acupuncture as part of an integrated approach to managing pain and edema and restoring immune function after radiotherapy.

An uncontrolled Soviet study by Bardychev of acupuncture and reflexotherapy for 141 breast and uterine cancer patients with late-onset radiation injuries to skin and soft tissue found that acupuncture was "an effective treatment for edema and pain. It also improved lymph flow, rheovasographic indexes and normalized hemostasis. The best results were obtained in stage I–II edema."[19] Another uncontrolled Soviet study by Kuzmina found that radiation edema was decreased 22% to 37% and immunological recovery was enhanced using laser acupuncture in conjunction with massage, application of DMSO (dimethyl sulfoxide, an anti-inflammatory), and routine drug therapy.[20]

Animal studies also support the benefit of acupuncture in enhancing immune function following radiation. A Taiwanese study of gamma-irradiated mice showed that handling acupuncture, electroacupuncture and laser acupuncture enhanced recovery of total leukocytes and differential white blood cells in the mice, with laser acupuncture having the greatest effect.[21]

Extending Survival with Cancer: Animal Studies

While most traditional Chinese medicine practitioners are extremely cautious with regard to any claims that acupuncture or other modalities may extend life, some animal studies suggest it might play a role in life extension. For example, an Israeli study looked at the effects of moxibustion in transplanted mouse breast carcinoma. The mouse breast tumors were surgically removed with and without the application of moxibustion. The protective effect of the moxibustion was remarkable:

> Surgical removal of the tumor 14 days after inoculation resulted in the deaths of 61% of the mice, compared with a 90.0% death rate in a sham operation, but only 37.5% with the addition of thermo-moxibustion therapy. Surgical removal of the tumor mass at day 17 post-inoculation resulted in a 70% mortality rate, while surgery supported by thermo-moxibustion protected the animals to the range of 40% mortality. Thermo-moxibustion as the sole treatment was effective when applied either before or very close to the tumor cell inoculation (35% and 33% mortality respectively, as compared to 61.7% in the control).[22]

Similar results were obtained in a study of the effects of combining radiation treatment and acupuncture-moxibustion in mice with subcutaneous Ehrlich ascites tumor: the group treated with moxibustion and electroacupuncture had the best therapeutic results while, interestingly, the group given electroacupuncture alone had no significant clinical results.[23]

Another provocative animal study from China looked at the effect of acupuncture on the growth of Ehrlich ascites tumor in mice who had been inoculated with the tumor cells. The mice who had acupuncture showed a slower weight gain than controls, "indicating the growth of tumor cells was inhibited in a certain degree by acupuncture treatment." Also, the treated mice survived a median 25 days compared to control survival of a median 16 days.[24]

Herbal Therapies for Cancer

Although I have focused up to this point on acupuncture, moxibustion, and acupressure, the scientific literature on traditional Chinese herbal therapies is even more intriguing. It is important to remember Eisenberg's point that, contrary to American preconceptions, herbal therapies, not acupuncture, are the principle remedies in traditional Chinese medicine. As you read the often astonishing claims for the herbal remedies, keep in mind two thoughts: first, clinical trials in China are frequently not randomized controlled clinical trials. And even when they are, the methodology is often suspect by Western scientific standards. So the human trials reported below should be seen as suggestive and intriguing but by no means definitive.

On the other hand, it is important to note Kaptchuk's suggestion that traditional Chinese herbal therapies may often be more effective in traditional clinical combinations than when single components are isolated in Western scientific analysis and then simply administered as new chemotherapeutic agents in conventional medical practice. So while poorly designed studies may overstate the potential benefit of traditional Chinese herbal remedies in some respects, the transformation of elements from ingredients in a complex holistic traditional medicine to pharmacological agents in a Western medical system may cause us to underestimate the benefits of the intact traditional therapies.

With these cautions, it is important to recognize that traditional Chinese herbal therapies have already yielded a significant number of anticancer drugs, including indirubin from *dang gui lu hui wan*, irisquinone from *Iris lactea pallasii* and Zhuling polysaccharide from *Polyporus umbellata*.[25] There is no question that the ingredients of many traditional Chinese herbal remedies are pharmacologically active in cancer. According to a extensive analysis by Eric J. Lien and Wen Y. Li at the University of Southern California School of Pharmacy, Chinese herbs and plants from 120 species belonging to 60 different families have been used to treat cancer. Their highly technical text, *Structure Activity Relationship Analysis of Anti-Cancer Chinese Drugs and Related Plants*,[26] groups the drugs according to their bio-organic structure and chemistry and gives each plant's name, the active biochemical principle it contains, and the research evidence for its specific anticancer activity.

The Promise of Juzentaihoto

Juzentaihoto, or JT-48 or JTT, which is spelled and labeled variously in different translations, appears to be one of the most thoroughly studied and promising of Chinese herbal remedies. Its traditional use was in anemia, anorexia, and extreme exhaustion and fatigue. Researchers now suggest it "may now provide new advantages with little toxicity in combination with chemotherapy or radiation therapy [as well as] preventing leukemia in cancer patients who take antitumor agents."[27]

Juzentaihoto has been reported to be effective against the toxic side effects of the chemotherapy *cis*-diamminedichloroplatinum (CDDP) in mice with bladder tumors, inhibiting tumor growth and prolonging survival.[28] It has been reported to be protective in animal studies against the side effects of the chemotherapies mitomycin C and cisplatin and "markedly changed survival curves" for the animals, suggesting that the herbal therapy "may be a new way to prevent or minimize the toxicity" of both chemotherapies.[29] It potentiated a combination of chemotherapy and hyperthermia in mice with experimentally induced sarcoma tumors, while reducing or eliminating the chemotoxicity of mitomycin C.[30]

Juzentaihoto also helped strengthen the biological recovery of mice following radiation treatment.[31] It enhanced immunological and fatty metabolic parameters in postoperative patients with gastrointestinal cancer, causing a "remarkable elevation" in natural killer cell activity.[32] It also was reported to extend survival in a randomly controlled clinical trial with advanced gastrointestinal cancer patients. Patients given the herbal remedy had 3- to 10-year survival rates, "significantly higher than commonly anticipated." Patients who received palliative surgery were given a combined herbal therapy said to "strengthen the patient's resistance and dispel the invading evil" in combination with chemotherapy. Control groups were given one of two chemotherapy regimens, 5-fluorouracil (5-FU) or MMF. "The combination of traditional Chinese medicine with chemotherapy was better than chemotherapy regimen alone . . . Immunological studies of the survivors revealed an enhancement of both humoral and cellular immunity."[33]

Finally, and most important, the herbal therapy in combination with chemotherapy and hormonal therapy was reported to have *extended life and improved quality of life for metastatic breast cancer patients*. In a controlled clinical trial at the National Cancer Center Hospital in Tokyo, advanced metastatic breast cancer patients were given either chemotherapy and endocrine therapy alone or in combination with juzentaihoto. There were 58 patients who could be evaluated in the group receiving the herbal remedy and 61 in the control group. The survival curves were not significantly different for the first 38 months of the study, but beyond that *the survival rate was significantly higher in the group receiving juzentaihoto*. Quality of life was also better for those receiving the herb, including physical condition, appetite, and coldness of hands and feet. Herbally treated patients also were protected from bone marrow suppression associated with chemotherapy. The authors at the National Cancer Center Hospital concluded, "Treatment with Juzentaihoto is better than without Juzentaihoto in treatment for advanced breast cancer patients."[34]

A prospective randomized controlled clinical trial at the Chinese Academy of Medical Science in Beijing in 1989 combined a traditional Chinese herbal remedy with radiation in *nasopharyngeal carcinoma* (a cancer of the pharynx) and reported a striking increase in survival, as well as reduced local recurrence in the herbally treated group. Ninety patients were given a well-known "destagnation" herbal remedy (to disperse stagnant blood) with radiotherapy, while 98 controls received radiotherapy alone. The 5-year success rate (measured in this study as the number of patients surviving minus the number with recurrences salvaged by retreatment) was 53% in the herbally treated group vs. 37% in the control group—a statistically significant result. The herbally treated group also had far fewer local recurrences (14% vs. 29%), but the metastatic rate for both groups was the same (21%). The last finding was welcomed by the researchers because it seemed to refute the belief that destagnation promotes the spread of cancer by circulating blood.[35]

A 1989 Chinese clinical trial on *squamous cell carcinoma of the esophagus* showed two herbal therapies to be superior to chemotherapy, according to histological analysis of tumor tissue, but the study did not assess survival. The study compared three types of traditional Chinese herbal medicines in 42 patients given the herbs together with cyclophosphamide (a chemotherapeutic agent) prior to surgery with 100 patients who received only surgery. Examination of surgical specimens from all patients were then studied. The researchers found that infiltration of lymphoid cells into tissues and cancer tissue degeneration were more prominent in patients treated with the herbs *Menispermum dehuricum* D.C. or *Chelidonium majus* L., and were less clear in patients treated with the herbs plus chemotherapy or surgery alone. The author commented that the herbal treatments may work by activating an immunological rejection mechanism, while the chemotherapy may diminish the immunological response of the host without obviously damaging the cancer tissue.[36]

Another 1989 Chinese study (not a controlled trial) assessed combining conventional and herbal therapies for *small cell lung cancer* and reported extended survival, apparently in comparison with published survival statistics. The authors conclude that "by long-term combined modality [chemotherapy, radiotherapy, immunotherapy, and unspecified Chinese herbs], the survival rate has obviously improved and the possibility of cure has evidently increased."[37]

Still another uncontrolled Chinese clinical trial assessed combining chemotherapy and herbal therapy in *liver cancer* and showed good short-term results. Thirty patients were given the herbal immunostimulator bai nian le in combination with the chemotherapies levamisole and cimetidine. The authors reported increased natural killer cell activity with "expansion of tumor mass checked and with clinical conditions obviously improved."[38]

Astragalus membranaceus and Ginseng

A 1990 study at the Department of Clinical Immunology and Biological Therapy at the University of Texas System Cancer Center in Houston and the Chinese Academy of Medical Sciences in Beijing found that a fractionated extract of the herb *Astragalus membranaceus* increased the anticancer activity of killer cells potentiated by the well-known experimental substance, low-dose recombinant interleukin-2. The study found a "10-fold potentiation" of the interleukin activity when it was used in combination with the herbal extract. Used with the herbal fraction, a smaller and far less toxic dose of interleukin had the same tumor cell killing activity as a dose ten times larger when used alone. The authors pointed out that high-dose recombinant interleukin-2 has proved excessively toxic and that future work with the substance may require strategies to potentiate lower doses. An extract from *A. membranaceus* has that potentiating capacity.[39]

A second study using a fraction of the same herb (fraction F3) showed that the fraction reversed the immunosuppression caused by the chemotherapy cyclophosphamide and represented a "rational basis for the use of *Astragalus* in immunotherapy."[40]

A 1989 Japanese study of an extract from *Panax schinseng* found that the substance inhibited growth of liver cancer cells in culture and stimulated protein synthesis in these cells, "thus converting the cell characteristics both functionally and morphologically to those resembling original normal liver cells. . . . We have called such a phenomenon 'reverse transformation' or 'redifferentiation' which can be regarded as decarcinogenesis. In this report, the results of our recent investigations are presented with particular reference to reverse transformation of B16 melanoma cells induced [by the ginseng extract]."[41]

This kind of redifferentiation of cell lines toward the structure and function of healthy cells is also caused in certain cell lines by specific nutrients, as we saw in chapter 12.

Traditional Methods of Treating Cancer with Chinese Herbs

In real life, of course, most practitioners of traditional Chinese medicine do not make use of the scientific studies. Indeed, most practitioners in my experience are largely unaware of how remarkable the scientific studies are; they simply offer what they have learned to be the most appropriate therapy for the patient's particular situation.

One interesting but, some specialists report, somewhat dated book on the traditional system of cancer treatment with traditional Chinese herbs is *Treating Cancer with Chinese Herbs,* by Hong-Yen Hsu. Hsu headed the Taiwan Pharmaceutical Association for 34 years and served as the chief of the Food and Drug Control Bureau of the National Health Administration in Taiwan, as well as chairing the department of botany at a Taiwan university before founding the Oriental Healing Arts Institute in Los Angeles. In classic Chinese medicine, Hsu says, there is no specific concept of cancer. Some tumors are simply considered more dangerous than others:

> Those that can be cured are probably Western medicine's equivalent of a benign tumor. The Chinese have perfected over the years many, many formulas that reduce or arrest swelling and alleviate pain. They have also learned much about nutrition and are extremely aware of the benefits to be derived from nutritive supplementary tonics. These are the medicines that are discussed in this book. The formulas and herbs don't propose to cure cancer as such, but many of them do alleviate pain and prolong life by supplementing and strengthening the body's life force and by arresting the progression of tumors.[42]

The various herbal remedies for different types of cancer are said to work by circulating the blood and dissipating "stagnation," detoxifying and "dissipating hard lumps," "breaking accumulations," "treating coagulation," "treating weak vitality," "dispersing heat," and so forth.[43] Beyond the many specific remedies for different types of cancers and different individual conformations related to cancer, Hsu recommends two general anticancer remedies: the "C-C Combination" and the Japanese formula "W.T.T.C."[44] He cites studies by Nakayama

Koumei of Chiba University in Japan showing that W.T.T.C. enhanced post-surgical survival in patients with esophageal and stomach cancer by about 10% and enhanced relapse-free survival by larger amounts, although "the data base is not sufficiently scientific."[45]

A sense of the Chinese view on specific cancers can be sampled by reviewing the chapter on breast cancer. After reviewing the Western view of breast cancer, Hsu describes Chinese thinking:

> The general Chinese medical view is that women's breast cancer is caused by the accumulation of melancholic anger, depression, obstruction of spleen vitality, reversal of liver vitality, deficiency of blood and vitality, stagnation of blood in the muscles, accumulation of sputum over several years, and internal bursting. Thus breast cancer is linked to the seven passions and the exhaustion of blood in the liver meridian, the melancholic accumulation of liver vitality, and obstruction of *ch'i* [Qi, vital energy]. . . .
>
> Chinese medical treatment during the initial stage is aimed at detoxifying, relieving melancholy, softening the hardness, supplementing the blood, and dissipating stagnant blood.[46]

Hsu then gives numerous specific herbal formulas, which have ingredients like "ten baked fresh crab shells" and "juice pressed from fresh asparagus taken with yellow wine." One of my favorites from a purely lyrical point of view recommends:

> Equal portions of wasp's nest, stools of a male rat, and melia are lightly baked and ground into powder for treating bursting. This powder is spread on the cancerous site.[47]

Broffman suggests that while the diagnostic sections of Hsu's book remain valid, the herbal formulas for cancer treatment have changed with time and research.[48]

Two more recent texts recommended by Broffman are *The Treatment of Cancer by Integrated Chinese-Western Methods* by Zhang Dai-zhao, and *Chinese Herbal Therapies for Immune Disorders* by Subhuti Dharmananda.

Dharmananda's book outlines a treatment strategy for tumors that a practitioner of traditional Chinese medicine might employ. It uses traditional Chinese herbs to protect, restore, and enhance the immune system; antitoxin therapies, preferably selecting those herbs containing alkaloid components that have antitumor activity; a mass-resolving (tumor-resolving) formula, used even in conjunction with Western therapies, since the Western treatment will eventually convert the malignant mass into a mass of dead tissues, much like an abscess that is ready to burst; and adjunctive therapies to treat specific symptoms, such as nausea, that accompany a Western therapy. The first three steps are followed throughout the period of cancer therapy. When the tumor is resolved, the immune-enhancing therapy is maintained for a period of several weeks to assure complete normalization of the body functions. The adjunctive therapies are used only as required by the presence of symptoms. The therapeutic plan is followed for a brief period (e.g. 1 month) every 6 months for the purposes of *preventing* the recurrence of tumors.[49]

Zhang Dai-zhao has written an accessible book that includes specific formulas for use by practitioners of traditional Chinese medicine. His section on breast cancer, for example, differentiates and classifies three different kinds of breast cancer: "Qi stagnation due to liver depression," "phlegm dampness due to spleen deficiency," and "stagnant toxins." Each type of breast cancer is characterized by a different clinical picture and requires a different therapeutic strategy. Each requires a different common herbal prescription.[50]

Qi Gong

Qi gong is the most mysterious of all the major components of traditional Chinese medicine and is possibly the oldest and most important of the martial arts. Says Eisenberg:

> The practice of Qi Gong involves some of the key elements found in Western relaxation training. These include paying attention to one's breathing, establishing a passive disregard toward one's thoughts, and—unique to Qi Gong—instructions in techniques to sense the source of one's Qi (vital energy) at a point below the navel and to learn to move it through one's body. . . .
>
> It is said that anyone can learn Qi Gong exercises and that it takes approximately three to six months before one can "feel one's Qi" (in the form of heat or fullness) and begin to move it at will.

The practice of Qi Gong, when analyzed from a Western perspective, may be thought of as a combination of behavioral techniques. These are typically performed for 30 to 60 minutes every day of the year. The behavioral components of Qi Gong include the elicitation of the relaxation response and/or other aspects of relaxation training, aerobic exercise, progressive muscle relaxation, guided imagery, and elements of the placebo effect. In China, where an estimated 50 million persons practice Qi Gong every day, there is an unprecedented opportunity to investigate the impact of behavioral (that is, non-pharmacological, cognitive) therapies as they relate to a multitude of illnesses.[51]

The most reassuring thing to notice, as Eisenberg points out, is that the basic practice of qi gong, *like the basic practice of yoga,* involves the practitioner in a "behavioral package" of health-promoting practices that have been tested and refined over thousands of years.

The concept of qi is central to Chinese medicine and numerous other traditional medicines. It is the prana of yoga: the vital charged energy of feeling alive that many sensitive people and any moderately regular practitioner of a psychophysiological discipline comes to know as an experiential truth. This qi or prana is often depleted by excesses in the activities of life: excessive sexual intercourse, excessive eating, excessive time in front of the television, excessive work, excessive talking. These and many other activities, especially if undertaken in an unbalanced psychological state, deplete prana or qi. Ordinary people can *feel* the reality of this statement—not just the Chinese, but Westerners who learn to notice these things. *Subjectively or experientially, the reality of qi is profoundly experienced by millions of people.*

The problem is that scientifically we still do not know what qi really is, although that is one of the most intriguing questions on the frontier of scientific "energy medicine." According to the Chinese view, Eisenberg explains:

"Qi" is said to be that which differentiates the animate from the inanimate. The body is viewed as a complicated series of conduits through which the "Qi" flows. These conduits are the acupuncture meridians referred to in Chinese diagrams depicting human anatomy. Pathogenesis relates to the excess or deficiency inextricably linked to the force of Yin ("female," "cold," "hollow," etc.) and its opposing force, Yang ("male," "hot," "solid," etc.)

The Chinese clinician's task is to identify where the Qi exists in excess or is deficient. This is done chiefly by means of taking a history, observing and using pulse and tongue diagnosis. The diagnostic label used by the Chinese clinician refers to the specific imbalance which has been noted on physical examination. Each therapy, whether it includes needles, herbs, changes in diet or meditation, is aimed at reestablishing the balance of Qi.

There is one more point of traditional Chinese terminology which is worth remembering. "Internal Qi Gong" or "Soft Qi Gong" refers to an individual's ability to sense and move his/her own Qi within his/her own body. "External Qi Gong" or "Hard Qi Gong" refers to the (alleged) ability of some Qi Gong practitioners to emit their Qi externally so as to influence other animate or inanimate objects.[52]

This is the precise point at which we move decisively into an area which requires suspension of disbelief for many Westerners. As Eisenberg describes it: "These individuals claim to have practiced qi gong from early childhood and proudly displayed their seemingly supernatural powers to audiences as large as 50,000 persons. Qi gong masters split stones with their hands and their foreheads, had trucks driven over them, had massive stone slabs lowered on their bodies by cranes, claimed to be able to see within human bodies and to move inanimate objects at will."

When they were "emitting qi" some research studies claimed to have documented heat changes in the skin surface of practioners:

Thermally sensitive films suggested that when Qi Gong masters emitted energy, the energy tracked down lines in the forearms and legs which were similar to classical acupuncture meridians.

A second series of publications were more fantastic still. Professor Feng Li Da of Beijing published an article pertaining to the *predictable change of bacterial cell growth* in response to external Qi emission by Qi Gong masters. Her paper reported on the ability of several Qi Gong masters to *increase or decrease bacteria cell growth in a variety of common bacteria*. Dr. Feng claimed to have replicated these experiments on numerous occasions in multiple laboratory settings and seemed confident of her results [emphasis added].[53]

The literature on Therapeutic Touch, described in chapter 18, gives us some sense of the scientific basis for these claims. In Therapeutic Touch, even under carefully blinded conditions, practitioners who, like qi gong masters, did not touch the patient, envisioned themselves transmitting vital energy into the patient. Test results showed that Therapeutic Touch brought about physiological changes in the patient. But qi gong goes far beyond Therapeutic Touch. While attending a conference in Beijing in October 1988, Eisenberg invited a qi gong master to his hotel room:

> He came equipped with an electrical volt meter and a simple wiring device. The device was no more than a plug attached to two wires with live ends. He put the plug in the wall and demonstrated its current by lighting lightbulbs, and then tested the current on his hand-carried volt meter. He then licked his thumb and forefinger of both hands and grasped the two live wires. I was horrified and worried he would quickly be electrocuted. He was not. Moreover, he convinced me that he could light a lightbulb by touching it with other fingers of both hands. More curious still was his ability to regulate voltage across his hands, at will, simply by touching the volt meter with the ground in one hand, the meter device in the other. On several attempts he regulated the voltage from 0 to 220 volts, or held the voltage constant, at will, upon my request.

> Because I have grown increasingly skeptical of such provocative claims, I asked him how I could be certain he was in fact conducting electricity and not simply fooling me by means of some high technology trick. He offered to touch me with his hands while he was connected to the wall socket. I declined, but a colleague with me at the time volunteered. When touched on the shoulder by the Qi Gong master, my colleague's trapezius and biceps muscles went into spasm. Moreover, the Qi Gong master could control the electrical current so as to induce the spasm or not. I allowed the Qi Gong master to touch me for a split second, long enough to feel the live current emanating from his forefinger. He was "live" all right.[54]

As a final proof, the qi gong master produced two metal skewers and a pork chop, which he cooked on the skewer by means of the electrical current running through his hands. "I was astounded," said Eisenberg, "and have no adequate explanation for why the qi gong master did not injure his skin or cause a serious heart irregularity, seizure, or other damage to his person."[54]

These stories, however well vouched for by multiple observers, would be of no great moment for us were it not that qi gong is regularly used to treat large numbers of biopsy-proven malignant cancer patients. They are treated with a combination of internal and external qi gong. Qi gong is also used as a treatment for a variety of other illnesses, typically chronic neurologic and musculoskeletal diseases, including multiple sclerosis.

One medical account of the use of qi gong in cancer is a study by Meizhen Gao and Yongmo Liu, of Hunan Medical College. Their subject is a new approach to qi gong taught by the late Guo Ling, a famous qi gong master who was reported to have had cancer of the uterus and undergone six operations without recovery, and who then "began to probe ways of modifying Qi Gong to cure her own disease." She reportedly recovered from cancer using her "new qi gong" method, which she has taught to many advanced cancer patients in Beijing with "significant results."[55]

Meizhen Gao, one of the authors of the study, is a physician who was cured of severe insomnia using "new qi gong" and then proceeded to coach four cancer patients. "These results were astonishing. At this writing, three of the four have survived for more than seven years." The cases included a 31-year-old woman with lung carcinoma (biopsy- and x-ray-confirmed) who was treated with radiation therapy in November 1979. She returned for treatment with an abdominal mass for which she received additional radiation in April 1980, and began practicing "new qi gong" in May.

> There was improvement of general well-being after four months of practice. Then the patient switched to another type of Qi Gong in October. By April, 1981, her general condition deteriorated with reduction in physical strength, as well as loss of appetite and weight. Chest films showed multiple patchy shadows of various densities in both lung fields in addition to the original shadow. Blood streaks were found in the sputum. She resumed and has continued practicing Quo Ling's Qi Gong since May 1981. Chest [films] show absorption of the shadows in both fields and the original tumor shadow is no longer evident. There was a thickening of the pleural shadow in the left superior mediastinal region. Chest films taken in September 1984 showed no evidence of recurrence. She was living and well during a recent follow-up visit in October 1986.[56]

The second case was that of a 50-year-old man diagnosed in April 1979 with adenocarcinoma of the right lung, grade II, with metastases to adjacent lymph nodes. He received radiation therapy and two courses of cyclophosphamide. After starting "new qi gong" his condition and appetite improved and edema in the legs subsided. In October 1986 he was alive and well.

The third case was that of a 37-year-old woman diagnosed in September 1978 with lymphosarcoma of the mediastinum (the tissues separating the two lungs) with metastasis to the bone marrow and distant lymph nodes. She received chemotherapy and began to practice "new qi gong" in July 1980. Follow-up x-ray films showed the tumor shadow no longer visible, and she was alive and well in July 1986.

The fourth case was that of a 49-year-old woman diagnosed in November 1981 with inoperable metastatic adenocarcinoma of the lung who was discharged without treatment. She began to practice the "new qi gong" in November 1981. Chest films in January 1982 showed a reduced shadow in the lung, and the cough and other symptoms had disappeared. "Her family did not tell her the true diagnosis [and] consequently she stopped practicing Qi Gong after her symptoms subsided. Her condition rapidly deteriorated, and she became bedridden. She was unable to resume Qi Gong therapy and died in October 1982."

In their discussion of these four cases of advanced cancer with distant metastases or recurrences, in which the patients were apparently not cured by conventional therapies, the authors note that three patients survived more than 7 years with roentgenologic evidence of reduction or disappearance of the tumors. They also observed that the most outstanding common effect of qi gong was the improvement in the general condition of the patients, as evidenced by increase in appetite, gain in weight, increased vigor, better physique, and increased activity. Further, according to the authors, qi gong appears to have a significant effect in promoting rapid recovery from adverse reactions to chemotherapy and radiotherapy such as lassitude, nausea, vomiting, loss of appetite, hair loss, loss of weight, and reduction in the number of leukocytes and platelets. They inferred that the effect of qi gong is not specifically anticancerous, but improves the patient's ability to deal with the cancer by mobilizing and regulating the vital energy.[56]

We should not be surprised that these physicians insist that it is essential that qi gong be practiced in precisely the right way—that it only works if it is the "new qi gong" and that a patient began to fail on some other form of qi gong. It is characteristic of most practitioners of health-promoting psychophysiological disciplines—or purely psychological or purely physical therapies—that they often believe that their *unique* approach is the only one that is effective.

Perhaps their belief in the unique benefits of their approach is part of what makes them effective with specific patients. Or perhaps in some cases, such as qi gong, only one kind of qi gong is effective and other kinds are much less so. We simply do not know. But, as a general rule, we know that many of the unusual cancer remission stories involve spiritual, psychological, nutritional, and physical approaches to cancer in widely differing combinations with widely differing specifics.

Conclusion

Traditional Chinese medicine is, in my judgment, one of the most intriguing of the adjunctive therapies for cancer. There is considerable evidence for its benefits in pain control and in alleviating the side effects of chemotherapy and radiation therapy. Patients frequently report these benefits, as well. There are also some reasons to believe that traditional Chinese medicine may help in the battle to extend life with cancer and to lower the risk of recurrence of cancer.

Notes and References

1 David Eisenberg and Thomas Lee Wright, *Encounters with Qi: Exploring Chinese Medicine* (New York: Penguin, 1987).

2 David Eisenberg, "Energy Medicine in China: Defining a Research Strategy which Embraces the Criticism of Skeptical Colleagues," *Noetic Sciences Review* 1990(Spring), 4–11.

3 Other scholars would divide traditional Chinese medicine into different components, but Eisenberg's approach is particularly helpful for the beginner.

4 Eisenberg, "Energy Medicine in China," 7.

5 Ibid.

6 Ibid., 8.

7 Ibid., 9.

8 Ibid., 6.

9 Ted J. Kaptchuk, *The Web That Has No Weaver: Understanding Chinese Medicine* (New York: Congdon and Weed, 1983), 3–4.

10 J.W. Dundee, "Belfast Experience with P6 Acupuncture Antiemesis," *Ulster Medical Journal* 59(1):63–70 (1990).

11 D. Stannard, "Pressure Prevents Nausea," *Nursing Times* 85(4):33–4 (1989).

12 Eisenberg and Wright, *Encounters with Qi*, 68–74.

13 Ibid., 74.

14 Ibid., 76–7.

15 T. Kondo, "Studies on the Management of Cancerous Pain of the Head and Neck Region," *Jibiinkoka-Rinsho* 73(9):1469–79 (1980).

16 I.A. Frid and D.G. Beliaev, "Treatment of Pain in Patients with Far Advanced Malignant Tumors," *Voprosy Onkologii* 26(7):76–81 (1980).

17 S.S. Iaritsin, et al., "First Clinical Trial of Acupuncture in the Complex Treatment of Patients with Breast Cancer and Bone Metastases," *Voprosy Onkologii* 25(5):110–2 (1979).

18 Eisenberg and Wright, *Encounters with Qi*, 77.

19 M.S. Bardychev, "Acupuncture in Edema of the Extremities Following Radiation or Combination Therapy of Cancer of the Breast and Uterus," *Voprosy Onkologii* 34(3):3–9–22 (1988).

20 E.G. Kuzmina, "Restoration of Immunologic Indices Following Reflexotherapy in the Combination Treatment of Radiation-Induced Edema of the Upper Limbs," *Meditsinskaia Radiologiia (Moskva)* 32(7):42–6 (1987).

21 D.M. Hau et al., "Comparative Study on Effects of Handling Acupuncture, Electro-Acupuncture, and Laser-Acupuncture on Counts of Various Leukocytes in Gamma-Irradiated Mice." Meeting abstract, Second International Conference on Anticarcinogenesis and Radiation Protection," Gaitherburg, MD, 8–12 March 1987.

22 M. Sternfeld et al., "The Contribution of Thermo-Moxibustion to Surgical Treatment in Transplanted Mouse Mammary Carcinoma," *Acupuncture and Electro-therapeutics Research* 10(1–2):73–8 (1985).

23 D.M. Hau, "Study of the Therapeutic Effects of Acupuncture-Moxibustion and Irradiation on Mice Bearing Subcutaneous Tumor." Meeting abstract, Second International Conference on Anticarcinogenesis and Radiation Protection," Gaithersburg, MD, 8–12 March 1987.

24 S.C. Lee and J.H. Lin, "An Inhibitory Effect of Acupuncture on the Growth of Ehrlich Ascites Cell Tumor in Mice," *Chinese Medical Journal (Beijing)* 22:167–71 (1975).

25 J. Han, "Traditional Chinese Medicine and the Search for New Antineoplastic Drugs," *Journal of Ethnopharmacology* 24(1):1–17 (1988).

26 Eric J. Lien and Wen Y. Li, *Structure Activity Relationship Analysis of Anti-Cancer Chinese Drugs and Related Plants* (Long Beach, CA: Oriental Healing Arts Institute, 1985).

27 H. Yamada, "Chemical Characterization and Biological Activity of the Immunologically Active Substances in Juzen-taiho-to (Japanese kampo prescription)," *Gan To Kagaku Ryoho (Japanese Journal of Cancer and Chemotherapy)* 16(4 Pt 2–2):1500–5 (1989).

28 S. Ebisuno, "Basal Studies on Combination of Chinese Medicine in Cancer Chemotherapy: Protective Effects on the Toxic Side-Effects of CDDP and Anti-Tumor Effects with CDDP on Murine Bladder Tumor," *Nippon Gan Chiryo Gakka Shi (Journal of Japan Society for Cancer Therapy)* 24(6):1305–12 (1989).

29 O.T. Iijima et al., "Protective Side Effects of the Chinese Medicine Juzentaiho from the Adverse Effects of Mitomycin C and Cisplatin," *Gan To Kagaku Ryoho (Japanese Journal of Cancer and Chemotherapy)* 16(4 Pt 2–2):1525–32 (1989).

30 K. Komiyama et al., "Potentiation of the Therapeutic Effect of Chemotherapy and Hyperthermia on Experimental Tumor and Reduction of Immunotoxicity of Mitomycin C by Juzen-taiho-to, a Chinese Herbal Medicine," *Gan To Kagaku Ryoho (Japanese Journal of Cancer and Chemotherapy)* 16(2):251–7 (1987).

31 Y. Ohnishi, "Preventive Effect of TJ-48 on Recovery from Radiation Injury," *Gan To Kagaku Ryoho (Japanese Journal of Cancer and Chemotherapy)* 16(4 Pt 2–2):1494–9 (1989).

32 T. Okamoto, "Clinical Effects of Juzendaiho-to on Immunologic and Fatty Metabolic States in Post-Operative Patients with Gastrointestinal Cancer," *Gan To Kagaku Ryoho (Japanese Journal of Cancer and Chemotherapy)* 16(4 Pt 2–2):1533–7 (1989).

33 G.T. Wang, "Treatment of Operated Late Gastric Carcinoma with Prescriptions of 'Strengthen the Patient's Resistance and Dispel the Invading Evil,' in Combination with Chemotherapy: Follow-up Study of 158 Patients and Experimental Study in Animals." Meeting abstract, First Shanghai Symposium on Gastrointestinal Cancers, 14–16 November 1988, 244.

34 I. Adachi, "Role of Supporting Therapy of Juzenthaiho-to (JTT) in Advanced Breast Cancer Patients," *Gan To Kagaku Ryoho (Japanese Journal of Cancer and Chemotherapy)* 16(4 Pt 2–2):1538–43 (1989).

35 G.Z. Xu et al., "Chinese Herb 'Destagnation' Series I: Combination of Radiation with Destagnation in the Treatment of Nasopharyngeal Carcinoma (NPC): A Prospective Randomized Trial on 188 Cases," *International Journal of Radiation Oncology, Biology and Physics* 16(2):297–300 (1989).

36 M.S. Xian, "Efficacy of Traditional Chinese Herbs on Squamous Cell Carcinoma of the Esophagus: Histopathological Analysis of 240 Cases," *Acta Medicinae Okayama* 43(6):345–51 (1989).

37 R.J. Cha, "Combined Modality Treatment of Small Cell Lung Cancer by Chemotherapy, Radiotherapy, Immunotherapy and Chinese Traditional Medicine," *Chung-Hua Chieh Ho Ho Hu Hsi Tsa Chih (Chinese Journal of Tuberculosis and Respiratory Disease)* 12(1)41–4, 63 (1989).

38 H.Y.Ling, "Preliminary Study of Traditional Chinese Medicine-Western Medicine Treatment of Patients with Primary Liver Carcinoma," *Chung Hsi I Chieh Ho Tsa Chih (Chinese Journal of Modern Developments in Traditional Medicine)* 9(6):325, 348–9 (1989).

39 D. Chu, "A Fractionated Extract of *Astragalus membranaceus* Potentiates Lymphokine-Activated Killer Cell Cytotoxicity Generated by Low-Dose Recombinant Interleukin-2," *Chung Hsi I Chieh Ho Tsa Chih (Chinese Journal of Modern Developments in Traditional Medicine)* 10(1):34–6 (1990).

40 D.T. Chu et al., "Immune Restoration of Local Xenogeneic Graft-versus-Host Reaction in Cancer Patients in vitro and Reversal of Cyclophosphamide-Induced Immune Suppression in the Rat in vivo by Fractionated Membranaceus," *Chung Hsi I Chieh Ho Tsa Chih (Chinese Journal of Modern Developments in Traditional Medicine)* 9(6):351–4, 326 (1989).

41 S. Odashima et al., "Induction of Phenotypic Reverse Transformation by Plant Glycosides in Cultured Cancer Cells," *Gan To Kagaku Ryoho (Japanese Journal of Cancer and Chemotherapy)* 16 (4 Pt 2–2):1483–9 (1989).

42 Hong-Yen Hsu, *Treating Cancer with Chinese Herbs* (Long Beach, CA: Oriental Healing Arts Institute, 1982), vii.

43 Ibid., 25.

44 Ibid.

45   Ibid., 251–2.

46   Ibid., 81–2.

47   Ibid., 88.

48   Michael Broffman, personal communication with the author, 1991.

49   Subhuti Dharmananda, *Chinese Herbal Therapies for Immune Disorders,* Institute for Traditional Medicine and Preventive Health Care, Portland, OR, 85–89.

50   Zhang Dai-zhao, *The Treatment of Cancer by Integrated Chinese-Western Medicine* (Boulder, CO: Blue Poppy Press, 1989), 81–3.

51   Eisenberg, "Energy Medicine in China," 8.

52   Ibid., 8.

53   Ibid., 9.

54   Ibid., 9–10.

55   Meizhen Gao, M.D., and Yongmo Liu, M.D., "Supplementary Treatment of Cancer by Quo Ling's 'New Qi Gong' Therapy." Typescript, Hunan Medical College, China, undated, 2.

56   Ibid., 8.

twenty

Unconventional Pharmacological Therapies—An Overview

Unconventional pharmacological therapies represent the largest and most diverse field of unconventional cancer treatments. Some are well-documented as being of value to cancer patients; others have no documentation whatsoever. In general, pharmacological therapies have attracted greater media attention than the quartet of spiritual, psychological, nutritional, and physical therapies that I have described in previous chapters. What differentiates pharmacological therapies most significantly from the quartet of health-promoting therapies is that *pharmacological treatments do not have any obvious intrinsic health-promoting benefits*. Prayer, psychotherapy and social support, eating healthy foods, relaxing, stretching, and exercising are all *intrinsically* health-promoting for most people. Taking a pill or an injection is neither intrinsically nor obviously good for your health, except insofar as the treatment is pharmacologically useful or engenders a positive placebo effect. (In fairness, this is also true of much of conventional cancer therapy.)

Thus pharmacological therapies, with no obvious direct health benefits, represent a much more complex and difficult field to evaluate than the health-promoting quartet of spiritual, psychological, nutritional, and physical therapies. It is a field where cancer quackery is not only more of a threat but in reality more prevalent. The proponents of alternative pharmacological therapies have also generated more intense opposition from mainstream medicine than have many of the proponents of "lifestyle therapies," which were the primary themes of the earlier chapters. On the other hand, pharmacological therapies lend themselves to evaluation by randomized controlled double-blind prospective clinical trials in a way that the quartet of lifestyle therapies do not.

The Profit Potential of Pharmacological Therapies

One crucial fact about pharmacological therapies is that *it is easier to make money from these therapies than it is from the quartet of health-promoting therapies.* Of course, spiritual healers, psychotherapists, nutritional counselors, and the like are paid, and some charge exorbitant amounts for their services. But we all have some general idea of what learning healthy ways of living is worth to us. Moreover, the health-promoting therapies generally represent *open* therapies in which there are no special secrets. Open therapies create open markets which tend to keep prices within a reasonable range.

The intrinsic value of a pill or injection, however, is much more difficult to assess. The pharmacological agent has a magic to it precisely *because* it is *not* obviously health-promoting and therefore we do not know how it works. It depends upon the efficacy of some mysterious inner properties of the pharmacological agent. The secret is what draws us. And, in a sense, the greater and more mysterious the secret, the more reasonable it may appear that obtaining this elixir of life involves a certain monetary expense.

Pills are more easily made into commodities than lifestyle-based health-promoting therapies. They can be marked up more easily for higher profit margins. And, through the modern miracle of patents, potentially therapeutic pills and injections for cancer can be *owned* by companies or individuals who can charge for these agents whatever the market will bear.

The pharmaceutical industry is, obviously, a very powerful force in American science, medicine, business, and politics. The industry must make large profits to realize a return on investment, particularly in a regulatory system where it costs $100 to $200 million dollars to bring a new drug to market. In this environment, drugs that *cannot* be patented are of little financial interest to the industry. They can, in fact, represent a tangible financial threat if they compete in cost-effectiveness with profitable patented products. Even if a drug can be patented, the prospect that it may only help either a small number of solvent people or a large number of impoverished people can keep a company from marketing the drug. Such small-return products are known as "orphan drugs," and Washington has worked hard to create incentives for bringing these drugs to market that counteract the natural market forces working in the other direction.

Producers of alternative cancer therapies that use pharmaceutical substances confront the same market forces that pharmaceutical companies do. Because the *capacity to patent* substances is not always available to the producers of some alternative therapies, many have reverted to the older medical tradition in which the critical ingredients of the medicine man's potions were a trade secret, passed down from master to student. Harry Hoxsey, who popularized the Hoxsey remedy, is an example of this. In other cases, patents have been a possible way to protect the producer's investment, and have been sought and obtained. The late Lawrence Burton in the Bahamas and Stanislaw Burzynski in Texas obtained patents for their treatments. Still other practitioners have offered an open pharmaceutical therapy which is available free, or at cost, or with only the smallest markup. Logically, one might think that treatments in this last category would be the most popular among alternative pharmacological therapies. But, in fact, it has been the secret therapies and the patented alternative pharmacological therapies that have attracted the most cancer patients, the most media interest, and the most mainstream opposition.

The "Great" Practitioners Who Claim Unique Success

A handful of practitioners of unconventional pharmacological cancer therapies are considered "great" by proponents and sympathetic analysts of alternative cancer therapies:

- The late Lawrence Burton, Ph.D., in the Bahamas, who claimed that his secret patented Immuno-Augmentative Therapy controls some cancers.
- Stanislaw Burzynski, M.D., Ph.D., in Texas, who claims that he has found a peptide fraction in human urine that controls some cancers.

- Joseph Gold, M.D., in Syracuse, New York, who believes that hydrazine sulfate can extend life with cancer.
- Emanuel Revici, M.D., in New York, who claims his "physiologically guided chemotherapy" is effective in curing or controlling some cancers.
- Gaston Naessens, in Quebec, who is known both for a remarkable microscope that he uses for diagnosis and for his claims of efficacy with pharmacological treatments for cancer and AIDS.

We have already discussed the work of two other "greats" of the alternative pharmacological therapy world in previous chapters: the double Nobel prize winner Linus Pauling, whose claims for the effectiveness of vitamin C in cancer are well known, and the late Virginia Livingston, who believed she had developed a cancer vaccine. These six men and one woman would generally be regarded as among the great minds of contemporary alternative pharmacological cancer therapies. There are certainly other candidates for this list, but this is a representative sample.

What do these practitioners of alternative pharmacological cancer therapies have in common? Some comparisons are of value, because collectively these practitioners seem to fit a deep archetypical need of many cancer patients to find an undiscovered genius with a *scientifically based* magic bullet that may cure or control their cancer. This is not to denigrate the need for a scientifically based cure in a culture that worships science. It is simply to acknowledge that many people in such a culture are unlikely to find spiritual, psychological, nutritional, physical, and traditional approaches to cancer sufficient.

What these seven practitioners have in common is that: (a) they are believed by their supporters to have developed a high-technology pharmaceutical treatment that is effective in curing or controlling at least some cancers; (b) with the important exceptions of Pauling, Gold, Livingston, and Burzynski, they have made relatively little recent effort to clarify their research for peer-reviewed medical journals; (c) despite (or possibly because of) the mystery or controversy surrounding their therapies, they are considered historical geniuses and are beloved by their patients and supporters; (d) they have or have had high media profiles in the alternative cancer press, the New Age press, and often the general media; (e) they have been placed (with the exception of Pauling and Gold) under extended legal challenge but, to date, have beaten back all efforts to stop them from practicing. Generally (the exceptions being Pauling and Gold) their therapies are very expensive or very inconvenient for most American patients to obtain.

"Open" and "Closed" Pharmacological Therapies

In chapter 8, describing a framework for evaluating alternative cancer therapies, I recommended that patients distinguish between "open therapies," in which everything about the therapy is known and available to any investigator for assessment, and "closed" or "partially closed" therapies, in which the practitioner says, in effect, "I have a secret or unique system for curing or controlling cancer, and if you come to my center I will provide it to you." Burton kept central components of his therapy explicitly secret. Naessens has explicitly kept his major diagnostic tool—a remarkable microscope—from being fully examined or reproduced. In contrast, Pauling, Gold, Livingston, and Burzynski have "scientifically open" therapies in the conventional sense of the term. Revici is a borderline case: while his frame of reference is so self-referential as to preclude simple evaluation, his therapy is sufficiently open to be called scientifically assessable.

Does this mean that practitioners who have closed or partially or "functionally" closed treatment systems have nothing to offer the informed cancer patient? Opinions differ. Advocates of these and other closed or partially or functionally closed therapies usually have elaborate rationales as to why the information which they claim could be invaluable to mankind is not being publicly shared. They point, for example, to the proprietary secrecy of pharmaceutical firms regarding some of their products. They say that, because of the hostility of mainstream institutions toward their favorite practitioner, he had no alternative but to protect his investment by a personal strategy of secrecy. Or else they argue that their favorite practitioner is protecting his therapy from a mainstream conspiracy to suppress cancer cures. They may also claim their favorite practitioner sought to offer his therapy for scientific evaluation but was ignored or persecuted (claims that are often true), so his current lack of interest in scientific evaluation is understandable. In some instances, as is the case for Revici, they may make the more justifiable claim that these practitioners have been willing to share their methods with the few physicians who have been willing to study intensively with them.

Most mainstream physicians and scientists, on the other hand, are disgusted by practitioners using unconventional pharmacological treatments who claim they have made a major advance in cancer therapy but are unwilling to submit their findings to the unmerciful scrutiny of full scientific review. Indeed, in my judgment, the "explanations" for why therapies must be kept secret—or are less than fully and completely described—lack a fundamental ethical basis. The arguments that justify a physician with a therapy that would genuinely help people with cancer in withholding it from scientific assessment are hard for most fair-minded people to comprehend. The fact that these arguments in support of secret "cancer cures" are so easily accepted by many proponents of alternative cancer therapies is, in my view, one of the most serious intellectual and moral deficiencies of the alternative cancer therapy culture.

Distinguishing between Therapy, Practitioner, and Service Delivery

In evaluating alternative therapies, I recommended in chapter 8 that one *distinguish between the plausibility of the therapy itself, the credibility and character of the practitioner, and the quality of the service delivery.* Rarely are these distinctions more useful than in evaluating a closed, expensive, or difficult-to-access alternative pharmacological therapy.

Lawrence Burton in the Bahamas—who thumbed his nose at the mainstream medical world and happily admitted to keeping part of his Immuno-Augmentative Therapy secret—had a very smooth and fairly expensive service delivery. Stanislaw Burzynski in Texas, who has sought to play the scientific game of open evaluation of his therapy, also has a smooth and very expensive service delivery. Revici in New York who, in his mid-nineties, long ago stopped publishing significant scientific articles in mainstream journals but who previously wrote an enormous scientific volume on his therapy, has a service delivery that is not expensive but that is described by many patients as being seriously disorganized. For many patients, such disorganization represents as serious an access problem as financial or geographical barriers. Naessens in Quebec, who has gone his own way in a small, remote Quebec town with Gallic disdain, makes a significant effort to explain many elements of his therapy to those who are interested, but holds the microscope as a proprietary device. In the face of legal challenges, his capacity to deliver services has been seriously compromised.

What is really fascinating about these practitioners is how extraordinarily *famous* their work is in the field of unconventional cancer therapies. In the preceding sections, we have seen that a considerable number of open and reasonably inexpensive "lifestyle therapies" are available to cancer patients. But many people with cancer are, understandably, seeking the magic bullet or the extra leverage beyond lifestyle therapy alone. Or they feel either disinclined or unable to follow the spiritual-psychological-nutritional-physical path.

Of profound interest psychologically is that, *for the most part, an inverse relationship exists between the openness of the alternative pharmacological therapies and the level of public interest in the therapy.* One would expect that the most open and most evaluated therapies would be the most interesting to patients. Pauling's work with vitamin C and Gold's work with hydrazine sulfate have received extensive independent assessment, both critical and supportive. What their therapies also have in common is that they make relatively modest claims about controlling cancer, yet their treatments generally draw less attention than the closed, expensive pharmacological treatments. At the other end of the spectrum, Lawrence Burton long resisted scientific assessment of his work, including an intensive effort by the Office of Technology Assessment in 1990 to develop a protocol acceptable to Burton for assessing his therapy. (Burton and his associates would have disagreed with my assessment on this point.) Despite the secrecy in which he enveloped his therapy, Burton was arguably the best known of all these practitioners.

Burzynski represents a partial exception to this postulated inverse relationship between scientific openness and fame: he has made his therapy available for independent assessment and he is almost as well known as Burton. Revici and Livingston represent middle cases. They make extensive claims for cure or control of cancer and have made their therapies available for scientific assessment, although relatively little has been done to evaluate their claims.

Lawrence Burton was also my favorite example of what a "secret magic bullet" therapy has to offer for people who do not look forward to lives of vegetarian diet, meditation, yoga, qi gong, acupuncture, and the rest. He told his patients that they can eat vegetarian diets if they like, because it means there will be more steak left for him and his friends, but that his therapy works as well or better with meat eaters. He encouraged his patients to enjoy their steaks, have a few drinks, and not to worry overmuch about smoking unless they have lung cancer. And since he was situated in the Bahamas, his patients were living in a resort setting. For a New York businessman diagnosed with a life-threatening cancer who has been a meat eater, social drinker, and smoker all his life, who believes in high-technology medicine, and who has little use for vegetarianism, meditation, and prayer, Lawrence Burton's clinic began to look pretty good when he considered the alternatives. And when the New Yorker went down to the attractive Bahamian clinic and found himself surrounded by patients who believed they were doing well on Burton's therapy, it was not difficult for him to feel encouraged, to have real hope, and to come to share the common perception of Burton's patients that Burton is a genius.

Because so much has been written—and is readily available for the interested reader—about all of these "great" proponents of alternative cancer therapies, I have used as a criterion for inclusion in this book the scientific *openness* of the therapies. For this reason, I do not discuss Lawrence Burton or Gaston Naessens, intriguing though they are. Others have written readily available accounts of their therapies. I have already discussed Linus Pauling and Virginia Livingston. In the following chapters I discuss Stanislaw Burzynski, Joseph Gold, and Emanuel Revici.

twenty-one

Stanislaw Burzynski—Antineoplastons on the Edge of Medical Credibility

A devoted scientist, Stanislaw Burzynski, M.D., Ph.D, is one of the prominent unconventional pharmacological practitioners of our time, and one who is completely committed to the open scientific evaluation of his therapy. While controversy continues to rage around his work, the promise is substantial that his therapy may be of benefit for some cancer patients.

Burzynski's work has been described in detail by several authors, most notably Ralph W. Moss in his excellent book *The Cancer Industry,*[1] which provides thorough accounts of many of the prominent figures in alternative cancer therapy. Moss is both a sympathetic investigator of many alternative therapies and a gifted science writer. He also describes in detail the politics surrounding unconventional cancer therapies and has made the most sophisticated statement available for the argument that the cancer establishment systematically suppresses independent scientific research on these therapies.[2] In what follows, I draw extensively on Moss's account, as well as on my visit to Burzynski's center in Houston in 1982; on a review of original scientific papers; and on my visit to Kurume, Japan, where I met with researchers who believe they have independently confirmed some of Burzynski's findings.

Burzynski was born in Poland in 1943, excelled in chemistry, and graduated first in his class from the Medical Academy of Lublin in 1967. The following year, at 25, he received his Ph.D. in biochemistry, and became one of the youngest recipients of both degrees in memory. He emigrated to the United States in 1970 and became a researcher and assistant professor at Baylor College of Medicine in Houston, Texas.

As a graduate student in Poland he had become intrigued with differential patterns of peptides—small chains of amino acids—in different human illnesses. At Baylor, he continued this work on his own under the supervision of a mentor who was also interested in peptides. He first worked with his own blood, then switched to urine as a peptide source. By 1974, he had isolated 119 peptide fractions in human urine, and published his results with two colleagues in a leading journal of physiological chemistry and physics.[3] Moss reports:

> Even when he was in Poland, Burzynski had suspected that some of these peptide fractions might have activity against cancer. The blood of one of the prostate patients had proved almost entirely lacking in one of the three faint peptide streaks. . . .
>
> Writing about Burzynski's early work, the DuPont scientists remarked: "They found some peptides could produce up to 97 percent inhibition of DNA synthesis and mitosis in the neoplastic cells of their tissue cultures."
>
> The active peptide fractions consisted of two groups. One was strongly acidic; the other, broad based and slightly acidic or neutral. The strongly acidic group had a very powerful effect on a . . . number of tumor cell lines, especially osteogenic sarcoma, a kind of bone cancer. But the other kind stopped the growth of many different kinds of cancer cells. With many backward glances, Burzynski decided to focus his attention on this broad-based peptide band. And it was this admittedly ill-defined substance that Burzynski now dubbed "Antineoplaston A." A new name was needed because these particular urinary peptides had never been described before. The name was derived from the Greek—*neoplasm* being a medical term for "new growth" or cancer. All subsequent forms of Antineoplastons derived from this substance.[4]

In a letter to me in November 1990, Burzynski gave a brief description of antineoplastons:

I always considered ^~~~~~~~~~~~~~~~~~~~ biochemical defense system in the body ~~~~~~~~~~~~~~~~~~~~~~~ ned cells. In my early work a ~~~~~~~~~~~~~~~~~~~~~~~~~~~ grant was awarded, we were screening peptides isolated from blood and urine for various important biological effects. . . . [I found it] necessary to concentrate heavily on cancer and the defense system in the body which parallels the immune system [see figure 21.1]. . . . This is the system which protects us from "the enemy within," contrary to the immune system which gives us the defense against invaders. Because of that, this is mostly a repair system, not aimed at killing misprogrammed cells. The errors in cell programming may lead to such diverse groups of disorders as cancer, benign tumors, certain skin diseases, AIDS, and Parkinson's disease [see figure 21.2]. . . . In each of these disorders, I have a theory how this system should work, as well as preliminary laboratory data. . . . We also have preliminary clinical experience in which we document objective responses in AIDS, Parkinson's disease, benign tumors, psoriasis and stimulation of wound healing . . . These patients came to us initially with cancer diagnoses, but at the same time, they were [also] suffering from these various disorders.[5]

The Turning Point—Burzynski Refuses to Do Research in the Medical Establishment

Max Gerson's fall from grace in the mainstream medical community did not occur until *after* he testified at a congressional hearing at which his cancer recoveries were touted as "miracles" and his colleagues recommended that Congress provide major funding for research into approaches similar to his but that Congress should *avoid* allowing existing medical organizations (a clear reference to the American Medical Association) to dominate the new inquiry. It was this direct affront to the authority of organized medicine that brought on the legal and professional harassment that destroyed Gerson's career. In Burzynski's history there is a parallel, although his challenge to the medical establishment was not as direct and his capacity to survive the subsequent harassment proved greater.

Moss reports that Burzynski's peptide discoveries were at first enthusiastically welcomed by fellow scientists and the media. He was invited to join the faculty of the department of pharmacology at Baylor, which would mean his leaving his position in the department of anesthesiology, where he had enjoyed complete freedom to conduct his research but where his work was obviously not closely connected to the department's basic mission. In a critical decision,

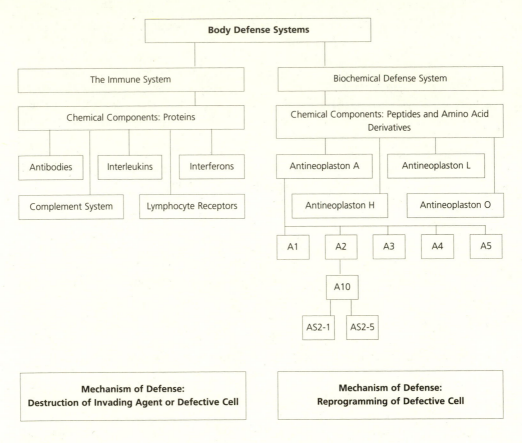

```
                          Body Defense Systems

           The Immune System              Biochemical Defense System

        Chemical Components: Proteins    Chemical Components: Peptides and Amino Acid
                                                        Derivatives

   Antibodies   Interleukins   Interferons    Antineoplaston A      Antineoplaston L

  Complement System   Lymphocyte Receptors       Antineoplaston H      Antineoplaston O

                                            A1   A2   A3   A4   A5

                                                   A10

                                                AS2-1  AS2-5

   Mechanism of Defense:                     Mechanism of Defense:
Destruction of Invading Agent or Defective Cell   Reprogramming of Defective Cell
```

Figure 21.1

Body defense systems. (Courtesy of Stanislaw Burzynski,
Burzynski Research Institute, Inc., Houston TX.)

Burzynski refused the offer to join the department of pharmacology. As Moss
reports:

> It looked like a promotion. There was one condition, however: he had to give
> up his budding private practice. Others might have grabbed at the chance and
> been happily absorbed into the cancer mainstream. There were, after all, ample
> rewards for doing so. But Burzynski hesitated. . . . Deep in his marrow, he
> feared institutionalization.[6]

This was, like Gerson's challenge to organized medicine, a critical turning
point in Burzynski's career. Burzynski, a central European immigrant like
Gerson, was being *welcomed* into the mainstream research establishment pre-

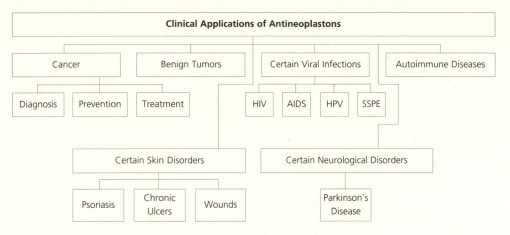

Figure 21.2

Clinical applications of antineoplastons. (Courtesy of Stanislaw Burzynski, Burzynski Research Institute, Inc., Hoston TX.)

cisely because of his exciting findings regarding antineoplastons. A man with the talents Burzynski was later to demonstrate—in his awesome personal effort to build a cancer research program entirely on his own—might have been expected to thrive in the intensely political atmosphere of large-scale cancer research, where political acumen is often as important to success as research brilliance and scientific good fortune. And yet, for better or worse, Burzynski refused the offer, despite clear warnings from his superiors of the likely political consequences. He later told Moss:

> "Most medical breakthroughs," [Burzynski said] with a sly touch of irony, "have happened because there was some lack of suppression by the supervisors of people doing some innovative work.". . . In addition, his private practice gave him financial independence. "If I should join them," he said, "I would do exactly what they were telling me to do, even though I would have a separate lab." When he refused their offer, these well-established cancer researchers turned against him and began to make life difficult. . . . Although he received an impressive certificate for meritorious service . . . his Chairman's last words were not auspicious: "Just wait, Burzynski. They're going to kick your ass."[7]

Because this was such a turning point, I asked Burzynski to review the reasons why he made this decision. Burzynski said that he was enjoying an ideal situation in the department of anesthesiology with a larger laboratory space than he would have had in the department of pharmacology; he had applied for a new $30,000 grant to continue his research; and, there was, he hoped, the prospect that he could develop a semiautonomous research unit loosely affiliated with the department of anesthesiology. By contrast, he said the reputation of the department of pharmacology was that it was autocratically run. He feared he would be unable to pursue his research. Burzynski says that at the time he refused the department of pharmacology offer he had no intention of leaving Baylor, and he expected to stay in his position with the department of anesthesiology. At a minimum, he misjudged the politics of the university. The situation "deteriorated," he said; his grant was not funded and he had to leave.

Reviewing his decision to leave Baylor, Burzynski offered his perspective:

> Regarding the issue of remaining at Baylor, I still believe that this would have led to disaster. One of the misfortunes of this country is that there is a big gap between basic scientists and clinicians. Contrary to the European situation, basic science researchers are despised by M.D.'s, and practicing physicians in medical schools are hated by basic researchers. A number of breakthroughs in medicine were done through the combination of basic science and clinical research in the same person. Well known examples are Louis Pasteur and Jonas Salk. When I initially came to the United States, I did not have any intention of practicing clinical medicine. I dreamed of being involved just in pure basic science. My enthusiasm quickly vanished after I noticed how biochemists are treated by clinicians. If I had stayed at Baylor after 1977, I would have had to rely on the mercy of proud clinicians using the same approach to Antineoplastons as to conventional chemotherapy. Such an approach would never have worked and the whole project would have been destroyed after the first unsuccessful clinical trial. I must admit, on the other hand, that it was my error to take "American democracy" too seriously. Coming from Poland, where everybody has a saintly opinion of the United States, I was convinced that this would be the country where democracy is everywhere. This may be true, but ultimately you have to prove this in court.[8]

Burzynski Attacked by the Medical Establishment

Moss describes in detail the extraordinary story—which will become scientific legend if antineoplastons ultimately prove to be a significant scientific discovery and the basis for an anticancer therapy—of how Burzynski set out virtually alone to develop, test, and win FDA (Food and Drug Administration) approval for a new anticancer drug—an effort that takes major pharmaceutical companies in good standing a decade and costs up to $100 million.[9] Burzynski undertook to do this with the cancer establishment pitted against him and with total assets of only $5,000. Historically, it is important to recognize the undeniable reality that he could have gone the other way, avoiding all of the massive opposition he has subsequently encountered. Whether the internal obstacles that the cancer establishment places before its own researchers would have proved greater than those Burzynski was to face as a maverick outsider, history cannot tell us. My own instinct—based on the strength of the scientific evidence that antineoplastons have promise and the entrepreneurial skills that Burzynski has subsequently demonstrated—is that he could have done better inside the American scientific establishment than outside it. Burzynski's assessment was that he would have been trapped by the bureaucratic and autocratic characteristics of the department and left without the freedom to pursue his research.

Having been forced out of Baylor, Burzynski faced a double-bind. Antineoplastons are largely *species-specific*. So, as Moss points out:

> Thus he was caught in a classic catch-22 situation. If he tested Antineoplastons in humans, the FDA was sure to come down on him eventually. But if he didn't so test them, he could never win FDA approval, since Antineoplastons, being species-specific, are not generally effective in animal treatment experiments [which the FDA was then using as a screen before authorizing human experiments]. His decision was thus to start treating patients, build up good records, let patient fees finance the future development of the drugs, and deal with the FDA later.[10]

Moss also notes that, "Financial considerations could not help but play their part. *It escaped no one's notice that an effective treatment, locked up in patents, would be worth a fortune*" [emphasis added].[11]

Had Burzynski gone inside the cancer establishment, on the other hand, I believe that there is a high likelihood that he could have found his way past the obstacle of the animal screen that FDA uses for anticancer drugs and made his way into human trials more quickly than he was able to on the outside. Once he had persuaded the FDA to allow him to conduct clinical trials, then by the curious logic of American cancer research *antineoplastons would have been a legitimate "experimental cancer therapy" instead of a dangerous unproven "alternative therapy" precisely because it was being conducted under the auspices of a recognized scientific institution instead of under the auspices of an independent center that had challenged the establishment.* He would have had the power to move the FDA around the problem of an ineffective animal screen precisely because he was developing a patentable therapy in conjunction with a major pharmaceutical house and a major university cancer center. All three players would have stood to benefit financially from his success. In case the FDA slowed clinical trials, he would also have been better placed to have antineoplastons tested in humans outside the United States because of his standing in the medical establishment and because of the standing and clout of his pharmaceutical industry partner.

Having made his decision, Burzynski proceeded to experience, as his Baylor department chairman had predicted he would, the full-scale legal and regulatory terror of county, state, and national authorities. He was investigated by the Board of Ethics of the Harris County Medical Society on the charge of using unapproved medications; he was refused research money by mainstream funders who had previously funded him.[12] Subsequently, he was to have his offices raided by the FDA, which seized 200,000 medical files and documents, and he was placed on the American Cancer Society's "unproven methods" list.[13] He was sued by an insurance company and investigated by a Federal grand jury.

Despite Burzynski's fall from grace, the NCI agreed to test three of his antineoplastons in its standard drug screen. Moss reports:

> Burzynski cooperated but was dubious. There were several test-tube and preventative models in which the drug had showed effectiveness, but the standard NCI pre-screen, P388 mouse leukemia, was not one of them. . . . As he had predicted, these compounds were not effective against mouse leukemia. Burzynski reasonably suggested that NCI try the Antineoplastons in cell-culture assays that were similar to "human solid tumors, especially adenocarcinoma of the breast" . . .

> Burzynski was hardly alone in voicing doubts about the P388 mouse model. Ironically, it was Dr. John Vendetti himself, chief of the NCI's Drug Evaluation Branch, who in 1983 coauthored an article in which he argued the limitations of this very mouse system. Scientists at NCI had found, for instance, that of seventy-nine drugs which had previously been judged negative in the P388, fourteen showed "significant activity" when retested in cell culture assays.[14]

Evaluating Antineoplaston Therapy

In 1982 a Canadian oncologist, David Walde, M.D., visited Burzynski in Texas. Moss quotes Walde's account:

> "I had no idea what to expect upon my arrival there and would not have been surprised to find a backdoor operation directed to the exploitation of patients for financial gain without the benefits of any therapeutic activity of the program. I also thought that documentation of the clinical cases would be poor and incomplete, making evaluation difficult if not impossible."
>
> What he found "was beyond my wildest expectations, and I had to rapidly backtrack on all my preconceived concepts of the situation."

Moss continues:

> Walde first visited the new antineoplaston production plant that Tad Burzynski [Stanislaw's brother] was busy assembling in a block-long building in nearby Stafford. The manufacturing guidelines were those suggested by the FDA and the entire operation—with its highly sophisticated, computerized control panels, its safety codes, and its sterile precautions—was the same as one might find in any modern pharmaceutical plant.
>
> "It was beyond my conception that an individual, without massive cash-flow funding from either commercial or governmental sources, would be able to single-handedly put together this sophisticated production capability. *My impression was that the entire program, both research and production, was built on the financial backs of the patients, supplemented by large personal bank loans by Dr. B*" [emphasis added].
>
> Walde's conclusion [Moss said] was that urinary peptides were an extremely promising area of cancer research.[15]

Stimulated by Moss's citation from the Walde report, I looked up the original and found it to be a model of the kind of balanced effort at evaluating an unconventional therapy that is so rarely found in the literature. Walde did say the positive things that Moss quoted, but he also said some other revealing things. For example:

> Dr. Burzynski does not and never has claimed he has the cure for all cancer. He never made any such claim to me. He tends to be readily and enthusiastically carried away about the possible theoretical extensions of his work, the ultimate

of which hopefully being the use of peptides in not only cancer therapy, but in a variety of biological modulations. *He can easily be misinterpreted as representing that he has the "cure"* [emphasis added].

He was very frank in his discussions. With malignancies such as ovarian, oat cell bronchogenic carcinoma and acute leukemias he has had dismal results. He cannot explain why hepatic and bony metastases of breast carcinoma seem to show a response, yet pulmonary and soft tissue disease often progresses even while the former regress, a situation contrary to standard chemotherapy, raising of course the later possibility of combined therapy once the role, if any, of peptides in cancer therapy is established.

The cancer processes that seem to respond best to chemotherapy show little response with his peptides. A good example is Hodgkin's, yet dramatic responses in some cases have been obtained with non-Hodgkin's lymphomas. The response data is far from complete, and preliminary. . . .

I had a chance to review a number of his charts, about 60 in all. Those that I was shown had excellent documentation. . . . The degree of response, complete remission, partial remission, stable and progressive disease has been assessed again by standard criteria. *Here I was in disagreement with a number of the assessments. Undoubtedly some interesting responses were occurring with a strong suggestion of an alteration in the natural history of the disease* [emphasis added]. However, I was only shown a small number of the total case load treated. Many were what I would term "dirty cases"; namely cases treated by some modality other than peptides, leaving open the criticism that the response was due to the prepresentation treatment, rather than peptides.[16]

Walde also noted that there was "an extremely high patient fallout" due to many factors, including high mortality related to the advanced stage of cancer in many patients; the fact that "the cost of the therapy is prohibitive, except for the very rich"; the fact that some patients become demoralized and leave treatment; the problems raised by assessing the effects of pretreatment; and the short duration of follow-up. Walde said: "One arrives at the situation of a major dilution in the number of assessable cases. The Phase II equivalent trials are therefore totally statistically invalid."

Walde also recorded telling conversations with Burzynski about Burzynski's use of the popular media to publicize his cause:

Politically, the situation at the moment over there is bordering on the impossible. I have stressed to Dr. Burzynski that he should avoid using the media to publicize his data. Dr. Burzynski retorts that this has been the only channel left open to him by repeated rejection of his submissions to journals and meetings. . . . He has to have patients to continue his research, as these fund the ongoing program. Public attention is therefore mandatory to maintain patient flow. This publicity inevitably ends up with the media Fed-bashing or accusations of a cancer-cure cover-up against the cancer societies. . . . I can appreciate the reasons for the criticisms launched against Dr. Burzynski. He proceeded with patient therapy, not only to investigate his peptides, but also to use the patients as a funding source.[17]

Yet with all these criticisms, Walde also came away with the powerful positive impressions that Moss cited above. He had looked up and read numerous articles in the historical and modern literature on urine therapy and concluded:

The whole concept of peptides in the modification of biological processes has been firmly established. . . . There is now enough data to necessitate us to look more closely at the nature and action of these peptides, as has been advanced by Dr. Burzynski, *even if these eventually do not result in any major therapeutic advances"* [Walde's emphasis].[17]

Whatever the faults of Walde's analysis, it was a genuine effort at a balanced assessment of an unconventional cancer therapy. Walde was a founding member of the investigatory drug subcommittee of the National Cancer Institute of Canada. He is also the leading Canadian authority on Essiac, a native Canadian alternative cancer therapy. I find him to be a remarkable example of an oncologist with a balanced and open interest in effective assessment of unconventional cancer therapies. As we shall see, the next Canadian delegation arrived with less open minds.

Walde made his report to the health protection branch of Health and Welfare Canada. The Ontario Ministry of Health requested an assessment from two leading physicians of whether or not it should waive its standard practice of not paying for experimental cancer therapies in the case of antineoplastons. Bureaucratically, this would have been a major move for the Ontario Health Insurance Plan, and the fact that the possibility was entertained speaks volumes for the difference between the cultures of medicine in the United States and Canada.

Two Toronto physicians, Martin E. Blackstein, Head of the Division of Oncology at Mount Sinai Hospital and Daniel E. Bergsagel, Chief of Medicine at

Princess Margaret Hospital, visited the Burzynski clinic and research institute on November 15, 1982. Both were powerful and respected physicians in the Canadian cancer establishment. They returned with a blistering, critical report. The essence of their critique was that (1) there was little evidence that antineoplastons had significant antitumor activity against human or animal cancers; (2) Burzynski's argument that antineoplastons were species-specific created a line of argument for avoiding standard animal and tissue culture screens and required testing in humans; (3) four patients whom Burzynski had described as achieving remission in a test of antineoplastons had in reality not benefited from the treatment; and (4) a review of 12 of Burzynski's "best cases" showed results that were very questionable. They reported:

> We were surprised that Dr. Burzynski would show us such questionable cases. We were left with the impression that either he knows very little about cancer and the response of different tumors to radiation and hormonal measures, or else he thinks we are very stupid, and he has tried to hoodwink us. As we look back on the cases we were shown, we are left with the impression that the only patients who were still alive either had slowly growing tumors, or had received effective treatment before being referred to Houston.[18]

Moss has devoted a large section of his chapter on Burzynski to refuting this report, saying that the Canadian physicians' critique of Burzynski's cell line experiments was entirely inaccurate; that species-specificity is well-known in nature and independently demonstrated with respect to antineoplastons; and that they misread and misrepresented their review of Burzynski's 12 cases. Burzynski also wrote a detailed critique and called their visit "a complete failure and a great disappointment." He concluded:

> It is clearly evident that Dr. Bergsagel and Dr. Blackstein completely distorted the research, production and clinical data presented to them in Houston. One could expect that people who are medical doctors and who occupy important positions in two large hospitals in Toronto should not give false statements to their own countrymen. They should know that the delay in the approval of experimental treatment which they will create will cost lives of Canadian cancer victims.[19]

Reading the Blackstein-Bergsagel report and the refutation by Moss and Burzynski side by side is like listening to opposing attorneys offering drastically different accounts of the same event. Judging from the documents, the case made by Burzynski and Moss is somewhat more persuasive, particularly with the benefit of having read Walde's account of his visit to Burzynski, which is far closer to a model of how an open-minded oncologist can assess an unconventional cancer therapy than is the Blackstein-Bergsagel report.

On the other hand, I would emphasize that Burzynski—having gone to the public media to protect himself from medical regulatory opposition in Texas and to develop the patient flow he needed to finance his research program—made public various details of the negotiations for clinical testing of antineoplastons in Canada, to Walde's dismay and to Bergsagel and Blackstein's disgust. Although Walde presented a much more sophisticated, balanced, and thorough report than his colleagues, it is hard to fault mainstream oncologists for distrusting a practitioner who was breaking all the basic rules of the game in using an experimental therapy on patients without an FDA Investigational New Drug (IND) permit in either the United States or Canada, and whose public relations person was continuously going public on research issues that should not have been discussed. The fact that at that time it was still technically legal in Texas to use a new cancer drug with patients within the state without an IND permit is often pointed out in Burzynski's defense. But this legality did nothing to lessen the shock of such a practice to the medical establishment.

Moss describes Burzynski as having "moved swiftly" to follow Walde's suggestion to apply for IND clearance in Canada so that further studies could be undertaken there. He suggests that the Blackstein-Bergsagel report was the event that ended the prospects for any trials in Canada.[20] Walde remembers the events differently, and this is a critical point. According to Walde, the reason the studies did not go forward was that Burzynski refused to cooperate. The reason for Burzynski's failure to cooperate, according to Walde, was that "he was concerned about protecting his patents—that they would not be fully protected."[21]

If Walde's account is accurate, Burzynski again had an opportunity to reenter the research mainstream. He had a new chance to have antineoplastons tested and evaluated by independent researchers. It is clear from his subsequent record that Burzynski really does want independent evaluation of antineoplastons. But at this point, according to Walde, despite the tremendous pressure he was under in the United States, Burzynski was more concerned with protecting his patents than with moving forward as quickly as possible toward an open evaluation of his therapy. We can look at this from two points of view.

If we view Burzynski as a pharmaceutical entrepreneur protecting patents that could result in a vast fortune for his future research and himself, he was doing what many pharmaceutical companies would have done under the circumstances. If we accept the view of Burzynski as an embattled champion seeking to get a promising cancer therapy out to cancer patients as quickly as possible, one could certainly argue that the risk to Burzynski's patents was not too high a price to pay to regain mainstream research credibility. Here, after all, was a man who told alternative cancer therapy reporter Gary Null: "I'm going to fight no matter what they do, because I believe I'm doing the right thing. I believe that this is our obligation to the people. If you find something that's valuable, you must continue and I believe we've found something that may be able to save lives."[22]

Burzynski gives his own version of his reasons for not moving forward with the Canadian research:

> Dr. Walde is seriously mistaken regarding the approval in Canada. . . . I did not consider at all the problem of patent protection versus filing of an IND. First of all, the patent application was filed already, and, on the other hand, I did not have any reservation in sharing the details of production and treatment with Antineoplastons with any researcher all over the world. For instance, I gave the procedure on how to synthesize Antineoplaston A10 to the People's Republic of China, where I do not have any patent protection. In the future, the People's Republic of China could be a huge market for pharmaceuticals, much bigger than Canada. As a result of such sharing of technology, the doctors in China were able to synthesize Antineoplaston A10 a few years ago and are using their product successfully in their research.
>
> The initial approach from the Canadian authorities was extremely cooperative, but all of a sudden it changed, perhaps as the result of the second [Blackstein-Bergsagel] Canadian visit. Ultimately, Canadian authorities requested tremendous amount of data which were impossible to produce with our limited laboratory type production of Antineoplastons A2, A3, and A5. To deliver such data and comply fully with the requirements, it was necessary to have fully automatic urine processing plant. . . . This plant would have been finished many years ago, but it's not even finished today due to extreme expenses for our defense. Even today, we are not able to comply with Canadian requests.[23]

I believe in Burzynski's sincerity in saying this. The directors of many pharmaceutical companies would also speak truly of their desire to save lives. But when one enters the big business of cancer pharmaceuticals, either in mainstream or alternative medicine, the same business considerations are operating. No prudent pharmaceutical entrepreneur would move for more rapid studies and trials if he thought that the process might endanger his patents. Yet by Burzynski's account, patent problems had nothing to do with why the Canadian research opportunity did not go forward.

A Visit to Japan—My Own Reawakened Interest in Burzynski

The Blackstein-Bergsagel report cooled my interest in Burzynski for years, because I assumed that report was a good faith and neutral assessment. I had not yet read Walde's assessment. As a result of the Blackstein-Bergsagel report, I relegated Burzynski to the large category of alternative cancer therapists that I frankly did not know what to make of. The evidence of my senses had told me during my visit to Burzynski that he looked like a qualified scientist and that the therapy looked like perhaps the most promising and scientifically open of the pharmaceutical therapies I had seen. But how, I asked myself, could my reportorial assessment of Burzynski match a medically knowledgeable assessment by two very distinguished Canadian physicians who had made a site visit, examined case records, and seemed qualified to assess the science? But in more recent years, the consistent focus of some of the most knowledgeable advocate-analysts of alternative therapies on Burzynski, notably Ralph Moss and Robert Houston of New York, brought me back to take another careful look at Burzynski.

I had three personal friends who had come through the Commonweal Cancer Help Program and believed strongly that Burzynski "had something." One was a woman from New York with colon cancer with liver metastases. Her liver metastases had stabilized on the Burzynski program and she seemed to be enjoying life extension as a result of the therapy, but she was *profoundly* embarrassed by a side effect of the treatment that some patients experience which is not often cited by advocates: a strong odor that some people are sensitive to and others (like me) are not. The odor in her case was reminiscent of the odor of urine and made her feel like a "bag lady" who had soiled herself. In at least one instance, she was asked to leave a restaurant because of the smell. Because of the deeply isolating experience of cancer itself, this side effect was very troubling for my friend, even though she believed she was benefiting from the therapy.

A second friend from nearby Stinson Beach had gone to Burzynski with metastatic breast cancer: the therapy had not helped her, but she came away thoroughly convinced that other patients were being helped. A third friend from another nearby town had gone to Texas with metastatic prostate cancer and high hopes, since prostate cancer is one of the cancers for which the Burzynski therapy appears most promising. But he was not helped and subsequently died. A fourth friend and colleague, a health educator like myself with a strong professional interest in objective assessment of alternative cancer therapies, also visited Burzynski and came away with positive impressions.

My real sense that Burzynski possibly did "have something" came when, at the suggestion of Robert Houston, I visited Hideaki Tsuda, M.D., an anesthesiologist, and his colleague, a surgeon named Hiroshi Hara, M.D., at Kurume University School of Medicine in Fukuoka Prefecture. Tsuda had known Burzynski when they were both at Baylor University and had a friendly regard for him, but it was the high regard of a medical colleague, not a "true believer."

Tsuda had subsequently decided to do an independent evaluation of antineoplastons in both animals and humans. He and Hara and almost a dozen other colleagues formed the Antineoplaston Study Group. He had the advantage that Burzynski had foregone: a hospital setting and a university appointment. He had the further advantage that Japanese law made it much easier for him to proceed from animal studies to patient studies. Japan's enlightened universal system of health insurance pays for most of the costs of patient care for virtually all Japanese, so that the costs of observing a clinical series of patients given antineoplastons is relatively modest.

In the course of two studies with mice, in which they demonstrated both tumor prevention and inhibition, Tsuda, Hara, and their colleagues resolved to their own satisfaction the issue that had troubled the Canadian oncologists with respect to animal studies of antineoplastons. They acknowledged the discrepancies between animal and human studies regarding the effectiveness of antineoplaston 10, but speculated that the explanation might rest in the fact that antineoplastons are not naturally occurring in mice and are excreted rapidly, whereas humans show longer retention times. They therefore adopted a more frequent and larger dose in the athymic mouse study, reasoning that the smaller doses might be sufficient to prevent tumor formation, but not to inhibit an existing tumor. They concluded:

Antineoplaston A-10 and A-10 Injection are quite different from conventional chemotherapeutic agents because they are both naturally occurring in humans though not existing in animals. Accordingly in experimental studies, a larger and more frequent dose will be required to demonstrate quantitative antitumor effects. *An improved effect can be expected in clinical cases from the same dosage levels as evaluated experimentally"* [emphasis added].[24]

In other words, Tsuda and his colleagues were suggesting that the improved anticancer effects that might come with larger doses of the antineoplaston agents would go beyond tumor prevention to stabilization or reversal of existing cancers. The amounts required might seem very large by mainstream cancer therapy standards, but the substance involved was naturally occurring in humans and generally nontoxic.

Tsuda then presented to us ten case reports of patients with whom he and his colleagues had tried the antineoplaston therapies. These case presentations, which, with one exception, have not yet been reported in scientific journals, were what truly awakened me to the possibility that antineoplastons worked.

One case, which Tsuda has reported publicly, was described in the July-August 1990 issue of *Oncology News*. At a Swiss conference that is discussed further below, Tsuda reported that his group had administered a combination of cisplatin and antineoplastons to an elderly woman with inoperable metastatic ovarian carcinoma with massive ascites:

At the second-look operation following this therapy, the ovarian tumor could be removed easily, Dr. Tsuda reported. . . . "She is now enjoying her life very much without any side effects," he added. "By this kind of combination, we were able to augment the anticancer effect and reduce the miserable side effects of anticancer agents and keep up the patient's quality of life."[25]

Obviously, my report of the work of Tsuda and his colleagues at Kurume University Medical School in Japan is a reportorial account of the clinical impressions of a physician who was summarizing some early and limited case data. But in all my years of doing this work, rarely has an account had such an impact on me. Tsuda has, to the best of my capacity to discern, the kind of impeccable integrity that surrounds the Japanese cultural approach to science and many other things. He made clear that he had taken absolutely no money from Burzynski to conduct this research, nor would he, in part, he explained only half-jokingly, because he was a little older than Burzynski and in Japan the older colleague would never put himself in such a relationship with a younger colleague. Tsuda, like Burzynski, *welcomed* outside evaluation of his research, and asked me specifically to convey to Japan Cancer Institute authorities in Tokyo how much he would welcome constructive guidance.

Independent Laboratory Research Supporting Burzynski

In the United States, a review of independent assessments of antineoplastons by scientific researchers further deepened my sense that the promise of antineoplastons should be pursued. *Oncology News* for July-August 1990 gave a flavor of the excitement that the antineoplaston research was generating. Under headlines that read *Trials Underway at Several Research Centers* and *Antineoplastons: New Antitumor Agents Stir High Expectations,* an article led off with a report on independent studies by Dvorit Samid, Ph.D., at the Uniformed Services University of Health Sciences in Bethesda, Maryland, that had shown that "AS2–1 [the antineoplaston] profoundly inhibits oncogene expression and the proliferation of malignant cells without exhibiting any toxicity toward normal cells. . . . The Antineoplaston can actually induce terminal differentiation [reversion toward normal cellular structure]. . . . 'Such a dramatic phenomenon is seldom seen,' Dr. Samid noted."[26]

At the same conference, Burzynski reported a phase II trial of the antineoplaston AS2–1 (that Samid had tested) combined with the hormonal regimen DES (diethylstilbestrol) in 14 patients with prostate cancer resistant to hormonal therapy: "'By the end of the study we were able to identify two cases of complete remission, three partial remissions, seven objective stabilizations, and two cases of progressive disease.' Clinical improvement was accompanied by a drop in prostate cancer markers and by improvements in bone scans."[27]

Burzynski has now also completed but not yet published a phase II trial with astrocytoma (a nerve tissue tumor). While he is not free to talk of the trials until they are published, patients report that he is having really remarkable success with stage IV astrocytomas in children, and some interesting results with astrocytomas in adults, and with glioblastomas (brain cancers) in children and adults.

On March 16, 1989, the FDA approved Burzynski's request for an IND permit to do a phase II clinical trial at an independent institution on the effect of antineoplaston therapy on 15 patients with metastatic breast cancer.[28] But as of April 1991, the trial had not begun because Burzynski had not yet found the right pharmaceutical industry partner to underwrite the $400,000 to $600,000 cost of the trial.

The growing interest on the part of mainstream cancer researchers in Burzynski's work and increasing evidence of antineoplaston's effectiveness in some cancers led to the announcement in December 1991 of NCI-sponsored phase II trials of antineoplastons with brain cancer patients. On October 6, 1991, an NCI site visit team reviewed a best-case series of results using antineoplastons with brain tumors at the Burzynski Research Institute. As a result of this review, the NCI decided that phase II trials were indicated in order to confirm tumor shrinkage documented in this series and to determine the tumor response rate. The NCI will be conducting four independent phase II trials of antineoplastons A10 and AS2–1 with brain tumor patients having glioblastomas, astrocytomas, pediatric brain tumors, and low-grade astrocytomas.[29]

Burzynski's Current Impressions of the Effectiveness of His Therapy

Asking the developer of a new unconventional therapy for his own estimate of the efficacy of that therapy is a delicate but important step in assessing unconventional cancer therapies.

In our interview, Burzynski said he was clinically impressed, especially with the results with prostate cancer (which he has reported a phase II clinical trial on, described above) and brain cancers, specifically childhood gliomas, which he plans a phase II study on. After that, he said, in descending order, he is impressed with results with non-Hodgkin's lymphomas (80% of tumors reduced by 50%) and pancreatic cancers (70% of tumors reduced by 50%). Breast cancer follows, with lung cancer and colon cancer further down the list. I asked if he was referring to brief or sustained responses, and he replied that he was referring to sustained responses. Did this mean that the patients were cured? No, he said, the cancers could certainly recur. These figures, he added, were for responses using his synthetic antineoplastons. He is in the process of completing a production plant for production of a natural antineoplaston derived directly from urine. With the natural product, he said that he expected better responses with mesotheliomas and lung, bladder, breast, and colon cancers.

I pointed out that Tsuda in Japan had said that antineoplastons seemed to be more effective in keeping a tumor from growing, and therefore sustaining life, rather than in reducing the size of the tumor, which Burzynski was clearly describing in his estimates of objective responses described above. He replied that Tsuda had been largely limited to oral antineoplastons and that the injections were more effective. Burzynski then offered an interesting insight into the way he believes antineoplastons work:

> In humans, normal cells die off after 20 to 60 divisions. They enter a terminal differentiation at that point and die. In animals, they can sometimes revert back, but not in humans. Cancer cells become essentially immortal: they do not die, and so with the process of division the tumor grows. In highly malignant cells, those 20 to 60 divisions can happen very fast. So if you can force differentiation, they will die much more quickly and you will see the tumor reduction more quickly. That is why we can see better results with glioblastomas or pancreatic cancers, which are fast-moving cancers. In slower-growing tumors, like breast cancer, it can take longer to see results, unless you add some chemotherapy or interferon, which can shorten the course.[30]

This issue of the difference in efficacy between the synthetic and natural antineoplastons is one that troubles some of Burzynski's critics. Burzynski's early work with cancer patients used the natural antineoplastons, and they may be more effective. One scientist who stayed very close to Burzynski's research from its inception through 1985 reported:

> When Burzynski was using the natural product, I felt he had stumbled onto a really important discovery. The early cases suggested that. But when he started using the synthetic, my friend who worked there would say to me that the patients were dying. I think he had to make the move to synthetics for economic reasons—the natural product was too expensive to produce.

This scientist, who spoke on condition that I not identify him, had excellent access to the opinions of a dedicated staff member within the Burzynski Research Institute who *did* like and support Burzynski. This opinion of a loyal and longtime Burzynski staff member regarding the difference in efficacy between synthetic and natural antineoplastons, which parallels Burzynski's view that the two products work differently with different cancers, is thus worth recording. Burzynski offers a different view:

> The synthetic Antineoplastons are not less important than natural ones. They simply have a different spectrum of activity. . . . This could lead to misconceptions for somebody who has been associated with us for only a limited period of time. Knowing which types of cancer respond the best [to synthetic vs. natural antineoplastons], we are trying to make an appropriate selection of patients. We are trying to limit the admissions of patients with adenocarcinoma of the lung, because our production capacity of Antineoplaston A2 is very small. Once we have the automatic urine processing plant ready, we will be happy to accept a large number of lung cancer patients.[31]

Finances and Pharmaceutical Agreements

Two other subjects of concern that are often raised by critics of Burzynski are the financial workings of the Burzynski Research Institute and the question of whether Burzynski will ever consummate an effective agreement with a major pharmaceutical corporation that will take antineoplastons through the hugely expensive process of clinical trials and, if appropriate, commercial marketing for all cancer patients.

With regard to the question of whether or not the finances of the institute have been professionally run, Burzynski said quite candidly in our interview that the finances had been handled properly in the early years when he was personally responsible, from 1977 to 1981, but as the institute grew he hired "a succession of bad people" and only achieved what he regarded as good financial management 2 years ago.

But a more important financial question is an ethical one. I asked Burzynski whether or not he had always been careful to tell patients what he believed he could and could not offer, given the substantial patient flow he needed to finance the research program and the large and often unreimbursable burden that using the therapy imposed on patients.

Burzynski replied that in the early years, he did not know which cancers would respond and which would not, so in his view—and in the view of colleagues with whom he discussed this issue—the decision was properly on the patient's side. In later years, he said he has been more able to describe to patients whether or not he has had success with their kind of cancers, although some want to try the therapy even when the probability of success is not high (the same dilemma is well-known to conventional oncologists). He also responded that, in many cases, the effectiveness of the therapy can be determined within 6 weeks, which somewhat limits the financial burden to the patient.

The broader question of whether Burzynski will actually enter a working partnership with a major pharmaceutical firm to develop and market antineoplastons is also a question for critics and friends who note Burzynski's long-time distrust of large bureaucracies and organizations that he sees as trying to restrict his freedom.

The Burzynski Research Institute announced with some fanfare that Burzynski had signed a letter of agreement with Sigma-Tau, Italy's largest pharmaceutical company, authorizing them to conduct laboratory, preclinical, and clinical studies on A10 and AS2–1 in Europe.[32] But in August 1990, Burzynski's public information officer, Le Trombetta, expressed her frustration with the very slow pace of these announced studies and clinical trials. Sigma-Tau was also, Burzynski reports, originally interested in funding the FDA-approved phase II trial with metastatic breast cancer patients, but has since backed away from the agreement. Burzynski is said to be near agreement with another pharmaceutical firm that will finally take antineoplastons into the legal and commercial development that has eluded the agent for so long. The question is whether the successful agreement will always be around the next corner.

A Pattern of Distrust

Does Burzynski have a real pattern of distrust of large organizations, and has this pattern hampered the development of antineoplastons? This is a significant question.

It may be that Burzynski's early experience with the authorities in Poland provides an explanation of his aversion to bureaucracy. Burzynski was one of the youngest and most promising graduates of the Medical Academy of Lublin, but he refused to join the Communist Party, which Moss tells us was "the perquisite for academic achievement." As a result of this and the jealousy of classmates, "Burzynski suddenly found himself drafted in the Polish army—one of only two doctors from the academy drafted that year. . . . Finally, with the help of influential scientists, he was able to emigrate."[33] That was surely a formative experience for a brilliant young scientist: that his innate instinct to avoid the Communist Party bureaucracy resulted in a highly punitive military assignment.

He then came to America and became again an extraordinary academic success at Baylor as he had at the Medical Academy of Lublin. But when he was asked to do the equivalent of joining the Communist Party at Baylor—again a prerequisite for advancement—he again balked and went his own way. And, just as was the case in Poland, anyone could have told Burzynski that the consequences of what he planned to do would be as severe in the United States as they had been in Poland.

In more recent years, the pharmaceutical partnerships Burzynski has explored in the United States and abroad remain, for whatever reasons, just around the corner. The research and clinical studies continue to move forward simply because of the apparently compelling nature of the science that Burzynski has uncovered. The question for the coming years is whether or not Stanislaw Burzynski will actually sign up for and complete the major pharmaceutical agreements that are prerequisites for the large controlled clinical trials that will definitively evaluate the promise of antineoplastons. Skeptics claim that he does not actually want these trials. I believe that is entirely incorrect. But who knows whether he will, on the one hand, overcome a lifetime of distrusting partnerships with large bureaucracies and join forces with a pharmaceutical company or, on the other hand, ultimately try to win scientific acceptance of antineoplastons on his own?

I asked Burzynski whether there was anything I had not asked him that he would like to say:

> You have to understand all the attempts I have faced since Poland that were aimed at limiting my freedom. For the past fourteen years, I have been working under severe conditions with formidable enemies. The State Board of Medical Examiners, the FDA, the insurance companies . . . this has not been the ideal way to do research.[34]

Burzynski, like Max Gerson and Emanuel Revici—all great innovators in unconventional cancer therapy who immigrated to the United States as refugees from Central Europe—came from a medical tradition which tolerated and protected the integration of science and clinical practice. Permitting physicians to conduct extended clinical programs of experimentation with cancer patients, which the European system essentially allows physicians to do, brings both great risks and the potential of great benefits. Gerson, Burzynski, and Revici came to America believing that this was the land of freedom, and each was already trained in the permissive culture of European medicine. One can add to this that Burzynski, at least, like many scientists, was also by character antiauthoritarian. So all three pursued their unconventional cancer therapies in this new land, where perhaps they did not fully appreciate the cultural clues about the practice of medicine. And each faced the full force of opposition that organized medicine often visits on those who contravene the established norms—developed both for patient protection and for the trade-union interests of organized medicine—especially in the cancer field.

Practitioner, Therapy, and Service Delivery

In trying to find one's way through the morass of conflicting evidence on Burzynski and antineoplastons, let us return to the distinction between the *practitioner,* the *therapy,* and the *service delivery.*

The practitioner: Burzynski himself, most observers agree, is a brilliant man with a genuine scientific interest in the open assessment of his antineoplaston research, an attitude which is relatively rare among major practitioners of alternative pharmacological cancer therapies. Burzynski's commitment to open science in the face of extensive opposition deserves commendation. And yet, while Burzynski is unquestionably brilliant, while his commitment to science is profound, and while (most important) he may have made an important discovery in cancer therapy, legitimate questions persist about the wisdom of the decisions he made to go outside of mainstream institutions instead of inside them, decisions which have profoundly affected the course of the development of antineoplaston therapy and the prospects for its availability, proven and at reasonable cost, to cancer patients. Burzynski and his supporters have one view of these choices; his critics have another; the question remains an important and fair one.

The therapy: Antineoplastons as therapy—based on the current scanty research and clinical evidence—may well be recognized in coming years as having considerable benefit in the treatment of some cancers. The extent of this benefit is not yet clear, but it could be significant. More important, Burzynski has only been able to explore a small corner of the research that antineoplastons open up. At present, antineoplastons bring benefit to only a portion of patients seeking help at the Burzynski Research Institute, most of whom are suffering not only from advanced disease but also from the toxic side effects of previous treatment. Despite the laboratory evidence, the phase II clinical trials that Burzynski has reported, and the independent clinical studies of Tsuda in Japan, the history of science warns us emphatically that there is a long road to travel before we know the extent of the actual benefit of antineoplaston cancer therapy.

The service delivery: The largest legitimate doubts about antineoplaston therapy could be said to lie in the area of service delivery, broadly construed. I have already asked whether Burzynski made the right choice—from the point of view of the well-being of cancer patients—in turning down the offer to join the Baylor College of Medicine Department of Pharmacology to pursue his warmly welcomed line of research within the establishment. Was the extraordinary choice to build a major research program on high medical fees the ethical and necessary decision? Was Burzynski right to court major media attention to fend off the assaults on him and to keep the flow of patients coming in the early years so that the research could be continued? How strenuous an effort has the Burzynski Research Institute made to discourage cancer patients who are unlikely to benefit from antineoplaston therapy but who wanted to come out of desperation and who have the money to pay for the therapy?

There are no final answers, only the questions. I was impressed by Burzynski's frank advice to a friend of mine with metastatic ovarian cancer that she probably would not benefit from his therapy. Several other friends of mine have also been told not to come, and that is greatly to Burzynski's credit. One of the marks of less credible unconventional cancer treatment centers is that practitioners tell everyone to come who has money to pay for services.

Burzynski is far from alone in facing the issue of whether or not he should give expensive treatments to desperate patients who may not benefit. It is a perennial problem for practitioners of both conventional and experimental therapies. In experimental mainstream cancer therapies, the dilemma was most poignantly clear at the for-profit Biotherapeutics program in Franklin, Tennessee, which was run by former NCI researchers, who, like Burzynski, also charged very high fees for individually designed experimental research pharmaceuticals. (Now reorganized and called Response Technologies, the firm is no longer involved with experimental protocols, but now focuses on the outpatient delivery of "intensive" cancer therapies normally available only through hospitals.) Biotherapeutics had also faced the charge that it allowed patients to come who were very unlikely to benefit. Within the cancer establishment, outrage was expressed about the tactics of Biotherapeutics in offering experimental therapies for wealthy patients (often themselves physicians), both on the grounds that this contributes to a two-track medical system for the rich and the poor, and on the grounds that patients are paying for unproven therapies. Even if the credentials of the Biotherapeutics team were impeccable, the fear existed that the pay-for-individual-research scheme may allow the unwashed hordes of unconventional cancer therapy practitioners to breach the cordon sanitaire so carefully constructed to prevent cancer quackery in the United States.

There are currently many examples in mainstream medicine—coronary bypass surgery for patients who are unlikely to benefit is one of the most egregious—of expensive therapies that will help some patients, but are offered to many others who are unlikely to benefit. That Burzynski is asking patients to pay huge fees for an experimental therapy must be assessed in this context.

Presently, the Burzynski therapy costs $3,000 to $5,000 a month—or $36,000 to $60,000 a year—depending on the specific medications a patient is taking. Most patients cannot get their insurance companies to reimburse these expenses. And even if an insurance company is willing to pay, that raises the larger question of whether or not all patients in that insurance system should ultimately pay a higher premium for a very expensive therapy, the benefits of which may accrue largely only to certain subsets of cancer patients. Again, this is as real an issue for coronary bypass surgery as it is for antineoplaston therapy.

But ultimately, all the issues we have discussed will fade away. The awesome beauty of science is that in the end Burzynski is either right or wrong about antineoplastons. If he is right, he probably deserves at least a share of a Nobel Prize, because a *nontoxic* chemotherapy for cancer, even if only partially effective, would be a profound service to mankind. If he is wrong, if his phase II trial results do not hold up in more extended controlled trials, then this will be simply another tortured and unfortunate chapter in the long and often unedifying history of both conventional and unconventional cancer therapies.

Notes and References

1   Ralph W. Moss, *The Cancer Industry* (New York: Paragon House, 1989).
2   Another less favorable extended account of Burzynski's work is included in the *Report on Unconventional Cancer Therapies* by the Office of Technology Assessment.
3   Moss, *The Cancer Industry,* 289–91.
4   Ibid., 292.
5   Stanislaw Burzynski, personal communication with the author, 13 November 1990.
6   Moss, *The Cancer Industry,* 294–5.
7   Ibid., 295–6.
8   Burzynski, personal communication with the author, 13 November 1990.
9   Moss, *The Cancer Industry,* 297.
10   Ibid.
11   Ibid., 296.
12   Ibid., 298.
13   Ibid., 287–8.
14   Ibid., 299–300.
15   Ibid., 300–1.
16   David Walde, unpublished memorandum, 22 November 1982, 7–8.
17   Ibid.
18   M.E. Blackstein and D.E. Bergsagel, "The Treatment of Cancer Patients with Antineoplastons and the Burzynski Clinic in Houston, Texas." Report to the Ministry of Health, Province of Ontario, undated.
19   S.R. Burzynski, "Response to Site Visit to Burzynski Research Institute on November 15, 1982 and Report by Drs. M.E. Blackstein and D.E. Bergsagel," Burzynski Research Institute, undated.
20   Moss, *The Cancer Industry,* 301.
21   David Walde, telephone conversation with the author, 30 August 1990.
22   Gary Null, "This Man Could Save Your Life, But He Can't Get the Money to Do It," *Our Town* 13–19 May 1979. Quoted in Moss, *The Cancer Industry,* 297–8.
23   Burzynski, personal communication with the author, 13 November, 1990.
24   K. Hashimoto et al., "The Anticancer Effect of Antineoplaston A-10 on Human Breast Cancer Serially Transplanted to Athymic Mice," *Journal of the Japan Society for Cancer Therapy* 25(1):1–5 (1990).
25   *Oncology News* 16(4):1,6 (1990).

26   Ibid., 1.

27   Ibid., 6. For details, see abstracts in proceedings of 9th International Symposium on Future Trends in Chemotherapy, Geneva, Switzerland, 26–8 March 1990.

28   Moss, *The Cancer Industry,* 334.

29   Press Release, Burzynski Research Institute, 6 December 1991.

30   Stanislaw Burzynski, personal communication with the author, 13 November 1990.

31   Ibid.

32   Moss, *The Cancer Industry,* 333–4.

33   Ibid., 290–1.

34   Stanislaw Burzynski, personal communication with the author, 13 November 1990.

twenty-two

Joseph Gold—Does Hydrazine Sulfate Prevent Weight Loss and Extend Life with Cancer?

The story of Joseph Gold, M.D., makes a fascinating comparison with that of Stanislaw Burzynski. Like Burzynski, Gold made his discovery—of the anti-cancer effects of hydrazine sulfate—while working inside the medical establishment. But, unlike Burzynski, he stayed inside and faithfully played by the rules. Nonetheless, hydrazine sulfate spent 3 years on the American Cancer Society's (ACS) "unproven methods" list before becoming recognized as a promising experimental therapy.

Even today, after numerous preclinical and clinical studies have established its modest toxicity, its capacity for enhancing the nutritional status of cancer patients and helping them avoid weight loss (cachexia), and its consequent potential to extend life—at least with some cancers—hydrazine sulfate remains a drug that is difficult for cancer patients to get, even through the efforts of sympathetic oncologists.

Gold is the Director of the Syracuse Cancer Research Institute in Syracuse, New York. In 1968, he published a paper suggesting that a new approach to cancer might be to block the primary damage cancer does to the body.

Gold had studied the work of Otto H. Warburg, winner of the Nobel Prize for Medicine in 1931. Gold's innovation was based upon Warburg's controversial theory of the nature of cancer cell metabolism. In normal cell metabolism, energy is obtained through respiration—taking in oxygen and giving off carbon dioxide and water. But under some circumstances—such as when the muscles or brain require a quick burst of energy—that energy can be produced through fermentation, a primitive and wasteful process common in simple forms of life. Warburg postulated that cancer cells fulfilled their energy needs in this way.[1] Warburg's theory has remained controversial, although it is currently regarded as probably partially correct.

Extrapolating from Warburg's theory, Gold reasoned that if cancer cachexia— the weight loss often accompanying cancer—could be interrupted, the disease might be controlled.[2] Gold found that cachexia resulted from the cancer's recycling of its own wastes at the energy expense of the body. Cancer only partially metabolizes glucose, its fuel, producing lactic acid as a waste product. The body must then expend a great deal of energy to reconvert the lactic acid back into glucose. An ever-increasing amount of glucose then becomes available as fuel for the tumor, but only at great expense to the other tissues of the body.[3]

Working from this theoretical perspective, Gold began investigating ways of interrupting this "sick relationship." He experimented with various drugs and diets before finding a scientific paper in the early 1970s that provided the key: a substance called hydrazine sulfate could block an enzyme in the liver critical to the process of converting lactic acid to glucose.[4] Gold's report that a cheap and readily available chemical might be of help to cancer was not of great interest to the pharmaceutical industry, but it did have considerable appeal to many cancer patients. Soon it was picked up by advocates of unconventional cancer therapies and thousands of patients were trying it.

An early pilot study by Manuel Ochoa at Memorial Sloan-Kettering Cancer Center in New York evaluated hydrazine sulfate with 29 "adequately treated" patients with a wide range of tumor types. He reported no significant subjective or objective gains but, to the contrary, found "major neurological toxicity was observed in half of the patients."[5] Gold strongly criticized the methodology of the study—convincingly in my view.[6] Two other negative studies followed. Gold then published an article reporting positive effects of hydrazine sulfate in patients who were receiving the drug under the Food and Drug Administration (FDA) Investigational New Drug (IND) permits that had been given to a number of physicians.[7] He found subjective improvement in 70% of adequately treated patients and objective improvement, including tumor regression and cancer stabilization, in 17% of patients. But in March 1976, probably owing largely to the fact that it had become a favored alternative cancer therapy without undergoing conclusive testing within the scientific community, hydrazine sulfate was placed on the ACS's unproven methods list. Once the drug had been put on the ACS list, Gold's funding dried up.[8]

Soviet Studies of Hydrazine Sulfate

Fortunately for science and for cancer patients, scientists in the former Soviet Union were not deterred by the negative opinion of the ACS and continued to evaluate the drug. In large nonrandomized single-arm trials at the Petrov Research Institute of Oncology in Leningrad begun in 1975 and 1976, 356 patients were given hydrazine sulfate alone. The difficulties with such uncontrolled single-arm studies are well known, but the merit of the studies was that no concurrent or incompatible chemotherapy or medication clouded the picture. Gold reports: "Results of the nine-year study revealed the following: 50% subjective (anticachexia) response; 46% antitumor response; restoration of (previously lost) sensitivity to cytotoxics [e.g., agents toxic to cancer cells]; instances of long-term survival; and the absence of important clinical side-effects."[9]

Patients increased their weights and appetites and enjoyed improved strength and performance status. The cancer stabilized in 31% and regressed in an additional 15% of the sample. Says Gold: "Therapeutic effects were indicated as *frequently not appearing until the second or third course of therapy* [emphasis added], and their accrual in patients who were considered 'practically in the terminal phase' of their disease was cited as a 'factor' of potential clinical significance."[9]

It is important to remember that the Soviet studies used cancer patients with a wide range of different kinds of tumors and reported positive results across the whole range. Note that the Soviets reported actual antitumor as well as anticachexia affects. In Gold's view, hydrazine sulfate's antitumor and anti-cachexia effects may be related:

With the advent of a specific anticachexia agent, more effective cancer control becomes possible. For the devastating aspects of this disease are due to two principle causes: invasion of tumor into vital organs with consequent destruction of their function; and decay of the body by virtue of cachexia and its resultant effect on the integrity of all body systems. Each of these processes has its own metabolic machinery, each is amenable to its own therapy, and each is to some degree functionally interdependent on the other.[10]

The National Cancer Institute (NCI) noted the results of the Soviet studies without enthusiasm, contrasting them with two earlier negative studies from the United States. But interest among physicians and patients in the United States continued to grow, and, finally, through its complex and contradictory bureaucratic political process, the NCI formally expressed interest in metabolic and anticachexia research along lines that suggested a recognition of hydrazine sulfate's potential, but that placed obstacles in the way of additional funding for research. The struggle was more than one over hydrazine sulfate: it was a debate within the cancer establishment over how much emphasis should be placed on energy metabolism, cachexia, and nutritional factors in cancer. The antinutrition and anti-hydrazine sulfate forces were in the ascendancy, but the opposition had achieved mainstream respectability.[11] It is highly ironic that later—in 1990—cancer scientists would pronounce cachexia as the "sole cause" of two thirds of all cancer deaths.[12]

American Cancer Society Takes Hydrazine Sulfate Therapy Off the Unproven Methods List

In 1982, the ACS withdrew hydrazine sulfate from its unproven methods list. In fact, ACS officials began to wonder whether placing the drug on the unproven methods list in the first place had been their proudest hour. In the *Washington Post* on May 17, 1988, reporter Sandy Rovner wrote:

> What the circumstances were that actually got hydrazine sulfate onto the American Cancer Society's list of "unproven methods" are somewhat cloudy, even the ACS concedes. . . . Says ACS medical sociologist Helen Sheehan, who serves as director of Professional Education Programs for the ACS, "I suspect that because of the atmosphere created during the laetrile period there may have been some zealotry on the part of the committee. I think laetrile created a lot of that atmosphere and they [the patients using laetrile] were using

hydrazine. In fact," she notes, "they still are, and there are still all sorts of underground ways to get hydrazine outside of clinical trials." . . .

"From what I can understand of the past," [Sheehan continues] "many things were referred to this department that had real research potential, but because they were mixed in with things like herbs and teas and so forth, everything sort of got tainted," she said.[13]

Chlebowski Reports Life Extension in Lung Cancer

Hydrazine sulfate might well have remained in limbo in the United States for many years were it not for a young researcher named Rowan T. Chlebowski at the University of California, Los Angeles. Ralph Moss tells of the wonderfully ironic way in which Chlebowski came to conduct research on hydrazine sulfate:

Chlebowski is a bright, serious, and, by his own admission, loyal member of the cancer establishment. In 1980 he wanted to perform blood chemistry tests on cancer patients. Not surprisingly, few patients wished to volunteer for tests that did not hold out some hope for therapeutic benefit. *At the same time, people were calling the hospital where he worked, pleading for hydrazine sulfate* [emphasis added]. Chlebowski and his colleagues therefore decided to undertake a double-blind clinical trial of the drug while at the same time getting a chance to study blood chemistry."[14]

This study and subsequent studies by Chlebowski showed very substantial effects of hydrazine sulfate on controlling weight loss from cancer. In a 1987 study in *Cancer*, the Chlebowski team reported that they had previously demonstrated that hydrazine sulfate was metabolically active and reduced the increased glucose production rates seen in cancer patients with weight loss. They then reported that their clinical observations on "short-term hydrazine sulfate use" in cancer patients who suffered weight loss resulted in 71% of patients on hydrazine maintaining or gaining weight while only 53% of those on placebo did so. Sixty-three percent of those on hydrazine sulfate showed improved appetite, while only 25% on the placebo did so; 77% on hydrazine sulfate showed increased caloric intake, while only 53% on the placebo did so. Moreover, 71% of the patients receiving hydrazine sulfate experienced no toxic side effects whatsoever and most of the rest experienced only mild to moderate nausea and lightheadedness. Treatment was discontinued in 10% of patients receiving hydrazine because of "toxic effects." However, 6% of patients receiving placebo had treatment stopped for "toxic effects."[15]

But the truly important news was still to come. In a potentially historic study in the January 1990 issue of the *Journal of Clinical Oncology*, Chlebowski and his colleagues at Harbor-UCLA Medical Center reported hydrazine sulfate had significantly increased survival in a randomized controlled clinical trial of 65 patients with advanced inoperable non-small-cell lung cancer.[16] The hydrazine sulfate had been added to the best available conventional chemotherapeutic treatment for this very difficult cancer. Its life extension effect had been seen in patients who were "fully ambulatory": for such patients, hydrazine sulfate extended life to a median of 328 days, compared to a median of 209 days for patients who had received chemotherapy only. The authors admitted that the moderate sample size meant that their study was not definitive, but said that it provided support for the multi-institutional study of hydrazine sulfate presently underway.

An accompanying editorial in the *Journal* warned against making too much of the results, given the small sample size and the methodology[17]—a position which drew a biting critique from Gold in a succeeding issue. He pointed out that the editorial writer had not mentioned that over half of the other articles in the same issue of the same journal had used fewer patients than the Chlebowski study and had not been singled out for criticism.[18] "In focusing specifically upon the hydrazine sulfate study, this editorial in effect singles out this drug for continuing 'skepticism', despite the plethora of data indicating the opposite," wrote Gold.

Conclusion

In evaluating the Chlebowski study with non-small-cell lung cancer, it is important to recall that the Soviet studies found benefits with hydrazine sulfate across a wide range of tumor types, not only in one of the most difficult of all cancers, non-small-cell lung cancer. So the question legitimately may be asked: If, in a controlled clinical trial, hydrazine sulfate is shown to extend life by a substantial proportion in one of the most difficult cancers, is it not reasonable for cancer patients to assume that its benefit for other cancers (as suggested by the Soviet studies) may also be confirmed? Further, might that benefit also be proportional, so that patients with cancers with longer or more variable natural histories might experience much more extended benefits?

Gold believes that, based on the studies to date, the best course is to prescribe hydrazine sulfate from the very outset of treatment—even before weight loss occurs—because the metabolic pathways for weight loss are similar to those for tumor growth.[19]

The next step in the hydrazine sulfate debate will be triggered by the publication of the outcomes of three phase III studies presently being sponsored by the NCI. The first, a study of non-small-cell lung cancer patients, is a large multi-institution controlled clinical trial that was initiated in July 1989. The second, initiated in April 1990, also studying non-small-cell lung cancer patients, is being carried out by the Mayo Clinic and the North Central Cancer Treatment Group (NCCTG). The third, also undertaken by the NCCTG and the Mayo Clinic, and begun in August 1990, is examining data from the Mayo Clinics around the country. Significantly, this last study is being conducted with patients who have a colorectal cancer, which is resistant to 5-fluorouracil (5-FU) chemotherapy, and is the only study that will assess the effectiveness of hydrazine sulfate where there has been no adjuvant chemotherapy.

Hydrazine sulfate is inexpensive and is not a substance that is likely to make scientific reputations or large fortunes for pharmaceutical companies. Because it was available and gave hope without too much toxicity, some Americans with cancer began to use it because they, personally, could not wait another 20 years for the scientific community to render a decisive opinion on it. As a result, 20 years after it was proposed—despite considerable preclinical and clinical evidence of its benefit—it remains difficult for patients to obtain hydrazine sulfate by legal means, though it is relatively easy to get on the alternative therapy black market. Now, it is *finally* undergoing the large-scale NCI-sponsored studies necessary for full scientific evaluation.

I began this chapter by comparing the outside track that Stanislaw Burzynski took with the inside track taken by Joseph Gold. Gold, who stayed inside the cancer establishment and played by the rules, has received little if any scientific credit for the decades of work that has brought hydrazine sulfate this far. But although Gold has not received the credit that is his due, by staying within the cancer establishment and playing by the rules, he has brought hydrazine sulfate significantly further than Burzynski has brought antineoplastons. And antineoplastons had the great additional benefit that they had all the early markings of a highly successful pharmaceutical product.

As this book was going to press, reports of negative findings in the multi-institutional trials of hydrazine sulfate began to appear. Gold and other advocates of the treatment responded to the negative findings with charges that there had been serious deficiencies in the methodology of the studies, an accusation that the researchers involved have denied. Analyzing the facts in this dispute will occupy the next phase in the controversy over hydrazine sulfate.[20]

References

1   Ralph W. Moss, *The Cancer Industry* (New York: Paragon House, 1989), 188.

2   Ibid., 188–9.

3   Ibid., 189.

4   Ibid., 189–90.

5   Manuel Ochoa et al., "Trial of Hydrazine Sulfate in Patients with Cancer," *Cancer Chemotherapy Reports Part 1* 59(6):1151–4.

6   Moss, *The Cancer Industry,* 192.

7   Joseph Gold, "Use of Hydrazine Sulfate in Terminal and Preterminal Cancer Patients: Results of Investigational New Drug (IND) Study in 84 Evaluable Patients," *Oncology* 32:1–10 (1975).

8   Moss, *The Cancer Industry,* 194–5.

9   Joseph Gold, "Hydrazine Sulfate: A Current Perspective," *Nutrition and Cancer* 9(2&3):59–66 (1987).

10   Ibid.

11   Moss, *The Cancer Industry,* 200–1.

12   Brett C. Sheppard et al., "Prolonged Survival of Tumor-Bearing Rats with Repetitive Low-Dose Recombinant Tumor Necrosis Factor," *Cancer Research* 50:3931 (1990). See also, G. Darling, et al., "Cachectic Effects of Recombinant Human Tumor Necrosis Factor in Rats," *Cancer Research* 50:4011 (1990).

13   Sandy Rovner, "For Cancer Drug, A Long Road to Recognition," *Washington Post,* 17 May 1988.

14   Moss, *The Cancer Industry,* 206.

15   Rowan T. Chlebowski et al., "Hydrazine Sulfate in Cancer Patients with Weight Loss," *Cancer* 59:406–10 (1987).

16   Rowan, Chlebowski et al., "Hydrazine Sulfate Influence on Nutritional Status and Survival in Non-Small-Cell Lung Cancer," *Journal of Clinical Oncology* 8:9–15 (1990).

17   S. Piantadosi, "Hazards of Small Clinical Trials," *Journal of Clinical Oncology* 8:1–3 (1990).

18   Gold, "Hydrazine Sulfate in Non-Small-Cell Lung Cancer," Letter to the editor, *Journal of Clinical Oncology* 8:1117–8 (1990).

19   Joseph Gold, personal communication with the author, 12 November 1990.

20   Jeff Kamen, "Hope, Heartbreak and Horror," *Omni* (September 1993).

twenty-three

Emanuel Revici—Will His Unique Therapy Ever Be Scientifically Assessed?

Emanuel Revici, M.D., is a brilliant, unconventional cancer researcher and therapist who has offered the scientific community a scientifically "open" system of unconventional pharmacological cancer therapy. The scientific community, however, never took up the challenge of pursuing Revici's line of inquiry, so Revici went his own way, building a largely solipsistic scientific edifice the equal of which has rarely been seen in unconventional cancer therapies.

Revici is one of the most interesting of the "great men" of unconventional pharmacological cancer therapies. Born in Romania, Revici—now in his mid-nineties and still practicing in New York—has over decades developed a unique approach to illness that he has described in a major medical text he published in 1961 called *Research in Physiopathology as a Basis for Guided Chemotherapy with Special Application to Cancer.*[1]

Revici is a product of a particularly vibrant period of central European medical and scientific education. He received his medical degree from the University of Bucharest in 1920, became an assistant professor of internal medicine, practiced in Paris from 1936 to 1941, fled the Nazis to Mexico City where he directed a research institute from 1942 to 1946, and came to New York in 1947. In 1955, he purchased a small hospital in New York, Trafalgar Hospital, where he took the position of Chief of Oncology and consultant until it closed in 1978. The hospital prospered modestly for some time with an interesting research program and considerable patient demand until opposition from organized medicine and collaborating insurance companies forced its closure. An interesting and little known fact is that Revici gave Lawrence LeShan, the pioneering investigator of psychotherapy for recovery from cancer, the opportunity to conduct his ground-breaking psychological research with Trafalgar Hospital cancer patients after the leading hospitals in New York had uniformly rejected LeShan's requests for access to patients. LeShan is among many who believe that Revici definitely "had something" of value for some cancer patients in his unconventional cancer therapies.[2]

Revici's Biochemical Theory

Revici's theory is so complex that very few of his medical and chemical peers can understand it fully, which may partially explain why the scientific community did not pursue the testing of Revici's work, but most of those who do study him, like Professor Gerhard Schrauzer of the University of California, San Diego, consider him "an innovative medical genius, outstanding chemist and a highly creative thinker."[3]

Because Revici's theory is so broad, it applies not just to cancer but across the board to many other conditions for which he has devised treatments. He has therapies for itching, insomnia, vertigo, migraine, and hearing impairment.[4] He proposed a major therapy for radiation burns (very relevant to the needs of cancer patients) which Dwight L. McKee, M.D. describes as "today the only means that is efficient in healing radiation burns."[4] He developed therapies for osteoarthritis, rheumatoid arthritis, convulsions, variations in the pathogenesis of infectious diseases, the seventh-day postoperative bleeding in prostatectomies and nasal plastic surgery, and the seventh-day worsening of heart infections. He also found treatments that he claims are effective with AIDS, heart irregularities, Crohn's disease, colitis, unconsolidated fractures, prostate hypertrophy, and, very notably, drug addiction.[5]

The study of lipids was one of Revici's most creative contributions, and later research along these lines—which closely parallels Revici's research—resulted in a Nobel Prize for Bengt Samuelsson in 1982. Let us now consider Revici's theory and practice of cancer treatment. . .

Revici's description of how his cancer therapy works is highly complex. He describes his therapy as "biologically guided chemotherapy." He says that he uses lipids (forms of fats) or lipid substances with special properties as the biological guiding factors. The Office of Technology Assessment (OTA) report, *Unconventional Cancer Treatments,* summarized Revici's theory:

> He believes that tumor cells . . . share a common biochemical characteristic—an imbalance in the normal distribution of lipids—which he views not as the primary causer of cancer, but as the direct cause of its impact on the body's metabolism. He categorizes two general patterns of local and systemic effects of lipid imbalances, . . . one pattern resulting from an excess of fatty acids and the other pattern resulting from an excess of sterols [both constituents of lipids, or fats].

> A relative predominance of fatty acids leads to an electrolyte imbalance . . . and an alkaline environment in tumor tissues; Revici refers to this as a "catabolic" condition. In the opposite case, a predominance of sterols reportedly leads to a reduction in cell membrane permeability. . . . Revici refers to this outcome as an "anabolic" condition. Patients determined by Revici to have a predominance of fatty acids are treated with sterols and other agents with positive electrical charges that can counteract the negatively charged fatty acids. Those determined to have a predominance of sterols are treated with fatty acids and other agents that increase the metabolic activity of fatty acids.[6]

One of the best summaries of Revici's work is in a 1985 monograph by Dwight L. McKee, M.D., a young physician who worked with Revici for a number of years. McKee describes the law of organization Revici believes applies to all matter, wherein a primary electropositive part was bound to a secondary electronegative element at every level of biochemical organization. These entities form a hierarchic progressive series in an organism.[7]

Revici posits that there are two forces in biochemistry: *electrostatic* and *quantum* forces. Electrostatic forces move toward entropy (movement toward inertness and breaking down of order), while quantum forces balance the entropic tendency by moving toward organization. The *catabolic* tendencies of the organism are electrostatic or entropic, whereas the *anabolic* processes are quantum or negentropic (bringing an increase in order). Normal biological processes represent a balance of these forces while abnormal biology represents an excess of anabolic or catabolic processes.[7]

Revici was able to categorize the pathogenesis of diseases as either anabolic or catabolic. Revici's theory led to the recognition that two respective diseases may respond oppositely to the same agent depending on their anabolic or catabolic character. According to McKee:

> Revici devised a system which can be used to recognize the anabolic or catabolic character of a disease and can serve as a guide for pathogenically based therapy. Blood leukocytes, eosinophiles [a cell or structure readily stained by eosin], serum potassium, C reactive proteins, and especially different urine analyses such as surface tension, pH, specific gravity, calcium and chloride excretion are used in this way. . . . Separating the *agents* according to the anabolic or catabolic character, he introduced a new capitol concept in pharmacology."[8]

In further research, Revici demonstrated that anabolic and catabolic substances differed in their properties under ultraviolet light; anabolic agents emitted energy, whereas catabolic ones absorbed energy.[9] This correspondence between anabolic, light-emitting, negentropic agents and catabolic, light-quenching, entropic agents has deep resonances with the Oriental medical division between yin and yang, the female and male forces of the universe. As McKee notes:

> As a generality, Revici pointed to the *anabolic character of females* in any species, which he found to be rich in sterols, and the *catabolic character of males,* which he found to be rich in fatty acids. He showed that this proclivity applies in almost all biological processes, even in the *characters of tumors,* with a tendency for predominance of *sterols in females* and *fatty acids in males* [McKee's emphasis].[10]

Based on this theory of cancer causation, Revici employed anabolic or catabolic agents as antagonists in the treatment of neoplastic diseases. According to McKee, Revici got good results with a number of such preparations: "He found a specific antineoplastic action of *lipidic bivalent negative selenium* preparations . . . Revici obtained especially good results with selenium incorporated in tung oil, as well as incorporated in other unsaturated fatty acids as such or in their triglycerides" [McKee's emphasis].[11]

In further research, Revici was able to incorporate a wide range of elements in these "lipid envelopes" which, according to his theory, delivered the chemical agent directly to the tumor site because of the affinity of these lesion sites for concentrations of "free lipids." Says McKee,

> The result is an entire series of agents exceptionally low in toxicity. Due to their lipidic character, these agents act specifically upon the lipidic constituents of abnormal foci [such as cancer]. . . . Through this method, Revici has opened up an entirely new field for the therapeutic use of these elements, and especially those that are active but otherwise too toxic.[12]

After many tests for the specificity of a patient's cancer, Revici designs an individualized chemotherapy for each person. This is usually given orally, and by and large, is apt to have few side effects.

Revici agreed with nutritional cancer therapist Max Gerson on the avoidance of salt and the reinforcement of potassium supplies in the treatment of cancer, but disagreed with Virginia Livingston's claim that "cell wall deficient bacteria" in the form of *Progenitor cryptocides* is the cause of cancer, siding with Livingston's establishment critics in maintaining that the bacteria were "erroneously considered to be etiological factors in the disease when in fact they are only associated microbes fundamentally changed by the action of the lipids . . . present in the lesions."[13]

Assessments of Revici

There are relatively few independent scientists who have the ability to assess Revici's system and who also have gone on record with any significant statement about it. One of these scientists is Gerhard N. Schrauzer, Ph.D., Professor in the Department of Chemistry at the University of California, San Diego and one of the world's leading authorities on selenium. Selenium is one of the agents with which Revici claims success in treating cancer. Schrauzer, who dislikes the controversy associated with discussing unconventional cancer therapies, nonetheless felt obligated to write to the New York Board of Regents in 1986 when the board was considering revoking Revici's medical license.

> I am writing this letter today in my capacity as a cancer researcher who is well acquainted with Dr. Revici's research and accomplishments, hoping that you will decide not to revoke his medical license.

Dr. Revici has been engaged in research for more than half a century and has been practicing in New York for close to 40 years. He has seen and treated thousands of cancer patients, often for many years. If his methods of treatment differ from the currently accepted ones, this is due to a not insignificant extent to his vast experience in dealing with the desperately ill, with patients abandoned by conventional medicine in need of special care.

In his efforts to devise a more effective therapy, Revici conducted innumerable experiments in his Institute and published the results in a book in 1961. *After critically examining this book, I came to the conclusion that Dr. Revici is an innovative medical genius, outstanding chemist and a highly creative thinker* [emphasis added]. I also realized that few of his medical colleagues would be able to follow his train of thought and thus would be all too willing to dismiss his work. Because of my own professional interest in selenium, let me merely focus on this aspect of his work. Selenium containing medications were introduced into cancer therapy as early as 1911 by none less than the great physician August von Wasserman. Working with experimental animals, von Wasserman was able to show his selenium compounds produced liquefactive necrosis of solid tumors, an unheard of event at the time, hailed as a major success.

However, von Wasserman's compounds were too toxic and thus could not be employed in the treatment of human cancer. Dr. Revici deserves credit for having discovered pharmacologically active selenium compounds of very low toxicity. The same was achieved years later by one other great physician, Dr. Klaus Schwarz, in collaboration with a leading organic chemist, Dr. Arne Fredga, of Uppsala University. The National Cancer Institute has recognized the importance of selenium only within the past few years. Would one thus not have to conclude that Dr. Revici, in this one instance, was 40 years ahead of his time? The same could be said for many of his other researches which form the basis of his therapy.

For this activity, Dr. Revici is now to lose his license to practice medicine. If he does, the message to all physicians will be to avoid innovation at all cost and to treat strictly according to the currently accepted rules. . . . Thus, I beg you to reconsider your decision, also in the interest of his many patients whose lives depend on him.[14]

Robert G. Houston of New York, perhaps the foremost advocate-scholar of unconventional cancer therapies in the United States, writes in a 1987 review of Revici's work:

He [Revici] has been hailed by Schrauzer, . . . the world authority on selenium, as the foremost pioneer in its clinical application. Dr. Revici began its use in human cancer in 1948, and published a number of case histories of remission, along with x-ray evidence, in his medical textbook. . . .

Revici has [also] developed therapies for a wide range of medical challenges, including the treatment of pain, . . . drug addiction, radiation injury, . . . and AIDS. . . . His many significant contributions to medical science include publications in peer-reviewed medical journals regarding his discovery of the anti-hemorrhagic action of *N*-butanol in advanced cancer, . . . and of the diagnostic significance of changes in the surface tension of urine. . . . In 1950, Revici's paper on his investigations concerning the influence of irradiation on unsaturated fatty acids was delivered to the International Congress of Radiology in London; in this and in his medical monograph . . . he correctly described the inflammatory effects of leukotrienes (trienic conjugated fatty acids) and their derivation from arachidonic acid, research that was paralleled decades later by Bengt Samuelsson, . . . who won a Nobel Prize for the discovery. . . .

An independent clinical trial of Revici's therapy was conducted in Belgium by Prof. Joseph Maisin, the Director of the Cancer Institute of the University of Louvain. A foremost cancer authority, Prof. Maisin was the President of the International Union Against Cancer [a highly prestigious cancer research organization]. He reported that in 75% of 12 terminal cancer patients on whom the Revici medications were tried dramatic improvements occurred, including regression of tumors, disappearance of metastases, and cessation of hemorrhage. Amazingly, paralyzed patients were able to walk again (Maisin, 1965). . . .

Dr. Revici's findings of the anticancer value of cod liver oil fatty acids . . . received corroboration at the 1987 ACS [American Cancer Society] Science Writers Seminar, where Dr. Otto Plescia, Professor of Immunochemistry at Rutgers University, concluded that a diet with "inclusion of omega-3 fatty acids abundant in certain fish oils, reduces the risk of breast cancer."[15]

Houston's positive assessment of Revici was seconded by another American scientist with expertise in cancer and chemistry who was only willing to discuss Revici after expressing a strong preference for anonymity. The scientist is a European-born researcher who is internationally respected as one of the foremost authorities in his field.

The people who criticize Revici as he is today do not do him justice. He continues to practice medicine at the age of 95—and this is not a problem restricted to alternative therapy practitioners—how can he possibly be what he was in the 1960s at the height of his power? Revici has to be assessed in the context of the European traditions of medicine and cancer therapy from 1870 to 1960. In Europe, physicians have much more freedom to innovate. . . . Revici isn't an alternative therapy guy really. He is the inventor of a non-toxic chemotherapy. His crime was that he used chemicals that you can buy for $2 a pound, like epochlorohydrate, which are similar in many respects to more expensive alkylating agents.

His theory of anabolic and catabolic cancers, for example, is a very nice theory and not that peculiar. German research has shown that some cancers are in fact anabolic. What Revici is saying is that there are two kinds of cancer patients. One is a healthy guy in his fifties that weighs 200 pounds and looks almost too healthy. Revici says his cancer is often anabolic. The other is a pale wispy guy in his seventies and Revici says his cancer is often catabolic. Revici basically suggests that these two guys need different treatment. I find that compelling.

The tragedy is that Revici may take some of the best of his work with him when he dies because the therapy may not work as well in the hands of others as it does in his hands. The reason is that he is as good a physician as he is a chemist and so he is able to play with these medical-chemical relationships in a way that few others could without similar training and sensitivity.

But the reason I don't want to talk publicly about these things is that if I do, in the American climate, I end up with ketchup all over my tie. . . . I am tired of the closed-minded American perspective, which makes it almost impossible for an inventive physician like Revici to function as similar people do in Europe. Here physicians are supposed to just follow orders.

Of course the ultimate policy problem with Revici is that he is a man who prepares his own medications, and there are good reasons for the restrictions on that: suppose every physician was allowed to prepare his own medications. But in my judgment Revici is a kind of modern Paracelsus, and do you know how Paracelsus was finally evicted from Nuremberg? It was by the pharmacists guild, and the charge was that he was preparing his own medications.[16]

So Schrauzer, an internationally respected researcher, and my anonymous correspondent above, both of European background, both with impeccable scientific credentials, put Revici's work in a positive light, reinforcing the impression that Houston's favorable summary of Revici's accomplishments is worthy of further review.

Dwight McKee, M.D., the author of the monograph on Revici's work, which I quoted from above, worked with Revici for 6 years, between 1979 and 1985. McKee, a close student of unconventional cancer therapies, is also well-grounded in mainstream medicine. In a telephone interview in September 1990, I asked McKee to summarize his impressions of Revici's work.

McKee said that he believes that many of the pharmacological agents Revici works with are active in the treatment of cancer and are "orders of magnitude less toxic." He believes that Revici's dualistic model of the effects of pharmacological agents has validity and significance for understanding the responses of different patients to different chemotherapeutic agents, although Revici tries to extend the model too far. He believes that Revici is also correct in emphasizing the role of lipids in cancer biology and in his assessment of the importance of the lipidic aspects of medications and their interactions with malignant tumors.

During the years he worked with Revici, McKee thinks that he saw the best results in brain cancers—where he reports Revici achieved some complete remissions, some lasting 20 years. He reports that Revici also achieved impressive control in some pancreatic cancers, extending survival for up to 5 years. He also saw effective control, though not cure, of lung cancers, especially when the therapy was combined with radiation in small cell lung cancers. He saw clear responses of lymphomas to Revici's treatments. He did not see a large number of notable successes with breast cancer. "His lifework is a rich vein of gold waiting to be mined," McKee said.

Critiques of Revici

The major critique of Revici that one hears from some patients and from his colleagues in unconventional cancer therapies is that his service delivery system is not well organized. Using our distinctions among the practitioner, the therapy, and the treatment delivery system, one could argue that the practitioner is almost unquestionably a man of scientific genius; his therapy is scientifically intriguing and respected by many—including some leading scientists—but has not been systematically evaluated by independent researchers; and the service delivery of his therapy leaves a great deal to be desired.

Revici's patients describe waiting for hours to receive their medication in cramped offices under chaotic conditions. Some patients have reported poor results when they entrusted their medical care, as well as their pharmacological treatment, to Revici. Supporters of Revici, on the other hand, would point to the fact that he developed and operated a fully equipped hospital until organized medicine—in alliance with insurance firms—forced him to close the hospital down. Deprived of his hospital, Revici's only choices were to give up medical practice or to continue to practice as best as his means and age allowed him to. The fact that hundreds of patients continue to seek him out create the conditions of which patients complain.

A second critique comes from a well-known research-oriented scientist, a practitioner of an alternative pharmacological therapy *and* a physician who has studied his work closely. The criticism is that Revici keeps changing his formulations of therapeutic agents so that no single set of formulations has been reasonably evaluated. Said the scientist: "At some point you have to define a specific formulation and go through with a clinical trial." The physician, who knows Revici well, believes that these changes in medications are so frequent that sometimes he is "chasing placebo effects." This physician fully believes in the efficacy of some of Revici's therapies.

The third critique does not reflect on Revici exclusively, but on Revici and the American scientific system. Revici is, above all, a grand system builder, a man of staggering intellect who Robert Houston describes as the "Nicola Tesla of medicine" because of the sweep and breadth of his work.[17] Had Revici stuck with some of his most promising areas of research, and published repeatedly in the mainstream journals that were initially open to him, weaving a fabric of research of undeniable significance that attracted corroboration from other researchers, it seems highly likely that he would be recognized as a significant figure in medicine today.

Instead, Revici is a man driven by an inner passion to explore the farthest frontiers of medicine without the time or the patience to play the game of science. His masterwork, published in 1961, was evidence enough of the quality and breadth and depth of his intellect. But—perhaps in large part because of the political climate of opposition to his work from organized medicine—his work drew little effort at confirmation.

Gold's work on hydrazine sulfate now belongs to mainstream science. Burzynski's work on antineoplastons sits on the edge of mainstream science and is tilting into it. But Revici's monumental contribution remains almost entirely outside of the orbit of mainstream science. We may be the poorer for it.

References

1   Emanuel Revici, *Research in Physiopathology as a Basis of Guided Chemotherapy with Special Application to Cancer* (New York: American Foundation for Cancer Research, 1961).

2   Lawrence LeShan, personal communication with author, January 1988.

3   Gerhard N. Schrauzer, letter to the New York Board of Regents, 14 February 1986.

4   Dwight L. McKee, "Emanuel Revici: A Review of His Scientific Work," Institute of Applied Biology monograph, New York, NY, 1985, 4.

5   Ibid., 8–18 passim.

6   Congress of the United States Office of Technology Assessment, *Unconventional Cancer Treatments* (Washington, D.C.: U.S. Government Printing Office, September 1990), 115–6.

7   McKee, "Emanual Revici," 2.

8   Ibid.

9   Ibid.

10 Ibid., 10.

11 Ibid., 14.

12 Ibid.

13 Ibid., 9–15 passim.

14 Gerhard N. Schrauzer, letter to the New York Board of Regents, 14 February 1986.

15 Robert G. Houston, *Repression and Reform in the Evaluation of Alternative Cancer Therapies* (Washington, D.C.: Project Cure, 1989), 30–3. Vitamin A precursors such as those Revici used are now the subject of major research interest at the National Cancer Institute.

16 Anonymous, personal correspondence with author (1991).

17 Houston, *Repression and Reform*, 31.

PART SIX

Living with Cancer

twenty-four

Living with Cancer

From the earliest human times, wise men and women have concluded that living life skillfully is a high art, perhaps the highest art there is. Like all arts, the art of living is a creative act requiring the development of disciplined skills. And one of the greatest challenges of the art of living is to discover ways to face pain and misfortune. Learning to live with cancer skillfully, therefore, can become a challenge, often bringing with it a valuable new perspective on life.

A young woman named Avis, who attended a Commonweal Cancer Help Program retreat, had been living with recurrent thyroid cancer for many years. When she was first diagnosed with thyroid cancer as a 19-year-old college student, she had been told there was nothing to worry about—treatment was curative. But she suffered a series of increasingly severe recurrences, and her cancer was now at a life-threatening stage. She had undergone a series of increasingly painful medical procedures requiring medications that literally dissolved her sense of who she was for long periods of time.

Avis was a first-class athlete with a wide variety of athletic skills. One of the things that the cancer had taken from her was the capacity to participate in competitive athletics. At the same time, the prospect of more pain and more medical procedures was more than she thought she could bear. During the course of the weeklong program, she came to realize that there was a deep relationship between the courage and stamina that had made her a first-class athlete and the courage and stamina she needed in the struggle that faced her now. She realized that, just as her life as an athlete had been a supremely creative personal act, so her life with cancer called upon her deepest resources.

At some point in an encounter with cancer, many people recognize that what they face involves much more than dealing with choice of treatments and undergoing treatments. For most people who have had a serious cancer diagnosis, even if the treatment has been successful and the likelihood of recurrence is low, life will never be the same again. The art of life under these circumstances involves finding a way to live with the pain and losses that cannot be avoided, finding a way to cope with or even transform the fears and stresses that inevitably come, and finding out whether in the midst of the pain, loss, fear, and stress, anything of value—anything that enriches life—may also come out of all this hardship. The teaching of the perennial philosophy is that out of pain and hardship some of the greatest gains in life can come.

Problems of Living with Cancer

In what follows, I will try to chart a territory that is actually without boundaries or fixed landmarks—the territory of the problems that people encounter in living with cancer. Since every life is unique, a list of common problems is hard to design and harder still to discuss.

Nevertheless, I will try. Below is a list of the most common issues that people have described to me over the past 10 years. I have divided the list into two categories—problems directly associated with cancer and problems in living that may or may not be associated in the patient's mind with cancer or with its prognosis. This division is similar to, but somewhat different from, the distinction of the biological process of cancer as a *disease* and the human experience of cancer as an *illness,* which we discussed in chapter 2. The difference is that here both categories include problems related both to disease and illness, but the second category enlarges the frame of reference so that it involves the human experience of illness in interaction with the experience of other aspects of living.

Problems of living that relate to the cancer itself and treatment for it include:

1. How does one respond to the cancer diagnosis?
2. How does one face the difficulties of choosing between treatments?
3. How does one cope with the trauma of facing and undergoing treatment?
4. What is your relationship to your doctor and how do you deal with problems in communicating with him?
5. How does one live with the possibility of recurrence, or face a diagnosis of recurrence?
6. How does one live with the progression of cancer, either as shown on diagnostic tests or as physically experienced?

Problems of living that *may or may not* be linked by you to your cancer include:

1. *Current relationships:* with children, with spouse or partner, with parents, with friends, with co-workers; problems with sexuality and intimacy.
2. *Past relationships:* childhood unhappiness, trauma or abuse; past problems with parents, spouse, or partner; grieving the death of someone close; and grieving separation or divorce.
3. *Work:* attitudes of co-workers, attitudes of management, your satisfaction with work, keeping your job to keep insurance, job stress perceived as part of what contributed to cancer, and loss of cherished work.
4. *Finances:* loss of job, loss of income, loss of insurance, and dealing with insurance.
5. *Daily patterns:* restrictions in the ability to care for yourself or family; restrictions in exercise or other health habits; restrictions in daily pleasures—food, drink, smoking; and restrictions in mobility and energy.
6. *Environment and housing:* disruptive change of residence, separation from friends, living in a stressful or disliked home, and feeling one should live in a different home.
7. *Community:* sense of isolation from friends and interactive community, loss of community due to relocation, living in a disliked or stressful community, and feeling one should live in a different community.

8. *Creative life:* restriction or loss of capacities in areas in which you feel most creative or truly yourself.
9. *Psychological:* morale, self-esteem, capacity to think clearly, control of emotions, changes in values and perceptions, and living with a life-threatening illness.

Cancer Is Not Always the Greatest Problem

It took me some time after I started counseling people with cancer to realize that *cancer is not always experienced as the greatest problem facing a person with cancer.* Someone may be carrying a greater pain than the cancer, such as the death of a spouse, a divorce, a childhood trauma, the loss of a job, or some other issue that takes more time and energy to deal with than what might appear from the outside to be the central life issue—cancer.

I spoke earlier about the physician who came to Commonweal with a life-threatening recurrent bladder cancer that was not at all his major concern. What preoccupied him was grieving for a wife he had lost to a degenerative nervous disease. In order to nurse her he had deliberately chosen to forgo curative surgery, which would have kept him away from her during her last months, and chose a course of treatment that made it probable he would die of his cancer. When he came to Commonweal he had no fear of death and was, for the first time in his life, considering the possibility that he might be able to rejoin his wife after death. The loss of a mate or the loss of a child can leave a person with a permanently altered perspective on his own death. For some people, like this physician, death can in fact be experienced internally as the opening of a gate to a release from this life—and possibly the gate to another world—which they are ready to walk through.

The fact that *other problems in living may be more important than having cancer* is of great importance to patients and those who care about them in considering ways of healing. The first implication for any health professional, family member, or friend who wants to help a person with cancer—or indeed for the cancer patient himself—is that the most effective help one can provide may be addressing a problem that has little, if anything, to do with cancer.

Even in the more common situation where other problems are *less* important than cancer, help with the other problems of living may be more feasible.

Focusing attention on the soluble problems of living can reduce the stress on the cancer patient, giving him more energy to cope with his cancer. Since stress may, as we have seen, actually be a factor in the development and progress of some cancers, addressing problems contributing to stress may have an effect on the course of the disease.

Cancer as a Turning Point

In addition to the benefits of helping heal specific problems, there is an even greater benefit in identifying "metastrategies" that help a cancer patient shift his relationship to whole classes of problems of living. These metastrategies often involve the recognition by the patient that cancer can represent what Larry LeShan calls a "turning point." The cancer patient can discover his own ways to use the shock of the turning point as a signal that he now has permission to undertake a very fundamental reevaluation of what is important to him in life and what has become less important.

For many patients, this reevaluation happens spontaneously; they will say that many problems that used to preoccupy them no longer seem important; that many relationships that were difficult for them have healed; and that reassessment of their life priorities has in many respects improved their lives, giving them more strength to deal with the realities of the disease and treatment.

Most frequently, a change in life priorities following a cancer diagnosis is accompanied by what patients describe as a shift in consciousness. The cancer patient characteristically describes the change as one that brings a broader, higher, or more inclusive consciousness. We discussed this shift in chapter 9 on spiritual approaches to cancer. Whether or not one identifies this shift as spiritual is unimportant; the important thing is to recognize that the shift in consciousness is the essence of what makes the old problems in living accessible to resolution.

This shift in consciousness is different from a simple reevaluation of what matters in life. Often, the shift takes place shortly after the cancer diagnosis—or after diagnosis of a recurrence—and literally makes the world look different. As many people have described the experience, it is as though scales had fallen from their eyes and they were seeing the world absolutely fresh for the first time. They experience nature as radiant, family and friends as precious, life itself as sacred. This state of nonordinary consciousness encourages the reevaluation of one's life priorities. Then, when treatment achieves a possible cure or lasting remission, often the experience of nonordinary consciousness fades and the person moves back toward an ordinary experience of life. While the new orientation toward life priorities may survive the end of the crisis period, many patients mourn the loss of that nonordinary consciousness that came during their time of crisis when life seemed sacred.

In cases where the cancer recurs and the patient is told that there is no known cure, then the heightened sense of consciousness frequently returns. It may stay as long as life seems to hang in the balance, but if another lasting remission is achieved, the heightened sense of consciousness often subsides again.

Although some people are able to sustain the heightened state of consciousness, it usually goes up and down in waves on a continuing basis for the rest of their lives. To keep it steady usually requires developing a deep practice of meditation or participation in some psychophysiological discipline that continually renews the sense of life as sacred.

The fundamental point here is that, in this state of nonordinary consciousness, not only do priorities shift but the experience of problems in living can be transformed. The transformation does not always mean that problems weigh less heavily. When a loss or series of losses related to the illness is depressing in ordinary consciousness, it may even be experienced as *tragic* in nonordinary consciousness. The tragedy may be deeply experienced and expressed in tears and prolonged grieving. But it is more likely to be worked through precisely because it is experienced more profoundly.

As I have indicated, such changes often happen spontaneously. But for others who feel "stuck" in misery, anxiety, and depression with cancer, the skill of a friend, family member, or therapist may help them in finding ways to explore what a shift in consciousness might bring. This is a delicate issue, and often best left to a skilled psychotherapist experienced in work with people with cancer, through imagery, meditation, hypnosis, or other approaches to altered states. The important fact for the cancer patient is to recognize that deep and life-changing insights may lie just below the surface of anxiety, fear, and depression. If one is able to identify a process for accessing these insights, the experience of the illness and the capacity to resolve many major life problems can shift fundamentally.

Even when the shift in consciousness has taken place spontaneously, it is important to recognize that it can often be deepened by the use of some of these same approaches—such as meditation, imagery, or hypnosis—that can initiate access to nonordinary consciousness when people are stuck in fear, anxiety, or depression.

Problems in Relationships and Community

Probably the most common problems that cancer patients describe are those in relationships and community, past or present, with parents, children, spouses or partners, other family members, co-workers, and friends. The recurrent themes are not unique to people with cancer—rather, they are the themes of relational problems in modern life. But they have a special quality for the cancer patient because he often wonders whether there is some connection between the relational problem and the development of the cancer.

Childhood

Let us start with the issue of having experienced abuse, physical or psychological, as a child. It is well documented that a large proportion of American women have experienced some significant sexual abuse as children. This experience often has profound and lasting effects on psychological development and relationships for the rest of their lives. While the issue of whether tumors occasionally develop in some organ systems as a result of psychological or physical trauma to those systems remains highly controversial scientifically, I have seen too many women who have developed reproductive system cancers following childhood abuse to have any personal doubts that the correlation is sometimes real. I have met a considerable number of women who developed cancer in their reproductive systems who also *personally attributed* part of the development of these cancers to their experience of having been sexually abused as a child. That history of traumatic sexual abuse, in turn, made the experience of invasive and painful treatments for cervical or ovarian cancer even more traumatic.

Janis came on a Cancer Help Program retreat with ovarian cancer. She had experienced repeated sexual abuse during childhood with her father. She had not been able to tell anyone about the experience. She had made several efforts to tell her mother who denied that it was possible and threatened to punish her if she repeated the story. There are no scientific studies that can tell us whether the abuse was related to her cancer, but the important point for healing work was that she *attributed* her ovarian cancer in part to the experience with her father. During the course of the week, as she entered states of nonordinary consciousness through the repeated daily sessions of meditation and yoga, she experienced more deeply than she had before the memories of the abuse and her sense of how the ovarian cancer was a kind of repetition of the abuse. As she explored this great tragedy in her life, the experience of living with cancer began to shift. Precisely because she was able to put together memories and feelings and words, and to link these experiences deeply, an emotional healing took place in the face of the tragedy.

Sometimes the abuse is not sexual but psychological. The child received from one or both parents what Rachel Naomi Remen calls "don't live" messages. The child was told by the parent that the pregnancy was a mistake, that she was an unwanted child, that the parents had hoped for a boy, or that she was somehow wrong or disappointing in who she was in the world. Often, the child learned to suppress who or how she naturally was in order to please the parent, and developed a whole life pattern based on pleasing others and paying no attention to her own development or needs. Often a cancer diagnosis is the turning point that gives permission for the first time to explore being herself and what that would mean.

Sarah came on a Cancer Help Program with a recurrent cancer of the tongue. In the course of the week she remembered that when she was a boisterous and exuberant child, her mother used to pay her to be quiet for a while. She was told to hold her tongue. Again, no scientific studies can tell us whether this experience is related to the development of the tongue cancer. But Sarah experienced a connection. In the course of the workshop, she concluded that the recovery of her voice—in the sense of learning to say what she was feeling in present relationships instead of staying silent as she had been taught as a child—was an essential part of her healing.

Intimate Relationships

There are an infinite variety of ways in which marriage or intimate partnerships can interact both physically and symbolically with a cancer diagnosis. The stress of a bad marriage can be suspected of playing a part in the development of cancer, and the patient often faces a difficult decision over whether or not to stay in the marriage. A stressful divorce or separation, too, is frequently suspected by patients of playing a role in the development of their cancer.

Then come the issues of what the cancer diagnosis does to the marriage or relationship. In some cases it weakens or destroys it: the spouse cannot accept the cancer, the spouse (or patient) cannot rebuild intimacy and sexuality, or the marriage ends. In other cases, it strengthens the relationship, and problems that plagued both partners become resolved.

The end of a relationship following a cancer diagnosis is not necessarily negative. Sometimes a cancer patient recognizes that the cancer diagnosis has prompted a process of rapid internal growth and change within herself and that a relationship which had previously been tolerable—though rarely fulfilling—simply no longer provides an environment for the intensive healing work she has to do.

> Cynthia was an artist from Florida who had raised three children to adulthood and emotionally supported her businessman husband throughout his career. After she developed metastatic breast cancer and had a mastectomy, their intimate life ended and her husband was uninterested in therapy or in any sustained effort to re-create a sexual life together. With great courage and determination, Cynthia undertook a process of exploration of complementary as well as mainstream therapies, changed her diet, entered psychotherapy, came on a series of Cancer Help Program retreats, and fundamentally reinvented her life. She then discovered that her husband had been having an affair for a number of years. They divorced, a development that Cynthia found deeply painful but also liberating. Cynthia has now lived with her cancer for many years, leading a rich and fulfilling life.

Children

Problems involving children and cancer are often deeply poignant. Frequently, a young mother with a history of breast cancer in the family, herself now diagnosed with breast cancer, faces both the possibility that she may not live to raise her daughter *and* that her daughter may be at high risk for the same extraordinary suffering that she is undergoing. The mother often feels the pain of the child watching her go through this experience, and the pain of recognizing that the daughter is at risk of this same incredible assault on her self and her femininity that the mother is facing. If the prognosis is serious, the parent is often as concerned with the effect that her death will have on her children as she is with facing death herself.

> Jennifer was a computer programmer with metastatic breast cancer who came on a Cancer Help Program retreat. She had two children, a daughter age 5 and a son age 7 years. She was deeply involved in raising them. She had a good marriage, but her husband had lost a job shortly after the birth of their second child and she had had to return to work to support the family while he went through school to retrain himself for another position. He stayed home often, studying and caring for the children, and she felt bereft at having to work during these precious years. After 3 years at work supporting the family and agonizing over the time she was missing with her children, she developed breast cancer. Her husband had just finished school and was hired for a new job. He took over supporting the family and she returned to be with her children. A year later the cancer had metastasized. She came on the Cancer Help Program deeply grieving the possibility that she might not live to be with her children for the rest of their childhood, and that she had missed precious years already. She also faced the latest version of the exquisite dilemmas with which modern cancer treatments confront patients: she was being told that a bone marrow transplant was her "only hope." The procedure would not be reimbursed by her insurance, would cost $125,000, which she and her husband simply did not have, would be many times more difficult than the chemotherapy and radiation she had gone through already, and had not yet provided any significant evidence that it represented a cure for metastatic breast cancer. Nonetheless, she saw it as representing the best that scientific medicine had to offer in her situation.

Friends

Friends frequently pose a different set of problems. The most common dilemma is the difficulty the patient has with how friends react when they learn she has cancer. Many cancer patients describe how some friends simply cannot deal with the cancer and distance themselves; how others want to help, but act or speak in ways that are not helpful; and still other friends come forward and are of true assistance and support. The ability to educate friends concerning how they can actually be of most help is an important survival skill for people with cancer. There are many approaches to defining what helps and what does not help and communicating those facts to friends.

Sally was an older physician active in social circles in her southern community. She remembers being invited to a dinner party and discovering that all the other guests were offered drinks in elegant glassware while she was served her drink in a plastic cup—apparently on instructions from her hostess who had a phobic fear of contamination by "cancer germs."

Nancy was an interior decorator whose clients came from her wide circle of socially active friends. Her career, begun in middle life, was a very rewarding part of her life and she looked to it for support in the face of her cancer. Then she found that a number of friends who had discussed work with her had turned to other interior decorators out of concerns about whether or not she would be able to complete their projects or in distress at having to meet face to face with a friend with a serious cancer.

Another common problem in our highly mobile society—a problem that again particularly affects women—is when a woman has moved (often with her husband for career reasons) and develops cancer after several years in a community that she does not like as much as her old community and where she does not have a strong support network. Here the problem is not friends doing or saying the wrong things but the lack of friends close by who can really provide support.

The other side of these common problems is the frequency with which people with cancer report *positive* changes in many relationships. Their marriages may be better, their families closer, and they often experience extraordinary support from friends.

George was a carpenter, creative and athletic by nature, who noticed while running an increasing fatigue and shortness of breath. He was diagnosed with lung cancer and found that mainstream medicine had nothing to offer him. He undertook a very vigorous program of diet and complementary therapies, and found his already spiritually inclined life further transformed. But he also described himself as discovering that he was living in a circle of love created by a community of deeply supportive friends. He lived a deeply fulfilling life for several years and died in what he and his family considered a state of grace.

An experience like cancer tends to mobilize both the supportive and the negative potential in the social networks that surround each of us. The skill is in recognizing how critical relationship questions, positive or negative, can be in the face of cancer. Often help can be brought to bear by friends in ways that can transform the quality of life. Some clinicians and researchers would hypothesize, for reasons we have discussed, that the healing power of community may affect the course of the illness as well. Recall the studies reported in chapter 10, that people who have supportive networks have less mortality from all causes than those who do not, and specifically that women with metastatic breast cancer and strong social support tend to live longer than women with less support.

Problems in Work and Creative Life

Freud said that the essence of life was "love and work." Family and friends represent love, but what of work? For many Americans, work is profoundly central to our identities—our sense of ourselves. While true for both men and women, this is particularly true for men, who often have few meaningful relationships outside of work.

So work has many complex relationships to cancer. Often a cancer diagnosis follows a devastating disappointment in work life, and many people who have experienced this attribute the cancer in part to the stress of that disappointment. Cancer diagnoses also often follow retirement from a job that was central to a person's identity and life purpose.

When cancer is diagnosed, a new set of work-related problems may enter the picture. Some people are unfairly dismissed from jobs because of cancer and cannot find new positions or medical insurance because of the disease. Some are kept in their jobs but denied promotions or new opportunities in the organization. Still others find the primary problem is the reaction of co-workers to their illness—a reaction that they cannot escape in the work context. Some, who were never satisfied with their jobs, who believe the stress or disappointment of the job contributed to the development of the cancer, and who further believe that it is bad for their health to stay in the position, nevertheless feel they cannot leave because they need both the income and the insurance. This is a particularly painful dilemma.

> Celia was a librarian from New York who loved her work in libraries that directly served the general public. On her return from a year abroad, she took a job

with a specialized scientific library because it was the only position available at her advanced level of management skill and training. Following a painful divorce, she developed breast cancer. The diagnosis sharpened her awareness of how wrong her current position was for her, but her medical insurance and income seemed critical to her survival. She was caught in a job she believed was contributing to her illness.

Then there are work-related problems that result from physical or psychological changes that make it difficult for the cancer patient to continue to do the work that he enjoys—and sometimes the work on which his livelihood depends. Even if the financial situation is workable, the loss of capacity to function in a satisfying way—to be needed and useful—can be a great loss.

On the other side of the coin, a cancer diagnosis often gives people the courage to make work changes that they would not have risked before. With a sense that finding a satisfying work and creative life might really matter both in terms of quality of life and potentially in the course of the disease, some people transform existing work situations, find new meaning in what they are already doing, or leave work that does not fit in their lives, sometimes striking out in search of work that affirms them.

Sarah was a graphic designer from Washington who came on a Cancer Help Program. When I asked one of my favorite questions, what would you do if you did not have cancer and could do anything you wanted?, she responded: "I would leave my job, buy a van, travel across the country seeing friends, and then return to Virginia and found an artists' colony." I asked her what was keeping her from doing that. She considered the question for several days and concluded that she would leave her job and travel. She proceeded to do so, buying a van and traveling across the country as she had planned. She has not returned to Virginia yet to start an artists' colony, having stopped in California to attend art school, but I am waiting to hear the next chapter.

Living with Cancer

We could go through each of the areas described above in which problems in living with cancer come up and describe some of the huge variety of experiences that different people with cancer have. In the areas of love and work, the preceding two sections give at least a sense of what such a comprehensive review would reveal.

If living is an art, living with cancer often represents a challenge, whether it is accepted or not, to refine that art so that one can cope with difficulties scarcely imagined in the everyday world in which most people live.

To describe life with cancer as a high art does not mean that the challenge is necessarily to accept cancer with grace, or to achieve a level of consciousness where one is not touched by the vicissitudes of the illness, or any similar superficial ideas of what represents the art of life.

Some people are led, by their natures, to a beautiful grace and courage in the face of cancer. Others are led to an equally beautiful and honest expression of their fear, their grieving, their anger, their pain, and every other experience that comes to them.

One of the greatest lessons of the Cancer Help Program is that if you spend a week with a small group of people with cancer, you come to see and appreciate the beauty of each individual way of encountering cancer. Cancer directly encountered tends to strip one down to honesty and truth about one's life. Truth about a life, no matter how gnarled and twisted the life may be, makes that life intrinsically beautiful. The old Hasidic Jewish masters had a tradition that the light that came into the vessel of a human being who had sunk to the furthest reaches from God was of a power and quality that in some ways could not be matched by the great spiritual masters. God created sin, they reasoned, so that the return to God through repentance from this fallen state was possible, and so that this special light could be present in the creation.

That is a poetic way of saying what I have just said about how cancer directly encountered in any life can bring out the light in that life, and so transform lives that many cancer patients may have believed were hopelessly far from any creative or redeeming potential.

twenty-five

Controlling Pain

Pain is, naturally, one of the possibilities that people with cancer fear most. Yet cancer patients usually spend much less time considering how to control pain than they do researching choice in cancer therapies. There are seven very important points to remember about cancer pain, however:

1. Cancer is usually considerably less painful than people fear it will be.
2. An estimated 90% of cancer pain can be very adequately controlled.
3. Most physicians are *not* well trained in pain control, which is a real art and science.
4. The inadequate control of cancer pain is considered a scandal by pain specialists.
5. The probability of becoming addicted to opiate medications for pain is usually low, because the body metabolizes these drugs differently when it is in pain.
6. There are important nonpharmacological approaches to pain control, including psychological approaches and acupuncture.
7. The people who *know* how to control cancer pain in most communities—doctors and nurses—work with hospice organizations, and you do *not* have to be dying to get their help.

This chapter is about understanding and controlling cancer pain.

Understanding Pain

Pain is remarkable in that there are few—if any—words that express it adequately. Elain Scarry, Professor of English at the University of Pennsylvania, in her classic study *The Body in Pain,* describes fundamental observations about pain that may help us to understand it better:

> Physical pain has no voice, but when at last it finds a voice, it begins to tell a story. . . . Whatever pain achieves, it achieves in part through its unsharability, and it ensures this unsharability through its resistance to language. "English," writes Virginia Woolf, "which can express the thoughts of Hamlet and the tragedy of Lear has no word for the shiver or the headache.". . . True of the headache, Woolf's account is of course more radically true of the severe and prolonged pain that may accompany cancer or burns or phantom limb or stroke. . . . *Physical pain does not simply resist language but actively destroys it, bringing about an immediate reversion to a state anterior to language, to the sounds and cries a human makes before language is learned* [emphasis added].
>
> Why pain should so centrally entail, require, this shattering of language will only gradually become apparent . . . but an approximation of the explanation may be partially apprehended by noticing the exceptional character of pain when compared to all our other interior states . . . Our interior states of consciousness are regularly accompanied by objects in the internal world, that we do not simply "have feelings," but have feelings *for* somebody or something. . . . [By contrast] physical pain, unlike any other state of consciousness, has no referential content. It is not *of* or *for* anything. It is precisely because it takes no object that it, more than any other phenomenon, resists objectification in language . . . When physical pain is transformed into an objectified state, it (or at least some of its aversiveness) is eliminated. A great deal, then, is at stake in the attempt to invent linguistic structures that will reach . . . this area of experience.[1]

To put it more simply, pain tends strongly to elude our capacity to put it into words, and unlike our other internal states it has no object in the outer world to which it is attached. This is part of the reason pain is difficult to express. But when we do begin to put pain into language, it begins to tell a story, and that story often diminishes or erases pain. So the effort to find a language for pain is both important and healing.

Scarry describes the extraordinary work of Ronald Melzack and Patrick Wall, who created the celebrated gateway control theory of pain and also developed the McGill Pain Questionnaire.

> Melzack [recognized] that the conventional medical vocabulary ("moderate pain," "severe pain") described only one limited aspect of pain, its intensity; and that describing pain only in terms of this solitary dimension was equivalent to describing the complex realm of visual experience exclusively in terms of light and flux. Thus he and Torgerson, after gathering the apparently random words most often spoken by patients, began to arrange those words into coherent groups which, by making visible the consistency interior to any one set of words, worked to bestow visibility on the characteristics of pain.[2]

They developed sensory categories of pain that included: *temporal* dimensions (flickering, quivering, throbbing, beating sensations); *thermal* dimensions (hot, burning, scalding, searing); and *constrictive pressure* dimensions (pinching, pressing, gnawing, cramping, crushing). Other categories described dimensions of the *affective* (or emotional) and *cognitive* qualities of pain.

In contrast to physical pain, Scarry points out, psychological suffering is easily expressed in language. We can readily articulate our suffering, but for pain we have to use images, the language of "as if."

The great contribution of Scarry's work is that she counterposes the experience of physical pain and the possibility of human creativity. Pain, she suggests, *unmakes* us—it destroys our capacity to use language and takes over the content of consciousness in wordless agony. Finding a way to give pain a voice *reconstructs* or *remakes* us. Creativity, the act of *making* a voice for pain, makes us. Thus, for Scarry, the most profound relationship exists between the destructive power of pain (and pain is, after all, a signal that we are being destroyed) and the constructive power of creativity.

Now here we enter deeply into the real world behind the dry language of medicine and psychology with regard to what we can do with that aspect of cancer pain that can be worked with psychologically.

Imagery, Creativity, and Pain

Much of the most effective work in imagery and hypnosis with pain is quite literally in creating an opportunity that gives pain a *voice,* that enables it to express itself in the primordial and prelinguistic language of images. Thus the therapist may often, after inducing a state of relaxation, suggest: "Allow an image to form of your pain." A careful viewing of this image and a dialogue with it can often be both physically and psychologically transformative, frequently markedly diminishing pain.

Cristoff Müller-Busch, M.D., a pain specialist at the anthroposophical hospital at the University of Witten-Herdecke in Germany, has reported his strong impression that creative people often suffer less cancer pain than those whose creativity is blocked. And indeed, many activities that stimulate creativity are found by clinicians to alleviate both pain and suffering.

The fact that pain is resistant to language may also be related to the fact that physical pain is so difficult to remember. We are apt to remember more easily inner states that are stored in linguistic structures. On the other hand, there are symbolic structures that do store pain in us, and it often can be recovered through techniques of imagery and hypnotherapy.

After a patient has recovered from the initial shock of receiving a cancer diagnosis, one of his greatest fears is often that of being trapped in excruciating pain. This fear is rarely justified. Curiously, many intelligent people will expend great efforts on researching choice in both conventional and complementary cancer therapies and yet make little effort to understand the two possible outcomes of cancer that they fear most: pain and dying. Yet in pain, knowledge, choice, skill, and control are available that can make an enormous difference.

Why Cancer Pain, So Feared, Is Poorly Treated

"In a survey of public opinion on cancer . . . pain ranked next to incurability in people's fear. . . . *It has also been found that the general public believes cancer to be much more painful than it actually is,*" writes J.J. Bonica, Professor of

Anesthesiology at the University of Washington.[3] Moderate to severe pain, according to Bonica, is experienced by 30% to 45% of cancer patients at diagnosis, by 30% to 40% of patients with intermediate disease, and by 60% to 100% of patients with advanced or terminal cancer. This leads Bonica to pose a key question: "In view of the great advances in biomedical scientific knowledge and technology, and especially the great amount of interest in, and effort devoted to, cancer research and therapy, why is cancer *pain* inadequately relieved?" Bonica continues:

> Serious consideration . . . suggests that it is due to an inadequate appreciation or outright neglect of the problem of pain (in contrast to the problem of cancer) by oncologists, medical educators, investigators, research institutions, and national and international cancer agencies. . . . *Review of the curricula of medical schools reveals that few, if any, teach students the basic principles of the use of narcotics and other treatments that will effectively relieve cancer pain.* Moreover, many physicians in residency training for specialization in surgical, medical and radiation oncology receive little or no teaching about the proper management of cancer pain. . . . *Inadequate or total lack of interest or concern about the problem of pain by oncologists is further shown by the fact that very little, if any, information about the proper management of the pain problem is found in the oncology literature* [emphasis added].[3]

Foley's Classification of Types of Cancer Pain

One of the seminal articles on cancer pain was written by Kathleen Foley, M.D., a neurologist at Memorial Sloan-Kettering Cancer Center in New York, in the *New England Journal of Medicine* in 1985.[4] Foley is well known for her diagnostic division of types of cancer pain. Her categorizations of cancer pain are classic in the pain literature, and it is useful for the cancer patient and the family to know how a trained specialist in pain control might approach the specific type of pain a patient has.

Foley starts by differentiating between *acute* and *chronic* cancer pain. The onset of acute pain is well defined and it is associated with objective physical signs and hyperactivity of the autonomic nervous system that can be used by the practitioner to substantiate the patient's report of pain. Chronic pain, on the other hand, is pain that persists longer than 6 months, in which adaptation of the autonomic nervous system occurs. The objective signs common to acute pain are not present. Chronic pain leads to marked changes in personality, lifestyle, and functional ability: "*Such pain requires an approach that encompasses not only treatment of the cause of pain but also treatment of its psychological and social consequences*" [emphasis added].[4]

Starting with this distinction between acute and chronic pain, Foley then goes on to list five major types of patients with cancer pain.

The first group are those patients with acute cancer-related pain, in which the pain led to the diagnosis of cancer or where cancer therapy (surgery, chemotherapy, radiation) itself is the cause of the pain. Foley notes that for the former group, "pain has a special meaning as the harbinger of their illness. The occurrence of pain during the course of the illness, or after successful therapy, has the immediate implication of recurrent disease." For these patients, effective cancer therapy—such as irradiation of bone metastases—can bring dramatic pain relief. For those patients with acute pain related to treatment, "the cause of the pain is readily identified, its course predictable and self-limited. Such patients endure pain for the promise of a successful outcome."

The second group are patients with chronic cancer-related pain associated either with cancer progression or with cancer therapy. For those patients with chronic pain related to the progression of disease, combinations of pain strategies are often called for that may include direct antitumor therapies, analgesic drug therapies, anesthetic blocks, and psychological approaches to pain control. Psychological approaches, Foley emphasizes, may play a critical role with patients for whom palliative therapy may be of little value and would be physically debilitating:

> The sense of hopelessness and fear of impending death may add to and exaggerate the pain, which in turn contributes to the overall suffering of the patient. *Identification of both the pain and the suffering component is essential to the provision of adequate therapy.* Saunders has used the phrase "total pain" to describe the etiologic components other than the noxious physical stimulus, including emotional, social, bureaucratic, financial, and spiritual pain. *Those caring for this group of patients must be concerned with all aspects of distress and discomfort if the experience of physical pain is to be alleviated* [emphasis added].[5]

Patients with chronic pain associated with therapy are, Foley emphasizes, critical to identify:

> Treatment of the pain is often limited by the lack of available methods to remove the cause of the pain. . . . This group of patients closely parallels those in the general population with chronic, intractable pain. Identification of this group is imperative because recognition of the cause of the pain as independent of the cancer markedly alters the patient's therapy, prognosis, and psychological state. *Approaches other than drug therapy provide effective alternatives for pain management* [emphasis added].

The third group Foley identifies are those patients with preexisting chronic pain. These patients have a history of chronic nonmalignant pain in addition to cancer and its associated pain. Psychological factors play an important role for these patients, because their psychological and functional status is already compromised. They are therefore at high risk of further functional incapacity and escalating chronic pain. "However," says Foley, "*their history should not be used in a punitive way to minimize their complaints*" [emphasis added].

The fourth group is composed of patients with a history of drug addiction and cancer-related pain. These patients' history of drug addiction is compounded by cancer-related pain and the issues of medication. Active drug users represent a particularly difficult problem requiring consultation with drug-abuse specialists. Prior users can be treated just as other pain patients are, with the added recognition that they are at higher risk for recidivism.

The fifth group Foley identifies are dying patients. For these, maintaining the comfort of the patient is of paramount importance. The issues of hopelessness, death, and dying come to the fore, and the patient's suffering must be addressed. "*Inadequate control of pain exacerbates the suffering and demoralizes both the family and the medical personnel who feel they have failed in treating the patient's pain at a time when adequate treatment may matter most*" [emphasis added]. Foley concludes that rapid escalation of analgesic drug therapy and attempts to address symptoms should be employed.[6]

The type of cancer that one has obviously contributes greatly to the probability of pain. Foley found that 85% of patients with primary bone tumors had pain, compared with 52% of breast cancer patients, 20% of lymphoma patients, and only 5% of leukemia patients. Looking at cancer pain another way, the authors found that 78% of hospitalized cancer patients had pain due directly to tumor involvement, 50% had pain due to bone disease, in 25% pain was due to nerve compression, and in 19% it was due to treatment-related problems.[7]

Therapeutic Strategies in Pain Treatment

The first goal of the physician, according to Vittorio Ventafridda of the Italian National Cancer Institute, is to treat the cause of the pain. If this is not possible, treating the symptoms becomes the goal. The choice of methods for pain treatment should take into account the patient's degree of activity and the preferences of the patient. A patient for whom activity matters a great deal may prefer to accept more pain in order to maintain the preferred level of activity. In the same way, a patient who particularly values a clear mind may accept more pain in order to stay mentally clear. A patient who is actively fighting for life using immunosupportive adjunctive therapies may accept more pain in order to avoid the immunodepressive characteristics of many pain medications. But a patient whose enjoyment of life is being destroyed by pain may prefer a more active intervention in pain control.

Immediate relief of pain is the first goal of therapy, followed by ongoing control of pain for the rest of the patient's life. The ideal goal of this strategy—complete freedom from pain—is rarely possible, but pain can almost always be eased so that the patient can bear what was previously considered to be intolerable.

In planning the therapeutic strategy, it is necessary to pursue a series of objectives. Cancer pain may prevent the patient from getting adequate sleep, which will lower his pain threshold and result in constant tiredness and demoralization. This problem should be addressed first. Next, pain should be relieved when resting in bed or in a chair. Pain felt when standing and during activity should also be relieved. While the first and second aims are relatively easy to achieve, the third one requires a combined and sequential pattern of physical and psychosocial supports in order to be effective.[8]

This brings us to the greatest contribution of modern science to cancer pain management: the use of analgesic drugs and the concept of the analgesic ladder. The key points in analgesic pain management, according to Ventafridda, are:

- The drug must be administered at fixed hours and not on the patient's request to alleviate pain. Analgesics should be given regularly and prophylactically [with prevention as the goal]. The aim is . . . to gradually increase the dose until we obtain the maximum relief with the minimal interference with activity. The next dose is given before the effect of the first one has fully worn off. In this way it is possible to erase the fear of pain.
- The drug or drugs to be used should be selected and treatment . . . started at once. While the nature and cause of the pain are being assessed, therapy should be started with analgesic drugs, which should then be given on a regular basis.
- If a drug ceases to be effective, do not transfer to an alternative drug of similar strength but prescribe a drug that is definitely stronger.
- Use analgesic drugs primarily by mouth—the route of administration is important because it has a substantial impact on the patient's way of life. The patient taking oral medication is free to move around, travel as he wishes and, most important, be at home. Injections promote dependence on the person administering the drug. Oral administration eliminates muscle trauma and enables the patient to maintain control over his own drug administration.
- Use pure drugs, not compounds. With a compound an increase in the dose of one drug will automatically increase the dose of the other whether it is necessary or not.
- Check interaction with any other substances (chemotherapeutic, hormonal, etc.) which the patient is receiving.
- Control side effects.
- Learn how to use a few drugs well. The three basic analgesics are aspirin, codeine and morphine. Certain adjuvant drugs can also be helpful in certain specific cases. Learn to be familiar with one or two alternatives for each type of agent for use in patients who cannot tolerate the first choice drug. Your basic analgesic ladder, with alternatives, should include no more than nine or ten drugs in total [see figure 25.1 and table 25.1].[9]

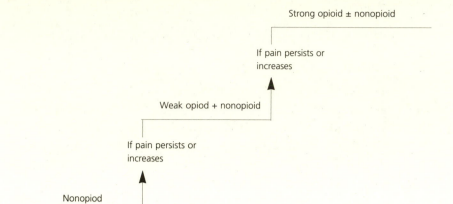

Figure 25.1

The "analgesic ladder." (Reproduced by permission of MTP Press Limited, Lancaster, England, from: M. Swerdlow and V. Ventafridda, eds., Cancer Pain, © *1987.)*

Table 25.1

Basic Analgesic Drug List

Type	First choice	Alternatives
Nonopioids	Aspirin	Paracetamol (acetaminophen)
Weak opioids	Codeine	Dextropropoxyphene Oxymorphone
Strong opioids	Morphine	Methadone Buprenorphine Levorphanol Standardized opium
Adjuvants		
Anticonvulsants	Carbamazepine	Phenytoin
Antidepressants	Amitriptyline	Clomipramine
Anxiolytics	Diazepam	Hydroxyzine
Corticosteroids	Prednisolone	Dexamethasone
Muscle relaxants	Diazepam	Baclofen
Psychotropics	Chlorpromazine	Haloperidol

Reproduced by permission of MTP Press Limited, Lancaster, England, from M. Swerdlow and V. Ventafridda, eds., *Cancer Pain*, © 1987.

Approximately 50% of cancer patients report good to excellent relief of cancer pain from medications alone.[10] Psychological approaches to cancer pain, as Foley indicated, offer an important complement to drug therapy. Tearnan et al. describe the important benefits of psychological approaches to cancer pain. First of all, psychological factors often color the perception of pain. Secondly, patients can be taught to manage pain through behavioral techniques, and this approach can be applied to other areas of patient distress, such as anxiety and depression. These approaches may also help to increase the patient's sense of mastery over his health environment. And finally, they have no negative side effects.[11]

According to Tearnan and colleagues a fascinating contrast between pain and life adjustment problems in patients with benign chronic pain and patients with chronic cancer pain is reported by some researchers:

> The relationship between pain and life adjustment problems for patients with chronic pain is well known. Many of these patients report difficulties in their marriages, work, and recreational activities. They also admit to significant levels of depression and other mood disturbance. *Surprisingly, cancer pain does not appear to be strongly correlated to psychosocial problems, negative mood in particular* [emphasis added].[12]

Many clinicians would find these data suspect based on direct experience with hundreds of patients who attribute their illness directly to life problems and emotional difficulties. Another explanation for this strange finding might be sought in the fascinating work of Lydia Temoshok with melanoma patients: some melanoma patients, Temoshok found, were extraordinarily out of touch with their emotional responses to life. Such patients might simply fail to report life adjustment problems and emotional difficulties that patients in pain with a benign chronic disease do report.[13] Other people with cancer may have developed cancer for reasons entirely unrelated to life adjustment or emotional problems, and so would logically not report the difficulties of most patients with benign chronic pain. However, many cancer patients do in fact consistently report serious life adjustment problems, and their pain is often responsive to psychological work that addresses these problems.

While researchers reasonably assure us that definitive controlled studies of' most psychological approaches to pain have not been done, there is no question in the minds of many clinicians who work with cancer pain that many of the psychological approaches described above routinely diminish, or sometimes even erase, cancer pain. In general, psychological approaches to pain work best with a therapist skilled in combining them as the individual patient requires. Thus a session may be part psychotherapy dealing with internal and interpersonal issues, part progressive deep relaxation and imagery or hypnotherapy, and part cognitive restructuring.

Tearnan and his colleagues[14] divide the psychological approaches to treating cancer pain into the following major categories[15]:

1. Psychotherapy as an approach to pain control "is based on the assumption that the perception of pain occurs within a personal and interpersonal context. The general assumption is that dealing with critical intra- and interpersonal issues will reduce the impact of pain."

2. Hypnosis is the oldest and most widely used approach. "Numerous clinical reports have appeared in the literature over the last three decades to support its efficacy in treating cancer pain. Hypnosis has also been reported to be effective in treating emotional distress, anxiety or treatment—related discomfort in cancer patients. Although the literature reports that 20%–50% of cancer patients benefit from hypnosis, this evidence is largely anecdotal and based on uncontrolled studies."[14]

3. Relaxation techniques and biofeedback, which are closely related to hypnosis, may also be useful. Relaxation training includes yoga, meditation, and progressive muscle relaxation, as well as autogenic relaxation techniques that use suggestions that the body is getting heavy, warm, or relaxed. Biofeedback uses instruments to induce physiologic awareness of the capacity to achieve responses such as relaxation.

4. Cognitive approaches include assessment of beliefs, expectations, and fears, and assistance to the patient in restructuring and reconceptualizing the pain.

5. Behavioral approaches focus on the role of environmental reinforcement of cancer pain. The authors suggest this approach is of limited value in cancer pain because the "the report of pain is important in the assessment of the disease process and should not be ignored."[14]

Virginia Veach's Work with Pain

The most effective psychological work with cancer pain that I have personally witnessed has been that of Virginia Veach, Ph.D., a psychotherapist and physical therapist who is also one of the senior co-leaders in the Commonweal Cancer Help Program. Veach is *frequently* able to help participants relieve pain, sometimes dramatically. I have watched her help participants in the Cancer Help Program reverse pain so frequently that I have come to trust her method. I have also tried her approach with others, and found that I too could sometimes—far less expertly—help with pain.

What Veach characteristically does is to elicit from the participant a detailed description of the pain. Is it sharp or dull? Pulsating or steady? Where exactly is it located? What shape is it? How wide, deep, and long is it? How big is it? Then she often asks whether the participant is *willing* to try to get out of the way of the pain and allow it to spread. This is usually a shocking idea to someone in pain. Veach reassures the participant that he can return to his effort to minimize the pain shortly. And, she emphasizes, she is not asking the participant to *make* the pain spread, but simply to see if it is possible to get out of the way and to *allow* the pain to spread.

Pain, Veach explains, acts like fire: it "wants" to spread. And often in the course of spreading it changes its character, becomes less intense, less sharp. The "hot" pain turns to warmth, and sometimes even to a tingling sensation that in many traditions is associated with healing.

The Story Pain Tells

We saw at the beginning of this chapter how few words adequately describe pain; how pain can "unmake" us. The other side of the coin is that the exploration of our inner lives—often prompted by pain—may shift our inner lives in relation to the pain. As we change, the pain may change. This phenomenon of pain shifting, when we pay attention to it, is deeply related to a distinction I introduced in chapter 2: the distinction between *pain* and *suffering*. Recall the diagram in which we contrasted:

Biomedicine (Science)	Biopsychosocial Medicine (Human experience)
Disease	Illness
Pain	Suffering
Curing	Healing

In each case, biomedicine is focused on the biological phenomena—disease, pain, curing—while biopsychosocial medicine attends both to the biological phenomena and the *human experience* of the biological phenomena. Thus, illness is the human experience of disease; healing is the human experience of the effort to recover health; and suffering is the human experience of pain.

So suffering is in large part the *story* that we tell ourselves about our pain. And that story can *sometimes* profoundly shift the experience of that pain. A widely cited example are the studies conducted in Korea and Vietnam of wounded American soldiers. Those who received lesser wounds that could be patched so that they could return to the lethal risks of the battlefield consistently reported *worse pain* than those with more serious wounds who were being sent home. The meaning of the wound amplified the pain for those being sent back in harm's way, and diminished the pain for those who knew they had escaped with their lives.

No Pain, No Gain?

In the face of serious pain, thoughtful people should learn to look beyond the initial simple and natural thought that the pain is always a direct result of the cancer, and that medication is the only response to the deeper messages that pain often elicits from us. The idea that we can benefit from pain is difficult to grasp, one that is often mocked or simplistically overstated. But consider this question: Have you learned more from the painful things in your life, or from the easy ones? Is it a mistake that Jesus was "a man of troubles and

acquainted with grief?" Or that Gautama Buddha's journey toward enlighten-
ment began with the direct perception of pain and suffering? One of my
favorite quotations from the *Yoga Sutras,* the greatest yoga text, says this: "The
acceptance of pain as an aid to purification, the study of holy books, and
complete surrender to the Divine within us, constitute yoga in practice."

Sometimes pain is too great to accept. In that case, medication is a great
blessing to bring the pain down to levels where we can work with it. At the
Lukas Klinik in Arlesheim, Switzerland, the great anthroposophical hospital
for cancer patients inspired by Rudolf Steiner, it is part of the creed of the
staff that the goal of pain medication is to make pain tolerable—but not
remove it completely—so that the patient can put it to spiritual use.

Morphine, Metastases, and Addiction

Not everyone can or does subscribe to the idea that pain has any benefits at
all. That is, after all, simply another one of the stories that pain may elicit
from us. Some people faced with pain simply want to be "snowed" with as
heavy a dose of pain medication as possible. One physiological disadvantage
to an excessive reliance on opioid drugs (like morphine) is that they may
depress the immune system. In some animal studies, morphine has been shown
to increase the rate of metastases in cancer-bearing rodents.[16] Other animal
studies show a cancer-*inhibiting* effect of opioids. No human studies have been
conducted on the important question of whether the best of pain killers are
a double-edged sword. But their known immunosuppressive effect makes that
a legitimate concern, and certainly justifies people who seek strategies to
shorten or minimize the need for opiates.

On the other hand, the old concern that use of opiates would cause cancer
patients to become drug addicts has been significantly reduced by recent
studies showing that opiates are metabolized differently by people in pain.[17]
Addiction turns out to be an uncommon phenomenon among pain patients
who take prescribed opiates. This may also put a different light on the rodent
studies showing increased cancer metastases in animals given opiates. The
treated animals were not, presumably, in pain. Perhaps the different way that
humans metabolize opiates when in pain lessens the threat of addiction. On

the other hand, some clinicians *do* report addiction problems with patients recovering from cancer who used large amounts of opiates.

Other Approaches to Pain

There are other approaches to pain worthy of careful consideration.

First, acupuncture is well known to help control many kinds of pain, and is very effective with some forms of cancer pain, as indicated in chapter 19.

Second, there are herbal medications that may be helpful with pain, particularly when the pain stems from tight muscles and a herbal relaxant would be effective.

Third, massage and acupressure can both be effective in reducing pain, especially (as above) pain associated with muscular tension.

Finally, physicians can prescribe the use of an electrical nerve-stimulating device that greatly reduces some kinds of pain. This device, called a TENS (transcutaneous electrical nerve stimulator; manufactured by the 3M company); looks like a miniature portable radio. The patient pastes wires coming out of it to the skin and adjusts the level and pulse of the electrical charge. Some patients take use of the device a step further and paste the wires to acupuncture points that their traditional Chinese medicine practitioner has identified as specifically related to the pain. One friend of mine was able to discontinue opiates for some time using this device.

Conclusion

Pain, the more one considers it, is a remarkable subject. We have reviewed seven key points about pain: (1) that cancer is generally less difficult than many people think; (2) that most cancer pain can be controlled; (3) that most physicians are not adequately trained in pain control; (4) that cancer pain is undertreated by most physicians; (5) that addiction to pain medication should not be a primary concern if you are in pain; (6) that there are important nonpharmacological ways to control pain; and (7) that the best pain control experts in most communities are doctors and nurses associated with hospice programs, and that you do not have to be dying to get their help with pain.

We looked at how wordless we are in pain and how pain "unmakes" us. We saw how being in touch with creativity may lessen pain. And we considered both the pharmacological and nonpharmacological approaches to controlling pain.

One potent pain reliever—acupuncture and traditional Chinese medicine—we did not discuss. Its potent benefits for some kinds of pain is discussed in chapter 19.

Notes and References

1   Elaine Scarry, *The Body in Pain* (New York: Oxford University Press, 1985), 3–6.
2   Ibid., 7.
3   J.J. Bonica, "Importance of the Problem." In M. Swerdlow and V. Ventafridda, eds., *Cancer Pain* (Boston: MTP Press, 1987), 3–8.
4   Kathleen M. Foley, "The Treatment of Cancer Pain," *New England Journal of Medicine* 313(2):85 (1985).
5   Ibid.
6   Ibid., 85–6.
7   K.M. Foley, "Pain Syndromes in Patients with Cancer." Cited in B.H. Tearnan et al., "Psychological Management of Malignant Pain." In C. David Tollison, ed., *Handbook of Chronic Pain Management* (Baltimore: Wilkins & Wilkins, 1989), 403.
8   Vittorio Ventafridda, "Therapeutic Strategy." In Swerdlow and Ventafridda, eds., *Cancer Pain,* 57–8.
9   Ibid., 58–61.
10 Tearnan et al., "Psychological Management of Malignant Pain." In Tollison, ed., *Handbook of Chronic Pain Management,* 402.
11 Ibid.
12 Ibid., 403.
13 Lydia Temoshok, "Repressive Coping Reactions in Patients with Malignant Melanoma as Compared to Cardiovascular Disease Patients," *Journal of Psychosomatic Research* 28(2):151–2 (1984).
14 Tearnan, "Psychological Management of Malignant Pain," 408–12.

15　See the Psychological Approaches to Cancer section of chapter 10 for more information on these techniques.

16　Edward W. Bernton, Henry U. Bryant, and John W. Holaday, "Prolactin and Immune Function." In Robert Ader, David L. Felten, and Nicholas Cohen, *Psychoneuroimmunology,* second edition (San Diego: Academic Press, 1991), 412–3.

17　Ronald Melzack, "The Tragedy of Needless Pain," *Scientific American* 262(2):27–33 (February 1990).

twenty-six

On Living and Dying

Even the wise fear death. Life clings to life.
Buddha

I write this chapter on death and dying with the greatest respect for the reader facing the possibility either of his own death or of the death of someone he cares about. I have had too many friends die of cancer to speak to you in any other way.

For those who may have difficulty beginning to read this chapter, I want to say right at the start that I believe there are 12 critical things to know about death and dying:

1. There is skill, choice, knowledge, and control in death and dying just as much as there is in the fight for life with cancer.
2. Some people believe that death is the end; others that life after death is a certainty. My own belief, as Rachel Naomi Remen puts it, is that *death is a mystery worth contemplating.* Death for me is a mystery in the deep sense of the term: a real possibility exists that life in some form continues after death, and intriguing scientific literature supports the spiritual writings and the experience of many

people who have had remarkable near-death experiences. Forceful arguments exist on the other side.

3. Whatever our beliefs about death, it is a fact that *there is such a thing as dying well,* and that we can consciously work toward dying well the way pregnant mothers work toward birthing well—and with the same uncertainty and absence of judgment about how we will actually fare in the event.

4. There is no single way of dying well, but an infinite variety of ways. A good death might be described mentally and emotionally as one in which—in the face of whatever biological experience we shall have—as much movement toward wisdom and healing as possible takes place for the one who is dying and for those who love him. A good death might be described physically as one in which pain and discomfort do not exceed what can be decently endured.

5. It is very useful to recognize the distinction between our *fear of dying and our fear of death.* This distinction then helps us focus first on specific fears we have about the dying process.

6. Most people are more afraid of being caught in interminable suffering during the dying process than they are of death itself. The reality, as we have seen in the chapter on pain, is that, in most cases, severe pain can be controlled and made tolerable.

7. Another fear people have is that they will remain alive when life no longer feels worth living, when they have become a burden to people they love, or when their dignity has been taken from them. This is a more complex set of concerns to respond to, but one important fact, emphasized by the great physician Eric Cassell, is that *many people with cancer die within a relatively short time of having truly decided that they are ready to die.*[1]

8. If death does not come to us at the point where we have truly decided that we no longer want to live, then we do have the option of taking our own life, if our religious beliefs allow it and if the suffering becomes intolerable. In the Netherlands, physician-assisted suicide for those facing a life no longer worth living is an acknowledged part of a public policy that requires the physician to follow a carefully prescribed protocol.[2] In the United States, a great debate is currently taking place over whether physician-assisted suicide should be legal. Many American physicians do assist patients in dying if all that remains is a painful existence

without dignity. Whether or not physicians are willing to assist us, many patients with life-threatening illnesses (AIDS patients have led the way in this) have simply learned what drug combinations are effective in suicide and have set those drugs aside for the day when life is no longer worth living.

9. *It is critically important to make sure that you have the best possible medical and nursing care while dying.* Those physicians who are wonderful when you are fighting for life may not be helpful when you are dying. The same is true of hospitals—a place that is superb for high-technology cancer therapies may not be the best place to die. One of the most difficult aspects of dying is the discomfort that may arise from many different sources. Helping a person relieve these symptoms and discomforts is a very high medical art that demands the interest, care, and attention of physicians, nurses, and care-givers. Finding the people in your community (they are often connected with a hospice) who are dedicated to this great human task can make a world of difference in the experience of dying. If you choose to die at home, the choice of home health care aides skilled in helping people die is at least as important as the physician and nurses you work with.

10. Some people are afraid that making practical estate arrangements or other arrangements for dying means that they have given up the fight for life. My general experience is that preparing for the possibility of death does not interfere with the fight for life at all—in fact it can enhance it, because you have taken away the worry of not having dealt with these very practical matters. Taking care of the things you want to take care of actually releases energy for the fight for life.

11. Part of preparing for death is giving some thought to helping loved ones with the grieving process. This can be tremendously important, because incomplete grieving often injures the rest of the life of a mate, a parent, or a child. In the process of a good death, a great deal of the mutual grieving of patient and loved ones takes place while the patient is still alive and participating. If this process takes place as consciously and fully as possible, the death can sometimes become, strangely, a great healing for all involved. While there is still grieving to do—a great deal of grieving, perhaps—it starts from a solid base. There are some excellent books on griev-

ing as well as good grieving support groups and therapists. I strongly recommend learning about these resources for survivors.

12. Our culture's attitude—in which death is a highly toxic subject and seen as a failure, either of the doctor or of the patient—is not only new historically but at odds with that of other cultures. In many cultures, dying is surrounded by rituals in which everyone participates. For many centuries in the West, this was also so. Death was often seen as the culmination of a life, and people gave great thought to how they might die well. It is possible in our culture to *detoxify death* by contemplating it, seeing what others have thought and said about it, and by giving ourselves time to be with it. In the face of sincere contemplation and prayer, the toxicity with which our culture has surrounded death often begins to dissolve.

All of this leads to exploration of what benefits we and those we love may receive from death and dying. We know all too well what the pain and losses will be. We know all too well that some people die with great difficulty and suffering, while others die peacefully. The question is whether or not we can find anything of value, in the midst of pain and loss, from death. The answer of some wise people over the centuries, and of many in our time, is that it is possible to find deeply meaningful and important experiences in the midst of facing death. In the rest of this chapter we explore some of these ideas in more detail.

The Literature on Death and Dying

One of the best ways to *detoxify* the subject of death and dying is to learn what wise people have had to say about their own experience with and meditations on death. In a sense, the classic and contemporary literature on death and dying provides a support group made up of some of the greatest saints, humorists, artists, cynics, and thinkers of all times. They speak across the ages to you—across time and space—with some very different ideas about how people have faced what William James called "the distinguished thing." I know they have helped me. Perhaps they may help you, too.

One of the best places to start an inquiry into death and dying is *The Oxford Book of Death,* a great collection of poems, other writings, and sayings about death. I have selected a number of quotations from *The Oxford Book of Death* to give you a sense of *how* reading what wise people through the ages have said about death can transform our own attitudes.

The editor of the collection, J.D. Enright, is a well-known poet and critic. "Reading for this anthology," he says, "I was moved to the thought that on no theme have writers shown themselves more lively." A survivor of one of the Nazi prison camps, quoted in the anthology, echoed this view with his observation, "when in death we are in the midst of life."[3]

"Death," said Arnold Toynbee, "is the price paid by life for an enhancement of the complexity of a live organism's structure."[4] There is a deep biological basis for this observation. As the Canadian naturalist David Suzuki explains, in primitive one-celled organisms, the original cell reproduced by dividing itself, so death was not inevitable. But complex organisms that could not simply divide developed sexual function as a means of reproduction. With the invention of reproduction, death appeared. Hence the very deep connections between birth, sexuality, and death.[5] Montaigne put it simply: "Make room for others, as others have done for you."[6]

Said Jung:

> Life is an energy-process. Like every energy-process, it is in principle irreversible and is therefore directed toward a goal. That goal is a state of rest. In the long run everything that happens is, as it were, no more than the initial disturbance of a perpetual state of rest which forever attempts to re-establish itself. . . . Thoughts of death pile up to an astonishing degree as the years increase. Willy-nilly, the aging person prepares himself for death. . . . It is just as neurotic in old age not to focus upon the goal of death as it is in youth to repress fantasies which have to do with the future.[7]

Many writers agree that dying is more difficult than death itself:

> PHAEDRUS: *But is death as horrible a thing as it's commonly asserted to be?*
>
> MARCUS: *The road leading up to it is harder than death itself. If a man dismisses from his thoughts the horror and imagination of death, he will have rid himself of a great part of the evil. In brief, whatever the torment of sickness or death, it is rendered much more endurable if a*

person surrenders himself to the divine will. For awareness of death,
when the soul is already separated from the body, is, I think, either non-
existent or else an extremely low-grade awareness, because before Nature
reaches this point it dulls and stuns all areas of sensation.[8]

Contemporary Views of Death

Some of the most interesting contemporary sociological views of death are
collected in a book edited by Edwin S. Shneidman, *Death: Current Perspectives.*
The first contribution is from Arnold Toynbee, who wrote a beautiful essay on
death in which he emphasized that:

> This two sidedness of death is a fundamental feature of death. . . . There are
> always two parties to a death; the person who dies and the survivors who are
> bereaved. . . . When, therefore, I ask myself whether I am reconciled to death,
> I have to distinguish, in each variant of the situation, between being reconciled
> to death on my own account and being reconciled to it on the account of the
> other party. . . . My answer to Saint Paul's question "O death, where is thy
> sting?" is Saint Paul's own answer: "The sting of death is sin." The sin that I
> mean is the sin of selfishly failing to wish to survive the death of someone
> with whose life my own life is bound up. This is selfish because the sting
> of death is less sharp for the person who dies than it is for the bereaved
> survivor.[9]

Ernest Becker won the Pulitzer Prize for *The Denial of Death,* which argued
that our whole lives are organized around fear and denial of death. Heroism,
Becker argued, is a "reflex of the terror of death":

> We admire most the courage to face death. . . . The hero has been the center
> of human honor and acclaim since probably the beginning of specifically human
> evolution. . . . The hero was the man who could go into the spirit world, the
> land of the dead, and return alive. . . . When philosophy took over from religion
> it also took over religion's central problem, and death became the real "muse
> of philosophy" from its beginnings in Greece right through Heidegger and
> modern existentialism.[10]

Summarizing the work and thought on death from religion, philosophy, and
science, Becker distinguishes between the "healthy-minded" argument that fear
of death is not natural to man, and derives from repressed or unfulfilled living,

and the "morbidly minded" argument that the fear of death is natural, what William James called "the worm at the core" of man's pretension to happiness.

> Jacques Choron goes so far as to say that it is questionable whether it will ever be possible to decide whether the fear of death is or is not the basic anxiety. In matters like this, then, the most that one can do is to take sides, give an opinion based on the authorities that seem to him most compelling, and to present some of the compelling arguments. I frankly side with the second school—in fact, this whole book is a network of arguments based on the universality of the fear of death, or "terror" as I prefer to call it, in order to convey how all consuming it is when we look it full in the face.[11]

Becker argues that the fear of death is biologically essential to the preservation of the species, and at the same time that continuous consciousness of this fear of death would be deeply counterproductive. He quotes the psychoanalyst Gregory Zilboorg: "If this fear were constantly conscious, we should be unable to function normally. It must be properly repressed to keep us living with any modicum of comfort."

And so, Becker says, "We can understand what seems like an impossible paradox: the ever-present fear of death in the normal biological functioning of our instinct for self-preservation, as well as our utter obliviousness to this fear in our conscious life."[12]

Another key point from this remarkable collection of contemporary views is Geoffrey Gorer's concept of *the pornography of death*. Gorer brilliantly argues that, while sex was pornographic to the Victorians, death has been the pornography of our time.[13]

Contemporary Psychospiritual Perspectives on Death and Dying

It is difficult in 1993 to realize what a transformation the last 30 years have brought in American attitudes toward death and dying. And indeed this transformation speaks volumes for the broader transformation of American consciousness over this period of time. As Phillipe Aries wrote in his classic book, *The Hour of Our Death*:

> Before 1959 when Herman Feifel wanted to interview the dying about themselves, no doubt for the first time, hospital authorities were indignant. They

found the project "cruel, sadistic, traumatic." In 1965 when Elisabeth Kübler-Ross was looking for dying persons to interview, the heads of the hospitals and clinics to whom she addressed herself protested, "Dying? But there are no dying here!" There could be no dying in a well-organized and respectable institution. They were mortally offended.[14]

Part of the best evidence for the transformation of the American mind through the 1960s, 1970s, and 1980s has been the opening of a substantial part of the population to an intense interest in learning from and caring for the dying. One of the foremost exponents of this work is Stephen Levine, author of a number of fine books on dying. Here is an excerpt from *Healing into Life and Death:*

> Our intention is not to keep people alive or to help them die either. Our work seems to be an encouragement to focus on the moment. To heal in the present and allow the future to arise naturally out of that opening. . . . We witnessed deep healings into the spirit of some who lived as well as miraculous healings in some who died . . . clearly healing was not limited to the body. The question "Where might we find our healing?" expanded. It was [about] the healing of a lifetime. The healing we took birth for . . . The deepest healing cannot be done solely in the separate. It needs to be for the whole, for the pain we all share. . . . Seeing it is not simply *my* pain, but *the* pain, the circle of healing expands to allow the universe to enter.[15]

Levine expanded on this theme in an interview in *Inquiring Mind:*

IM: *What do you mean by surrender?*

SL: *What we [Levine and his wife Ondrea] mean by surrender is softening and letting go of resistance, trusting the process. Many people misunderstand surrender as defeat. Surrender is actually the optimum strategy for living, including dying . . . Surrender is really about letting go of the last moment and opening to the next. Of course everyone's process isn't the same. Some people work wonderfully with mindfulness mixed with loving kindness. Other people have so much regret about the way they've led their lives that we encourage them to work with forgiveness, forgiveness of themselves, forgiveness of those they reacted towards . . .*

We have seen people in severe physical discomfort who when they started to surrender their resistance—to enter into contact with sensa-

tion—experienced that multiple changing quality of the pain that they thought was so solid. Then they could begin to direct their analgesics into the areas where they were needed . . .

IM: *How much difference does it make for someone who is dying to have done a lot of spiritual practice?*

SL: *When a person has a sense of something greater than themselves, whatever it might be, it is very helpful when they are dying. Also, someone who has done spiritual practice probably has a little more concentration to bring to the meditations for pain, for heavy states, or for forgiveness . . . People who have cultivated a willingness to go beyond safe territory—which means even beyond their practice—have an easier time with death.*[16]

We can see in the work of the Levines the idea that the process of learning to live well is also the process of learning to die well and that cultivating a relationship with our innermost being serves us well at the time of death. Dennis Leahy, M.D. expands upon the idea of surrender as a way of healing into death: "[We have all] spent much of [our] lives in the conscious and unconscious cultivation of uniqueness. This process does not end as we begin to die. We see herein that in the process of letting go, our individualization may become more, rather than less complete. In this sense there is great hope."[17]

The Questions Raised By Near-Death Experiences and Reports of Communications with the Dead

Many people who come on the Cancer Help Program have had near-death experiences that have changed their lives—experiences in which they almost died, or did die medically, and were then revived. Others have had experiences in which people they loved who died returned, after death, with messages that were deeply reassuring.

One of the most moving of these experiences for me happened with Kim and Sarah, the couple whose fight for life I described in chapter 1. I visited Sarah in the hospital shortly before she died. At one point I said to her: "It is absolutely not all right with me that this is happening to you, Sarah. But if you do die, I'd like to ask you a favor. It would make my life a lot easier if I heard from some friends who died that they were OK on the other side. So if you go, please try to come back and let me know you're OK." She promised she would.

Many months later I was getting a massage during a break in the late afternoon on the first day of a Cancer Help Program. I remarked to Jnani Chapman, the Cancer Help Program masseuse who was working on me, that I did not understand what was happening but that God seemed to be very present—that my body seemed to be filled with a strong charge of deep joyful and peaceful energy. It was a very unusual experience for me—I am not given to frequent experiences like this. Later that night, I got a message that Kim had called. I thought it might be to tell me of Sarah's death. It occurred to me immediately that if Sarah had died, perhaps that was connected to the extraordinary feeling I had had of the presence of God. Perhaps that was Sarah trying to keep her promise to me. I called Kim, reached him, and during the conversation I told him of my experience. He said Sarah had not yet been in touch with him, but that he very much hoped she would.

The next morning I received a faxed letter from Kim as follows:

Dear Michael:

Sarah died at 2:15 P.M. on February 19. The night after her death I had the most extraordinary and vivid dream. I was in a hospital being restrained by three doctors. They were pleading with me not to go into Sarah's room. They said her body had decomposed and that if I saw her in that condition it would leave me with a very unpleasant final vision. I became angry and pushed them aside and told them I had to see her. I ran to her room and opened the door. Sarah was reclining unclothed on her side, in the way of the odalisque in the painting by Ingres. Her body was radiant, full and perfect. Her hair shined like golden threads and her lips and cheeks were pink and glowing. I stared at her in amazement. The doctors were wrong: she had become perfect. I went to her bedside and sat down. Her eyes were closed and her limbs hung limp. I embraced her and as I did her chest heaved, her eyes and mouth opened, her lungs filled with air and she came alive. My heart soared and my eyes filled with tears of joy. Sarah looked up at me and said "Kim, I am not alive." I paused and then asked her, "Is it good or bad where you are?" She looked at me and rolled her eyes in the way she would when I said something really dumb. She said, "Good and bad do not apply here." I said, "Well, is it OK? Are you OK?" Sarah's lips tightened and her eyes squinted as if to say, let me think about that one. Then slowly she nodded her head and said, "Yes, it's OK, but I need some time to get used to it." I held her shoulders and looked into her face and asked, "Sarah, when I die, will I be able to be with you?" She very simply said yes. Then her eyes closed and her body went limp again. I panicked and ran into the corridor and began a desperate search for the doctors. The halls were deserted. I decided to go back to Sarah's room, but could not find my way. I began opening the doors in the corridor, but all the rooms were empty. I then awoke sitting straight up in bed.

Waves of sorrow, sadness, incompleteness and emptiness flow over me on a regular basis. But when I think of this dream it gives me a deep sense of comfort.

I wanted to share it with you.

Peace and Love,

Kim

It could well be that Kim's dream was the vivid fulfillment of the wish of a grieving husband to know that his wife was well on the other side, particularly after I had suggested that perhaps my experience had been Sarah's attempt to keep her promise to communicate with me. But anyone with an open and inquiring mind who works for sustained periods of time around people facing death cannot help confronting the significance of near-death experiences, based on both reports from patients and on the clinical and empirical literature.

Joan Borysenko provides a beautiful personal experience in her book *Guilt Is the Teacher, Love Is the Lesson:*

Many years ago . . . I sat with a young woman who was dying. Her name was Sally, and she had been living with a rapidly growing and rare rectal cancer for the year or so that we knew each other. We worked on meditation and imagery techniques that helped relieve treatment side effects and brought Sally some peace. We talked of emotions, finishing old business, forgiveness, and grieving. We also talked of Sally's concept of death . . . that consciousness died with the brain rather than surviving in any way beyond the body.

When the day of Sally's death came, I was visiting her in the hospital. I was scared because I'd never been with a dying person before and didn't have any notion what to expect. Her parents had gone off to have lunch when I came, so I had about 45 minutes to sit alone with Sally. To my great relief, she seemed comfortable as she drifted in and out of consciousness. We just sat together in the silence. Then after a while I screwed up my courage and asked "Where do you drift off to, Sally? Your face looks so peaceful." She opened her eyes and turned to look at me. Her eyes were full of love and wonder.

In a tiny, soft, and very amused voice, she said, "Well, you may have trouble believing this, but I've been floating around, touring the hospital. I've just been to the cafeteria, watching my parents eat lunch. Dad is having grilled cheese. Mom is eating tuna. They are so sad they can barely eat. I will have to tell them that my body may be dying but *I'm* certainly not. It's more like I'm being born—my consciousness is so free and peaceful." Sally faded out for a while and when she came back she told me: "It's so *beautiful,* Joan. I'm drifting up out of my body toward a kind of living light. It's very bright. So *warm,* so loving." She squeezed my hand a little, "Don't be afraid to die," she said looking at me with so much kindness. "Your soul doesn't die at all. You know? It just goes home. It just goes on from here" [emphasis added].[18]

I have wrestled for years with the question of whether I personally trust these beautiful accounts of the soul surviving death. For me the scientific literature on near-death experiences has deepened the question considerably, and tilted me toward a belief that there is a good chance that these accounts reflect a transcendental mystery.

The Scientific Literature on Near-Death Experiences

I find it intriguing that, at present, the scientific support for the survival-of-death hypothesis is much stronger than the scientific evidence supportive of any decisive "cure" for cancer among the unconventional cancer therapies. In other words, the evidence that we may survive death, while not conclusive, is certainly far better developed, and empirically more persuasive, than the evidence that any unconventional cancer therapy *reliably* leads most people to recover from cancer.

In addition, you cannot read the literature on near-death experiences and communications with the dead without slipping into realms of parapsychology that are difficult to evaluate and strain ordinary norms of credibility. That is, the *science* as reported is often reasonably good; but the *implications* of the scientific reports, if we credit them, lead toward a whole transpersonal reality that many of us (myself included) are not sure whether we can actually credit.

For many, the question of the survival of the personality after death is a key question. One perspective, often voiced by writers in the physical sciences, and one which echos many of the great spiritual traditions, is elaborated by Sir James Jeans in *Physics and Philosophy:*

> When we view ourselves in space and time, our consciousnesses are obviously the separate individuals of a particle-picture, but when we pass beyond space and time, they may perhaps form ingredients of a single continuous stream of life. As with light and electricity, so may it be with life; the phenomena may be individuals carrying on separate existences in space and time, while in the deeper reality beyond space and time we may all be members of one body.[19]

Gertrude Schmeidler, an emeritus professor of psychology at the City University of New York, has contributed a sober evaluation of "Problems Raised by the Concept of the Survival of Personality After Death" to a multidisciplinary discussion of the subject.

Historians and anthropologists, she points out, tell us that the majority opinion of mankind has overwhelmingly held that the personality survives death, but an important minority has thought otherwise. Yet there is great diversity of view cross-culturally regarding what form this future existence takes. Still, Schmeidler finds "one common thread running through all the discrepant ideas of future existence: the idea that the surviving spirit is recognizable."[20] Says Schmeidler:

> The only self-consistent and complete set of answers, so far as I know, consists of attributing all that occurs to the will of God and then stating that the will of God is unknowable and out of reach of science. This means that from the scientific point of view, the commonly held belief that a recognizable personality survives death has no coherent theory to support it. But this does not necessarily mean that the belief is false.[21]

Schmeidler then turns to some of the types of data that address different specific questions regarding the personality surviving death:

> One large set [of data] answers the question of whether the self can, without the intervention of its own body, interact directly with other bodies. This is a

subject studied by parapsychologists, who often divide it into two subtopics: ESP [extrasensory perception], or information obtained without use of the senses, and PK, [psychokinesis], or physical changes produced without bodily intervention. *There is by now clear evidence that such interaction can occur. I will cite a single example, chosen from many others that seem to me equally strong* [emphasis added].[22]

The example Schmeidler cites is of a technique of studying psychokinesis using an instrument called a random number generator (RNG), which records events that physicists consider truly random:

In RNG research, a subject is asked to push a button on a machine so that the next recording will show a particular change (e.g., a faster rate of particle emission on some trials; a slower rate on others.). This is an impossible task for our bodies. Our sense cannot tell us what the next random event will be and our effectors cannot change it. . . .

Radin, May and Thomson . . . summarized the data of all published RNG research with binary targets from the time this method was introduced . . . to 1984. They found 75 reports, describing 332 experiments. When those experiments were evaluated as a whole, they showed success at rates astronomically higher than chance . . . I suggest to you that this demonstrates that some nonbodily part of ourselves can interact with an object in the external world.

This in itself tells us nothing about survival, but it and other evidence for ESP and PK seem to legitimize the concept that our self (whatever it is) includes something that has properties which our body does not have. This in turn seems to legitimize queries about the possibility of nonphysical existence after the body's death, and thus the survival concept.[23]

Schmeidler then discusses the other lines of research that consider the survival hypothesis more directly "but do not give such clear-cut results."

Two of the methods study living persons. One is the near-death experience. . . . Of those who revive after being considered clinically dead, perhaps half report having had vivid experiences while apparently dead. The experiences they report tend to have a good deal in common but are far from a complete overlap. Perhaps most impressive are the occasional cases where a person revived describes accurately events that occurred in a distant place during the time of apparent death.

The second method with living persons tests those who claim to have out-of-body experiences, that is, experiences of being at a location distant from one's body. Some have accurately described events at that distant place. . . .

One method studies the dying. . . . Fairly often a dying person claims that a dead relative has come to help with the transition to an afterlife. . . .

Other methods study the dead. . . . Apparitions sometimes give information that is later found to be correct . . . At least one careful investigation has found that many messages gave correct and specific information known to no one who was present. And psychics and mediums, trying to obtain messages from a dead person, have often reported accurate information that was unknown to anyone present and (more rarely) that was known to no one alive until an attempt to check the message confirmed its correctness.

Each of these lines of evidence can be explained away by one or another counterhypothesis. The commonality among near-death experiences is explained as a combination of physiological change and wishful thinking. All the cases of accurate information are explained as extraordinary examples of effective ESP. . . . The explanations are ad hoc and seem forced; they often postulate more effective ESP than has otherwise been found. They are more intellectually satisfying than the survival interpretation, but whether they are more intellectually satisfying than the thesis of a spirit, separable from the body and surviving death, is still controversial.[24]

The beauty of this summary of the literature on near-death experiences and the survival of death is its neutrality. Schmeidler states the case exactly as I have come to see it: the solid ESP and PK literature clearly suggest that a part of us can function outside ourselves; this in turn is consistent with, but does not demonstrate, the legitimacy of the literature on out-of-body experiences; and both literatures then support, but do not demonstrate, the possibility that near-death experiences are more than simply physiological hallucinations; and this in turn suggests, but does not demonstrate, a rationale for accurate information coming from departed souls.

A number of separate investigators, as Schmeidler suggests, have found that between 35% and 48% of people who come close to death have near–death experiences suggestive of an afterlife. Poll data by George Gallup have also supported these figures.[25]

Karlis Osis and Erlendur Haraldsson did some of the pioneering scientific studies of near-death experiences of dying patients, reported in *At the Hour of*

Death. They studied over 1,000 death or near-death experiences of patients in the United States and northern India in order to achieve a cross-cultural comparison of these experiences from two very different cultures.

They found, first, that the psychological experiences that patients had that were suggestive of postmortem existence were of shorter duration than hallucinations concerned with this life—just as ESP phenomena in general are of shorter duration than imagery related to this world. Second, they found these deathbed visions were mainly of dead and religious figures (by a 4:1 ratio), while only a minority of hallucinations in the general population concern dead and religious people.

> This finding is loud and clear: *When the dying see apparitions, they are nearly always experienced as messengers from a postmortem mode of existence.* Of the human figures seen in visions of the dying, the vast majority were deceased close relatives. This is in agreement with our hypothesis that close relatives would be the natural guides in transitions to an afterlife. Hallucinations of mental patients and drug-induced visions seldom portray close relatives. The pilot survey revealed the most dramatic characteristic of deathbed apparitions: the ostensible intent to take the patient away to the other world. *This was again found to be the dominantly stated purpose of the apparitions of the dying, as well as of come-back cases, in both American and Indian cultures.* . . .

> In the pilot survey, it was noted that patients responded to the otherworldly apparitions in a most surprising manner. They wanted to "go"—that is, to die. Some even bitterly reproached those who resuscitated them. Again, we encountered cases of such resentment in both countries. Nearly all the American patients, and two-thirds of the Indian patients, were ready to go after having seen otherworldly apparitions with a take-away purpose. *Encounters with ostensible messengers from the other world seemed to be so gratifying that the value of this life was easily outweighed* [authors' emphasis].[26]

Patients who saw apparitions concerned with this world did not experience peace and serenity, while those who experienced "messenger" apparitions did. Patients who saw heaven or beautiful gardens reported strongly predominant feelings of peace, serenity, or religious feelings, while a small portion had negative experiences. Qualities of the scenes reported included brightness, intensity of colors, and great beauty. Some patients who saw no visions also became as serene and elated as those who saw messenger figures. And patients who were physiologically close to death had much more "complete" near-death experiences than those who experienced themselves as coming psychologically close to death.

> We found that mood elevation near death resembles those ESP cases where a person will respond with emotions appropriate to a distant event, even though he is not consciously aware of what happened there. . . . . There were some cases where patients ceased to feel pain. According to our afterlife hypothesis, the mind or soul may disengage itself from awareness of bodily pain and discomfort, as if gradually separating from its physical frame.[27]

The authors then review some of the alternative explanations of near-death imagery and experience. These include theories that the experiences are drug-induced; that they are related to brain disturbances caused by disease, injury, or uremic poisoning; that they are caused by lack of oxygen, or psychological factors associated with severe stress, or by cultural factors. In response, they argue that only a small minority of patients with these experiences had received hallucinogenic pain medications, and those that did had no greater frequency of afterlife visions than others. Brain disturbances in general either decreased or did not affect these experiences. Military research on oxygen deprivation, the authors state, does not support the anoxia hypothesis. And psychological factors, which can cause hallucinations, were not found to be related to phenomena associated with postmortem life.[28]

Cultural background, on the other hand, does influence near-death experiences. Indian patients, for example, saw a predominance of elderly male messenger figures while Americans predominantly saw younger female figures. But:

> The phenomena within each culture often do not conform with religious afterlife beliefs. The patients see something new, unexpected, and contrary to their beliefs. Christian ideas of "judgement," "salvation," and "redemption" were not mirrored in the visions of our American patients. Furthermore, while we had many reports about visions of Heaven, visions of Hell and Devils were almost totally absent. . . . We reached the impression that cultural conditioning by Christian and Hindu teaching is, in part, contradicted in the visionary experiences of the dying. It seems to us that besides symbolizations based on inculcated beliefs, terminal patients do "see" something that is unexpected, untaught, and a complete surprise to them.[29]

The core elements described above by Osis and Haraldsson give only a general sense of the near-death experience. Here is a composite near-death experience described by Kenneth Ring, another influential researcher, from his popular *Heading Toward Omega: In Search of the Meaning of the Near-Death Experience:*

The experience begins with a feeling of easeful peace and a sense of well being, which soon culminates in a sense of overwhelming joy and happiness. This ecstatic tone, although fluctuating in intensity from case to case, tends to persist as a constant emotional ground as other features of the experience begin to unfold. At this point, the person is aware that he feels no pain nor does he have any other bodily sensations. Everything is quiet. These cues may suggest to him that he is either in the process of dying or has already "died."

He may then be aware of a transitory buzzing or windlike sound, but, in any event, he finds himself looking down on his physical body. At this time, he finds that he can see and hear perfectly; indeed his vision and hearing tend to be more acute than usual. He is aware of the actions and conversations taking place in the physical environment, in relation to which he finds himself in the role of a passive, detached spectator. All this seems very real—even quite natural—to him; it does not seem at all like a dream or a hallucination. His mental state is one of clarity and alertness.

At some point, he may find himself in a state of *dual awareness*. While he continues to be able to perceive the physical scene around him, he may also become aware of "another reality" and feel himself being drawn into it. He drifts or is ushered into a dark void or tunnel and feels as though he is floating through it. Although he may feel lonely for a time, the experience here is predominantly peaceful and serene. All is extremely quiet and the individual is only aware of his mind and the feeling of floating.

All at once he becomes sensitive to, but does not see, a presence. The presence, who may be heard to speak or who may instead "merely" induce thoughts into the individual's mind, stimulates him to review his life and asks him to decide whether he wants to live or die. This stock-taking may be facilitated by a rapid and vivid visual playback of episodes from the person's life. At this stage, he has no awareness of time or space, and the concepts themselves are meaningless. Neither is he any longer identified with his body. Only the mind is present and it is weighing—logically and rationally—the alternatives that confront him at this threshold separating life from death: to go further into this experience or to return to earthly life. Usually the individual decides to return on the basis not of his own preference, but on the perceived needs of his loved ones, whom his death would necessarily leave behind. Once this decision is made, the experience tends to be abruptly terminated.

Sometimes, however, the decisional crisis occurs later or is altogether absent, and the individual undergoes further experiences. He may, for example, continue to float through the dark void toward a magnetic and brilliant golden light from which emanates feelings of love, warmth and total acceptance. Or he may enter into a "world of light" and preternatural beauty, to be (temporarily) reunited with deceased loved ones before being told, in effect, that it is not yet his time and that he has to return to life.

In any event, whether the individual chooses or is commanded to return to his earthly body and worldly commitments, he does return. Typically, however, he has no recollection of *how* he has effected his "reentry."[30]

A crucial question is whether or not these near-death experiences are simply hallucinations of the dying brain. This suggested a fascinating line of research, part of which was initiated by the cardiologist Michael Sabom, who was initially a skeptic regarding near-death experiences, in his classic *Recollections of Death*. Sabom took special note of the fact that one aspect of the near-death experience is that it is simultaneously an out-of-body experience. Ring summarizes:

Sabom made a diligent search for detailed OBE (out-of-body experiences) accounts from NDErs [those who have had near-death experiences] on the grounds that such reports provide one of the few avenues through which to secure data about NDEs that can be independently corroborated. . . . If [for example] a patient whose eyes, let's say, are taped shut, suffers cardiac arrest and has an OBE during which he later claims to have seen two physicians, one of them black, whom he has never met before, hurriedly enter the operating room to assist in the defibrillation procedure whose details he then describes in correct sequence, this is obviously an account that does not depend for its veracity on the patient's say-so. . . . This is precisely what Sabom has done in a half dozen incidents where his respondents have given him highly specific and sequential accounts of their OBEs while near death. By interviewing members of the original medical team involved in these cases, talking to family members who had pertinent information, and checking the medical records directly, Sabom was able to produce impressive if not conclusive evidence of apparently accurate perceptions during OBEs. In short, according to Sabom, patients were describing events they could not have seen given the position of their body and could not have known given their physical condition.[31]

The work of Stanley Grof, a highly innovative psychiatrist who did careful research using LSD in psychotherapy with dying cancer patients, gives further interesting insight into the phenomenon of near-death experiences. In Grof's work, the patients he worked with, who were given LSD after very careful preparation and watched through the procedure, went through a set of phases that began with the very difficult experience of physical death and ended in an ecstatic experience of rebirth. When these patients had completed the death-rebirth experience, they were characteristically convinced that at the time of actual death their souls would survive, and they had no further fear of death.

The Great Art of Making the Dying Physically Comfortable

It is an expression of the malady of our time that while many people want to attend lectures on transcendent experiences in death and dying, far fewer people take the time to visit and sit with the dying, and fewer still are interested in the practical matters of making a dying person as comfortable physically as possible so that he and his family members have some chance to enjoy the last months, weeks, or days of life.

The reality is that practical knowledge is as important, and often more important, than an ungrounded spiritual impulse to assist the dying. As Sylvia Lack, M.D., told a training conference for physicians concerned with the care of the dying:

> There is far too much talk in death and dying circles in this country about psychological and emotional problems, and far too little about making the patient comfortable. Any group concerned with service to the dying should be talking about smoothing sheets, rubbing bottoms, relieving constipation, and sitting up at night. Counselling a person who is lying in a wet bed is ineffective . . . If people are cared for with common sense and basic professional skills, with detailed attention to self-evident problems and physical needs, the patients and the families themselves cope with many of their emotional crises. Without pain, well nursed, with bowels controlled, mouth clean, and a caring friend available, the psychological problems fall into manageable perspective.[32]

One of my favorite books on the practical aspects of dying is by Deborah Duda, *A Guide to Dying at Home*.[33] In the chapter called "Getting on with It: Preparations and Homecoming," Duda covers what you need to die at home. Here she lists everything from the doctor, medicines, and bed to such essential details as hot-water bottles, a dishpan for bathing, and drinking straws that bend.

Duda covers in detail how to choose a physician who will honor your wishes, how to work effectively with a physician, pain control, and giving shots or injections.[34]

One of the best health professional guides I have seen in this area is *The Physician's Handbook of Symptom Relief in Terminal Care,*[35] by Gary A. Johanson, M.D. of the Home Hospice of Sonoma County, California. The *Physician's Handbook* is a loose-leaf binder with color tab–coded sections that cover common problems the physician, patient, or family member may encounter. In offering this compendium, Johanson writes:

> The degree of success achieved in skilled symptom control will greatly influence how effectively caregivers and families will be able to assist patients in realizing their emotional, spiritual and social comfort in the final days of their lives.
>
> The greatest asset in terminal care is a listening/caring approach. The greatest skill is knowing when it is appropriate to apply which palliative measure.
>
> No matter how much we deny it, the fact is that conventional treatment often becomes inappropriate, and therefore poor medicine in the terminal patient. We who care for these patients are not off the hook simply by plugging along on conventional treatment pathways when it is no longer appropriate. . . .
>
> There is always something that can be done for terminal patients. None of us can expect to know all the techniques that have been developed in the area of terminal care. For our patients' benefit and our own education, we should not hesitate to consult a reference or a colleague for assistance.[36]

This handbook is not only useful for physicians but also for patients and family members who want to be knowledgeable about the options that physicians and nurses are (or should be) considering. Many physicians have relatively little interest in or knowledge of how to provide the best possible support for a dying person. It is a very high and, in fact, noble skill of the healer. Having this information represents another area in which the patient or family member is able to work more effectively in partnership with physicians and nurses.

While Johanson's *Physician's Handbook* does an excellent job of covering the more technical aspects of symptom relief in dying, Duda provides a practical introduction to making the senses comfortable and to providing enjoyable experiences wherever possible.

Her discussion covers touch (massage, hair care, hugging, holding, and cuddling), moving the person, smells, cleanliness, creating beautiful environments, hearing (sound, music, reading), and taste and diet. The issues of intravenous (IV) feeding and dehydration represent an example of a critical area in which knowledge and forethought can make a vital difference in the dying experience. Says Duda:

> IVs are used to nourish people who can't eat or drink enough to stay alive. The decision whether or not to use IVs in terminal care raises again the question of the quality of life versus the quantity. Feeding the body cells by means of IVs often prolongs the life of the body. The cost is discomfort, less ability to move and the need to have a nurse. Dad said, "When I have all those tubes in I feel like a patient. When I don't, I feel like me."

> The result of not taking enough fluids into the body is dehydration. *The chemical imbalance created by a lack of fluids often causes a person to have a sense of well-being or euphoria* [emphasis added]. It's a relatively comfortable death. The main discomfort, dryness of the mouth and thirst, is helped by sucking on ice chips and clean moist washcloths. It generally takes only a few days for a debilitated person to die from lack of fluids.[37]

Duda is supported by medical experts in this opinion on dehydration. Johanson suggests a policy for IV fluid therapy:

> In the terminal patient, the benefits of dehydration can be many, including sedation, decreased vomiting, and decreased urine output and secretions. IV fluids should only be used if hydration seems like it will improve alertness, decrease nausea, prolong life in a positive way, or otherwise provide true comfort.

> Conscious withholding of intravenous and other supportive measures is not a question of "non-treatment." Instead, it is a matter of what is appropriate treatment from a biologic, humane and spiritual point of view. Some patients suffer as much from inappropriate treatment as they do from the underlying illness itself.

> In other words, IV infusion should be looked upon as primarily a supportive measure for use in acute or acute-superimposed-upon-chronic illnesses to assist a patient through a temporary period toward some recovery of health. To use such measures in the terminally ill, without such expectation of return to health, is generally inappropriate and therefore not good medicine. Such measures should ethically only be used if the treating physician is convinced they are clearly contributing to the comfort of the patient.[38]

Dying and Grieving

Dying and grieving are deeply interconnected, so it makes sense to treat them together. The dying person must engage in *anticipatory grieving* for the loss of himself. The family and friends who will be left behind have what is often as sharp—and sometimes even sharper—a grief to deal with. They, too, may do anticipatory grieving, and they will also grieve later.

Grieving is something that one can learn how to do. It is something that can cripple a life experience—or a dying experience—if it is drastically incomplete. Many cultures prescribe elaborate and effective systems of grieving. In the United States, we have lost most of these rituals—a very great loss, indeed. And so it has been the psychiatrists and other modern shamans who have taken on the job of helping us grieve our own deaths or the deaths of those we love.

One of the best known theories of the dying process has been presented by Elisabeth Kübler-Ross. In her famous book, *On Death and Dying,* she presents a theory of a series of stages in the human response to dying. The first stage of the dying process, according to Kübler-Ross, is *denial and isolation:*

> Denial, at least partial denial, is used by almost all patients, not only during the first stages of illness or following confrontation, but also later on from time to time. . . . These patients can consider the possibility of their own death for a while but then have to put this consideration away in order to pursue life. . . . Denial functions as a buffer after unexpected shocking news, allows the patient to collect himself and, with time, mobilize other, less radical defenses.[39]

Actually, Kübler-Ross notes that the very first reaction may be a temporary state of shock, which is then followed by this initial response of denial.

The second stage for Kübler-Ross is *anger.*

> The next logical question becomes: "Why me?". . . In contrast to the stage of denial, this stage of anger is very difficult to cope with from the point of view of family and staff. The reason for this is the fact that this anger is displaced in all directions and projected onto the environment at times almost at random.[40]

The third stage is *bargaining:*

> The third stage, the stage of bargaining, is less well known but equally helpful to the patient, though only for brief periods of time. If we have been unable to face the sad facts in the first period and have been angry at people and God in the second phase, maybe we can succeed in entering into some sort of an agreement which may postpone the inevitable happening: "If God has decided to take us from this earth and he did not respond to my angry pleas, he may be more favorable if I ask nicely."[41]

The fourth stage is *depression:*

> When the terminally ill patient can no longer deny his illness, when he is forced to undergo more surgery or hospitalization, when he begins to have more symptoms or becomes weaker and thinner, he cannot smile it off any more. His numbness or stoicism, his anger and rage will soon be replaced with a sense of loss. This loss may have many facets: a woman with a breast cancer may react to the loss of her figure; a woman with a cancer of the uterus may feel she is no longer a woman. . . . With the extensive treatment and hospitalization, financial burdens are added; little luxuries at first and necessities later may not be afforded any more. . . . All these reasons for depression are well known to everyone who deals with patients. What we often tend to forget, however, is the preparatory grief that the terminally ill patient has to undergo in order to prepare himself for his final separation from this world. If I were to attempt to differentiate these two kinds of depressions, I would regard the first one as a reactive depression, the second one as a preparatory depression. The first one is different in nature and should be dealt with quite differently from the latter.[42]

In Kübler-Ross's view, we can respond to the reactive depression with action—seeking to ameliorate the losses with word or deed. The preparatory depression, on the other hand, should not be met with any attempt to "fix it":

> The patient should not be encouraged to look at the sunny side of things, as this would mean he should not contemplate his impending death. It would be contraindicated to tell him not to be sad, since all of us are tremendously sad when we lose one beloved person. The patient is in the process of losing everything and everybody he loves. If he is allowed to express his sorrow he will find a final acceptance much easier, and he will be grateful to those who can sit with him during this state of depression without constantly telling him not to be sad.[43]

The fifth and final stage is *acceptance:*

If a patient has enough time (i.e., not a sudden, unexpected death) and has been given some help in working through the previously described stages, he will reach a stage during which he is neither depressed nor angry about his "fate.". . . Acceptance should not be mistaken for a happy stage. It is almost void of feelings. It is as if the pain had gone, the struggle is over, and there comes a time for "the final rest before the long journey" as one patient phrased it. . . . While the dying patient has found some peace and acceptance, his circle of interest diminishes. He wishes to be left alone or at least not stirred up by news and problems of the outside world. Visitors are often not desired and if they come, the patient is no longer in a talkative mood. . . . He may hold our hand and ask us to sit in silence. Such moments of silence may be the most meaningful communications for people who are not uncomfortable in the presence of a dying person. We may together listen to the song of a bird from the outside. Our presence may just confirm that we are going to be around until the end. We may just let him know that it is all right to say nothing when the important things are taken care of and it is only a question of time until he can close his eyes forever.[44]

While these are the five stages of dying for Kübler-Ross, it is often forgotten that she also accords a special place to *hope* throughout the five-stage process.

We have discussed so far the different stages that people go through when they are faced with tragic news. . . . These means will last for different periods of time and will replace each other or exist at times side by side. The one thing that usually persists through all these stages is hope. . . . In listening to our terminally ill patients we were always impressed that even the most accepting, the most realistic patients left the possibility open for some cure, for the discovery of a new drug or the "last minute success in a research project.". . . It is this glimpse of hope which maintains them through days, weeks or months of suffering.[45]

Other Views of the Process of Dying

Kübler-Ross's vision of the stages of dying has many virtues, but it has been strongly criticized by many thoughtful professionals. Edwin S. Shneidman is one:

In the current thanatological scene there are those who write about fewer than a half-dozen stages lived through in a specific order—not to mention the even more obfuscating writing of a life after death. My own experiences have led me to rather different conclusions. In working with dying persons I see a wide range of human emotions—few in some people, dozens in others—experienced in a variety of orderings, reorderings, and arrangements. The one psychological mechanism that seems ubiquitous is denial, which can appear or reappear at any time. Nor is there any natural law that an individual has to achieve closure before death sets its seal. In fact, most people die too soon or too late, with loose threads and fragments of agenda uncompleted.

My own notion is more general in scope; more specific in content. . . . My general hypothesis is that a *dying person's flow of behaviors will reflect or parallel that person's previous segments of behaviors, specifically those behaviors relating to threat, stress or failure.* There are certain *consistencies* in human beings. Individuals die more-or-less characteristically as they have lived, relative to those aspects of personality which relate to their conceptualization of their dying. To oversimplify: The psychological course of the cancer mirrors certain deep troughs in the course of the life—*oncology recapitulates ontogeny* [Shneidman's emphasis].[46]

Another special observer of the dying process was Erich Lindemann, Professor of Psychiatry at Harvard, who studied loss and grieving for years before he developed cancer. Lindemann described his own process of *anticipatory grieving* in the face of his impending death from cancer.

First, he wanted *information* from his physicians, and he wrestled with all the complex questions about what a physician should and should not tell a patient and how the news should be transmitted. Second, he struggled with what to do with the feelings that his impending death brought up for him. Third, he found that the agreement with family and friends on *the ways in which he would be remembered* was of critical importance to him:

It can only be represented by symbols, such as a book, or—there is a building named for me in Boston, the Lindemann Mental Health Center, which means an awful lot. So you have something which continues your identity's existence by a global attribute, a book or a building which then allows the survivors to remember those things which are pertinent to *you,* the particular person, just as at various stages of your anticipatory grieving you think about various aspects of that life which you are now reconstructing.

Now [this] . . . was a revelation to me and led me to wonder, in looking at grief in patients, if they have similar tasks. They don't write books, but with members of their families, or the nurse, they have confidential exchanges about the sort of things they did with other people. They like to be visited by a lot of friends, so long as they don't feel too embarrassed about sharing their emotions, and would like to pick up items of their lives which they shared with the future survivors. And they will rub in these experiences with the family and friends, so they will be sure to remember when they are gone. So this constructing of a collective survival image of oneself which will still be there when one happens not to be there any more in the flesh is the core of grieving, which, if it is done well, is apt to be an admirable process—a fascinating process if one is lucky enough to witness it.

Then Lindemann comes to a beautiful and rarely described issue:

Every once in a while one hears about some person who is confronted with a severe illness and is not going to live, who is an inspiration to somebody else. And from our observations, it is these people who do such a good job of recalling their own lives and their own shared experiences, constructing an image which is a tenable image of a human being. . . .

[Sometimes] there is not enough contact between the patient and his family. The family gets into a conflict over whether to stay or not, how much to share in the patient's illness; whether these sometimes trite things which the patient brings up are worth the time of the patient and everybody else. And for the family, a very important problem may come up . . . namely, that one does one's grieving so well that one emancipates oneself from the person who is going to die and then has no relationship anymore. The [family] don't know whether to visit or whether to stay away; if they try to pull themselves out of the bondage they will feel they are disloyal. This problem of a relationship which may be severed too successfully becomes a difficult one for the anticipatory griever. Sometimes patients who have a terminal illness come to terms with this illness, are all settled; and then when people still come, they don't want to see them anymore. One wonders what is the matter with them unless one is aware of the fact that a process has been going on, and one has to tap at what phase this process is now.[47]

Lindemann describes how important to him it was to go and visit places that had had great meaning to him:

I really became hypermanic, in the sense that I raced around and wanted to do all the things that would be wonderful to do once more. In other words, see that people who are confronting death are not in an environment which is restrictive of *doing* possibilities; that they are still as mobile as is compatible with their ailments, and still as rich in possible experiences for a little while. I guess it isn't silly to make up for the things you won't have any more of later, and token fulfillment along that line can make an enormous difference.[48]

Grieving for Survivors

"A person's death is not only an ending: it is also a beginning—for the survivors," writes Shneidman. Studies of widows who have recently lost a husband show a heightened likelihood of death from alcoholism, malnutrition, and other conditions. It seems "grief is itself a dire process, almost akin to a disease, and that there are subtle factors at work that can take a heavy toll unless they are treated and controlled."[49]

The death of someone we love can induce a response very similar to that found in those who have experienced a disaster such as an earthquake or explosion:

> Martha Wolfenstein has described a "disaster syndrome": a combination of emotional dullness, unresponsiveness to outer stimulation and inhibition of activity. The individual who has just undergone disaster is apt to suffer from at least a transitory sense of worthlessness; his usual capacity for self love becomes impaired."[50]

Lily Pincus was a distinguished social worker who lived in England and wrote a book called *Death and the Family: The Importance of Mourning.*

> All studies agree that *shock* is the first response to death. . . . It may find expression in physical collapse . . . , in violent outbursts . . . , or in dazed withdrawal, denial, and inability to take in the reality of death.

> Mourners often complain that they were not prepared for what it would be like: "Why did nobody warn me that I would feel so sick . . . or tired . . . or exhausted?"; "Nobody ever told me that grief felt so like fear"; "I wish I had known about the turmoil of emotions . . ."[51]

The acute shock, says Pincus, usually lasts only a few days, followed by a *controlled phase* during which the mourner is supported by relatives and friends.

> The real pain and misery makes itself felt when this controlled phase, and the privileges that went with it, is over, and the task of testing reality, coming to terms with the new situation, and the painful withdrawal of libido from the lost person begin. It is then that the mourner feels lost and abandoned and attempts to develop defenses against the agonies of pain. *Searching* for the lost person, an almost automatic universal defense against accepting the reality of loss, may go on for a long time. . . .

Most people are not aware of their need to search but express it in restless behavior tension, and loss of interest in all that does not concern the deceased. These symptoms lessen as bit by bit the reality of the loss can be accepted and the bereaved slowly, slowly rebuilds his inner world. . . .

As the bereaved becomes more relaxed, and tension, frustration, and pain decrease, *searching* may lead to *finding* a sense of the lost person's presence. . . .

There are no timetables for what have been called the phases of mourning, nor are there distinct lines of demarcation for the various symptoms of grief which find expression during these phases. For the bereaved, the most alarming and bewildering aspects of grief are those in which he can no longer recognize himself, for example, the often irrational anger and hostility, which may be quite alien to the mourner's usual behavior and may make him feel that he is going insane. . . . They express the ambivalence of the mourner toward all these people but most especially, and painfully, toward the lost person who is causing him so much distress by his abandonment.[52]

For the shock that may immediately follow death, warmth and rest and a nourishing protective environment can be a real help. For the controlled period that Pincus mentions above, the support of friends and relatives can make a great difference.

The great challenge takes place as we begin to face life without the person we loved, and here the truth seems to be "the fundamental importance of being able to mourn and to 'complete the mourning process'." But, like the fight for life with cancer, there are no firm guidelines for how to complete the mourning process; each must be "allowed to mourn in his own way and his own time."[53]

The mourning process, like the process of physical healing, involves the healing of a wound, a new formation of healthy tissue. In mourning, however, the cause of the injury, the loss of an important person, must not be forgotten. Only when the lost person has been internalized and becomes part of the bereaved, a part which can be integrated with his own personality and enriches it, is the mourning process complete. With this enriched personality the adjustment to a new life has to be made.[54]

Conclusion

Of all the chapters in this book, this has been the most difficult to write. Writing this chapter immersed me in the awesome and varied literature on death, dying, and mourning. On the one hand I felt grateful for the experience because I learned in greater depth things that I can pass on to others in the Cancer Help Program and through this book.

But the simple fact is that as I write these words, death, in my eyes, has not lost its power. It may well be that the soul survives death. I was skeptical of this years ago, but now believe it to be as likely as not. It is certainly true that we can detoxify death—that we can remove the taboos of thinking and feeling about it, and that great comfort and understanding can come from this process.

But even if I knew for a fact that my soul and the souls of those I love will survive death, I am not sure the pain of death and loss would be gone. I remember the story of an enlightened Eastern teacher who lost his child to death. His students came to see him the next day and found him crying.

"Master," one said, "you teach us that all life is an illusion. How is it that you are crying because of the death of your child?"

"It is true that life is an illusion," the master responded. "But the death of a child is the greatest illusion of all."

I go back to the words I started the chapter with, the words of the Buddha: "Even the wise fear death. Life clings to life." We have read, and can read, of those who overcome this fear. But most of us fear death. There is no shame in this. Death remains a great mystery, the central problem with which religion and philosophy and science have wrestled with since the beginning of human history. Acknowledging this, we can, perhaps, come to face it with greater understanding, more preparation, and greater love.

References

1   Eric J. Cassell, *The Healer's Art* (Cambridge, Mass.: MIT Press, 1989), 210.

2   Peter A. Singer and Mark Siegler, "Euthanasia—A Critique," *New England Journal of Medicine* 322(26):1881 (1990).

3   D.J. Enright, "Introduction." In D.J. Enright, ed., *The Oxford Book of Death,* (Oxford: Oxford Press, 1987), xi.

4   Arnold Toynbee, "Life After Death." Ibid., 3.

5   Maria Monroe, "Before There Was Death," letter to the editor, *Inquiring Mind* 6(2):2 (1990).

6   Montaigne. In Enright, ed., *The Oxford Book of Death,* 2.

7   C.G. Jung, "The Soul and Death." In Enright, ed., *The Oxford Book of Death*, 45.

8   Desiderius Erasmus, *Colloquies,* trans. Craig R. Thompson. In Enright, ed., *The Oxford Book of Death*, 46.

9   Arnold Toynbee, "The Relation Between Life and Death, Living and Dying." In Edwin S. Shneidman, ed., *Death: Current Perspectives* (Mountain View, Calif.: Mayfield Publishing Company, 1984), 10–4.

10 Ernest Becker, "The Terror of Death." In Shneidman, ed., *Death*, 15–6.

11 Ibid., 18.

12 Ibid., 19.

13 Geoffrey Gorer, "The Pornography of Death." In Shneidman, ed., *Death*, 26.

14 Philippe Aries, *The Hour of Our Death* (New York: Vintage Books, 1982), 589.

15 Steven Levine, *Healing into Life and Death* (Garden City, N.Y.: Anchor Press, Doubleday, 1987), 4–15.

16 Steven Levine, interview in *Inquiring Mind,* 6(2):1–6 (Spring 1990).

17 Dennis R. Leahy, "The People." In Eric Blau, *Common Heros: Facing a Life-Threatening Illness* (Pasadena, Calif.: New Sage Press, 1989).

18 Joan Borysenko, *Guilt Is the Teacher, Love Is the Lesson* (New York: Warner books, 1990), 15–7.

19 Sir James Jeans, *Physics and Philosophy.* In Larry Dossey, *Beyond Illness: Discovering the Experience of Health* (Boston: New Science Library, 1984), 139.

20 Gertrude R. Schmeidler, "Problems Raised by the Concept of the Survival of Personality After Death." In Arthur Berger et al., ed., *Perspectives on Death and Dying: Cross-Cultural and Multi-Disciplinary Views* (Philadelphia: Charles Press Publishers, 1989), 201–2.

21 Ibid., 205–6.

22 Ibid., 206.

23 Ibid., 206–7.

24 Ibid., 207.

25 Kenneth Ring, *Heading Toward Omega: In Search of the Meaning of the Near-Death Experience* (New York: Morrow, 1985), 35.

26 Karlis Osis and Erlendur Haraldsson, *At the Hour of Death* (New York: Hastings House, Publishers, 1986), 186. © 1977 by Karlis Osis and Erlender Haraldsson. Reprinted with permission of the publisher, Hastings House.

27 Ibid., 188–9.

28 Ibid., 189–90.

29   Ibid., 191–3.

30   Ring, *Heading Toward Omega,* 36–7.

31   Ibid., 41–2.

32   Sylvia Lack, quoted in Deborah Duda, *A Guide to Dying at Home* (Santa Fe, N.M.: John Muir Publications, 1982), 150. Reprinted with permission from the publisher John Muir Publications. © Deborah Duda.

33   Deborah Duda, *A Guide to Dying at Home* (Santa Fe, N.M.: Hohn Muir Publications, 1982).

34   Duda, *A Guide to Dying at Home,* 102–10.

35   Gary A. Johanson, M.D., *Physician's Handbook of Symptom Relief in Terminal Care* (Sonoma County, Calif.: Home Hospice of Sonoma County, 1988).

36   Ibid., iii–iv.

37   Duda, *A Guide to Dying at Home,* 128–9.

38   Johanson, *Physician's Handbook* appendix 1.

39   Elisabeth Kübler-Ross *On Death and Dying*, (New York: Collier, 1970), 38–9. Reprinted with permission of Macmillan Publishing Co. Copyright © 1969 by Elizabeth Kübler-Ross.

40   Ibid., 50–1.

41   Ibid., 2.

42   Ibid., 85–6.

43   Ibid., 87.

44   Ibid., 112–3.

45   Ibid., 13–39.

46   Edwin S. Shneidman, "Some Aspects of Therapy with Dying Persons." In Shneidman, ed., *Death: Current Perspectives,* 275–6.

47   Erich Lindemann, "Reactions to One's Own Fatal Illness." In ibid., 262–3.

48   Ibid., 265.

49   Edwin S. Shneidman, "Postvention and the Survivor-Victim." Ibid., 412–3.

50   Ibid., 414.

51   Lily Pincus, "The Process of Mourning and Grief." In Shneidman, *Death: Current Perspectives*, 402–3. Copyright © 1974 by Lily Pincas. Reprinted by permission of Pantheon Books, a division of Random House, Inc.

52   Ibid., 405.

53   Ibid., 408.

54   Ibid., 409.

Making Your Choices

We come to the end of this book. This last chapter is an informal review of points we have discussed throughout the book organized around the question of how you approach making your choices. Following this chapter is an appendix, Choice in Resources, that discusses numerous specific options in both conventional and complementary therapies. You may wish to review that appendix after reading this chapter.

Remember, your choices do not have to be made all at once. That would be overwhelming as well as unwise. So do not think too far ahead—only as far as you need to. Many months may pass before the next choice needs to be made.

Obviously I cannot describe all the permutations you may face at each step of the way, but I would like to map out for you the critical moments of choice in the chronological order in which most patients face them.

At each point in facing cancer, you are given an opportunity to develop new knowledge, skills, and control. However, if you like, you can also make the choice not to learn too much. Some people feel they would like to leave most of the choices to their physicians.

Choice Points

Prevention

Although the audience for this book is primarily people with cancer and the health professionals who care for them, the issue of prevention is painfully important to many people with cancer who are concerned that their children may be at risk. Perhaps the most common concerns are voiced by women with breast cancer—sometimes themselves the daughters of mothers who had breast cancer—who are deeply concerned for their own daughters. In fact, there are some very important things that can be done when children are young to lower their lifetime risk of cancer, such as providing them information concerning sane approaches to carcinogen exposures, diet, exercise, and mental health.

Prediagnosis

At this point you may have identified a lump or some other warning sign of possible cancer but have not yet seen a doctor. Enter the medical system carefully by selecting a physician who has a good reputation for both the competent and humane handling of diagnosis and for his skills in treatment. You might prepare yourself by making a list of questions and suggestions about, for instance, how you want to be told if the diagnosis is cancer; how long the test results will take to get back; and how much time you would have to make a decision on therapy, if the tests prove positive.

Diagnosis

This is a critical point. The delivery of a cancer diagnosis by a physician is, as we have seen, a considerable art. If the delivery of the diagnosis is done badly, you may need to recover not only from the shock of diagnosis but from the way the doctor told you. Many people literally go into shock when they are given a cancer diagnosis. They may not hear anything the physician says after the word "cancer." Bringing a tape recorder to the session is one possibility (some physicians even provide tapes of the diagnostic session precisely because recall is often so distorted by shock). In the period in which you are in shock,

References

1   Eric J. Cassell, *The Healer's Art* (Cambridge, Mass.: MIT Press, 1989), 210.

2   Peter A. Singer and Mark Siegler, "Euthanasia—A Critique," *New England Journal of Medicine* 322(26):1881 (1990).

3   D.J. Enright, "Introduction." In D.J. Enright, ed., *The Oxford Book of Death,* (Oxford: Oxford Press, 1987), xi.

4   Arnold Toynbee, "Life After Death." Ibid., 3.

5   Maria Monroe, "Before There Was Death," letter to the editor, *Inquiring Mind* 6(2):2 (1990).

6   Montaigne. In Enright, ed., *The Oxford Book of Death,* 2.

7   C.G. Jung, "The Soul and Death." In Enright, ed., *The Oxford Book of Death*, 45.

8   Desiderius Erasmus, *Colloquies,* trans. Craig R. Thompson. In Enright, ed., *The Oxford Book of Death*, 46.

9   Arnold Toynbee, "The Relation Between Life and Death, Living and Dying." In Edwin S. Shneidman, ed., *Death: Current Perspectives* (Mountain View, Calif.: Mayfield Publishing Company, 1984), 10–4.

10 Ernest Becker, "The Terror of Death." In Shneidman, ed., *Death*, 15–6.

11 Ibid., 18.

12 Ibid., 19.

13 Geoffrey Gorer, "The Pornography of Death." In Shneidman, ed., *Death*, 26.

14 Philippe Aries, *The Hour of Our Death* (New York: Vintage Books, 1982), 589.

15 Steven Levine, *Healing into Life and Death* (Garden City, N.Y.: Anchor Press, Doubleday, 1987), 4–15.

16 Steven Levine, interview in *Inquiring Mind,* 6(2):1–6 (Spring 1990).

17 Dennis R. Leahy, "The People." In Eric Blau, *Common Heros: Facing a Life-Threatening Illness* (Pasadena, Calif.: New Sage Press, 1989).

18 Joan Borysenko, *Guilt Is the Teacher, Love Is the Lesson* (New York: Warner books, 1990), 15–7.

19 Sir James Jeans, *Physics and Philosophy.* In Larry Dossey, *Beyond Illness: Discovering the Experience of Health* (Boston: New Science Library, 1984), 139.

20 Gertrude R. Schmeidler, "Problems Raised by the Concept of the Survival of Personality After Death." In Arthur Berger et al., ed., *Perspectives on Death and Dying: Cross-Cultural and Multi-Disciplinary Views* (Philadelphia: Charles Press Publishers, 1989), 201–2.

21 Ibid., 205–6.

22 Ibid., 206.

23 Ibid., 206–7.

24 Ibid., 207.

25 Kenneth Ring, *Heading Toward Omega: In Search of the Meaning of the Near-Death Experience* (New York: Morrow, 1985), 35.

26 Karlis Osis and Erlendur Haraldsson, *At the Hour of Death* (New York: Hastings House, Publishers, 1986), 186. © 1977 by Karlis Osis and Erlender Haraldsson. Reprinted with permission of the publisher, Hastings House.

27 Ibid., 188–9.

28 Ibid., 189–90.

29   Ibid., 191–3.

30   Ring, *Heading Toward Omega,* 36–7.

31   Ibid., 41–2.

32   Sylvia Lack, quoted in Deborah Duda, *A Guide to Dying at Home* (Santa Fe, N.M.: John Muir Publications, 1982), 150. Reprinted with permission from the publisher John Muir Publications. © Deborah Duda.

33   Deborah Duda, *A Guide to Dying at Home* (Santa Fe, N.M.: Hohn Muir Publications, 1982).

34   Duda, *A Guide to Dying at Home,* 102–10.

35   Gary A. Johanson, M.D., *Physician's Handbook of Symptom Relief in Terminal Care* (Sonoma County, Calif.: Home Hospice of Sonoma County, 1988).

36   Ibid., iii–iv.

37   Duda, *A Guide to Dying at Home,* 128–9.

38   Johanson, *Physician's Handbook* appendix 1.

39   Elisabeth Kübler-Ross *On Death and Dying,* (New York: Collier, 1970), 38–9. Reprinted with permission of Macmillan Publishing Co. Copyright © 1969 by Elizabeth Kübler-Ross.

40   Ibid., 50–1.

41   Ibid., 2.

42   Ibid., 85–6.

43   Ibid., 87.

44   Ibid., 112–3.

45   Ibid., 13–39.

46   Edwin S. Shneidman, "Some Aspects of Therapy with Dying Persons." In Shneidman, ed., *Death: Current Perspectives,* 275–6.

47   Erich Lindemann, "Reactions to One's Own Fatal Illness." In ibid., 262–3.

48   Ibid., 265.

49   Edwin S. Shneidman, "Postvention and the Survivor-Victim." Ibid., 412–3.

50   Ibid., 414.

51   Lily Pincus, "The Process of Mourning and Grief." In Shneidman, *Death: Current Perspectives,* 402–3. Copyright © 1974 by Lily Pincas. Reprinted by permission of Pantheon Books, a division of Random House, Inc.

52   Ibid., 405.

53   Ibid., 408.

54   Ibid., 409.

Making Your Choices

We come to the end of this book. This last chapter is an informal review of points we have discussed throughout the book organized around the question of how you approach making your choices. Following this chapter is an appendix, Choice in Resources, that discusses numerous specific options in both conventional and complementary therapies. You may wish to review that appendix after reading this chapter.

Remember, your choices do not have to be made all at once. That would be overwhelming as well as unwise. So do not think too far ahead—only as far as you need to. Many months may pass before the next choice needs to be made.

Obviously I cannot describe all the permutations you may face at each step of the way, but I would like to map out for you the critical moments of choice in the chronological order in which most patients face them.

At each point in facing cancer, you are given an opportunity to develop new knowledge, skills, and control. However, if you like, you can also make the choice not to learn too much. Some people feel they would like to leave most of the choices to their physicians.

Prevention

Although the audience for this book is primarily people with cancer and the health professionals who care for them, the issue of prevention is painfully important to many people with cancer who are concerned that their children may be at risk. Perhaps the most common concerns are voiced by women with breast cancer—sometimes themselves the daughters of mothers who had breast cancer—who are deeply concerned for their own daughters. In fact, there are some very important things that can be done when children are young to lower their lifetime risk of cancer, such as providing them information concerning sane approaches to carcinogen exposures, diet, exercise, and mental health.

Prediagnosis

At this point you may have identified a lump or some other warning sign of possible cancer but have not yet seen a doctor. Enter the medical system carefully by selecting a physician who has a good reputation for both the competent and humane handling of diagnosis and for his skills in treatment. You might prepare yourself by making a list of questions and suggestions about, for instance, how you want to be told if the diagnosis is cancer; how long the test results will take to get back; and how much time you would have to make a decision on therapy, if the tests prove positive.

Diagnosis

This is a critical point. The delivery of a cancer diagnosis by a physician is, as we have seen, a considerable art. If the delivery of the diagnosis is done badly, you may need to recover not only from the shock of diagnosis but from the way the doctor told you. Many people literally go into shock when they are given a cancer diagnosis. They may not hear anything the physician says after the word "cancer." Bringing a tape recorder to the session is one possibility (some physicians even provide tapes of the diagnostic session precisely because recall is often so distorted by shock). In the period in which you are in shock, it is unwise for you to make choices about therapies or to allow yourself to be rushed into treatment. The best treatment for shock is to be in a warm, safe place with a caring friend and nourishing food. When you begin to emerge from shock, you will begin naturally to think about choices that need to be made. Pressing choices before that is a serious error.

Choosing a Physician and Therapy

There is no rule that the doctor who gives you your diagnosis need be your physician for treatment. Choosing a treatment physician and the initial therapy are two of the most critical choices you can make. Here are a number of points to think about:

- Do you want a physician you can trust who will make all the decisions? A physician who will explain options but guide you to the choice he believes best? A physician who will explain options but be willing to share the choice with you? Or a physician who will be your consultant as you do extensive research and choose for yourself? All are legitimate approaches.
- Do you want to select as your physician the first physician you contact? Do you want to get two or three opinions before you select a physician? Or do you want to shop extensively for a physician? You may have a choice among the many specialists—surgeons, radiologists, chemotherapists—as well as other therapists. A good approach is to find an oncologist that you can trust to set out your options and coordinate the other specialists.
- Just how much reading and research do you want to do before choosing a therapy? Do not let anyone rush you into treatment, unless necessary (not very frequent in cancer) until you have completed your investigations.

Coping with Treatment

Coping with treatment often involves developing skills that most physicians do not discuss. One of the best resources for developing skills in coping with treatment is an independent support group where patients are supported by the facilitator in exchanging information with one another on methods for handling cancer and treatment. Patients should be able to discuss both complementary therapies and mainstream treatments. A support group is a very good place to start. One young man, who was connected with the Wellness Community in Santa Monica, decided to organize his own support group before entering a particularly severe treatment—interleukin-2—for a recurrence of his malignant melanoma. He talked with them about ways they could help him best with the 6 weeks of excruciating treatment. They were then able to organize visiting times and to respond to his requests "to talk to me" or "just play me some music" or "just sit here, saying nothing," etc. Pain and disorientation can be greatly diminished when friends and family know just how they can help best.

Complementary Cancer Therapies

Choices in complementary therapies are even more difficult than choices in conventional therapies because of the relative scarcity of evidence with which to assess different options. Complementary cancer therapies include spiritual, psychological, nutritional, physical, pharmacological, herbal, traditional, and the other approaches I have described in previous chapters.

Since I have already discussed complementary therapies at length in this book, here I will simply remind you of a few rules of thumb in searching for these therapies:

- Never try to force an alternative or adjunctive therapy on a family member or friend who is not interested. Remember, this is *their* cancer, not yours, and the point is not to convince them that they should do what you might do. Find out how you can help *them*. You may think that the way for you to help is to convince your parent or friend to try macrobiotics or visualization. But, for your mother, it might be more meaningful for you to come home for weekends while she goes through therapy. Ram Dass's book *How Can I Help?* is an exquisite discussion of this point.[1] We rarely help by forcing our vision on others. We often help simply by listening carefully, by asking how we can be of help, and by responding to the needs we are able to respond to.

- If you are choosing for yourself, or helping an interested friend or family member choose, remember the distinctions I have made between *open and closed therapies*, between *intrinsically health-promoting therapies and those that are not obviously good for you in some reasonable way*, and between *the therapy, the practitioner, and the service delivery*. The safest choices are among open therapies that are intrinsically health-promoting. The safest practitioners are credentialed practitioners charging reasonable fees who deliver the promised therapy effectively and professionally. These are what you might call "no regrets" therapies—practices that you would not regret having undertaken whatever the outcome. As you go out from this safe inner circle into riskier areas, such as closed therapies that involve secret formulas, therapies that are not intrinsically health-promoting, therapies that operate by less validated principles, therapies where you do not fully trust the practitioner or for which he is not credentialed, or therapies where the service delivery is expensive or unprofessional or both, you move into areas where choices should be much more carefully weighed.

- If you are considering one of the more expensive therapies offered at one of the well-known alternative clinics in Mexico, the Bahamas, Germany, or elsewhere, I believe it is usually worth going there first and checking out the clinic or practitioner *before* agreeing to enter the therapy. This enables you to talk to the patients who are using the therapy, and to take a few days to think about it, as opposed to signing up for an expensive therapy that you have only read about. Ask the practitioner for the names and phone numbers of some patients you can talk with, and try to get some other names and numbers independently, either from the list of those previously treated by the practitioner or from one of the alternative cancer information networks. I am particularly put off by clinics that follow up your initial contact with them with repeated phone calls and a hard sell, sometimes using scare tactics.

- It is also worthwhile, especially for those who tend to be enthusiastic about alternative therapies, to check out what the mainstream cancer organizations have to say about the therapy. I would ask the American Cancer Society and the National Cancer Institute for their statements, if any, on a therapy I was considering. The Office of Technology Assessment (OTA) report *Unconventional Cancer Treat-*

ments is a major resource, describing many of the therapies more objectively than any mainstream organization has in the past. Then go to a medical library, and ask the research librarian to do a search of the cancer literature under the name of the practitioner or the therapy, which may yield both positive and negative reports in the peer-reviewed medical literature.

- A guide like *Third Opinion* by John Fink, perhaps the most comprehensive "tour guide" to alternative cancer therapies presently available, may be the best starting point. While Fink's general orientation is in favor of the complementary therapies, this book contains a great deal of useful information and was used extensively by OTA researchers in the preparation of their report on unconventional cancer treatments.

- Because there is no reliable cure for cancer among the unconventional cancer therapies, it should go without saying that one should be sure that mainstream therapies do not have an efficacious treatment for the kind of cancer you have before embarking on a purely unconventional course of treatment. From time to time I meet people with cancer (Hodgkin's disease, for example, or early-stage breast cancer) who could have achieved a highly probable cure, but spent months or years pursuing alternative therapies at great risk to their health. Most people instinctively take the wiser course of seeking to integrate the best of conventional and unconventional cancer treatments, only turning to purely unconventional treatments if potentially curative conventional therapies are not available.

- If you do undertake an unconventional cancer therapy, it is wise to keep yourself under the care of a competent mainstream oncologist. An increasing number of oncologists are willing to monitor patients while they undertake unconventional courses of treatment, especially when they are convinced that the curative conventional treatments have been exhausted and that the unconventional therapy seems unlikely to do harm. The oncologist will also be aware of palliative conventional options that you may wish to keep in reserve as you explore the unconventional course.

- Knowing when to *stop* an unconventional course of treatment is very important. In psychological therapies, a psychotherapy that does not instinctively feel right to you is rarely helpful. And it is a very poor sign when a psychotherapist insists that you "caused" your cancer and can therefore just as surely reverse it if you want to. In nutritional therapies, as indicated repeatedly in the chapters on this subject (see part IV), uncontrolled weight loss that does not result in a stabilization of weight at some reasonable level— like high-school or college weight—is reason for real concern. It is also reason for concern when an alternative therapist repeatedly re-assures you that every worsening of your physical condition is a "healing crisis" that is to be expected as a positive result of treat-ment. The theory of healing crises as elements in naturopathic treatments is accepted by many alternative therapists, but it is a perilous theorem that can be exploited at great hazard to your health by the unknowledgeable or unscrupulous practitioner.

Having urged these cautions for unconventional therapies (just as I have for mainstream therapies), the bottom line for me remains that the exploration of ethical complementary cancer therapies remains a viable option for people with cancer who want to do so. I have a strong belief that spiritual, psycho-logical, physical, nutritional, and sometimes traditional therapies can enhance quality of life, and possibly extend life, for people who believe that they may be helpful.

Pain Control

Most cancer pain—either from treatments or from the cancer itself—can be controlled, and the fear of being caught in unendurable pain is largely un-founded. To this end, it is worth exploring both conventional and complemen-tary systems. Here are the principle guidelines:

- Most cancer pain is not as well controlled by doctors as it should be. Doctors receive little education in pain control in medical school, and the underuse and unskillful use of pain control medica-tions by physicians is widely considered a national scandal in medicine.
- Physicians associated with hospice programs are likely to be the most expert in the effective use of pain control medication, and

you do *not* have to be dying to get their assistance in designing an effective pain control program. Call your local hospice office to see if you can make an appointment with one of their doctors.

- Unconventional approaches to pain control can also be very useful and often have fewer side effects than drugs. These approaches include traditional Chinese medicine (acupuncture and acupressure), visualization, meditation and breathing techniques, psychological counseling, and behavioral training.

- Understanding the difference between physical pain and human suffering can make a difference in the best response to both. Suffering is the psychological experience of loss that can create or enormously augment physical pain. Suffering is just as real, and just as important, as the physical basis for pain. When suffering is directly addressed, and expressed as fear or anger or grief, it tends over time to move and change, and the physical pain associated with it often diminishes or can disappear. I cited the example of soldiers in Korea and Vietnam who received large wounds and suffered relatively little pain because they knew they were going home, while others who suffered smaller wounds experienced great pain because they knew they were going back to face death on the battlefield again. The difference between the two was the difference in the meaning of the wound, and the meaning of the wound was what dictated the level of suffering. The wound of a life-threatening cancer can cause huge suffering, and if that suffering is not addressed, then unnecessarily high levels of pain medication may be used for a pain that is deeper—not lesser—than a purely physiological pain.

- Spiritually, it is wise to remember that pain can be a great teacher. Most of us know that we have grown most during the painful times of our lives. On the other hand, too much pain can overwhelm the capacity to learn from it. Given that we cannot escape pain and suffering, which comes to all of us, the wisest course is to discover how we can learn from it: how we can accept it and make use of it. I do not say this lightly or easily, nor is it a teaching that any of us can always make use of. But it is something to remember, and strive toward, for those of us who resonate to this old idea.

Healing

Healing essentially involves choices in how one seeks to create the inner and outer conditions that maximize the possibilities of physical, mental, emotional, and spiritual well-being in the face of cancer. Healing can take place whether one is recovering physically or facing recurrence or even death. Healing, I believe, tends to optimize the chances for physical recovery and certainly transforms the quality of life.

The great value of healing, as Larry LeShan has put it, lies in using cancer as a turning point in one's life. For most people cancer is an extremely unwanted and unhappy development. The pain should be deeply acknowledged. The question is whether the pain can also be used to open up a space in your life to reflect on who you are, what you truly want for the rest of your life, where you are going, what matters to you now, and how you can change your life in ways that make sense to you.

People who find a way to use cancer as a turning point often seem able to expand some of the best parts of their lives at the very moment that they are facing one of the worst crises of their lives. Therefore, their lives improve even in the face of the trauma of cancer.

This inner work of healing can be done by the patient himself; with a support group; with a psychotherapist; with a minister, rabbi, or spiritual counselor; with a network of supportive friends; within one's family; at work; and in a thousand uniquely personal ways. It certainly *expands life* to seek this kind of healing and it may possibly *extend life* for some people by stimulating the immune function and other resilience factors. The search for healing can also transform one's relationship with events that used to feel stressful, so that they feel less stressful. Stress, as we have seen, is known to enhance the growth of many cancers.

Fear of Recurrence

Living with the fear of recurrence is one of the most anxiety-provoking problems that a person who has had an initial successful treatment faces. The quarterly or annual checkups for recurrence can be terrifying, as can the question of whether or not a new health problem signals the return of cancer. One of the best ways to deal with this fear is through a support group or with a psychotherapist who works extensively with cancer patients. If this fear is talked over with other patients living with the same problem, it often diminishes. It is also a part of the process that leads one to a deeper appreciation of life, which can diminish the fear of death and therefore the fear of recurrence.

Recurrence

Facing a recurrence can be as difficult—or even more difficult—than facing the initial diagnosis, primarily because recurrent cancer is generally metastatic and mainstream medicine does not have many definitive curative treatments for metastatic cancer. For people who have been actively using complementary therapies or living a consciously healthy life since the initial diagnosis, the recurrence can be doubly devastating because they often feel their efforts were in vain. Recurrence renews the whole cycle of choices about physicians and therapies. It also plunges many people deeper into choices in complementary therapies. And it raises many of the issues of pain control and dying.

Dying

We all die. Whether or not we die of cancer, we all face the prospect of death someday. For most of human history, death has been a part of life. Contemporary Western cultures have marginalized and hidden the experience of death more successfully than any previous culture. The idea of death has become more *toxic* than it was in earlier times. Faced with the prospect of death, there is knowledge, choice, skill, and control about how, where, and when we will die. Here are some key points to think about:

- Some people think they know death is "the end." Others believe they know that life after death is certain. My belief is that death is a great mystery, a mystery worth contemplating.
- Some people think they have to be "positive" all the time, and that allowing themselves to think about death will hasten their dying.

My belief—and that of most experienced therapists I know—is that this is a profound misreading of what "fighting for life" is all about, and that thinking about death is for many (by no means all) a critical part of *both* fighting for life and preparing to face death. It is a critical part of the deeper healing process.

- The antipodes that many people experience in facing death are the wish to fight intensively for life and the wish to achieve a peaceful acceptance of death. Neither of these attitudes is "better" or "worse" than the other. Many people switch back and forth between the two.

- The fear of death is natural and common, although I have met many people—older people and people with cancer—who have lost all fear of death. Some people even look forward to death as a release or as a way to join a partner who has died before them. But fear, which is the most common human response, is amplified in our culture by the toxicity we have created around death. We can diminish the toxicity of the Western experience of death by doing what other cultures have naturally done: face death, think about it, learn about it, talk about it, and recognize the knowledge, choice, skill, and control that goes into the kind of death each of us would choose.

- The kinds of choices we have include: whether to die in a hospital or at home, finding quality care, and considering hospice services, either at home or at one of the centers. We also need to ask whether we want to extend life at all costs or to allow a relatively painless natural process to take us out of life when the time comes, and whether to wait for death or meet it by taking our own lives, with or without the assistance of a physician. Each of these choices requires care and preparation.

- There is a certain amount of negotiating room for most people about when they actually die. It is well documented that many people wait to die until after an especially meaningful holiday or wait for a child to arrive to be at the bedside or for a grandchild to be born. Less well documented experimentally, but often experienced by clinicians, are people who put off death for months or even years to see a child graduate from school or marry. In fact, we really never know when someone is going to die. I knew a woman who was expected to die without leaving the hospital, who unhooked herself from the intravenous (IV) lines, walked out of the hospital, and lived for several more years. Another friend described how, at one point in her illness, she knew she was breaths away from death, and chose to continue to breathe to see her daughter in a few days, and then recovered for a period of many months before dying. Death is much more "negotiable" than we sometimes think. To a surprising degree we may be able to choose when and where we die.

- Those who have been at the edge of death often report that the actual process of dying can be, for some, surprisingly easy. I am not talking about the physical discomfort surrounding death, but the process of actually letting go into death. Many poets and writers throughout the ages have recorded this experience—often with their last words.

- I have found that reading the great writers on the subject of death has deeply transformed my own relationship to it (see chapter 26, On Living and Dying). That, and meeting so many friends through the Commonweal Cancer Help Program who are facing death. I started the Cancer Help Program with a great fear of death, but the last 8 years of work with people who were facing death has deeply changed my relationship to it. I do not fear death nearly as much as I once did. And facing the fear of death has had a deeply positive effect on my own life. So I commend to you the possibility that reflecting on death may be of benefit to you as well.

In conclusion, I will try to answer a question I am often asked: What would I do if it were me?

I do not know the answer to that question. I do not think anyone can know that unless he actually faces the experience of cancer. But here are my thoughts:

I would be paying a great deal of attention to the *inner healing process* that I would hope that the diagnosis would trigger in me. I would be giving careful thought to what had meaning for me *now*—just what in my life I wanted to let go of and what I wanted to keep.

I would give careful thought to choosing a mainstream physician. I would be looking less for someone with wonderful empathic skills than for someone who had a reputation for basic kindness who would also be willing to take the time I needed to answer my questions. Above all, I would be looking for someone who really stayed on top of the technical aspects of my treatment and who recognized that I was the kind of patient who wanted to share in making the decisions. I would also look for someone who was willing to stick with me if I embarked on alternative therapies. If possible, I would want someone who had a good reputation for staying with his patients medically and emotionally if they were facing death.

I would use mainstream therapies that offered what seemed to me a real and meaningful chance for recovery, and I would use them with gratitude and work to augment their effectiveness. But I suspect that I would be somewhat unlikely to undertake experimental therapies or therapies with a very low probability of success that were very toxic and would compromise my capacity to live and die as I chose.

I would use complementary therapies. My first choices would include psychotherapy with a therapist experienced in work with people with cancer; a first-rate support group; and a healer with a good reputation. I would deepen and augment my regular nutritional program and I would strengthen my meditation and yoga practices. I would spend a lot of time in nature, walking in the woods, along the ocean, and in the mountains.

I would unquestionably use traditional Chinese medicine.

I would explore whether any of the high-tech alternative therapies appeared to have anything to offer me.

I would be deeply grateful for all the training I had received from friends in the Cancer Help Program in how to face cancer as best as one humanly can. I would recognize the months or years of active battle for recovery that lay ahead, followed either by living with the possibility of recurrence or facing recurrence and death as a fundamentally new part of my life. I would go for life, for recovery, with every possible tool and resource I could find. But I would also seek to face death with the same recognition of the challenge and the possibilities.

I would spend time with people I care a lot about, and with books, with writing, with music, with nature, and with God. I would do everything I could that I had not yet done and did not want to leave undone. I would not waste time with old obligations or conventions, although I would seek to extricate myself from them decently. I would be off into pure life, following its lead.

I can say none of these things with certainty. How can any of us know what he would actually do?

In cancer, there is no single right choice for all of us, but there are surely right choices for each of us. There are no certain courses of action, but there are certainly educated and wiser choices, as opposed to uneducated and more foolish ones. The skill is in the movement from ignorance toward knowledge and from knowledge toward wisdom. In wisdom, we choose what we are least likely to regret. Accepting the pain and sorrow inherent in the fate we have been given, we can seek also the beauty and the joy.

Reference

1   Ram Dass and Paul Gorman, *How Can I Help? Stories and Reflections on Service* (New York: Alfred A. Knopf, 1987).

Appendixes

Choice in Resources

Writing this discussion of resources for cancer patients has been one of the most difficult tasks I have faced. The reasons for these difficulties are instructive, and worth considering at the outset.

The *easiest* resources for me to describe are those that simply provide information. Whether or not I agree with the bias of the information source, I can describe and assess the kind of information you will get.

The *hardest* resources to describe are those that identify specific sources of conventional or unconventional cancer *treatments*.

Why is this? Consider mainstream treatment first.

We can (and do) list the Comprehensive Cancer Centers selected by the National Cancer Institute. But while the latest technology and treatments are provided in these centers, many other hospitals offer treatments for most cancers that are equally good, and the human side of the treatment may be *decidedly* better than in some of the Comprehensive Cancer Centers.

Identifying the best *practitioners* is even more difficult. We certainly know many oncologists, radiotherapists, surgeons, psychiatrists, and psychologists across the country who have been highly recommended by patients. But many of the best mainstream practitioners *do not want to be listed* in a resource guide. They are known by word of mouth and by professional referrals. Their practices are already overflowing. And a lovely, if endangered, ethic still holds sway in some medical circles that self-advertisement does not fall within the great traditions of medicine or healing.

Even if we choose to disregard the preference of these practitioners not to be listed, other difficulties remain. First, we know only a tiny fraction of the good practitioners in the United States and abroad. Listing the one we know but not the hundred we do not know is unfair. Second, when good practitioners grow too busy, the quality of their service drops—often dramatically. Third, and most important, is the whole question of what a "good" practitioner is. Setting aside the issue of incompetence, one could evaluate a practitioner in terms of technical skills, humanistic qualities, and preferences for different "styles of risk" in therapy (e.g., does the oncologist prefer an aggressive or conservative approach to treatment?). *Ultimately, what makes for a good "fit" between patient and practitioner encompasses technical, humanistic, and stylistic factors that cannot be summarized in an abstract formulation.* Simply put, the oncologist who is good for one patient may be wrong for another.

For all of these reasons, I have chosen not to list mainstream physicians and other practitioners. In chapter 6, I described how to find the practitioners that will work best with you: Ask other cancer patients; ask other physicians who work with these doctors; ask nurses who work closely with surgeons, radiation therapists, and oncologists in hospitals and can compare them.

Now, let us consider the problems involved in describing resources in unconventional or complementary cancer therapies.

All the problems involved in deciding whether to identify specific mainstream hospitals and doctors remain problems for some unconventional centers and practitioners: well-known centers are by no means necessarily the best; many of the best practitioners do not want to be listed because their practices are already full; those that become too busy often provide lower-quality services; and the problem of "fit" between patient and practitioner remains.

Nonetheless, while it is not common practice in mainstream medicine to list preferred individual practitioners, it is common practice in the literature on unconventional treatments to list individual practitioners as resources. Here another set of problems emerge. The "pro-alternative therapy" publications provide glowing reports of these practitioners and their centers; the "anti-alternative therapy" publications condemn them. In the chapters on individual practitioners in this book, you have seen how difficult it is to evaluate fairly even a handful of the most interesting practitioners, if one moves beyond the "true believer" position. So my dilemma has been acute.

For all these reasons, I urge *caution* in using this resource section, particularly with respect to the unconventional cancer treatments. I describe resources as best I can. Evaluating them is up to you and your physician and those whose judgment you trust.

Information Sources for Mainstream and Complementary Therapies

Public Services

> National Cancer Institute
> Hot line: 1-800-4-CANCER

The National Cancer Institute (NCI) publishes a wide range of useful pamphlets and brochures on many types of cancer and cancer treatments. The NCI hot line can give you a great deal of specific information on different types of cancer treatments—both mainstream and complementary—research programs, and treatment institutions. The information on mainstream treatment is usually excellent. The information on unconventional treatments is usually a rehash of information from the American Cancer Society's "unproven treatments" list. This can be a useful starting point for your researching an unconventional therapy, provided you understand the strong skepticism of the NCI about these therapies.

> American Cancer Society (ACS)

The American Cancer Society (ACS) is a significant resource. You should distinguish between the central office and the local chapters around the country. The central office is criticized by some practitoners of mainstream cancer therapy for its particular biases in funding cancer research. It is also vilified by advocates of alternative therapies for the lead role it has played in marginalizing unconventional cancer therapies in the United States. Whatever one's view of these criticisms, ACS also has local chapters all over the country that can provide patients with information on cancer and cancer treatment, as well as referrals to a variety of support services and agencies that provide individual counseling and support groups, equipment and supplies, home care for patients, financial assistance, legal services, rehabilitation services, nursing home care, and hospice care. Some of these local ACS chapters are excellent. For many years, one of the best support groups in Northern California was sponsored by a local ACS chapter.

But, in evaluating unconventional cancer treatments, ACS has rarely lived up to the standard that would be of greatest assistance to patients and practitioners alike. It has tended to lump truly dangerous and bizarre alternative therapies with creative and compassionate experimental approaches to cancer that simply had not come up through the mainstream credentialed research system. [See discussion of the ACS "unproven cancer treatments" list, below.]

R.A. Bloch Cancer Foundation
4410 Main Street
Kansas City, MO 64111
Hot line: 816-932-8453

The R.A. Bloch Cancer Foundation is an unusual organization. It was created by Richard Bloch, cofounder of the tax preparation service, H&R Block. He funds it entirely, seeking no contributions from elsewhere.

The foundation has local services for Kansas and Missouri residents, and national services. The local services in Kansas City include support groups, biofeedback, and free second opinions from a panel of oncologists.

Nationally, the foundation offers a hot line staffed by volunteers. They do not discuss therapies but send out information packets. They can also refer you to counselors, who will call you collect but whose service is otherwise free. The foundation also operates a computerized cancer information network called "Cancer Forum" through which you can communicate free of charge with other cancer patients or with volunteer researchers. The cancer hot line also provides newly diagnosed cancer patients with the opportunity to talk with persons who have had cancers similar to their own.

Computer Database Searches

For cancer patients who like to see what their physicians have read (or should have read), nothing surpasses computerized database searches of the literature describing treatments for your cancer. If you have a computer with a modem, you can subscribe to one of the medical databases, such as BRS Colleague (1-800-955-0906). You then have access to the entire cancer literature of the world. With a few simple search words you can track down in seconds the articles on virtually any subject in the medical literature that has been written about in recent years. You can then display the titles of these articles on your screen, print these titles out, look at them, and circle the titles from which you want to read brief abstracts. You can go back into the database and ask for these abstracts, which you can print out. You can read the abstracts and then order the full text of any article you want from the service. In some instances, the database has the full text available for immediate printout through your computer.

The same computer database also gives you access to two NCI databases: the PDQ database on treatment choice for patients and the PDQ database for physicians on current clinical trials involving your type of cancer. The PDQ physician database is more interesting, and you can gain access to it as a layman. It lists all current clinical trials for your type of cancer, including complete details about who can qualify, what the investigational therapy is, possible side effects, etc. It gives the name of the chief investigator and a contact phone number.

The initial subscription fee for BRS Colleague is $95. The fee per hour for the use of the NCI CANCERLIT database is $32 during prime time (day) and $22 at other times. There is a $20 minimum monthly charge. A typical search might take 15 minutes; an extensive one would require half an hour or longer.

Medical School Libraries

Medical school libraries provide you with a wealth of information on cancer treatments at virtually no cost, except for photocopying. Often it is possible to do the same kind of computerized literature search described above. You simply ask the medical reference librarian to perform the search for you. You can then go to the stacks for the articles of interest to you. Libraries have the added advantage of having medical texts as well as journal articles.

As I have mentioned before, one of the best starting places for gathering basic information on your cancer and possible treatments is *Cancer: Principles and Practice of Oncology*, edited by Vincent T. DeVita, Samuel Hellman, and Steven A. Rosenberg (New York: Lippincott, 3rd ed., 1989). You may want to copy the chapter on your illness so you can take it home and read it with a medical dictionary. Starting with DeVita et al. will make the computerized literature search much more comprehensible.

Hospital Libraries

Many major metropolitan hospitals have special libraries specifically designed for patients interested in educating themselves about their condition. Others have libraries for their medical staffs that patients can use, although some, quaintly, require a patient to have his physician's permission to research his own disease. Some hospital cancer centers even have libraries devoted specifically to resources for cancer patients, including books, articles, video- and audiotapes, and community resources. The staffs of these libraries are available to help patients with their research. Many are also equipped for a fee to do computer literature searches on the more specialized questions you may have.

A model for this kind of patient information library is the Planetree Health Resource Center. The first Planetree Center opened in 1981 at the Pacific Presbyterian Medical Center (now California Pacific Medical Center) in San Francisco. Currently, four Planetree Health Resource Centers are in operation around the country (see below) and numerous other centers have adopted the model. Each Planetree Resource Center provides a range of services to patients, including a lending library, clipping file, computer database search service, and a customized in-depth health information packet which contains information about the range of conventional and complementary treatment options, articles, a bibliography, excerpts from medical texts, and a list of support groups and organizations.

Planetree Health Resource Centers are currently located in:

California Pacific Medical Center
2040 Webster Street,
San Francisco, CA 94115
415-923-3680

Mid-Columbia Medical Center
200 East 4th Street
The Dalles, OR 97058
503-296-8444

San Jose Medical Center
98 North 17th Street
San Jose, CA 95112
408-977-4549

Beth Israel Hospital
1st Avenue at 16th Street
Silver Building, 8th Floor
New York, NY 10003
212-420-2958

Consultants for Mainstream and Complementary Therapies

CanHelp
3111 Paradise Bay Road
Port Ludlow, WA 98365-9771
Tel: 206-437-2291
Fax: 206-437-2272

CanHelp is a resource service for people with cancer which has been directed by medical writer Patrick McGrady since 1983. It is a controversial service, praised by many users interested in unconventional treatments and criticized by others for a variety of reasons discussed below. Says McGrady, "I can help guide you through the maze of claims, counterclaims and putdowns regarding conventional and alternative therapies. I am not a doctor; I do not prescribe therapies; and I have no stake in any particular school of therapy or philosophy. In trying to locate your best options, I work with the best doctors I can find. As a medical writer, I am used to translating medical jargon into plain English and simplifying abstract concepts. When my search is completed, you are invited to discuss the options with me."

Clients receive: a computer printout of research and treatment information from medical databases; a personal interpretation of this information; copies of relevant reports from CanHelp's files; and a synopsis of conversations concerning your case with CanHelp's medical advisors.

Clients must submit a series of medical documents, including pathology reports, surgical reports, blood work, and imaging reports such as computed tomography (CT) scans.

The fee for this service is $400 for American clients. In-person consultation costs $250 per hour. An initial brief telephone consultation is free of charge.

McGrady's service, widely used by cancer patients interested in alternative treatments, is criticized on several grounds. For one thing, McGrady has been outspokenly critical of the American cancer establishment in his journalistic writing and in speeches, so physicians and patients who do not share his perspective do not like his service. Second, McGrady recommends a number of unconventional cancer treatments in many of his letters to patients that are on the "unproven treatments" list of the ACS. Third, at least one medical writer has written a detailed critique of the CanHelp Program arguing, among other things, that McGrady is involved in medical decision making beyond an appropriate level.[1] Overall, the service appears to be appreciated by many patients who use it. I regard him as one of the most knowledgeable resource people in the field.

The Health Resource
209 Katherine Drive
Conway, AR 72032
Tel: 501-329-5272
Fax: 501-329-8700

The Health Resource is a medical information service founded in 1984 by Janice Guthrie. Guthrie describes the importance of her own research as a cancer patient: "The information I gathered helped me to locate a specialist interested in my particular type of tumor and enabled me to discuss intelligently my condition with him and to be an active participant in the decisions regarding my treatment. My research was so important to me in enabling me to make informed decisions, choose a combination of conventional and alternative therapies, and regain a sense of control over my personal health that I decided I wanted to do similar research as a service for other people with medical problems. This goal was compatible with my formal training in research and computer technology . . ."

Guthrie's clients receive an in-depth research report that contains: information on conventional and alternative treatments for their specific cancer; profiles of cancer patients with the same type of cancer who have either recovered or outlived their life expectancy; a computer search of the medical literature on their cancer; a list of relevant clinical trials; copies of the latest medical journal articles discussing treatments for their cancer type (including the author's address); information on coping with chemotherapy and radiation therapy (e.g., herbal, nutritional, and psychological techniques); suggestions for immuno-stimulation; and a list of recommended books on cancer.

Bound reports 110 to 150 pages in length cost $225 plus shipping. "Rush" service is available for an additional $75. Clients not satisfied with the report can return it within 30 days for a full refund.

Guthrie researches both mainstream and complementary therapies but does not have a strong advocacy stance that orients her clients toward a specific type of therapy. I regard Guthrie as a highly knowledgeable resource for people with cancer.

National Advocacy and Support Organizations

> National Coalition for Cancer Survivorship
> 1010 Wayne Avenue
> Fifth Floor
> Silver Spring MD 20910
> 301-650-8868

The National Coalition for Cancer Survivorship (NCCS) is a remarkable resource. It was founded in 1986 by Fitzhugh Mullan, M.D., a senior Public Health Service officer and cancer survivor, as a resource and advocacy group for cancer survivors. (Disclosure: I was on the founding Advisory Board.) NCCS provides support for persons wishing to locate or form self-help groups; assists survivors with insurance and employment problems; provides speakers on a wide range of topics; promotes the interests of survivors through the media; testifies in state and federal hearings; and provides a variety of publications of interest to survivors, including The *National Networking Directory of Cancer Support Services*. The NCCS also publishes the *Networker,* a quarterly newsletter that discusses issues affecting survivors.

NCCS is generally conservative on unconventional cancer treatments and more active on traditional issues of cancer survivors such as insurance, employment, and other social and bread-and-butter issues.

Individual memberships are $25, or less for those unable to pay the full amount.

Corporate Angel Network
Westchester County Airport
Building One
White Plains, NY 10604
Tel: 914-328-1313
Fax: 800-328-4226

Founded in 1981, the Corporate Angel Network is a nationwide service that transports cancer patients and a family member or friend free of charge to or from a "recognized cancer treatment," using empty seats on corporate aircraft. When possible, transportation from the airport to the hospital is also arranged, along with hotel accommodations.

The only requirements of the service are that the patient be able to walk unassisted and that no life support or other special services be required. Flights are not guaranteed and backup plans are needed.

National Alliance of Breast Cancer Organizations
Second Floor
1180 Avenue of the Americas
New York, NY 10036
Tel: 212-719-0154
Fax: 212-719-0263

The National Alliance of Breast Cancer Organizations (NABCO) is a savvy information and advocacy umbrella group for the numerous grassroots breast cancer action and support groups that have blossomed nationwide. Its brochure describes it as "a non-profit, central resource that provides individuals with accurate, up-to-date information on all aspects of breast cancer, and promotes affordable detection and treatment . . . NABCO is also active in efforts to influence public and private health policy on issues that directly pertain to breast cancer—such as insurance reimbursement, health care legislation and funding priorities."

NABCO is generally conservative on unconventional cancer treatments, and active on issues like improving insurance and funding breast cancer research.

A $40 annual membership in NABCO includes a subscription to the quarterly *NABCO News,* which monitors new developments relating to breast cancer, and NABCO's annually updated *Breast Cancer Resource List.* The *List* is an extensive compilation of written and audiovisual materials from various sources and also contains regional listings for major support organizations. Free customized information packets addressing individual patients' needs are also available upon request.

> Y-Me Breast Cancer Support Organization
> 18220 Harwood Avenue
> Homewood, IL 60430
> 708-799-8338

Y-Me was founded in 1978 as a "not-for-profit organization that provides information, Hotline counseling, educational programs and self-help meetings for breast cancer patients, their families and friends."

Y-Me has a toll-free hot line at 1-800-221-2141 (9 A.M.–5 P.M., CST) or 24 hours at 708-799-8228. Upon request, trained volunteers, all of whom have had breast cancer, are matched to callers with similar backgrounds and experiences. Presurgical counseling and practitioner referral are also available through the hot line.

Local chapters hold meetings with experts on various subjects of concern to breast cancer patients. Trained volunteers and staff members are available to present workshops to organizations and businesses stressing the importance of early diagnosis.

Y-Me has chapters in ten states and offers information and support to persons wishing to establish local support programs.

Y-Me is very conservative on unconventional cancer treatment issues. Chapters vary greatly in the quality of the service they provide.

Patient Advocates for Advanced Cancer Treatments
PO Box 1656
Grand Rapids, MI 49501
Tel: 616-453-1477
Fax: 616-453-1846

Patient Advocates for Advanced Cancer Treatments (PAACT) is a remarkable resource for prostate cancer patients that provides an iconoclastic and intelligent ongoing review of the latest developments in prostate cancer treatment.

It is a patient-oriented organization that was formed in 1987 "to act as a support and advocacy group for prostate cancer patients, their families, and the general public at risk." PAACT's founder, Lloyd Ney, is a former prostate cancer patient who rejected conventional therapy for his worsening condition in favor of an experimental therapy in Canada that was then unapproved for use in the United States.

Membership in PAACT requires a $50 yearly donation (or statement of inability to pay) and entitles the member to a subscription to the monthly *Cancer Communication* newsletter, which contains "the latest and most up-to-date information on treating prostate cancer." However, a comprehensive packet of information on prostate cancer will be sent to anyone who requests it. The *Prostate Cancer Report,* updated periodically to include the latest research and treatment information, is also available. PAACT maintains a listing of prostate cancer support groups in 26 states.

In its role as patient advocate, PAACT takes an active role in promoting expedited new drug evaluation and approval by the Food and Drug Administration (FDA).

National Brain Tumor Foundation
323 Geary Street
Suite 510
San Francisco, CA 94102
Tel: 415-296-0404
or 1-800-934-CURE
Fax: 415-296-9303

The National Brain Tumor Foundation was founded in 1981 and has as its stated goals "improving the quality of life of brain tumor patients and finding a cure through research."

In contrast to PAACT, the iconoclastic patient-driven review of what is happening with prostate cancer treatment, the National Brain Tumor Foundation tries to meet the needs of both patients and professionals, with a resultant tone of caution that almost always characterizes patient-professional cancer support and research advocacy organizations.

The foundation funds basic research and clinical trials at major research institutions throughout the United States, and also supports research in quality-of-life issues that face brain tumor patients. The foundation also offers assistance directly to patients and families, including: *GUIDE,* a comprehensive publication intended to educate patients and facilitate informed decision making; *SEARCH,* a newsletter that keeps patients in touch with advances in treatment and support options; nationwide referrals to support groups; and a volunteer-staffed phone line (1-800-934-CURE) that connects patients with professional caregivers and brain cancer survivors.

Leukemia Society of America
733 Third Avenue
New York, NY 10017
212-573-8484 or 1-800-955-4LSA

The Leukemia Society of America is a "national voluntary agency dedicated solely to seeking the cause and eventual cure of leukemia and allied diseases [lymphoma, Hodgkin's disease, and multiple myeloma] . . . The Society supports five major programs: research, patient-aid, public and professional education, and community service." The society has 56 chapters in 36 states.

A wide range of written and audiovisual material about leukemia and current treatments is available through local chapters of the society. The society also places a high priority on maintaining local resource and referral materials for patients and their families. Many local chapters offer free support groups for patients and their families and friends.

The Leukemia Society also funds a patient assistance program for people unable to meet the high costs of treatment. The program provides up to $750 per year to patients for specific tests and procedures, drugs, and transportation.

The Leukemia Society is similar in tone to the ACS: it provides strong support for mainstream research and is very skeptical of unconventional cancer treatments.

Candlelighters Childhood Cancer Foundation
7910 Woodmont Ave.
Suite 460
Bethesda, MD 20814
1-800-366-2223

Candlelighters is a nonprofit international network for support groups of parents of children with cancer that includes parents and other family members, health care professionals, and educators. Its goals include providing support systems for family members affected by children's cancers; facilitating an exchange of information on research, treatment, medical, and community resources; identifying patient and family needs so that medical and social service systems respond adequately; and seeking consistent and sufficient research funding. The foundation also seeks to provide resources that link, on demand, professional services to family needs. There are no fees for Candlelighters membership or services.

Among its other activities, the national group issues quarterly and youth newsletters and various other publications and educational materials; acts as an information clearinghouse, including library and database searches; provides speakers; and helps in forming new local groups.

Candlelighters is a remarkable organization that tends to be conservative about unconventional cancer treatments for several reasons. First, it is primarily a mainstream group and most mainstream cancer support and advocacy groups take conservative positions on unconventional cancer therapies. Second, one of its leading organizers, Grace Monaco, is an attorney with an informed and generally skeptical perspective on unconventional cancer treatments (her views are widely criticized by proponents of many alternative therapies). Third, to a significant degree, childhood cancers have been responsive to advances in mainstream cancer treatments, and therefore advocacy of alternative treatments for children is even more controversial than advocacy of alternative treatments for adults.

Mainstream Treatment Centers and Comprehensive Cancer Centers

The NCI has selected a number of Comprehensive Cancer Centers throughout the country to act as leaders in laboratory, clinical, and cancer control and prevention research. These centers are also intended to be important resources for the communities in which they are located. Although, many metropolitan areas and some states do not have Comprehensive Cancer Centers, and many hospitals not designated as centers offer excellent care for cancer patients.

In order to be designated a Comprehensive Cancer Center, facilities must meet a number of criteria, including: having a strong program of basic research and research in cancer prevention and control; demonstrating an ability to transfer findings into clinical practice; conducting clinical studies and participating in high-priority clinical trials; providing training for health professionals; and offering a wide range of information and educational services for patients and health professionals in the community. The following is a list of currently designated Comprehensive Cancer Centers:

Alabama
University of Alabama at Birmingham Comprehensive Cancer Center
Basic Health Sciences Building
Room 108
1918 University Boulevard
Birmingham, AL 35294
205-934-6612

Arizona
University of Arizona Cancer Center
1501 North Campbell Avenue
Tucson, AZ 85724
602-626-6372

California
The Kenneth Norris Jr. Comprehensive Cancer Center
University of Southern California
1441 Eastlake Avenue
Los Angeles, CA 90033
213-226-2370

Jonsson Comprehensive Cancer Center
University of California at Los Angeles
200 Medical Plaza
Los Angeles, CA 90027
213-206-0278

Connecticut
Yale University Comprehensive Cancer Center
333 Cedar Street
New Haven, CT 06510
203-785-6338

District of Columbia
Lombardi Cancer Research Center
Georgetown University Medical Center
3800 Reservoir Road, N.W.
Washington, D.C. 20007
202-687-2192

Florida
Sylvester Comprehensive Cancer Center
University of Miami Medical School
1475 Northwest 12th Avenue
Miami, FL 33136
305-548-4800

Maryland
The Johns Hopkins Oncology Center
600 North Wolfe Street
Baltimore, MD 21205
301-955-8638

Massachusetts
Dana-Farber Cancer Center
44 Binney Street
Boston, MA 02115
617-732-3214

Michigan
Meyer L. Prentis Comprehensive Cancer Center of
Metropolitan Detroit
110 East Warren Avenue
Detroit, MI 48201
313-745-4329

University of Michigan Cancer Center
101 Simpson Drive, Ann Arbor, MI 48109
313-936-9583

Minnesota
Mayo Comprehensive Cancer Center
200 First Street Southwest
Rochester, MN 55905
507-284-3413

New Hampshire
Norris Cotton Cancer Center
Dartmouth-Hitchcock Medical Center
2 Maynard Street
Hanover, NH 03756
603-646-5505

New York
Memorial Sloan-Kettering Cancer Center
1275 York Avenue
New York, NY 10021
1-800-525-2225

Columbia University Comprehensive Cancer Center
College of Physicians and Surgeons
630 West 168th Street
New York, NY 10032
212-305-6905

Roswell Park Cancer Institute
Elm and Carlton Streets
Buffalo, NY 14263
716-845-4400

Kaplan Cancer Center
New York University Medical Center
462 First Avenue
New York, NY 10016
212-263-6485

North Carolina
Duke Comprehensive Cancer Center
PO Box 3814
Durham, NC 27710
919-286-5515

Lineberger Comprehensive Cancer Center
University of North Carolina School of Medicine
Chapel Hill, NC 27599
919-966-4431

Cancer Center of Wake Forest University at the Bowman Gray School
of Medicine
300 South Hawthorne Road
Winston-Salem, NC 27103
919-748-4354

Ohio

Ohio State University Comprehensive Cancer Center
410 West 10th Avenue
Columbus, OH 43210
614-293-8619

Pennsylvania

Fox Chase Medical Center
7701 Burholme Avenue
Philadelphia, PA 19111
215-728-2570

University of Pennsylvania Cancer Center
3400 Spruce Street
Philadelphia, PA 19104
215-662-6364

Pittsburgh Cancer Center
200 Meyran Avenue
Pittsburgh, PA 15213
1-800-537-4063

Texas

University of Texas M.D. Anderson Cancer Center
1515 Holcombe Boulevard
Houston, TX 77030
713-792-2553 or 1-800-345-6324

Vermont

Vermont Cancer Center
University of Vermont
1 South Prospect Street
Burlington, VT 05401
802-656-4580

Washington

Fred Hutchinson Cancer Research Center
1124 Columbia Street
Seattle, WA 98104
206-467-4675

Wisconsin
Wisconsin Clinical Cancer Center
University of Wisconsin
600 Highland Avenue
Madison, WI 53792
608-263-8090

Unusual Oncology Practices (Variations in Medical Practice)

This section gives four *examples* of what is sometimes referred to as "variations in medical practice." The four practitioners listed below are credentialed physicians, oncologists, or hematologists, who have oncology practices that differ substantially from the norm. Some of them give consultations or workshops for patients who are visitors.

Keith Block, M.D.,
899 Sherman Avenue
Suite 515
Evanston, IL 60201
708-492-3040

(See chapter 17 for a full description of the work of Keith Block).

Keith Block has his clinical practice in Evanston, Illinois, and is Medical Director of the Cancer Treatment Program and Medical Chief of Nutritional and Behavioral Oncology at the Edgewater Medical Center in Chicago. He is also a Clinical Instructor at the University of Illinois.

Block treats a wide variety of cancers and other catastrophic diseases using a multifaceted approach. His private practice and hospital programs include conventional treatment along with individualized adjunctive components, including nutrition, body maintenance, stress care, and psychological support. Block also conducts training workshops designed to give apparently healthy patients—as well as those suffering from more extreme, difficult-to-treat diseases—the tools and support necessary to meet the challenges of living with disease.

William Buchholz, M.D.,
851 Fremont Avenue
Suite 107
Los Altos, CA 94024

Tel: 415-948-3613
Fax: 415-948-0871

William Buchholz graduated from Stanford Medical School and is board certified in internal medicine and hematology. He has been in the private practice of medicine and oncology in Los Altos since 1978. His wife, Susan Buchholz, Ph.D., a clinical psychologist, works with him. The Buchholzes summarize the principles of their practice as follows:

1. "The whole person and his or her family and friends are affected physically, emotionally, and spiritually [by cancer]. A comprehensive treatment program recognizes this and addresses the unique needs of each individual, treating the person as well as the disease."
2. "Conventional Western medicine has very powerful and useful treatments for certain cancers. Other aspects of treatment are better addressed by complementary therapies. Psychological techni-ques likewise are important in dealing with attitudes and emotions and their effects on recovery. A comprehensive program considers all of these systems and is inclusive rather than exclusive."
3. "Developing a strategy to deal with cancer requires knowing not only what treatments to use but when to use them. Patients may correctly conclude that they must change their diet or deal with spiritual concerns. Such changes may have to be delayed, however, while surgery to prevent a bowel obstruction takes precedence. Fighting cancer alone is too exhausting—patients should use all their resources and support."
4. "Although not everyone is cured, the potential for becoming whole again is possible for all of us. Each of us has the potential to be a hero, to grow wiser. We need to take care of ourselves, honor what is most precious within us, and at the same time become more forgiving of our own humanity. What makes cancer a heroic journey is the style in which it is done. What makes being doctors so rewarding is the chance to be with so many heros."

Dr. Buchholz also offers workshops at his office on various subjects of interest to cancer patients.

Northwest Oncology Clinic
Cabrini Medical Tower
901 Boren Avenue, #901
Seattle, WA 98104
Tel: 206-292-2277
Fax: 206-292-2015

Glenn Warner, M.D., founder of the Northwest Oncology Clinics, is a board-certified radiation oncologist and immunologist. The clinic is a "'total care' facility combining a full range of medical, therapeutic, and support services for the treatment of cancer . . . Your questions will be answered and you will participate in the decision-making process from the very beginning. The primary factor in treatment planning is the quality of the patient's life. Our objective is to control the cancer without making the treatment worse than the disease."

Warner's view is that cancer is a systemic disease usually requiring more than one type of therapy. Among those available at the clinic are: surgery; radiation; chemotherapy, used within the overall goal of keeping the immune system active; immunotherapy, through the use of bacteria vaccines or other drugs; nutrition, vitamins, and exercise; and support therapies, such as individual and family counseling, relaxation techniques, imagery, and stress reduction.

In keeping with his belief in the importance of the immune system in fighting cancer, Warner believes that "the treatment program must be guided so that the person's resistance is not suppressed. It is far better to come to our clinic before any therapy begins, rather than as a last resort."

Dr. Warner does see people from all over the United States, but he also requires that patients make periodic visits to the clinic when necessary.

> Falk Oncology Centre Limited
> 2nd Floor
> 890 Yonge Street
> Toronto, Ontario M4W 3P4, Canada
> 416-921-2525

Rudy Falk, M.D., is a Professor in the Department of Surgery at the University of Toronto, and was for 8 years Head of the Division of General Surgical Oncology at Toronto General Hospital. In 1985, he formed the Falk Oncology Centre, an outpatient practice in Toronto. (Pat McGrady of CanHelp [see section I under Consultants for Mainstream and Complementary Therapies, above] often recommends Falk.)

Falk describes his practice as a "combination therapy" that "emphasizes total patient care, including psychological and nutritional support."

Falk says of his treatments: "There is an ongoing attempt for improvement; drugs that are more effective with less toxicity, treatments that will produce responses in patients where previous therapies have failed; improved equipment, technique, and methods." Falk describes the rationale behind his approach:

> When an abnormal situation arises in the body, prostaglandins are released, and although these are necessary in the body as a cytoprotective agent, when they are produced excessively they de-activate or block the function of the macrophage cell. The macrophages are the first line of the immune defense system and it is essential that these function. Nonsteroidal anti-inflammatories [NSAIDs] have been known for a long time to block the excessive production of prostaglandins; however, unless they are combined with the carrier molecule, sufficient quantities of NSAIDs cannot be taken by patients without serious side effects.

The present therapy offered at the Falk Centre consists of low doses of chemotherapy combined with a carrier molecule, sodium hyaluronate, plus NSAIDs. Intravenous vitamin C is also given as a free radical scavenger to help rid the body of broken down cells, and hyperthermia is occasionally used as an adjuvant therapy to "stress" the cancer.

Spiritual, Religious, and Healing Resources

Many churches, synagogues, and other places of worship provide prayer services for people with serious illnesses. Some of these prayer services are rote activities, but others are authentic and powerful and are run by counselors trained in both spiritual and psychological therapies. Indeed, many medical centers today include psychological and spiritual counseling as vital elements in their programs. Churches and synagogues often provide psychological as well as spiritual approaches in the counseling they offer. Often such services are free of charge. Trained pastoral counselors may offer an attractive alternative to psychotherapy for those who prefer counseling in a spiritual context or cannot afford a psychotherapist.

The national professional organization that sets standards for some religious counselors is the American Association of Pastoral Counselors, 9504 A Lee Highway, Fairfax, VA 22031, 703-385-6967. The association certifies pastoral counselors and accredits pastoral counseling centers. The latter are usually independent nonprofit organizations or are connected with churches, seminaries, or hospitals. All counselors certified by the association have both psychological and theological training. The association can refer you to a counseling center or individual counselor in your area.

Healers

Many kinds of healers practice inside and outside traditional churches or religious institutions. Some churches offer laying-on-of-hands services for sick people, and often welcome people in need who have not previously attended the church. Tastes vary, but some of these services are authentic and powerful.

Few formal networks exist for locating healers. Tapping into the network of people in your community knowledgeable in this area is the most important first step. Cancer support groups are a good source of referrals to virtually any kind of practitioner, healers included. Inquiries through churches, listings in the local New Age directory, or natural food store bulletin boards are also good first steps. Ask as many questions of the practitioner as you need to in order to be assured that he is the right one for you. If he is not, he may be able to refer you to someone else.

The choice of a healer is a very individual matter, and it is extremely important that the fit be right. In order to realize the benefit of the relationship, you must have full confidence in the person and in the technique. If you do not, keep looking until you find a person you do trust and who can help you mobilize your own innate healing capacity.

Psychological Services and Support Groups

Psychotherapists

Psychiatrists (physicians trained in the diagnosis and treatment of the mentally ill), psychologists, licensed clinical social workers, medical social workers, and marriage and family counselors are all licensed to provide psychotherapy, but not all practitioners are specifically trained to understand and provide for the concerns of people with cancer and their families.

Finding the right therapist requires time and careful research. The field of health psychology is a new one, only recently recognized as a specialty by the American Psychological Association (APA). However, it is currently the largest category of psychologists in the APA. People with mental illness traditionally seek out psychiatrists, and they are the only mental health professionals licensed to prescribe medications for depression and anxiety. But most cancer patients are not mentally ill, and some psychologists are extensively trained in dealing with issues confronted by people with life-threatening illnesses.

If you live in a major metropolitan area, it can be relatively easy to find a therapist skilled in dealing with the psychological needs of people with cancer.

Outside of metropolitan areas it is harder to find people so trained. One ῀
to locate both therapists and support groups is through the local branch of ῁
ACS, which often runs groups and makes referrals. Oncology centers in lar᷁
hospitals often have departments of social work or psychiatry staffed wit᷁
therapists. Hospitals can often make referrals, as well.

The local or state branch of the American Psychiatric Association or the
American Psychological Association can be contacted to make referrals to
members who have experience with cancer patients. Also, the American Society
for Psychiatric Oncology/AIDS at Memorial Sloan-Kettering in New York (212-
639-8010) has a national membership, and will give you the names and phone
numbers of members in your area. The Association for Humanistic Psychology
has a referral service (415-346-3246) in the San Francisco Bay Area which is
expanding its base nationwide.

These are the more formal avenues for locating therapists. In reality many,
perhaps most, people locate practitioners though less formal routes, often with
good results. The physician managing your case may be able to direct you to
a therapist. Many patients locate therapists simply by asking other cancer
patients or members of support groups they attend. You can also contact
hospices and other organizations that offer cancer support groups to get
referrals.

A key point to remember is that you do have more than one choice: it is wise
to interview more than one therapist and to ask about credentials and experience. It is also important to ask about the therapist's training and experience
in working with people with cancer. But training is not the whole story. In
interviewing someone as a potential therapist, determine whether the therapist's beliefs and attitudes are congruent with your own. Ask about the person's
philosophy of care, how he views illness and its causes, how he views body
change, and even what his thoughts are about spiritual realities. Be sure to
ascertain if he is available by phone nights and weekends, if he makes hospital
visits, or conducts sessions on the phone.

If after three to five sessions your relationship with your therapist does not
seem beneficial to you, do not be afraid to seek out another therapist. You
have every right to expect the same sense of comfort, safety, and understanding
with your therapist that you experience with a good friend.

Psychologists and psychiatrists are able to bill your insurance so that you may
be partially reimbursed for their services. However, many insurance companies
do not reimburse as completely for this kind of service as they do for physical
health care, and some insurance policies do not cover these costs at all. It is

important to read your policy carefully to see what services and what providers are covered by your insurance contract.

Generally speaking, therapists trained at the masters degree level are not able to bill insurance companies, whereas those with doctorates can. Exceptions to this are those therapists with a Marriage, Family, and Child Counselor degree (MFCC), who can often bill for insurance reimbursement.

If you are on Medicare, you may be able to have a psychologist's expenses partially paid if your oncologist or primary care physician prescribes psychological therapy for you. Check with your local Medicare office and with your oncologist.

Support Groups

Many hospitals now offer cancer support groups. They vary greatly in quality. For information on which hospitals in your area may offer cancer support groups, look up "Hospitals" in the Yellow Pages of your telephone book. Call the department of oncology or the department of social services at the hospital and ask whether the hospital provides support groups for people with cancer and their families. The regional branch of the ACS is also a good source of information on local support groups.

The American Self-Help Clearinghouse (201-625-7101) is a national organization that can refer you to national self-help groups, as well as to state and regional clearinghouses that have information on local groups that are not members of national networks.

If you think that a support group might be useful to you, do not be discouraged if the first one you find does not suit your needs. Keep looking until you find the right one. Support groups vary widely depending upon the skills and orientation of the leader and the experiences and concerns of the members.

Often people find a support group most helpful when they are first diagnosed or are undergoing active therapy. However, participation in a group may become less useful over time. Review your experience of what you are receiving and do not hesitate to leave if you feel that the group is no longer beneficial to you.

There are also support groups for family members, spouses, and children which may be useful in some cases. People with cancer sometimes even organize their own personal support groups made up of their friends and family.

If no group exists that meets your needs and you are interested in starting one, the Self-Help Clearinghouse (see above) can provide information on model groups in other parts of the country and may also be able to connect you with others who have an interest in starting a group. Local clearinghouses are also good resources for starting groups.

The Consumers Union (1-800-272-0722) publishes a useful guide for cancer patients called *Practical Resources for Cancer Survivors* edited by Fitzhugh Mullan, M.D., and Barbara Hoffman, J.D., of the National Coalition of Cancer Survivors, which goes into considerable detail about how to find a suitable support group and also about how to organize a peer-support group yourself.

National Support Groups with Local Affiliates
> The Wellness Community
> National Office:
> 2190 Colorado Avenue
> Santa Monica, CA 90404
> 310-453-2300

The Wellness Community is an excellent national network of cancer support centers imbued with the sane philosophy of its founder, Harold Benjamin, Ph.D. (see chapter 6).

The goal of the Wellness Community is to "provide a free program for people with cancer and their families where educational, emotional, and social support create an atmosphere of hope in which patients can actively participate in their fight for recovery."

The Wellness Community seeks to provide a homelike setting for people with cancer where they can come to be with others in the same situation. These centers offer informal sharing groups, ongoing weekly groups facilitated by psychotherapists, family groups, relaxation and visualization sessions, workshops and lectures conducted by experts in a variety of topics, exercise and nutrition classes, social events, and groups designed to facilitate the exchange of information in specialized areas of concern to cancer patients.

The Wellness Community is expanding nationwide; and currently has centers in the following cities:

> **Los Angeles/Westside**
> 2200 Colorado Avenue
> Santa Monica, CA 90404
> 310-453-2300

Los Angeles/South Bay
109 W. Torrance Blvd.
Suite 100
Redondo Beach, CA 90277
310-372-2094

Los Angeles/Foothills
100 No. Hill Avenue
Suite 107
Pasadena, CA 91106
818-796-1083

Valley/Ventura
5655 Lindero Canyon Road
Suite 104
Westlake Village, CA 91362
818-597-9777

Orange County
1924 E. Glenwood Place
Santa Ana, CA 92705
714-258-1210

San Diego
3760 Convoy Street #320
San Diego, CA 92111
619-467-1065

San Francisco/East Bay
350 No. Widget Lane #101
Walnut Creek, CA 94598
510-933-0107

Chicago
1110 Jorie Blvd.
Suite 102
Oakbrook, IL 60521
708-572-6370

Greater St. Louis
12 South Hanley
St. Louis, MO 63105
314-721-4664

Greater Cincinnati
Towers of Kenwood
8044 Montgomery Road #385
Cincinnati, OH 45236
513-791-4060

Knoxville
1844 Terrace Avenue
Knoxville, TN 37916
615-546-4661

Baltimore
P.O. Box 65247
Baltimore, MD 21209
301-832-2719

Philadelphia
Balapointe Office Center
111 Presidential Blvd.
Suite 235
Bala Cynwyd, PA 19004
215-664-6663

Greater Boston
1146 Beacon Street
Brookline, MA 02146
617-232-2300

Center for Attitudinal Healing
19 Main Street, Tiburon, CA 94920
415-435-5022

The Center for Attitudinal Healing was founded in 1975 by Gerald Jampolsky, M.D., the author of the internationally known *Love Is Letting Go of Fear*.[2] The center's aim is to "supplement traditional health care through an environment in which children, youth, and adults faced with life-threatening illness can actively participate in the process of attitudinal healing. The Center is not about illness or dying, but rather about the quality of life no matter what the circumstances." It has a strongly spiritual orientation.

"The concept of attitudinal healing is based on the belief that it is possible to choose peace rather than conflict, and love rather than fear . . . Attitudinal healing is the process of letting go of painful, fearful attitudes. When we let go of fear, only love remains. At the center of our definition of health is inner peace, and healing is the process of letting go of fear."

The center offers a wide variety of support programs for children, youth, and adults. In addition to serving people with life-threatening illnesses, the center also provides support for people dealing with long-term illness, caregivers and family members, and those dealing with bereavement. Workshops and training programs in attitudinal healing are also available. The center publishes a quarterly newsletter and also has a catalogue of books, videos, and audiotapes.

The Center for Attitudinal Healing office in Tiburon, maintains an extensive listing of Attitudinal Healing programs and other centers in the United States, Canada, and Australia whose philosophies and approaches are similar to its own. The list is available upon request.

Major Metropolitan and Regional Support Groups
The following is only a sampling of some of the better-known regional support organizations for people with cancer. The local chapter of the ACS can provide a more exhaustive list of support groups in your area.

New England
The Behavioral Medicine Program for Cancer Patients
New England Deaconess Hospital
185 Pilgrim Road
Boston, MA 02215
617-632-9529

The Behavioral Medicine Program for Cancer Patients is a highly regarded medical outpatient clinic designed to help patients deal with the stress of the disease and of the side effects of treatment, and to help the patient take an active role in his care.

Patients are trained in the practice of the relaxation response, which "is elicited by mental focusing techniques, which bring about measurable physiological changes, including decreases in heart rate, blood pressure, and muscle tension. These changes can counteract many of the physical effects of stress." Stretching exercises, awareness training, breathing techniques, nutrition information, and use of "creative imagination" in a state of deep relaxation are also employed.

The staff includes psychologists, a social worker, and support personnel. The program is offered in groups of 12 to 15 in order to allow participants to realize the benefits of interacting with others who have had a similar experience. Groups run for 9 weeks and each session lasts 2 hours. Follow-up programs are available for patients completing the program, in order to help them maintain the practice of the techniques learned to provide continuing support.

The fee for the initial assessment is $300 and each of the group sessions is $60. The discharge assessment fee is $150. Coverage of services by insurance policies varies. For some patients there is an interest-free installment payment program and scholarship support is available in selected cases.

Stress Reduction Clinic
University of Massachusetts Medical Center
Worcester, MA 01655
Tel: 508-856-2656
Fax: 508-856-1977

Jon Kabat-Zinn, Ph.D., Director of the Stress Reduction Clinic, is one of the outstanding pioneers of meditation-based programs for people with cancer and other illnesses. He describes the clinic program as "an eight-week-long course designed to teach people with a wide range of chronic medical diagnoses and varying degrees of chronic stress, pain, and illness how to take care of themselves as a complement to the care and treatment they are receiving through more traditional routes. The core of the program is a relatively intensive training in mindfulness meditation and its application in daily living to coping with stress and pain."

A physician referral is required for a patient to be considered for the program. Patients with cancer—as well as other medical conditions—are evaluated individually, and then, if appropriate and sufficiently motivated, enrolled in the program. Thirty people attend one $2^{1}/_2$ hour session per week, plus an all-day Saturday session during the sixth week. Participants are required to devote a minimum of 1 hour daily, 6 days a week, to the practice of mindfulness techniques, with guidance from audiotapes.

Kabat-Zinn's book, *Full Catastrophe Living*,[3] provides a detailed description of the program and its orientation.

Wellspring Center for Life Enhancement
3 Otis Street
Watertown, MA 02172
617-924-8515

Wellspring Center provides services for people with life-threatening and chronic illnesses as well as those who care for them. These include support groups, consultations to discuss relevant resources and referrals, an audiovisual lending library, and a program in which persons with illness and family members can receive support and instruction in relaxation and visualization either at home or in the hospital.

Training and consultations are also available to hospitals, hospices, churches, and professional organizations.

Exceptional Cancer Patients
1302 Chapel Street
New Haven, CT 06511
Tel: 203-865-8392
Fax: 203-497-9393

Exceptional Cancer Patients (ECaP) was founded in 1978 by Bernie Siegel, M.D., author of *Love, Medicine and Miracles* and other books.[4] Siegel is one of the most famous, and still controversial, advocates of mind-body approaches to cancer which "help people find the strength to grow and change in the face of serious health problems."

According to the organization's literature, the ECaP therapeutic model, used as an adjunct to mainstream medical therapies, is intended to encourage patients to participate in their own process of healing. "Individuals are supported in making emotional and spiritual changes which may lead to a better quality of life and, secondarily, to an extension of their lives."

ECaP offers group sessions, psychotherapy for individuals, couples, and families, education and support for AIDS patients, an extensive mail-order catalog of books, cassettes, and videotapes which convey the ECaP philosophy, and a health professional training program.

ECaP groups meet once a week for 2 hours, and are facilitated by two psychotherapists. Individuals must submit an application, followed by a 2-hour intake consultation with a therapist. The individual is then assigned to one of the eight ongoing groups according to his unique needs. Fees are based on a sliding scale, and patients are encouraged to participate in groups for a minimum of 3 months.

ECaP also maintains a referral service to groups with similar philosophies nationwide.

New York
SHARE: Self-Help for Women with Breast Cancer
19 W. 44th Street
Suite 415
New York, NY 10036
Tel: 212-719-0364
Hot line (English): 212-382-2111
Hot line (Spanish): 212-719-4454
Hot line (Chinese): 718-296-7108

SHARE is a highly regarded center that offers support groups for women with breast cancer, including groups in Spanish and Chinese, and a number of special groups, such as newly diagnosed patients, seniors, and patients with ovarian cancer. SHARE also operates a patient hot line (also multilingual) and presents an ongoing educational series on issues of interest to breast cancer patients. Generally, it has an outstanding reputation among women who use the service in New York.

San Francisco Bay Area
Cancer Support Community
401 Laurel Street
San Francisco, CA 94118
415-929-7400

The Cancer Support Community in San Francisco is an excellent example, as is SHARE in New York, of the benefits of a quality-oriented independent support program for cancer patients. It offers a variety of programs for cancer patients, their families, and caregivers. All services are provided free.

Support programs include groups, grief counseling, individual, couple, and family counseling, and home and hospital visits. Classes in relaxation and stress reduction, pain management, guided imagery, biofeedback, nutrition, and exercise are also available. The organization has a library and information and referral center.

Women's Cancer Resource Center
3023 Shattuck Avenue
Berkeley, CA 94705
510-548-9272

The Women's Cancer Resource Center is another example of a high-quality, independent support program. It provides a number of free (donations requested but not required) services to women with cancer, including support groups, yoga and relaxation classes, educational events, and a library, referral, and information service.

Cancer Support and Education Center
1035 Pine Street
Menlo Park, CA 94025
415-327-6166

The Cancer Support and Education Center offers a intensive course for cancer patients and family members in which "you will learn how to turn hopelessness and helplessness into a strong will to live. You will learn how to feel empowered to work in partnership with your physicians. We will teach you techniques to work with your medical treatment as an ally, to enhance its effectiveness. You will be assisted in discovering untapped resources for healing and living more fully."

The self-help intensive course is presented in two formats: 1 day a week for 7 hours over a 10-week period, or 10 consecutive weekdays.

Nutritional consultation, medical consultation, massage, and individual, couples, and family counseling are also available on a fee basis.

Washington, D.C. Area
Medical Illness Counseling Center
Chevy Chase Metro Building, Suite 530
Two Wisconsin Circle
Chevy Chase, MD 20815
301-654-3638

The Medical Illness Counseling Center is a high-quality counseling program in the Washington, D.C. area, with an excellent local and national reputation. It "specializes in helping families with medical problems. [Its] professional services are directed toward decreasing emotional stress, physical symptoms, disability, and the undesirable side effects of various treatments." It also works with people who have been recently diagnosed with a serious illness, are experiencing chronic pain, preparing for major surgery, have a terminal illness, or have recently experienced the loss of a loved one.

The staff at the center includes psychiatrists, psychologists, social workers, nurse clinicians, and registered nurse therapists. They refer, when appropriate, to self-help groups and spiritual counseling. The center works with children, adolescents, and adults. Involvement by the entire family is encouraged.

After an initial visit, a treatment plan is developed which may include: psycho-therapy, group therapy, family therapy, biofeedback, hypnosis, guided imagery, physical therapy, sex therapy, or medication.

Fees for various services can be obtained by telephoning the center, and a sliding scale is available for qualifying individuals. When services are covered, the center also accepts Medicare.

Residential Programs for People with Cancer

> Commonweal Cancer Help Program,
> PO Box 316
> Bolinas CA 94924
> 415-868-0970

Founded in 1985, the Commonweal Cancer Help Program (our program) offers six weeklong retreats each year for people seeking physical, mental, emotional, and spiritual healing in the face of cancer. This is a nonmedical, education program for patients under the care of a physician. The retreats are intended to provide participants with the opportunity to reduce the fear and stress associated with cancer, to examine personal beliefs and behaviors that do not contribute to well-being, and to explore the ways of living and choices in treatment that may be of benefit.

The retreats include experiences with yoga, meditation, imagery, progressive relaxation, massage, vegetarian diet, art therapy, poetry, classes on informed choice in cancer therapy, daily support group meetings, and opportunities for people with cancer to learn from one another. Each retreat is limited to a total of eight cancer patients and/or support people. The fee is $1,280. Some scholarships are available.

> Simonton Cancer Center: New Patient Program
> PO Box 890
> Pacific Palisades, CA 90272
> 310-459-4434

The New Patient Program is a 5-day educational and psychotherapeutic session for cancer patients and their spouses conducted by O. Carl Simonton and the staff of therapists at the Simonton Cancer Center. Simonton is co-author of the widely read *Getting Well Again* and other books.[5] He and his former wife, Stephanie Simonton, pioneered mental imagery as an adjunctive approach to cancer.

The program focuses on the influence of belief systems. Participants learn techniques for enriching their lives in order to promote their health, lifestyle counseling, and relaxation and mental imagery exercises. Patients also explore the importance of gentleness, the role of stress, secondary gain from illness, and other contributing factors to disease. The issues of recurrence and death are also examined.

Because of the importance of emotional support for the patient, spouses or "most significant others" must attend the program.

The total cost of the program is $3,250, which may be fully or partially covered by some insurance policies.

Optimum Health Institute
6970 Central Avenue
Lemon Grove, CA 92045
619-464-3346

The Optimum Health Institute offers a 3-week course in "rejuvenation" through diet, various health practices, and attitudinal adjustment. (See Optimum Health Institute under Unconventional Nutritional Programs, below).

The cost of the program per week for a private room is $365.

Vega Study Center
1511 Robinson Street
Oroville, CA 95965
916-533-7702

The Vega Study Center offers a 12-day "Cancer and Healing" program every other month. The fee for the program is $1,095, or $995 for registration 1 month in advance. (See Vega Study Center, under Unconventional Nutrition Programs, below).

Bristol Cancer Help Centre
Grove House
Cornwallis Grove
Clifton, Bristol BS8 4PG, England, United Kingdom
011-44-0272-743216

The Bristol Cancer Help Centre offers a weeklong residential course which employs group support, meditation, visualization, and self-help techniques to assist patients in adjusting to the experience of cancer and cancer treatment. (See Bristol Cancer Help Centre, below).

The cost of the residential course is £350. Scholarships are available.

The Yarra Valley Living Centre
PO Box 77G
Yarra Junction
Victoria 3797, Australia
Tel: 011-61-059-67-1730
Fax: 011-61-059-67-1715

The Gawler Foundation (see the discussions of Ian Gawler in chapters 10 and 13) conducts two residential programs for people with cancer at its Yarra Valley Living Centre, both conducted by Ian and Gayle Gawler.

The initial 10-day program focuses on developing self-help techniques and coping skills. Other aspects of the program are: transforming fear into positive action; developing peace of mind; personal pain control techniques; improving communication skills; personal development through disease; and a workshop using drawing to gain personal insight. A 5-day follow-up program focuses on problem solving and application of the techniques.

Nutritional Therapies—Mainstrean, Complementary, and Unconventional

Complementary and Mainstream Nutritional Therapies

Good mainstream and complementary nutritional counseling for cancer patients is not always easy to find. If you are interested in incorporating a nutritional component in your treatment and health-promotion regimen, you may wish to locate a mainstream dietitian or nutritionist to assist you. Or you may wish to seek out an experienced complementary nutrition educator. Cancer support groups are possible sources of referral to dietitians and nutritionists who have worked with cancer patients, as are physicians and nurses.

Referrals to mainstream dietitians in your state can be obtained through the American Dietetic Association (1-800-366-1655). Dietitians have received training based on current mainstream research on nutrition and have had at least 4 years of undergraduate training, participated in an internship, and have passed a registration test. Some states also have licensing requirements for dietitians.

Standardized educational requirements do not yet exist in most states for nutritionists or nutrition educators, so there is great variability in the kind of training they bring to their work with people with cancer. Some are university caliber researchers. Others have no business offering advice to cancer patients or anyone else. Inquire about the level of formal training that the nutritionist has completed and the nature and extent of his training with other practitioners in the field. Lack of standards for training does not necessarily mean that many nutritionists are not qualified to work with people with cancer. On the contrary, many have masters degrees or doctorates and bring a very broad perspective to their work. But it is important for the person with cancer seeking nutritional guidance to be cautious.

Like the search for any health care practitioner, consider training, but also look beyond it for someone who listens carefully and is willing to support your independent efforts to heal yourself. When you interview nutritionists or dieticians, be specific. Ask what kind of diet the practitioner would recommend for you and why. Describe your ideas for an anticancer diet and ask what he thinks of it. Also ask the practitioner to refer you to other cancer patients that he has worked with, and for a bibliography of nutrition resources that the nutritionist respects.

In assembling a team to work with you on a treatment and health maintenance program, it is important to understand that dietitians and nutritionists are *not* primary care providers and so do not treat cancer. They are able, however, to translate diet theories into practice, a skill which most physicians do not have. Many nutritionists are also capable of helping you implement a nontraditional nutritional therapy if you choose to pursue one, since many of these therapies are inherently health-promoting when carried out in a sensible manner. In any case, it is wise to arrange a conversation between your physician and nutritional consultant to ensure the best possible coordination of your care.

Unconventional Nutritional Programs

The following unconventional nutritional programs are not supported or recommended by mainstream medical experts. They represent a reasonable sampling of some of the better-known "alternative" nutritional programs.

The Kushi Institute
PO Box 7
Beckett, MA 01223
413-623-5741

(See chapter 15 for a discussion of macrobiotics.)

The Kushi Institute's curriculum on macrobiotic diet and lifestyle ranges from "the practical basics of natural, whole foods cooking to the comprehensive studies of macrobiotic healing arts. It is offered to individuals who want to establish their health and deepen their comprehension of the relationship between body, mind, and spirit."

The Macrobiotic Residential Seminar is a weeklong residential program that includes daily cooking classes and lectures on the theory and practice of macrobiotics. The cost is $895 and the course is limited to 18 people.

The institute also offers a more intensive "Leadership Training" program in three 5-week sessions, each of which covers the following five subject areas: "order of the universe, macrobiotic cooking, shiatsu and ki-energy adjustment, macrobiotic health evaluation, and macrobiotic health care." The cost of a 5-week session is $2,495.

Other Beckett, MA, seminars and an annual, summer weeklong conference in rural Vermont are described in the Kushi Institute's program brochure, which is available on request.

Vega Study Center
1511 Robinson Street
Oroville, CA 95965
916-533-7702

The Vega Study Center and the affiliated George Ohsawa Macrobiotic Foundation were founded by Herman and Cornellia Aihara. The center offers a number of residential courses ranging from 3 to 12 days in length. Courses in basic macrobiotic theory are offered, as well as cooking classes and more specialized workshops.

A 12-day "Cancer and Healing" program is offered every other month. Included in the schedule are instruction in preparing low fat, low cholesterol, sugar-free meals; the macrobiotic perspective on healing, emotions, and overcoming fear; communication with medical practitioners; and demonstrations of "home remedies."

Regular fees are: $150 per day, $595 per week, and $1,095 for 2 weeks, all inclusive.

Gerson Institute
PO Box 430
Bonita, CA 91908
619-472-7450

(See chapter 14 for a description of the Gerson therapy; see also Centro Hospitalario del Pacifico S.A. under Mexico in section XII, below.)

Ann Wigmore Foundation
196 Commonwealth Avenue
Boston, MA 02116
617-267-9424

The Ann Wigmore Foundation is popularly known for its wheat-grass and alternative nutritional therapy. It offers a 1- or 2-week residential course called "Living Food Lifestyle" for "people with allergies, heart disease, and other 'incurable' conditions." Ann Wigmore describes her beliefs about and approach to cancer in the foundation literature:

> The role of nutrition in cancer has been confirmed by new scientific observation which shows that the cause [of cancer] is twofold: 1) The blood is lacking in organic mineral elements and true nutrients out of which healthy, vibrant cells are created, and 2) the blood and consequently the tissues have become so saturated with waste and foreign matter that the life of the individual is being threatened. As a safety measure, the body builds at a rapid pace cancerous cells from the blood pollutants and reduces the impurities of the blood. My work with cancer patients has proven beyond the shadow of a doubt that constipation is the greatest crime against health and is the cause of cancer in many instances. Important steps such as enemas, colonics, and wheatgrass implants must be taken in order to get the colon back to health. And, of course, letting go of fear enables the body to heal.

The course ". . . assist[s] you in making lifestyle changes necessary for self-healing. We emphasize reversing the aging process with exercise, affirmation, visualization, yoga, relaxation and transformational activities."

The curriculum includes: internal cleansing; growing greens and wheat-grass; composting and soil management; indoor gardening; sprouting; food-combining; energy soup; rejuvelac (a fermented wheat preparation); dehydration; fermentation; recipes; traveling with living food; weight loss; and sessions with Ann Wigmore.

The cost for the 2-week course is $1,150 for a private room, $850 for dormitory accommodations, and $550 for day students.

The Living Food Lifestyle program is also offered at the affiliated Ann Wigmore Institute, PO Box 429, Rincon, Puerto Rico 00677, 809-868-6307).

Ann Wigmore is the author of a number of books sold though the institute, which also sells a video about the program and numerous "accessories" such as juicers, dehydrators, sprouters, and water filters.

Optimum Health Institute
6970 Central Avenue
Lemon Grove, CA 92045
619-464-3346

The Optimum Health Institute was formerly affiliated with Ann Wigmore's Boston organization, which at the time was called the Hippocrates Institute. The philosophical basis of both institutions is quite similar in that both emphasize the rejuvenation of the body through a diet of "living foods," employment of various health practices, and attitudinal adjustment. Raychel Solomon, founder of the Optimum Health Institute, describes her approach to health in her book *Coming Alive with Raychel,* available through the Institute.[6]

The Optimum Health Institute offers a 3-week residential course, though 1- or 2-week stays are possible, but not recommended. The program includes daily exercise and sessions on food combining, organic gardening, rejuvelac, sauerkraut, sprouting, growing and using wheat grass, recipes, menu planning and kitchen setup, natural beauty care, pain control and relaxation techniques, and training in self-esteem and mental and emotional "detoxification."

The cost of the program per week for a private room is $365.

Nicholas Gonzalez, M.D.
737 Park Avenue
New York, NY 10021
Tel: 212-535-3993
Fax: 212-628-9085

Dr. Gonzalez completed his undergraduate work at Brown University and graduated from Cornell University Medical College in 1983. As a senior student at Cornell he became interested in alternative approaches to the generally accepted means of treating cancer. One of these alternative approaches was to try to treat cancer by nutritional means. While a student pursuing a senior elective, Gonzales decided to study the cancer treatment developed by a radical alternative practitioner, William D. Kelley.

During this period and in subsequent analysis while a fellow training in clinical immunology and bone marrow transplantation, Gonzalez conducted an extensive review of case histories of patients he found had done well on the Kelley nutritional and psychological program.

The treatment Gonzalez offers, based on Kelley's work, consists of an intensive nutritional program which involves three parts: diet, supplementation, and detoxification. The program is highly individualized, with diets ranging from vegetarian to diets high in animal protein. Supplements consist of vitamins, minerals, glandular concentrates, and enzymes. A patient may be required to take as many as 150 capsules a day as part of the regimen.

The detoxification protocol involves coffee enemas which "help clear the body of metabolic wastes." Patients must be able to eat and do the coffee enemas in order to benefit from the treatment.

All patients are treated on an outpatient basis. The fee for the initial evaluation, consisting of two lengthy sessions, is $1,500. During the first session—usually lasting about $1\frac{1}{2}$ hours—Gonzalez takes a complete patient history and performs the physical examination. During the second session—usually $1\frac{1}{2}$ to 2 hours long—Gonzalez reviews the results of the evaluation and tests with the patient and describes the treatment program. Phone consultations during the course of treatment are free of charge, but blood tests require an additional fee.

The supplements are sold through a separate mail-order source. Their cost varies from patient to patient but can be expected to average about $400 per month during the course of treatment.

Livingston Foundation Medical Center
3232 Duke Street
San Diego, CA 92110
Tel: 619-224-3515
Fax: 619-224-6253

(See chapter 16 for a discussion of the work of Virginia Livingston; see also Livingston Foundation Medical Center, under Alternative and Complementary Treatment Centers, below.)

Physical Therapies—Mainstream and Unconventional

Massage

(See chapter 18 for a discussion of massage.)

Massage can be a relaxing and revitalizing experience for people with cancer. Many different styles of massage or bodywork are available. *Therapeutic touch* does not involve actual physical touch at all, while *Swedish massage* (perhaps the most common style) can range from light stroking to deep tissue work. *Acupressure* is based on the same traditional Chinese medical model that acupuncture uses, except that it involves the use of finger, palm, or elbow pressure on the meridian points, rather than needles. Jin shin jitsu, jin shin do, and jin shin are also varieties of acupressure. *Shiatsu* is a traditional form of acupressure that involves working with meridians (lines of "qi energy" in the human body, as yet unproven by Western medicine) as well as points on the meridians and which also uses range-of-motion techniques.

Beyond basic technique, practitioners vary in their gifts, skills, and training; how they combine styles; how sensitive they are to the needs of their clients; and how experienced they are in working with people with cancer. Be prepared to talk to a variety of practitioners and to have an introductory massage with several. Consider whether the practitioner is certified by a school licensed by the state and accredited by a major organization such as the American Massage Therapy Association.

For the cancer patient interested in massage, the best source for referrals is a support group where other cancer patients can recommend a practitioner who is competent and understands the needs of people with cancer. The American Massage Therapy Association (AMTA) (312-761-2682) can give you a number to call in your state for referrals to an AMTA member in your area who practices the style of massage you are interested in. However, membership in the association is not required to practice, and many competent massage therapists are not members. In the same way, the American Oriental Bodywork Therapy Association (516-365-5025) can supply a list of acupressure practitioners nationwide or can refer you to a state representative.

While massage is often helpful, it can also be harmful. Inappropriate massage technique can break a bone weakened by cancer metastases, especially a vertebra in the spine. This danger is known and described in the literature on chiropractic as discussed in chapter 18. It is usually possible to minimize this danger by telling your masseur where any bone metastases are and having him avoid deep pressure in those areas. Ideally, you would find a massage practitioner who has worked with people with cancer. You might arrange a conversation between your physician and the massage practitioner to discuss any contraindications to massage. It is also worth noting that the massage practitioner could conceivably be the first person to notice new tumors. You may wish to discuss this possibility with the practitioner in advance and decide how he would communicate such a finding.

Therapeutic Touch

(See chapter 18 for a discussion of Therapeutic Touch.)

Therapeutic Touch, as discussed in chapter 18, is a modern version of the ancient system of "laying-on-of-hands" except that the hands are kept slightly above the body. Some kind of scientifically unexplained interaction between the practitioner and the patient has been shown in a number of studies to beneficially change blood chemistry values and to be associated with other physical benefits.

Therapeutic Touch is often valuable for people who dislike or should not experience direct touch—and even for those who can. Many nurses are trained in Therapeutic Touch. Some hospitals allow nurses to use it in the hospital. It is an approach to mind-body healing worth exploring for those who wish a modern approach associated with a research literature.

Referrals to Therapeutic Touch practitioners nationwide can be obtained through the Center for Human Caring at the University of Colorado (303-270-6157).

Reiki

Reiki is culturally "farther out" than Therapeutic Touch, but it is a widely disseminated system and hence worth noting here because of its accessibility. Reiki teacher and practitioner Beth Gray describes the technique as "involving the laying-on of hands to channel energy in a particular pattern. It is entirely gentle and stimulates the body's own innate wisdom to cure at the cause of the problem, promoting a holistic balancing of the body, mind, and spirit."

Reportedly an ancient technique, it was "rediscovered" in the 1800s by Dr. Mikao Usua, a Christian minister in Kyoto, Japan. Reiki practitioners, or "channels," have completed a process of "attunement" or "fine-tuning" with a Reiki master. "Once a Reiki channel has been 'turned on,' it is simply a matter of using the energy. It is used to bring balance and aid healing in others, but the channel can also direct energy to himself or herself."[7]

Treatments involve the placing of the practitioner's hands on various parts of the body, often for an hour or more:

> The Reiki channel does not really attempt to "diagnose" or "treat" the subject person. . . . From the experience of giving Reiki, the channel may make some intuitive guesses as to the subject's underlying condition. However, there is no need to diagnose, because the channeler will cover all parts of the subject's system anyway—and the apparent symptoms are often not really the root cause. As for the treatment, it is more a question of the subject's own system being opened up and allowed to get involved in the healing process. . . . There is no clear, rational explanation of how Reiki energy works.[8]

Reiki practitioners can often be found listed in the New Age directory for your area, if there is one, or through the Reiki Alliance at PO Box 41, Cataldo, ID 83810; 208-682-3535. However, according to Heather Riley of the Reiki Center in Woodside, California (408-997-1758), any person interested in long-term Reiki work can simply receive training from a Reiki master (typically over a weekend) and perform Reiki on himself.

Yoga Classes and Retreats

(See chapter 9 for a discussion of yoga.)

Yoga is an approach to stress reduction that many cancer patients have found useful in increasing their capacity to manage stress. The greatest danger of yoga to a person with cancer is the same as the greatest danger of massage, chiropractic, or other forms of bodywork. Some yoga poses could add physical stress to bones weakened by cancer metastases and contribute to a bone breaking. The danger is particularly great with metastases to the spine, since yoga works to increase the flexibility of the spine.

Many systems of yoga are currently taught in the United States. Though they all arise out of a common tradition, they can vary considerably in their relative emphasis on the physical, breathing, and meditation practices and even on their approach to each of these elements of yoga. Most beginner-level classes focus on the physical poses but also introduce students to the breathing practices, meditation, and sometimes relaxation techniques, as well.

It is important to find a method and teacher that suit your needs. You may have to attend several different classes in order to find one that is right for you.

Locating a yoga teacher can be quite easy in most cities. The Yellow Pages has listings under "Yoga" of individuals and organizations that offer classes. Organizations also tend to offer, in addition to the basic beginner's classes, more specialized workshops or course classes that will allow you to explore aspects of yoga that are particularly useful to you. Some also offer extended retreats where participants can immerse themselves for a period of time in a yogic lifestyle, an experience that can be restful, and even transformative.

The *Yoga Journal*, 2054 University Avenue, Berkeley, CA 94704, 510-841-9200 or 1-800-359-YOGA, publishes an annual directory of yoga teachers and organizations nationwide which can be useful for finding teachers and also yoga retreats. Natural foods stores often have notices for classes, as do local New Age directories often found at these stores. Of course, a personal recommendation—especially from another cancer patient—is probably the best way to locate a good yoga teacher who is sensitive to the needs of people with cancer.

Until you are very familiar with the style of yoga you have chosen—regardless of the gentleness of the practice—it is *very important* to inform the teacher of your physical condition and to ask if there is any part of the class that you should not participate in. Among its other benefits, yoga brings about a gradual deepening of your awareness of your body, including its strengths and limitations. It is important for anyone, but especially for people with cancer, to be very gentle with the practices as this awareness is developing.

These are some of the yoga systems that people with cancer have found useful:

Integral Yoga Institute
Route 1, Box 1720
Buckingham, VA 23921
804-969-3121

The Integral Yoga Institute has branches in many cities, with major institutes in New York and San Francisco. Most of these centers offer beginner and advanced beginner-level classes in yoga. Both drop-in and 4- to 6-week course classes are offered. These are fairly standardized and vary only slightly from center to center.

The 1^1/$_2$ hour drop-in classes focus on a very gentle and meditative style of hatha yoga and also include a guided deep relaxation, instruction in basic yogic breathing practices, and a brief instruction in meditation. Because it is such a gentle practice and because the classes provide at least an introduction to several components of yoga, many people have found Integral Yoga to be a good introduction to yoga, even if they choose to incorporate elements of other styles as they gain in proficiency.

Most Integral Yoga institute centers also offer workshops or course classes in subjects such as meditation, vegetarian cooking, and the philosophy of yoga.

The institute also offers two silent yoga retreats approximately 1 week in length, one in the summer at its Virginia center and between Christmas and the New Year in California. (Personal disclosure: I was trained in Integral Yoga.)

Iyengar Yoga Institute
8233 West 3rd Street
Los Angeles, CA 90048
213-653-0357

The approach to yoga in the Iyengar method differs markedly from that of Integral Yoga. Iyengar yoga is considered rigorous, even by people whose health and stamina is good. Because of this, it is particularly important that you discuss your physical condition with the teacher before you join a class. On the other hand, Iyengar teachers may offer special programs for people with health problems.

The focus in Iyengar yoga is on physical, or hatha yoga, practices. As the method is described in the institute's literature, "Mr. Iyengar's approach is marked by dynamism and precision. Iyengar yoga is unsurpassed as a way to build strength, stamina, and flexibility while cultivating a sense of graceful purpose and well-being . . . Iyengar yoga is meditation in action; the self is explored through the discovery and release of tension patterns and psychological resistances. As practice continues, a student's ability to relax and concentrate generally improves markedly, and his or her inner awareness is enhanced."

Iyengar teachers receive extensive training and Iyengar yoga is probably taught by more teachers than any other method in the country.

Viniyoga
1258 Mansfield Avenue N.E.
Atlanta, GA 30307
404-875-7110.

Viniyoga is taught by Desikachar, a yoga teacher based in Madras, India, with students around the world. While both integral yoga and Iyengar teach standard sets of yoga poses and practices, Desikachar teaches his yoga teachers to individualize the poses and other practices that each student undertakes. A well-trained teacher in Deskikachar's method can be a great gift to a yoga student with special needs, such as a person with cancer.

Kripalu Center for Yoga and Health
Box 793
Lenox, MA 02140
413-637-3280

The Kripalu Center for Yoga and Health was founded by Yogi Amrit Desai in 1971 and currently has a residential staff of 350 people serving 12,000 guests a year. Kripalu is situated in a wooded country setting and offers, in addition to its programs, vegetarian meals and spa facilities.

Kripalu has a full schedule of workshops and programs of varying lengths, most from 3 to 14 days in length. These are described in detail in *The Kripalu Experience,* a program guide issued twice yearly. Subjects range from 3-day program like "Gentle Yoga," "Women and Yoga," and "Relationships that Work" to "The Art of Stress-Free Living" and a more intensive meditation retreat lasting 1 week. The cost of a 3-day program ranges from $240 for the dormitory to $540 for deluxe accommodations. Six-day programs range from $465 for the dormitory to $1,035 for deluxe lodgings.

Kripalu also offers a less structured "Rest and Renewal" program, where you may come and create your own schedule from among a number of possible activities, including stretches and postures, meditation sessions, videos, workshops, and use of the Kripalu facilities.

Teachers of kripalu yoga can also be found in many areas of the country. This is a very gentle style of hatha yoga, quite easy for beginners, though teachers of more rigorous forms can also be found. Classes last approximately 1 hour and include postures, guided relaxation, and breathing practices. Kripalu Center can refer you to a teacher in your area.

Qi Gong

(See chapter 19 for a discussion of qi gong.)

Qi Gong is a psychophysiological discipline like yoga or tai chi. The aim of qi gong is to reestablish the flow of chi (energy) which revitalizes the body and all of its systems. It is a component of traditional Chinese medicine widely used in China as an adjunct to mainstream cancer treatment. It has gained increasing popularity in the United States.

Qi gong instructors range along a relatively wide spectrum of practice, from a highly pragmatic, no-frills, contemporary approach to a more metaphysical, ritualistic, or "religious" one. The choice you make along this range is a matter of personal taste.

The practitioners of traditional Chinese medicine at the Pine Street Benevolent Society in San Anselmo, California, suggest that a competent instructor should have at least 10 years' experience as a qi gong practitioner. Individuals who have had many years' experience in the practice of tai chi or internal martial arts may have practiced qi gong for a shorter time, but may nevertheless be quite skilled as instructors.

Other cancer patients are probably the best resources for locating qi gong instructors. Practitioners of traditional Chinese medicine in your community would also be able to make referrals.

Traditional Medicines

Most traditional medicines can be used in conjunction with mainstream therapies with no ill effects. If you are undergoing any mainstream therapies, be sure to check with both your doctor and a traditional practitioner about the possibility of any conflicts in the treatments.

Traditional Chinese Medicine

(See chapter 19 for a discussion of traditional Chinese medicine.)

It is not difficult to find practitioners of traditional Chinese medicine in most parts of the United States. The easiest way to locate the practitioners in your community is to look under "Acupuncture" in the Yellow Pages. Cancer support groups are also an excellent resource for finding referrals to acupuncturists who treat cancer patients.

The challenge is to find a practitioner who knows his craft well. The practitioners at the Pine Street Chinese Benevolent Association in San Anselmo, California, have developed a series of guidelines for cancer patients who are looking for capable acupuncturists. These are:

- *Credentials and licensing examinations:* The most reliable indication that a practitioner of Chinese medicine has attained an acceptable level of training is possession of a license granted by the state of California, which has very rigorous entrance requirements. Practitioners from all over the world travel to California to take the examination. Other states vary considerably in the standards they set for licensing. The National Commission for the Certification of Acupuncturists (NCCA) is also a very prestigious credential.
- *Location of training:* There are acupuncture schools in many parts of the United States. "Certified" schools are those that have qualified their programs to meet the standards of the state of California or the NCCA. Most Chinese, Japanese, and Korean practitioners have received fairly high levels of training in those countries. Most European schools that lead to the state of California license or NCCA certification have credible programs. *Chinese or Hong Kong 3-month courses or various workshop trainings tend to be inadequate. This is also true for physicians who have taken a "short course" program.*
- *Experience:* Inquire about the length of time the practitioner has been in full-time practice. "Full-time" is minimally defined as 500 patient visits per year. Look for a practitioner who has had at least 5 years of full-time practice.
- *Scope of practice:* A general practice of traditional Chinese medicine should include acupuncture techniques, herbal remedies, complementary supplements, general nutritional guidelines, general exercise guidelines, and general stress management guidelines.
- *Experience with cancer:* The practitioner should have treated a minimum of 100 cancer patients and should have experience with your type of cancer as well—5 to 15 cases for unusual cancers and at least 25 cases for more common types. The practitioner should also provide you with patient contacts.

  The acupuncturist or herbalist you choose should also be familiar with Western medical protocols so that he does not prescribe a treatment that contradicts your primary program (e.g., antioxidants that will interfere with radiation treatments).
- *Other interview questions:* How does the practitioner assess the success of treatment? What criteria are used for this assessment? How accessible is the practitioner both for office visits and phone

consultations? What kind of sterile procedures are used? What is the fee structure? Is there a sliding scale? If not, the first visit might range from $40 to $100 (the latter is justified if the intake interview lasts at least an hour and the practitioner has an hour of research and preparation before the next visit). Subsequent visits may range from $20 to $50.

Ayurveda

Ayurveda is one of the principle traditional medicines of India, which has in modern times been only partially eclipsed there by Western medicine. Ayurveda arose from the same ancient tradition that gave birth to yoga. Deepak Chopra, M.D., an eloquent practitioner of Ayurveda,[9] describes the ancient practice as follows:

> The ancient doctors of India were also great sages, and their cardinal belief was that the body is created out of consciousness. A great yogi or swami would believe the same thing. Therefore, theirs was a medicine of consciousness, and their way of treating disease pierced the body's matter and went deeper, into the core of mind. When you look at Ayurveda's anatomical charts, you don't see the familiar organs pictured in Gray's Anatomy, but a hidden diagram of where the mind is flowing as it creates the body. This flow is what Ayurveda treats.[10]

Dr. Vasant Lad, Director of the Ayurvedic Institute in Albuquerque, New Mexico, and author of *Ayurveda: The Science of Self-Healing,* explains the process of healing according to Ayurveda:

> Throughout life, there is a ceaseless interaction between the internal and external environment. The external environment comprises the cosmic forces (macrocosm), while the internal forces (microcosm) are governed by the principles of [the three elements]. A basic principle of healing in Ayurveda holds that one may create balance in the internal forces working in the individual by altering diet and habits of living to counteract changes in his external environment.[11]

A practitioner of Ayurveda uses various diagnostic techniques, such as examination of the pulse, tongue, face, lips, nails, and eyes to monitor the disease process, which is, in turn, a reflection of an imbalance among the three basic principles.

The maintenance of a diet compatible with the individual constitution is considered of basic importance to the recovery and maintenance of health.

Yoga, breathing practices, and meditation are also employed in a therapeutic program, as are herbal preparations. Other components of a treatment program may be emotional release (the recognition, understanding, and release of negative emotions), therapeutic vomiting, and the use of purgatives, enemas, and fasting.[12]

Unlike Chinese medicine, Ayurveda is not recognized in the United States as a licensed treatment modality. Various training programs in Ayurveda do exist in the United States, but state laws vary as to whether practitioners can use their training to treat patients. The names and locations of some of the Ayurvedic practitioners in the United States who have received classic training in Ayurveda in India can be obtained through Dr. Lad's Ayurvedic Institute (505-291-9698).

Homeopathy

According to homeopathic educator Dana Ullman, M.P.H., homeopathy "is a natural pharmaceutical science that utilizes extremely small doses of substances to stimulate a person's immune and defence system. Each medicine is individually prescribed according to the 'law of similars'—that is, a substance which creates in overdose a specific set of symptoms in a healthy person will cure these similar symptoms in a sick person when given in very small doses." Homeopathy is largely dismissed by Western medicine, although it is widely practiced in Europe and India. Some rigorous scientific studies supportive of homeopathic principles have been conducted, but none with cancer that I am aware of.

Ullman is director of Homeopathic Educational Services, 2124 Kitteredge Street, Berkeley, CA 94704, 510-649-0294, which is a mail-order source of information and educational materials on homeopathy and homeopathic products for health professionals and the general public.

The National Center for Homeopathy, 801 North Fairfax Street, Alexandria, VA 22314, 703-548-7790, fax: 703-548-7792, issues an annual directory of homeopathic practitioners, study groups, pharmacies, and resources.

American Cancer Society List of Unproven Methods of Cancer Treatment

The ACS maintains a list of unproven methods of cancer treatment and monographs describing these therapies and the centers that offer them. The list can be obtained by calling your local ACS office. The NCI also provides information about specific unproven methods, and this can be obtained by calling the hot line at 1-800-4-CANCER.

Basically, the list of unproven methods represents the best effort of the ACS to deal with the problem of unconventional cancer treatments. The list has been criticized both by advocates of alternative cancer therapies and by mainstream researchers and policy specialists on the grounds that it fails to differentiate between some of the more bizarre therapies and some interesting therapies that have not come up through the standard mainstream credentialing process.

It is also worth comparing the unproven methods list with the accounts of unconventional cancer treatments contained in the Office of Technology Assessment (OTA) report, *Unconventional Cancer Treatments*.[13] The OTA report is widely regarded as providing a much more sophisticated analysis of these therapies.

According to the ACS, in many cases "unproven methods of cancer treatment" have some or all of the following characteristics:

1. They tend to be isolated from established scientific facilities and associations.
2. They often do not use regular channels of scientific and clinical communications.
3. They claim the established medical and scientific organizations, political and governmental agencies have conspired against them.
4. Their clinical and scientific records are weak and sometimes nonexistent.
5. They sometimes discourage or refuse consultation with reputable physicians or scientists.
6. Their treatments are sometimes secrets, or secretly prepared.
7. They sometimes discount biopsy verification in cancer diagnosis.
8. They may have multiple, unusual degrees from obscure institutions of higher learning or even correspondence schools.
9. Their chief supporters tend to be prominent statesmen, actors, writers, lawyers, even members of state and local legislatures—persons not trained or experienced in the natural history of cancer, in the care of patients with cancer, or with accepted scientific procedures and methods.

The ACS ranks unproven methods according to how effective the method is; how likely the method is to cause harm to the patient; and how much the method is used. According to these criteria, the unproven methods of "highest concern" are: antineoplastons (Stanislaw Burzynski's therapy; see chapter 21); the Committee for Freedom of Choice in Medicine, Inc.; the Contreras method; the Greek cancer cure of Hariton Alivizatos; Immuno-Augmentative Therapy; laetrile; Livingston therapy (see chapter 16); macrobiotic diet (see chapter 15 and the Kushi Institute and Vega Study Center in section VIII, above); the

National Health Federation; the Revici method (see chapter 23); and the techniques of O. Carl Simonton (see chapter 10).

"Of high concern" are dimethyl sulfoxide (DMSO); the Gerson diet (see chapter 14); Hoxsey herbs (see Bio-Medical Center below); the International Association of Cancer Victors and Friends, Inc.; Iscador (see below); Dr. Kelley's nutritional and metabolic therapy (see Unconventional Nutritional Programs, above); live cell therapy; the metabolic therapy of Dr. Harold Manner; and psychic surgery. "Of concern" are Vlastimil Brych; electronic devices; and chaparral tea.

Probably the most striking current anomaly on this list, even accepting the controversial assumptions of the ACS, is the inclusion of O. Carl Simonton's psychological imagery techniques in the category of "highest concern."

Alternative and Complementary Treatment Centers: United States, Canada, Mexico, Bahamas, Britain, and Europe

This resource section does not attempt to provide a comprehensive list of alternative cancer treatment centers. The reader interested in a wider list and fuller descriptions can consult three documents: the ACS list of "unproven methods of cancer treatment" described above; the OTA report, *Unconventional Cancer Treatments;* and the valuable resource book by John Fink, *Third Opinion,*[14] which describes most of the leading unconventional cancer treatment techniques used by American cancer patients today. Fink is generally supportive of these treatments; the ACS is generally critical; and the OTA report is somewhere between the two. Ralph Moss's *Cancer Therapy*[15] and Richard Walters' *Options*[16] are also valuable, generally pro-alternative sources of information on these therapies.

United States

> Livingston Foundation Medical Center
> 3232 Duke Street
> San Diego, CA 92110
> Tel: 619-224-3515
> Fax: 619-224-6253

(See chapter 16 for a discussion of the work of Virginia Livingston.)

The Livingston Foundation Medical Center was established in 1971 by Dr. Virginia Livingston. The clinic provides immunological treatments based on the models developed by Dr. Livingston, including vaccines, diet and nutrition, supplements, psychological counseling, detoxification, antibiotics, and conventional drug therapies (as long as the latter are seen as consistent with the goal of immune enhancement).

The Livingston Foundation Medical Center offers two programs for patients. The first is a 10-day clinical immunotherapy program designed for patients suffering from an advanced debilitating illness. The second is a 2-day annual diagnostic program designed to evaluate the status of a patient's immune system. The latter program is designed for persons who wish to use these techniques to maintain optimal health, for persons with chronic health problems, or for those who have a strong family history of immunodeficiency conditions. This program involves vaccines, diet, and lifestyle changes.

The 10-day program provides the basis for selecting and implementing an immunotherapy regimen which will be continued by the patient at home. Upon arrival, all patients are interviewed by a staff physician and a comprehensive medical history is compiled, including a family history record. The interview is followed by a complete physical examination using conventional diagnostic techniques. Selective diagnostic tests are then used to evaluate the status of the patient's immune system and to identify any underlying microbial or bacterial infections. If the immune system is found to be inadequate by these measures, an immune enhancement program may be initiated. This might involve the administration of one or more vaccines, antibiotics, and antibodies (such as gamma globulin), as well as stimulation and restoration of liver function, detoxification, dietary adjustment, and nutrient supplementation.

Patients and family members are instructed in the administration of the various immunological therapies, nutrition planning and meal preparation, use of supplementary immune enhancement techniques, and detoxification procedures to be used by the patient after leaving the clinic.

The medical center also offers group and individual counseling designed to help individuals and families cope with the stress of illness. Visualization and stress reduction techniques believed to enhance immune response are also taught to patients.

In addition to cancer, the medical center treats patients with other potentially life-threatening diseases such as lupus, arthritis, and scleroderma. The clinic operates on an outpatient basis only.

The cost of the 10-day program is approximately $5,500. A deposit of $2,500 must be made in advance and the balance must be paid at the time of checkout. Additionally, laboratory work sent outside typically costs $500 to $800. The medical center estimates that the average patient pays between

$600 and $1,000 per month for an ongoing program at home during the first year.

The 2-day prevention program requires an initial deposit of $600 toward the total cost of approximately $1,200, which must be paid in full upon completion of the program.

Institute of Applied Biology
26 East 36th Street
New York, NY 10015
Tel: 212-685-0111
Fax: 212-685-0112

(See chapter 23 for a discussion of the work of Emanuel Revici.)

According to patient literature supplied by Dr. Revici's office, all substances administered as part of Dr. Revici's therapies are "carefully and thoroughly demonstrated to be non-toxic. Therefore patients under his care suffer no significant adverse reactions from his medications. This general lack of toxicity permits Dr. Revici to administer his medicines in doses much higher than ordinarily used, sparing healthy cells and the immune system from harm."

An initial consultation with Dr. Revici costs $200 (paid by traveler's check or money order), and the patient must bring all previous pathology reports with diagnoses, results of any current laboratory tests, x-ray films, computed to-mography (CT) scans, and magnetic resonance imaging (MRI) tests. The patient must also bring the names of current medications being taken currently and a history of previous therapies for the cancer.

Follow-up consultations with Dr. Revici are $95 and injections of medications are $50. Fees for laboratory tests are billed directly to the patient.

Dr. Revici stresses that the best results are obtained with his therapy when he has sufficient information to guide the therapy individually so that dosages can be adjusted and medications altered when necessary. Therefore, his office recommends that all patients participate in the chronic disease management program, run by Dr. Bijan Khoshbin, to provide regular and close monitoring of symptoms and the effects of medications. The charge for this service is $150 per month and includes physical examinations, urine analysis, adjuvant nutri-tional treatment, prescription of diagnostic tests, and referrals to specialists when necessary. This fee and service are separate from any charged by Dr. Revici for his services.

Nicholas Gonzalez, M.D.
737 Park Avenue
New York, NY 10021
Tel: 212-535-3993
Fax: 212-628-9085

(See Unconventional Nutritional Programs, above for a description.)

Burzynski Research Institute
6221 Corporate Drive
Houston, TX 77036
713-777-8233

(See chapter 21 for a discussion of the work of Stanislaw Burzynski.)

All patients visiting the Burzynski Research Institute are treated on an outpatient basis. The treatment is self-administered and, according to the institute, usually free of side effects. Dr. Burzynski also believes that the treatment does not interfere with surgery, radiation therapy, or most chemotherapies and immuno-therapies. In some cases, small doses of conventional chemotherapy or immu-notherapy agents are used along with the antineoplaston treatments.

At the time of initial contact, a detailed medical history is taken over the phone, and after a review of the patient's history, one of the medical staff calls the patient to discuss whether or not the treatment may be of help.

Patients are monitored closely during the first 2 weeks of treatment, with appointments typically scheduled twice weekly during this period. After the initial 2-week stay, follow-up visits are scheduled every 4 to 8 weeks. Follow-up visits average 2 to 5 days in length.

Initial patient response is evaluated by standard medical tests, usually within the first 3 to 6 weeks of treatment. At a minimum, treatment usually lasts 4 months to 1 year.

For most patients, the fee for antineoplaston treatments range from $135 to $315 per day. The initial consultation with Dr. Burzynski, without treatment, is $125. Follow-up appointments are $60. Other expenses include the usual diagnostic tests (radiographs, CT scans, MRI) and standard blood and urine tests which are used to monitor the patient's progress. If intravenous administration of the therapy is necessary, additional supplies must be procured outside the clinic at a cost of $4,200 to $6,300.

An initial deposit of $5,000 is required from all patients prior to the start of treatment. For patients receiving antineoplaston therapy intravenously, a monthly deposit of $2,500 is charged beginning with the second month of treatment. For patients taking capsules, no further payments are required until the tenth month of treatment, when an additional $5,000 deposit is made.

After the first week of treatment, the institute begins filing insurance claims to the patient's insurance carrier. If insurance payments are forthcoming, the patient does not have to make further monthly payments, and the $5,000 deposit is refunded once insurance has paid the entire bill.

Accommodations in nearby furnished apartment complexes can be arranged in advance through the clinic.

Mexico

Mexican alternative cancer treatment centers all operate in a frontier cultural context that defies easy description. To some people, the treatments at these centers appear to be the quintessence of cancer quackery and sleaze. To others, the operators of these centers are folk heroes and courageous cancer treatment pioneers. You pay your money (often a lot of money) and take your choice.

If you are considering treatment in Mexico, you would be well advised to travel to the Tijuana area and spend some time visiting the clinics that interest you and talking to patients about their experiences before signing up for treatment. There are motels and trailer parks just north of the border on the American side where many cancer patients live while undergoing treatment. The grapevine there about what is happening at the clinics is strong and well-informed.

> Bio-Medical Center
> PO Box 727
> Tijuana, B.C., Mexico
> Tel: 011-52-66-84-90-11
> 011-52-66-84-90-81
> 011-52-66-84-90-82
> 011-52-66-84-93-76
> Fax: 011-52-66-84-97-44

The Bio-Medical Center is one of the best-known Tijuana cancer clinics. It is an outpatient clinic that treats all types of malignancies using the Hoxsey therapy, immunotherapy, chemotherapy (in serious cases), homeopathy, and chelation therapy.[17] The treatment also includes supplements and dietary restrictions. The Hoxsey therapy has long been regarded as an archetype of cancer quackery by the American Medical Association and the ACS.

The legend is that the origins of the Hoxsey therapy date back 150 years to veterinarian John Hoxsey who observed a horse cure its cancer by eating certain wild plants in the pasture. Hoxsey gathered these herbs, added ingredients from home remedies for cancer, and successfully treated other animals with cancer. His descendants used the same preparation to treat cancer in humans.[18] Hoxsey did not claim to know how or why the treatment worked.[19]

The OTA, in its evaluation of the Hoxsey therapy, reports:

> The data indicate that many of the herbs used in the Hoxsey internal tonic or the isolated components of these herbs have antitumor activity or cytotoxic effects in animal test systems. The complete Hoxsey herbal mixture has not been tested for antitumor activity in animal test systems, with human cells in culture, or in clinical trials, however. It is unknown whether the individual herbs or their components that show antitumor activity in animals are active in humans when given in the concentrations used in the Hoxsey tonic. It is also unknown whether there might be synergistic effects of the herbs used together.[20]

Initial x-ray films and examination run from $250 to $450. The cost of the Hoxsey therapy itself, for as long as it is necessary, is $3,500. A down payment of at least 30% must be paid on the first visit. (The clinic claims that inability to pay does not prevent a patient from receiving therapy.)

American Biologics-Mexico S.A. Hospital and Medical Center
United States Admissions Office
1180 Walnut Avenue
Chula Vista, CA 92011
Tel: 619-429-8200 or 1-800-227-4458
Fax: 619-429-8004

Clinic: 15 Azucenas Street, Tijuana, B.C., Mexico

American Biologics-Mexico is one of the most efficiently operated of the Mexican alternative cancer treatment centers. Its founder, Robert Bradford, is a long-time veteran of the alternative cancer therapy wars and an accomplished businessman who knows his product (alternative cancer therapies) and his clients. Bradford offers one of the broadest lines of alternative therapies available in any Mexican clinic, with one of the most polished presentations of his product.

Although American Biologics-Mexico treats all kinds of cancer, the staff claims that adenocarcinomas of the lung, colon, and breast are their best overall responders. The staff claims also that they do well with leukemias, lymphomas, and localized sarcomas. They report that extensive liver metastases and pancreatic cancer are their most difficult cases.

American Biologics-Mexico claims symptom-free or mostly symptom-free 5-year survivals in roughly 20% of their cases. They do not promise to "cure" cancer. Writing in their literature, Michael Culbert, Vice-President of American Biologics-Mexico, states, "Our maximum claim is that, under the best of conditions, we will place cancer under 'control' so that a patient may live out his/her appointed genetic lifespan without cancer being a major problem."

American Biologics-Mexico implements individualized, integrated metabolic and eclectic programs developed by its sister organization, the Bradford Research Institute. American Biologics-Mexico offers a comprehensive range of services. According to Culbert, "Our sole interest is in the disease-free survival of the patient, not the proving of a concept or theory. To this end, we may use any combination of vitamins, minerals, enzymes, amino acids, endocrine balancing, immune enhancement, gastrointestinal detoxification, alkaline diet, herbs, oxidative therapies, and even antibiotics, chemotherapy, surgery or low-grade radiation or synthetic hormones." American Biologics-Mexico also offers "live-cell" therapies.

American Biologics-Mexico S.A. Medical Center and Hospital describes itself as a fully accredited and licensed general hospital and teaching facility. Both in- and outpatient services are available; there are beds for a maximum of 27 inpatients and the clinic can serve approximately 40 outpatients per day.

Prices range from $1,900 for 1 week for outpatients to $4,500 per week for inpatients with private rooms. The average stay is between 3 and 4 weeks.

Hospital Ernesto Contreras
P.O. Box 43-9045
San Ysidro, CA 92143-9045
Tel: 1-800 326-1850 or 1-800 LAETRYL
Fax: 011-526-680-2709

Hospital: Paseo Playas de Tijuana No. 19, Playas de Tijuana, B.C. 22700, Mexico

The Hospital Ernesto Contreras is one of the oldest unconventional cancer therapy centers in Tijuana. Dr. Ernesto Contreras, Sr., was among the first practitioners to offer laetrile as a treatment for cancer.

Contreras reports that his hospital treats about 1,000 patients a year, 80% of whom are considered advanced or terminal cases. The hospital treats all kinds of cancers. Contreras claims a subjective response rate among hospital patients of 65% and an objective response rate of 35% (i.e., cases in which the tumor has decreased in size by at least 50%).

Contreras and his staff believe that cancer is a systemic rather than localized disease, calling for a three-pronged emotional, spiritual, and physical approach. The hospital offers a varied metabolic therapy, including amygdalin (laetrile), detoxification, proteolytic enzymes, nutritional regimen, intravenous amino acid and vitamin solutions, high-dose vitamin C, and oxygen, for most carcinomas and lymphomas.

For primary brain tumors and sarcomas, the hospital utilizes the Alivett treatment, "a process which kills the abnormal cells and inhibits their reproductive rate while selectively feeding normal cells to re-establish their normal reproductive rates. . . . Inasmuch as the ingredients of the treatment are found in the human cell, the resultant product is non-toxic even when administered in quantities well above those recommended." The treatment consists of a series of injections (normally 20) administered daily.

The Warburg therapy, which is known in the United States as the Cone cancer therapy system, is employed for tumors of the head and neck, pulmonary metastases, myelomas, and any other tumors resistant to the treatments described above. This therapy is considered experimental in the United States, but may be available by patient request with informed consent. The therapy consists of a low fat, high carbohydrate nutritional regimen and three nontoxic medications—Lente insulin (an insulin zinc preparation), quercetin, and thyroid hormone. In theory, these components combine to starve tumor cells and boost acidity to lethal levels within the targeted cells.

Immusyn C is also available at the Hospital. According to hospital literature, Immusyn C is a chemotherapeutic agent selectively toxic only to cancer cells that can be used alone or in combination with other chemotherapies or radiation. 714-X, the therapy developed by Gaston Naessens in Canada, is also available at Hospital Ernesto Contreras.

In addition to the 50-bed, standard hospital facilities on the first floor, Hospital Ernesto Contreras maintains 20 motel rooms on the second floor. Outpatients are encouraged to stay at the International Motor Inn in San Ysidro on the U.S. side of the border. The hospital provides frequent van service to the facility.

The average stay is 3 weeks. The cost typically ranges from $8,500 to $10,000 including meals and lodging for both patient and a companion. Costs for patients receiving either the Alivett or Warburg therapies on an outpatient basis may be slightly less. A minimum $6,500 deposit is required upon initiation of services, with the balance due on departure.

Take-home medications typically cost $1,500 to $2,000. Surgical procedures, chemotherapy, radiation, and antibiotics are charged separately.

Centro Hospitalario del Pacifico S.A.
449 Nubes
Playas de Tijuana, B.C., Mexico
and the Gerson Institute
PO Box 430
Bonita, CA 91908
Tel: 619-472-7450
Fax: 619-267-6441

(See chapter 14 for a discussion of the Gerson therapy.)

The Gerson Institute in Bonita, California is associated with the Centro Hospitalario del Pacifico S.A. (CHIPSA) in Tijuana, which offers the Gerson program. Some patients like the experience at CHIPSA and others do not. Like most of the Mexican cancer clinics, the program experiences changes with time and personnel changes. If you are considering participating in the program, it is certainly worth visiting the hospital and talking with patients before signing up.

CHIPSA recommends a minimum initial stay of 21 days, and 4 to 6 weeks for more seriously ill patients. The hospital requires a deposit of $3,990 at the time of admission, and a $3,990 deposit in advance for each subsequent week. Additional charges may be incurred, especially by patients who are very ill. Companions pay $308 per week, which includes room and board and training in the Gerson therapy.

After leaving the hospital, the therapy is continued at home for upward of 18 months with periodic adjustments. This regimen consists of a vegan diet (plant products only), juices taken hourly, and detoxification. Once a routine is established, the patient can usually leave home two times each day for 5 hours, though an extended lunch period is required. A 3-month supply of Gerson medications costs $550 (not including adjuvant medications) and a juicer costs a minimum of $240. Specialized food requirements may entail substantially higher costs (from $200 to $500 per week) and much greater efforts to obtain needed items.

Canada

> C.O.S.E. Inc.
> 5270, Fontaine
> Rock Forest, Quebec, J1N 3B6, Canada
> Tel: 819-564-7883
> Fax: 819-564-4668

Gaston Naessens, a French-born biologist, utilizes an apparently powerful microscope of his own invention, called the "Somatoscope," to examine live blood for the purpose of diagnosing cancer and monitoring treatment.

Naessens theorizes that harmless microorganisms arising within the body could, under some conditions, become lethal. This theory places him in the tradition of researchers whose work has been eclipsed by Pasteur's belief that organisms originating outside the body were responsible for disease. Naessens' theory is parallel to that of the late Virginia Livingston (see chapter 15) and other exponents of the existence of entities called "cell wall–deficient bacteria" said to play a role in cancer and other diseases.

Using the Somatoscope, Naessens believes that he is able to view the cycle of the "somatid," a pleomorphic (form-changing) organism in the blood which is "a transitional link between matter and cosmic energy. It may well be the first manifestation of life." In people with fully functional immune systems, the somatid cycle consists of three stages, whereas an impending diseased state is indicated by the presence of successive 13-stage cycles.[21]

In the literature describing his therapy, Naessens states that healthy bodies develop and fight off small cancers regularly, but that a deficient immune system allows the cancer to reach a critical point where it withdraws nitrogen from the body for its own use, and in the process paralyzes the immune system. Naessens utilizes a camphor derivative called 714X which reportedly inhibits the formation of the substance produced by the tumor that makes nitrogen available to the tumor and suppresses the immune system.

According to the clinic, it is not necessary to have the results of a blood test initially when giving 714X. However, a fresh blood test is recommended after 3 months in order to evaluate the success of the treatment. Few practitioners have the necessary equipment to accomplish this, but the clinic can supply the names of those who do.

714X is said to be nontoxic and to have no known side effects. It is injected daily into the lymph nodes (preferably in the groin). In average cases, three series of 21 injections are required, each followed by a "booster shot." It is recommended that the patient continue the treatment until no more signs of the disease are present.

A quantity of 714X sufficient for one series of injections (21 days) costs $300. The protocol and injection instructions are included with the shipment. Payment must be accompanied by a medical prescription.

Bahamas

> Immuno-Augmentative Therapy Centre, Ltd.
> PO Box F-2689
> Freeport, Grand Bahama
> Tel: 809-352-7455
> Fax: 809-352-3201

Immuno-Augmentative Therapy (IAT) was developed by the late Lawrence Burton, Ph.D., and has been used with patients at his Bahama center since 1977. The IAT Centre remains open after his death. IAT is one of the best-known and controversial unconventional treatments for cancer. The effort to evaluate the effectiveness of IAT was the original impetus behind the OTA's *Unconventional Cancer Treatments* report. The OTA was unsuccessful in its effort to reach agreement with Burton on an objective assessment of his therapy. Burton kept key elements of his therapy a proprietary secret. His critics believe his therapy is pure quackery; his supporters believe it is pure genius, and patients keep coming to fill his Bahamian treatment center.

The IAT literature describes the reported theoretical basis of the treatment:

> During the 1960's, Lawrence Burton, Ph.D., with a team of scientific and medical investigators, pursued a means to reduce or inhibit tumor growth. An accepted assumption was that animals have one or more components in their blood which control mitosis (cell division) and growth . . . and, therefore, there existed an anti-cancer immune defense mechanism. They further assumed that a *balanced proportion* of these components results in normal mitosis and cellular growth, but an imbalance may result in malignant neoplasms. They believed, too that these components could be

isolated without deactivating them. . . . Their hypothesis indicated that administration of such growth components . . . would cause the host's natural immune defense mechanism to function, and result in reduction and/or remission of neoplastic tissue [emphasis in original].[22]

The treatment regimen is based on reported assessment of the patient's immunocompetence. The patient's blood is then tested twice daily for the relative concentration of four basic factors. Patients inject themselves daily with processed blood products to maintain the proper balance of these factors. The dose levels are determined by a proprietary computer system which is also used to monitor results and project necessary dosages once patients leave the center. The self-injection protocol continues at home indefinitely.[23]

All IAT patients must be accompanied by an adult companion. The center is an outpatient facility, so patients must stay in local hotels or apartments that have kitchen facilities. Patients stay an average of 12 weeks in Freeport.

Four weeks of therapy cost $5,000, and thereafter the cost per week is $500. This fee includes all routine tests, services, and other components of the therapy. The cost of the home maintenance prescription is $50 per week.

Switzerland

Lukas Klinik
CH-4144 Arlesheim, Switzerland
011-41-061-701-3333

(See chapter 3 for a discussion of anthroposophical medicine.)

The Lukas Klinik is perhaps the most beautiful cancer hospital I have visited in my travels. Founded by followers of the anthroposophical thinker Rudolf Steiner, I found it to have a deep aesthetic appeal. The clinic uses mainstream therapies in combination with anthroposophical therapies including vegetarian diet, movement therapy, color therapy, art therapy, speech therapy, herbal therapy (including Iscador; see section XIII, below), and special baths. The disadvantage of the clinic for Americans, at least at the time of my visit, was that most staff did not speak English and most discussion was in Swiss German. For German-speaking cancer patients with a proclivity toward the anthroposophical spiritual tradition, the Lukas Klinik is well worth exploring.

Germany

Hans A. Nieper, Dr. med.
Paracelsus Klinik at Silbersee
Oertzeweg 24
3012 Langenhagen, Germany
Tel: 011-49-511-348-08-08
Fax: 011-49-511-318417

Hans Nieper is a controversial German alternative cancer therapist who receives mixed reviews from American cancer patients who visit him. His therapies for cancer are based on "the principle of assisting the body's own defense mechanisms, which exist in every human being." He postulates that in the 40% of the population whose defenses are not sufficiently strong to ward off cancer, it is important to strengthen the immune system as a preventive measure through a diet containing large amounts of carotene, selenium, vitamins C and D_2, magnesium, and molybdenum. In cases of existing cancer, these substances can be utilized along with others, such as bromelain—an enzyme obtained from pineapple—to combat the cancer. The latter is one of a number of enzymes used to "deshield" the tumor cell membrane and to "deblind" immune cells so that the tumor becomes susceptible to action by the immune system.

Dr. Nieper uses radiotherapy and chemotherapy only for short-term alleviation, since he believes that these are injurious to the body and do not address the underlying cause of the cancer, the deficient immune system.

A number of methods are claimed to restore the immune system, depending upon the point in the system where the disturbance lies. One of the therapies Dr. Nieper uses to restore immune function is "desodification" (elimination of sodium) "By this method, cancer cells are 'detoxified' from the inside. Which method is actually applied depends on the clinical picture of the individual patient. However, the basic principle is always the administration of certain natural substances which do not destroy but which restore."[24] Nieper also uses BCG (bacille Calmette-Guérin), Wobe-Mugos enzymes, and laetrile in his therapy.

In addition, Nieper uses a "gene repair" therapy which is based on his theory that "gene 'instabilities' (not true mutations) may play a pivotally important role in cancer. The elimination of such gene instabilities seems feasible. This would then result in a normalization (or re-differentiation) of the cancer cell—or its elimination. Starting from investigation of so-called anti-cancer surveillance steroids to which belong Tumosterone and DHEA [dehydroepiandrosterone], Dr. Nieper introduced plant-derived gene surveillance substances into the clinical management of cancer."[25]

Patients normally remain at the hospital for 9 to 21 days. Fees for inpatient therapy normally range from DM 450 to 550 per day, including all doctors' fees and treatment costs.[26]

Robert Janker Klinick
Fachklinik für Tumorerkrankungen
Baumschulallee 12-14
5300 Bonn 1, Germany
Tel: 011-49-228-7291-0
Fax: 011-49-228-631832

The Janker Klinik is one of the most popular German cancer clinics for American cancer patients seeking an "unconventional/conventional" treatment outside the United States. It is strongly recommended by writer-researcher Patrick McGrady (see section I, under Consultants for Mainstream and Complementary Therapies, above). The program makes use of intensive chemotherapies and other protocols not available in the United States.

England

Bristol Cancer Help Centre
Grove House
Cornwallis Grove
Clifton, Bristol BS8 4PG, England, United Kingdom
011-44-0272-743216

Since its founding in 1980, the Bristol Cancer Help Centre has been a pioneer in the development of psychosocial support programs for people with cancer. According to the center's description of its work, "Our approach is not an alternative to medical treatment. The holistic model promoted at Bristol is patient-centered, targeting the disease at the level of the body, mind and spirit. Counseling, group sessions, meditation, visualization, and a range of creative therapies are used to help individuals develop their own resources to cope with threats to quality of life and potential recovery."

The Bristol Centre offers an "Introductory Day" which can be complete in itself, but they strongly recommend that patients continue with the weeklong "Residential Course" and subsequent "Follow Up Days." All programs are led and supervised by physicians with support by therapists and other staff members. The center also recommends that spouses, support people, and caregivers attend along with the patient.

In the residential course, group support, meditation, visualization, and self-help techniques are employed to help patients in adjusting to the experience of cancer and cancer treatment. Patients are assisted in assessing their own needs, establishing personal goals, setting up a network of support, and creating a self-help program. They also learn about holistic medicine and its possible effect on the course of the disease.

The cost of the residential course is £350, although the center states that its policy is that no one be denied a place because of lack of funds.

Alternative Pharmaceutical Treatments

Hydrazine Sulfate

(See chapter 22 for a full description.)

Hydrazine sulfate is an inexpensive drug of mild toxicity that studies have shown can, in some cases, enhance the nutritional status of cancer patients and help them avoid weight loss—thus possibly extending life. In the United States, it is currently available to cancer patients through their physicians. The physician must obtain the substance through the FDA's Investigational New Drug compassionate (IND) program. For information on obtaining hydrazine sulfate in this way, ask your physician to contact the Syracuse Cancer Research Institute Inc., Presidential Plaza, 600 East Genesee Street, Syracuse, NY 13202, 315-472-6616.

The compound is also sold through several of the Mexican clinics.

Iscador

According to the Swiss Society for Oncology, Iscador is a fermented extract of mistletoe that was first proposed as a treatment for cancer in 1920 by Rudolph Steiner, the founder of anthroposophy. It is the most widely used unconventional pharmacological agent for the treatment of cancer in Europe. It is less widely used in the United States. Iscador is thought by proponents to have anticancer activity and to increase immune function. The toxicity of Iscador varies according to its preparation and method of administration, but in the hands of a knowledgeable practitioner it is relatively nontoxic. There is a considerable research literature on Iscador and related mistletoe products, some of it demonstrating antitumor activities or immunostimulation in experimental systems. I am not aware of any clinical studies showing significant antitumor activity in controlled human clinical trials.

According to Immaculada Marti, M.D., an anthroposophical physician at Davies Medical Center in San Francisco, Iscador is not available from sources in the United States, but must be obtained by a physician from European suppliers. In the anthroposophical tradition, Iscador is not used as an isolated pharmaceutical treatment, but is usually administered as part of a combination therapy along with other anthroposophical medicines, external therapies (such as baths), and movement therapies.

Dr. Marti is one of about 35 anthroposophical physicians practicing in the United States. She is able to provide patients and interested physicians with information about anthroposophical approaches to cancer care and to direct them to the nearest anthroposophical practitioner: call 415-565-6000. The Lukas Klinik (see Treatment Centers above) in Switzerland is the leading anthroposophical treatment center in the world and the source of much of the research on Iscador and other anthroposophical medicines.

Laetrile

Laetrile (also known as amygdalin) is a controversial cancer treatment found naturally in the seeds of apricots and other members of the Rosaceae family. Its use was fairly widespread in the mid-1970s, but it has become less sought-after as a cancer treatment since that time. According to the OTA report, *Unventional Cancer Treatments*:

> Laetrile proponents claim that laetrile kills tumor cells selectively, while leaving normal cells alone. In support of this, Ernst Krebs, Jr. [one of the developers of laetrile], hypothesized that normal cells produce an enzyme, beta glucosidase, that breaks down laetrile, releasing cyanide, which is then converted by a second enzyme, rhodanese, to the less toxic thiocyanate molecule; cancer cells, however, lack the enzyme rhodanese, according to Kreb's theory, and are therefore killed by free cyanide.[27]

In contrast to the early years of laetrile's use, when claims for antitumor activity were made, proponents more recently have cited laetrile's effectiveness as part of a wider metabolic regimen, including DMSO, vitamins, enzymes, and other substances.[28] Many clinics in Mexico use laetrile in this way, including American Biologics-Mexico and Hospital Ernesto Contreras described above. Mainstream clinical trials of laetrile showed no significant antitumor activity, but these studies have been (predictably) criticized by proponents of laetrile on methodological grounds.[29]

According to the OTA report, the most common adverse side effects of laetrile ingestion are nausea, vomiting, headache, and dizziness. Laetrile itself is about

6% cyanide by weight and cyanide toxicity has been observed in people taking it. Lethal doses of cyanide can be reached if an excessive amount of laetrile is ingested or if something is done to accelerate the release of cyanide, such as eating foods high in the enzyme that promote this release (e.g., nuts, lettuce, celery, or mushrooms).[30]

The use of laetrile is illegal in many states. The Cancer Control Society (213-663-7801), an advocacy organization for alternative cancer therapies, can provide information about laetrile, lists of practitioners who prescribe it, and the circumstances under which it may be legally obtained.

Immuno-Augmentative Therapy:
Immuno-Augmentative Therapy Centre, Ltd.
Freeport, Grand Bahama
Tel: 809-352-7455
Fax: 809-352-3201

(See Immuno-Augmentative Therapy Centre above.)

Antineoplastons:
Burzynski Research Institute
6221 Corporate Drive
Houston, TX 77036
713-777-8233

(See chapter 21 for a discussion of the work of Stanislaw Burzynski; see Alternative and Complementary Treatment Centers above.)

Autogenous Vaccines:
Livingston Foundation Medical Center
3232 Duke Street
San Diego, CA 92110
Tel: 619-224-3515
Fax: 619-224-6253

(See chapter 16 for a discussion of the work of Virginia Livingston; see also Alternative and Complementary Treatment Centers: United States, Canada, Mexico, Bahamas, Britain, and Europe above).

Notes and References

1   David Zimmerman, "How Pat McGrady's 'Can Help' Helps Patients with Cancer," *Probe: David Zimmerman's Newsletter on Science, Media, Policy and Health,* November 1, 1991.

2   Gerald G. Jampolsky, *Love is Letting Go of Fear* (New York: Bantam Books, 1970; Berkeley, CA: Celestial Arts Publishing Co., 1988).

3   Jon Kabat-Zinn, *Full Catastrophe Living: Using the Wisdom of Your Body and Mind to Face Stress, Pain, and Illness* (New York: Dell Publishing, 1990).

4   Bernie S. Siegel, M.D. *Love, Medicine and Miracles* (New York: Harper & Row, 1986; HarperCollins, 1990).

5   O. Carl Simonton, Stephanie Matthews-Simonton, and James Creighton, *Getting Well Again* (Los Angeles: Jeremy P. Tarcher, 1978).

6   Raychel and Mark Solomon, *Coming Alive with Raychel* (San Diego: Raymark Books, Inc., 1986).

7   Michael Hollingworth, "Everyday 'Miracles'" *Australian Wellbeing* March/April 1986, 94.

8   Ibid.

9   Dr. Chopra is the author of several informative books on Ayurveda: *Creating Health: Beyond Prevention, Toward Perfection* (Boston: Houghton Mifflin Company, 1987); *Return of the Rishi: A Doctor's Search for the Ultimate Healer* (Boston: Houghton Mifflin Company, 1988); and *Quantum Healing: Exploring the Frontiers of Mind/Body Medicine* (New York: Bantam Books, 1989).

10 Deepak Chopra, *Quantum Healing: Exploring the Frontiers of Mind/Body Medicine* (New York: Bantam Books, 1989).

11 Dr. Vasant Lad, *Ayurveda: The Science of Self-Healing* (Wilmont, Wis.: Lotus Press, 1984), 29.

12 Ibid., 52–68.

13 U.S. Congress Office of Technology Assessment. *Unconventional Cancer Therapies* (Washington, D.C.: Government Printing Office, September 1990).

14 John Fink with Sue Carlan, *Third Opinion: A Guide to Alternative and Adjunctive Therapies, Clinics and Physicians in the Treatment and Prevention of Cancer,* second edition (Garden City Park, NY: Avery Publishing Group, 1992).

15 Ralph W. Moss, *Cancer Therapy: The Independant Consumer's Guide to Non-Toxic Treatment and Prevention* (New York: Equinox Press, 1992).

16 Richard Walters, *Options: The Alternative Cancer Therapy Book* (Garden City, NY: Avery Publishing Group Inc., 1993).

17 Bio-Medical Center literature.

18 Office of Technology Assessment, *Unconventional Cancer Treatments,* 75.

19 H.M. Hoxsey, *You Don't Have to Die* (New York, NY: Milestone Books, 1956). Cited in Office of Technology Assessment, *Unconventional Cancer Treatments,* 76.

20 Office of Technology Assessment, *Unconventional Cancer Treatments,* 79.

21 Christopher Byrd, "Gaston Naessens' Symposium on Somatidian Orthobiology: A Beachhead Established" *Townsend Letter for Doctors* October 1991:797–99.

22   Immuno-Augmentative Therapy Center literature.

23   Office of Technology Assessment, *Unconventional Cancer Treatments,* 131.

24   Dr. Hans Nieper, *New Biological Therapies* (Los Angeles: Paracelsus Hospital Corporation) p 7.

25   Ibid, 6.

26   John Fink, *Third Opinion,* 142.

27   Office of Technology Assessment, *Unconventional Cancer Treatments,* 103.

28   Ibid., 103.

29   Ibid., 106.

30   Ibid., 103.

Professional Training Programs in Spiritual and Psychological Approaches to Cancer

One of the critical questions for many health professionals is where they can find training and professional education programs in psychoeducational approaches to cancer. This appendix lists several resources in this field.

Health Training and Research Center
PO Box 7237
Little Rock, AR 72217
501-663-5369

Stephanie Simonton, Ph.D., one of the pioneers of imagery and related psychological approaches to cancer treatment, has trained many health practitioners in her psychological approach to cancer. She is a gifted educator with long experience in the field.

The Academy for Guided Imagery
PO Box 2070
Mill Valley, CA 94942
Tel: 1-800-726-2070
Fax: 415-389-9342

The Academy for Guided Imagery is one of the outstanding professional training organizations helping professionals to learn and incorporate imagery techniques into their work. It is co-directed by Martin Rossman, M.D. and David

Bresler, Ph.D. The academy was founded out of a concern "about standards of practice, clinical competency, and assessment skills on the part of clinicians seeking to use imagery with their patients."

The academy offers a formal professional certification program for health professionals in interactive guided imagery. The faculty is multidisciplinary and the students represent a cross section of health and mental health disciplines. The approach is "eclectic, holistic, humanistic and non-dogmatic, incorporating skills and approaches from many related disciplines and therapies, including hypnosis, Jungian psychology, psychosynthesis, self-actualization, and ego-state psychology, among others."

"Guided Imagery for Clinicians" is a three-day introductory workshop, and professionals wishing to complete their certification may continue with six additional workshops comprising 153 hours of training.

The cost of the certification program is $3,495 (payment plans are available), and courses currently rotate through metropolitan San Francisco, Los Angeles, and Seattle. Regional training centers are being established so that complete training may be obtained in each location.

Simonton Cancer Center
875 Via De La Paz
Suite C
Pacific Palisades, CA 90272
310-459-4434

O. Carl Simonton, M.D., and the staff of the Simonton Cancer Center conduct ongoing workshops for counselors, educators, clergy, hospice workers, nurses, and other members of the helping professions. Topics covered in the workshops include: counseling people with cancer; imagery, meditation, and visualization; the "Two Year Health Plan"; a research overview; the role of the support system; responsibility, guilt, and blame; death; play; and hope, trust, purpose, inner guide, and spirituality.

The course combines didactic presentation with small group processes and discussion. All workshops run Friday through Sunday and cost $295.

Institute for the Study of Health and Illness at Commonweal
PO Box 316
Bolinas, CA 94924
Tel: 415-868-2642
Fax: 415-868-2230

The Institute for the Study of Health and Illness at Commonweal (our program) is a training program for health professionals who work with patients or clients with life-threatening illnesses. Directed by Rachel Naomi Remen, M.D., who also serves as Medical Director of the Commonweal Cancer Help Program, the institute offers a curriculum of five weekend core workshops, advanced workshops, and clinical supervision seminars for past participants; public lectures; and personal and organizational consultations.

The institute's programs focus on introducing health professionals to a range of tools and techniques for using the healing power inherent in a therapeutic relationship. The spiritual needs of people with life-threatening illnesses are examined, along with effective strategies to meet these needs. Participants are also encouraged to examine personal beliefs and attitudes that may limit the effectiveness of therapeutic relationships, and to develop self-nurturing strategies.

Each of the institute's programs examines one of the basic issues in providing care that focuses on patients' needs. Each draws on theories and techniques developed in fields such as transpersonal psychology, theology, Eastern and Western spiritual traditions, imagery, the fine arts, and the art of medicine itself.

The fee for each workshop is $400, including room, board, and all materials.

National Institute for the Clinical Application of Behavioral Medicine
Box 523
Mansfield Center, CT 06250
Tel: 203-429-2238
Fax: 203-429-7949

The National Institute for the Clinical Application of Behavioral Medicine (NICABM) is "devoted to training and continuing education in behavioral medicine. Through practitioner-oriented conferences and products for health and mental health care providers, NICABM facilitates interdisciplinary communication and behavioral approaches to health and illness."

Among the program tracks that NICABM offers are: "strategies for working with cancer and other immune disorder patients"; "psychotherapy with medical patients"; "innovations in pain management"; and "marital and family therapy with medical patients." NICABM is recognized by the American Medical Association, American Nurses Association, American Psychological Association, the National Board of Certified Counselors, and the State Chapter of the National Association of Social Workers as a provider of continuing education credits.

Consciousness Research and Training Project, Inc.
315 East 68th Street, Box 9G
New York, NY 10021
212-879-9771

The Consciousness Research and Training Project offers 5-day residential seminars on healing based on the work of Lawrence LeShan, Ph.D. (see chapter 10).

The goal of the program is to enable participants to enter a "paranormal" state of consciousness "within which there is no individuation, rather an experience of *oneness* in the healer's consciousness, if only for an instant . . . Its primary and essential milieu [is] love, caring at an intense, deep, and profound level."[1] LeShan, having trained himself to achieve this state in his work with clients, found that frequently people with whom he worked reported physical or psychological changes that were of benefit to them.

Admission to the program requires the submission of an application, and a mixture of ages and professions is sought for each training group. Not all participants are health professionals.

Cancer Support and Education Center
1035 Pine Street
Menlo Park, CA 94025
415-327-6166

The Cancer Support and Education Center offers a 140-hour facilitator training program for those interested in learning the techniques used at the center in its work with cancer patients. (See chapter 27 for the description of the center's self-help intensive course under Major Metropolitan and Regional Support Groups, San Francisco Bay Area.)

Reference

1   Joyce Goodrich, "A Healing Training and Research Project." In James L. Fosshage and Paul Olsen, eds., *Healing: Implications for Psychotherapy* (New York: Human Sciences Press, 1978).

Glossary

Acupressure   A system of massage in which figure pressure on acupuncture points is used in place of needles.

Acupuncture   In traditional Chinese medicine, the practice of placing needles at key points along "energy pathways," or "meridians" on the body in order to "restore the energy balance." Best known in the West as a system of pain control.

Adenocarcinoma   A carcinoma of glandular origin.

Adjunctive therapies   Those unconventional cancer therapies generally considered more acceptable by mainstream standards, mostly notably the psychosocial interventions.

Amino acids   Organic compounds which are the building blocks of proteins. The body can manufacture nine of these but must obtain eleven others through food intake.

Analgesic   A substance that relieves pain without causing a loss of consciousness.

Antineoplastons   Substances originally isolated from human urine by Stanislaw Burzynski, which he believes have antitumor properties.

Ascites   Accumulation of fluid in the abdominal cavity.

Autogenous vaccine   A vaccine derived from the patient's own blood.

Ayurveda   The traditional Indian system of medicine that uses herbs, yoga, and various other techniques to bring the body into a state a harmony with its environment.

BCG   Bacille Calmette-Guérin—the attenuated bovine tubercle bacillus that Virginia Livingston used for cancer patients. Livingston described BCG as a close relative of *Progenitor cryptocides.*

Biofeedback   The use of instruments to induce awareness of the ability to achieve responses, such as relaxation, previously thought to be beyond conscious control.

Cachexia   Generalized weakening and malnutrition that often accompanies cancer and is often the cause of death in cancer patients.

Carcinoma   A malignant tumor originating in the tissues that line the organs of the body, such as the breast, intestines, uterus, etc.

Chromosomes   Structures in the cell nucleus containing DNA, the genetic material.

Clinical trials   Experiments involving humans.

Cohort study   A study in which a group is observed over a period of time.

Complementary therapies   Those approaches to the diagnosis, treatment, and care of cancer that fall outside conventional (or allopathic) cancer treatments, so called because they *complement* the intelligent use of conventional approaches. Complementary cancer therapies are also called "unorthodox" and "unconventional."

Control group   In a clinical study, a group identical to the one being examined, except for the absence of the one factor being evaluated. The results from the two groups are compared to assess the factor under study.

Controlled study   A clinical study which utilizes a control group.

Conventional cancer therapies   Those forms of cancer treatment widely practiced in major American cancer centers today: surgery, chemotherapy, and radiation.

Differentiation   The acquisition of particular structures and characteristics by cells or tissues which allows them to perform specific functions. Loss of cell differentiation is a defining characteristic of cancer.

DNA   Molecules in the cell nucleus that comprise the genes and which carry hereditary information.

Double blind   A method of minimizing bias in a clinical trial, where neither the patient nor those collecting and evaluating the data know what treatment the patient is receiving (e.g., whether the patient is a member of the study group or control group).

Dysplasia   Abnormal changes in cells, sometimes indicative of a precancerous state.

Edema   Accumulation of fluid in the connective tissue; swelling.

Endocrine therapy   The use of hormones, such as estrogen, in the treatment of cancer.

Endometrium   The membrane lining the uterus.

Epithelium   The tissue that lines the surfaces of the body's organs.

Essiac   A Native American herbal preparation obtained by Rene Caisse, R.N., in the 1920s. It is available in Canada on an experimental basis.

Etiology   The branch of medicine which examines the causes of disease.

Ewing's sarcoma   A tumor of the bone.

Free radicals   Chemical compounds that are byproducts of metabolism which damage cells and leave them vulnerable to the effects of carcinogens.

Genes   Individual units of hereditary material composed of DNA.

Grading   The classification of tumors according to the degree of differentiation of cancerous cells. Generally, the more differentiated the cells are, the better the prognosis. Grade I malignancies are the most differentiated, grade IV the least.

Hodgkin's disease   A malignant condition of the lymphoid tissues which results in the enlargement of the lymph nodes, spleen, and liver, and sometimes fever and weight loss.

Hoxsey herbs   An herbal formula developed by John Hoxsey in 1840. Reportedly based upon his observations of the plants his horse consumed prior to the disappearance of a cancerous tumor on its leg.

Hydrazine sulfate   An inexpensive chemical substance found by Joseph Gold to possibly be useful in treating cachexia, and which may also have anticancer properties.

Hyperthermia   The therapeutic application of heat, either locally, regionally, or systemically, based on the belief that tumors have a lower tolerance to heat than do healthy tissues. Ultrasound, radio-, and microwaves are among the techniques used in this process.

Imagery   The use of mental images which come to conscious awareness during a deeply relaxed state to motivate the body's healing response.

Incidence   The number of cases of a particular disease diagnosed; the rate of occurrence in the general population.

IND [Investigational New Drug]   Permits granted by the Food and Drug Administration for the use of new drugs with patients on an experimental basis.

In vitro   In an artificial environment, i.e., cell cultures, test tubes.

In vivo   In the body.

Iscador   A mistletoe extract used in anthroposophical medicine as an anticancer agent.

Lipids   Organic fatty substances that are insoluble in water but which are soluble in alcohol and some other fat solvents. They serve as fuel and are an important constituent of cell structure, along with proteins and carbohydrates.

Lymphoma   A malignant growth originating in the lymphoid tissues, specifically in the lymphocytes at a step in the differentiation process outside of the bone marrow.

Macrobiotics   Term coined by George Oshawa from the Greek for "large life." An approach to life derived from traditional Oriental philosophies whose goal is to live in harmony with the environment and whose principles are applied dietetically. The diet is grain-based and nondairy, primarily cooked, and can be vegetarian or nonvegetarian.

Macronutrients   Major components of food: fat, protein, carbohydrate, fiber, sodium, potassium, and calcium.

Maruyama vaccine   Perhaps the most widely used Japanese alternative cancer therapy. Similar to BCG, the attenuated bovine tubercle bacillus that Virginia Livingston used for cancer patients, it is derived from human tuberculosis rather than bovine tuberculosis.

Melanoma   A malignant form of skin cancer originating in the pigmented cells.

Meridians   "Energy pathways" believed by practitioners of traditional Chinese medicine to run through the body. Acupuncture needles are placed along meridians at "points" where the energy can be adjusted.

Metaplasia   The abnormal replacement of one kind of cells with another.

Metastases   Locations where cancer has spread from its primary site, usually via the lymph system, blood, or by invasive spread.

Micronutrients   Vitamins and trace minerals.

Mitosis The process which takes place in the dividing cell which results in the formation of two nuclei, each having the same number of chromosomes as the original nucleus.

Mortality rate The rate at which people die as a result of a particular cause in a given population.

Moxibustion The application of heat to acupuncture points.

Mutagen An agent that increases the frequency of mutation.

Myeloma A primary tumor of the bone marrow.

Neoplasm "New growth," or any abnormal growth of tissue that serves no physiological function; cancer.

Non-Hodgkin's lymphoma A family of lymphomas distinguished from Hodgkin's disease by the absence of the characteristic Sternberg-Reed cells.

Oncogene Genetic material normally present in cell (proto-oncogene) which has been triggered to cause uncontrolled cell growth.

One-arm study A study not employing a control group.

Palliative Treatment that provides relief from symptoms, as opposed to a cure for the condition.

Pathogen The specific agent or organism which causes a disease.

Pharmacological Pertaining to the use of an agent as a drug.

Placebo A substance or procedure with no intrinsic therapeutic value administered to a control group in a clinical study. Comparison with the results obtained from the study group determine the efficacy of the therapy being administered to the study group.

Pleomorphic A term used in microbiology to refer to bacteria that change in size and shape during their life cycle.

Progenitor cryptocides A bacterium, detectable through the dark-field microscope, which is postulated by Virginia Livingston to cause cancer.

Prospective study A study in which a group is monitored over a period of time and where results will be determined at a future date (as opposed to a retrospective or historical study). See Cohort study.

Qi In the traditional system of Chinese medicine, the vital energy or life force of the body.

Qi gong   An ancient Chinese martial art combining movement with meditation and breath awareness which has as one of its goals the conscious control of the body's energetic system.

Randomization   A method of minimizing bias in a controlled study, in which all subjects have an equal chance of being assigned to the study group or control group. In this way, all factors which might confound the results of the study can be considered to be equally present in both groups.

Reflexology   A system of therapeutic massage based upon the theory that pressure points affecting all of the body's organs and systems are located on the palms of the hands and soles of the feet.

Remission   The diminution or disappearance of disease; the period during which the disease is under control.

Retinol   The form of vitamin A found in mammals.

Retrospective study   A study where data are collected about events that have already happened.

Sarcoma   A neoplasm arising from the connective tissue, including bone, blood, muscle, fat, and lymph vessels.

Staging   The determination of the extent of cancer growth, a very important factor in the design of a treatment protocol. Systems vary by the type of cancer, but *generally* follow these steps:

> Stage I: localized cancer, probably without lymph node involvement.

> Stage II: local spread of cancer, possible lymph node involvement.

> Stage III: cancer has spread into adjacent tissues, definite lymph node involvement.

> Stage IV: cancer has metastasized.

Statistical significance   The mathematical measure of the probability that the results of a study are attributable to chance rather than to the effect of the therapy or agent being evaluated. If this probability is low enough, given the size of the study and strength of the results, the results are considered to be "statistically significant."

Survival rate   The percentage of people with a particular cancer who have survived a given length of time.

Therapeutic Touch   A modern version of laying on of hands in which the practitioner seeks to rebalance "energy fields" that are postulated to exist within and around the body.

Yoga A philosophical school of Hinduism that elaborates a system of physical, psychological, and spiritual approaches to the integration of the individual with the transpersonal. Yoga is best known as a physical discipline, including stretching exercises, breathing and relaxation techniques, and meditation practices.

Acknowledgments

Many people, and a number of extended networks or communities, have contributed to the evolution of *Choices in Healing*. First, I acknowledge above all my Research Associate, Don Flint, who has worked for years with me, through countless revisions of this book, with intelligence, energy, dedication, humility and good humor. Frank Urbanowski, my publisher, Harriet Harvey and Katherine F. Arnoldi, my editors, and Nadine Parker, my Administrative Assistant, have contributed to the book beyond measure.

Philip R. Lee, long-time Chairman of the Commonweal Advisory Board, has been my mentor in the health care field for many years. This book owes him a great debt for his advice and counsel.

Rachel Naomi Remen, Virginia Veach, Asoka Thomas, and Jenepher Stowell have been invaluable comrades in the world of psychological and spiritual work with people with cancer through our joint work in the Commonweal Cancer Help Program.

The whole book has been reviewed by the late Jenifer Altman, Bill Buchholz, Harris Dienstfrey, Tom Ferguson, John Fink, Robert Houston, Richard Grossman, Adam Lerner, Edna Lerner, Steve Lerner, Max Lerner, and the late Brendan O'Regan. I owe a special debt to Dienstfrey, Ferguson, Houston, and Edna Lerner for the detailed reviews and support they provided.

Chapter reviews were provided by Jeanne Achterberg, Keith Block, Michael Broffman, Stanislaw Burzynski, James Carter, Marcus A. Cohen, Alistair Cunningham, David Eisenberg, Bernard Fox, Joseph Gold, Gar Hildebrand, Alex Jack, Gary A. Johanson, Yola Jurzykowski, Lawrence Kushi, Marion Nestle, Julia Rowland, Gordon Saxe, William Redd, Le Trombetta, Patricia Spain Ward, Gary and Julie Wagner, Arthur D. Alexander III, and David Walde.

Kate Strasburg was of special assistance during the time this book was written. She helped research quotations for the book and created an invaluable bibliography, "The Quest for Wholeness," that informed much of this book. She also developed an exceptional library in patient-centered care at Commonweal.

Choices in Healing owes a special debt to several extended communities.

First and foremost, it has been inspired by the participants and staff of the Commonweal Cancer Help Program, and all those who have attended my Tuesday night talks in the Cancer Help Program through which this book developed. The core staff includes or has included Asoka Thomas, Jenepher Stowell, Marion Weber, Nadine Parker, Christine Boyd, Jnani Chapman, Holly Bronfman, Robin Lysne, Monica Kaufer, Christine Schultz, Shanti Soule, Jeanne Bel, Purusha Doherty and co-leaders Rachel Naomi Remen (who is also Medical Director), Virginia Veach, Nischala Devi, Shannon McGowan, and Lenore Lefer. I also wish to acknowledge the other staff members who joined us for the early Cancer Help Programs held at Yogaville in Buckingham, Virginia. Swami Satchidananda, Nischala Devi, Holly Bronfman, Madhuri Honeyman and Jan Abruzzo deserve special thanks for their contributions to the Virginia programs.

Second, it owes a great intellectual debt to the participants in the annual Lloyd Symington Foundation Conference on New Directions in Cancer Care at Commonweal. This community includes or has included Rachel Naomi Remen, Virginia Veach, Marion Weber, Lucy Waletzky, Larry LeShan, Joan Borysenko, Barrie Cassileth, Sandra McLanahan, Nischala Devi, Barry Flint, Grace Monaco, Shannon McGowan, Keith Block, William Buchholz, Jeanne Achterberg, Frank Lawlis, Irving Berg, Harold Benjamin, Michael Samuels, Richard Grossman, Leo Stolbach, John Fink, Toby Symington, Wendy Schain, Ursula Brandt, Alistair Cunningham, W.M. Gallmeier, Herbert Kappauf, Gerwin Kaiser, Stephanie Simonton, Anna Halprin, Dawn Lemanne, Michael Hawkins, Julia Rowland, Dale Borglum, Jim Spira, Lydia Temoshok, Jan Abruzzo, Dean Ornish, Mark Renneker, Shunsacu Fukuda, Fawzy Fawzy, Jon Kabat-Zinn, and many others.

Third, it also owes a great debt to the overlapping intellectual communities of the Institute for the Advancement of Health, the Fetzer Institute, the Institute of Noetic Sciences, and the Center for the Advancement of Health, where some of the foremost clinicians and researchers concerned with mind-body health have gathered. Eileen Growald of IAH, Rob Lehman of the Fetzer Institute, the late Brendan O'Regan and Winston Franklin of IONS, and Charles Halpern of the Nathan Cummings Foundation, who founded the Center for the Advancement of Health, had the foresight to create and nurture these formative intellectual communities.

Fourth, it owes a great debt to the remarkable intellectual community of researchers, scientists, clinicians, and advocates of both mainstream and complementary cancer therapies that came together to produce the Office of Technology Assessment report *Unconventional Cancer Therapies,* for which I served as Special Consultant.

Fifth, the book also owes an immeasurable debt to the extended Commonweal community— friends across the country, staff, participants in Commonweal programs, individual and foundation donors—without whom Commonweal's work would not be possible. Peter Almond, Carolyn Brown, Arthur Carpenter, Colleen Hicks, Winifred Mauzy, and Arthur Okamura as members of the Board of Directors, and David Parker, Executive Vice President and General Manager, deserve special acknowledgment.

Finally, I want to acknowledge my great debt to those who taught me useful things about the life of the spirit: to Swami Satchidananda, who taught me the yoga practices that have been the ground of my inner life; to Desikachar, who deepened and broadened my understanding of yoga; to Dharmawara, who taught me Vipassna meditation; to Harada Roshi, who taught me the precepts of Zen Buddhism by living example; to the friends who have also been real teachers; to my family, which enjoys the special grace of caring for each other; to my son Joshua, who teaches me humility; and to Sharyle Patton, wife, friend, and partner beyond compare.

About the Author and Commonweal

The Author

Michael Lerner, Ph.D., is President and founder of Commonweal. His interests include mind-body health, with a special interest in cancer; high-risk children and young people; and the architecture of an environmentally sustainable future. Lerner is the founder of the Commonweal Cancer Help Program, described below. He received his B.A. from Harvard in 1965 and his Ph.D. in political science from Yale in 1971. After serving as an assistant professor with a joint appointment in the Department of Political Science at Yale Graduate School and Yale Medical School, Lerner was named a founding associate of the Carnegie Council on Children. He came to California in 1972 and in 1973 founded Full Circle, a residential treatment center for children with learning and behavioral disorders in Marin County. In 1976 he founded Commonweal. In 1983 he received a MacArthur Prize Fellowship for his contributions to public health, and in 1990 was named a United States–Japan Leadership Fellow. In 1988–90, he served as Special Consultant to the Office of Technology Assessment for its landmark study, *Unconventional Cancer Treatments*. He also serves as President of the Jenifer Altman Foundation.

Commonweal

Commonweal is a health and environmental research institute located in Bolinas, California. Founded in 1976, it has three major program interests: serving high-risk young people, their families, and the professionals who work with them; helping people with cancer, their families, and the professionals who work with them; and supporting movement toward a just and ecologically sustainable global future.

The major current programs related to cancer include: (1) the Commonweal Cancer Help Program, which conducts weeklong support and learning programs for people with cancer; (2) the Commonweal Cancer Project, which investigates informed choice in the integration of mainstream and complementary cancer therapies; and (3) the Institute for the Study of Health and Illness, which conducts training programs for health professionals interested in reclaiming access to the great traditions of healing in medical practice and health care.

For information on the Commonweal Cancer Help Program, please contact Asoka Thomas, Program Coordinator of the program.

For information on the Commonweal Cancer Project or the Institute for the Study of Health and Illness, please contact Don Flint, who divides his time between the two projects.

Commonweal, P.O. Box 316, Bolinas, California 94924, 415-868-0970.

Index

Note: Page numbers followed by "f" refer to figures, "t" to tables, and "n" to notes.

Affluence, and hormone-dependent cancers, 205

Afterlife, 489, 503, 530
 visions of, 504, 505

Agar, 213

Age, and success of chemotherapy, 50

Age-adjusted mortality, 52

Aggressive cancer therapies, 30, 31, 33, 37–40, 58, 59

Agonists, therapeutic, 337

AIDS, 400, 407, 444, 449
 and physician-assisted suicide, 491
 support group for, 559, 566

AIDS model of community response, 88, 89

AIDS treatment, unconventional, 88, 89, 96

Aihara, Herman and Cornelia, 573

Albright, Tenley, 358

Alcoholic beverages, 201, 323, 324, 326

Aldridge, David, 114, 128

Alexander-Jackson, Eleanor, 320–322

Alfalfa, 213

Alivizatos, Hariton, 588

Alkaloid-containing herbs, 387

Allergic response, and immune function, 245

Allergic stress, 244

Allergies, 242–245

Allopathic medicine
 American hegemony of, 83, 84
 in Japan, 41
 in pluralistic systems, 83, 84

Alopecia, vitamin E for, 101, 238

Alpha-tocopherol. See Vitamin E

Altered states of consciousness, 171, 175, 462

Alternative cancer therapies. See Cancer therapy(ies), alternative

Amaranth, 345

American Association of Pastoral Counselors, 557

American Biologics-Mexico, 593

American Cancer Society
 on nutritional interventions, 213
 as resource, 525, 539, 587, 588
 unproven methods list of, 435, 436, 539, 587, 588

American cancer therapies, 29, 30, 57–62

aggressiveness of, 30, 31, 37–40, 58, 59
choices in, 63–75
conventional, debate over efficacy of, 47–54
cultural influences on, 29, 57–62
unconventional, debate over efficacy of, 84–91

American culture, and approach to health care, 38

American Dietetic Association, 571

American Massage Therapy Association, 577

American Medical Association
 attack on Gerson, 264–266
 attitude toward unconventional therapies, 89
 list of cancer specialists of, 66

American medicine, mainstream, 29, 30

American Oriental Bodywork Therapy Association, 577

American Psychiatric Association, 559

American Psychological Association, 558

American Self-Help Clearinghouse, 560

American social policies, 38

American Society for Psychiatric Oncology/AIDS, 559

Ames, Bruce, 232

Amino acids, dietary restriction of, 207

Amitriptyline, 480t

Amputation, 33

Amussat, 176

Amygdalin. See Laetrile

Amyotrophic lateral sclerosis, 17

Anabolic conditions, 445, 446

Analgesia
 acupuncture for, 376–379
 for dying patient, 477

Analgesic drugs, 478, 479, 480t
 adjuvants to, 480t
 for chronic pain, 476
 coffee enemas and, 272, 273
 mindful direction of, 497
 oral vs. intravenous, 479
 prophylactic, 479

Analgesic ladder, 478, 479, 480f

Anderson, John, 321

Anemia
 herbs for, 381
 refractory, 8

Cameron, E., 225–230, 236, 245

Campbell, D. F., 145

Camphor derivative 714-X, 596, 597

Canadian herbal remedy (Essiac), 103, 107, 415

Cancer
  acceptance of, 470
  anabolic vs. catabolic, 445, 446, 450
  changing trends in, 47–52
  in children, 49
  control of, vs. cure, 110
  denial of, in Japanese medicine, 40
  electromagnetic hazards and, 104
  electromagnetic therapies for, 104
  emotional pain of, 457, 458
  experience of, 458, 532
  as "gift," 124
  as immunodeficiency condition, 322
  inner healing in, 529, 532
  Japanese theories of causation in, 40, 41
  Kushi's view of, 298
  leanness and, 357, 359
  living with, 457–470
    problems of. See Problems of living with cancer
  mental hygiene in, 137
  natural history of, 48
  New Age theories of, 303
  nutrition and, scientific view of, 197–199
  prediagnostic choices in, 522
  prevention of, 53
    choices in, 522
    natural approach to, 301
    nutritional approaches to, 199–202
    vitamin C and, 230–233
  recurrence of
    checkups for, 530
    fear of, 529
    response to, 529, 530
  regression of, nutrition and, 204
  remission of
    multimodal therapies and, 111
    psychological factors in, 183–188
  risk for, 465, 522
    in athletes, 357, 358
  screening for, 48
  spread of. See Metastasis
  as tragedy, 462
  trauma of, 529

  as "turning point," 461–463, 529
  ways of encountering, 470

Cancer: Principles and Practice of Oncology, 72–74, 201, 202, 541

Cancer as a Turning Point, 20, 138, 160

Cancer cells
  fermentation in, 434
  imagery of, 164–166
  lipid imbalance in, 445
  membrane polarization of, 268, 269
  nutritional deficiencies and, 207
  parasite within, 321
  redifferentiation of
    antineoplastons and, 422
    ginseng and, 384
  swelling of, 270
  vitamin C and, 233, 234

Cancer deaths, cachexia and, 436

Cancer diagnosis
  disruptions caused by, 140
  psychic, 104
  shift in consciousness after, 461–463
  shock of, 522
  taping during, 522
  withholding, 40

Cancer Forum, 72, 540

Cancer "germs," 467

Cancer Hot LIne, 72

Cancer incidence, trends in, 47

Cancer Industry, The, 405

CANCERLIT database, 541

Cancer literature. See Literature

Cancer mortality
  age-adjusted, 52
  interpretation of, 52, 53
  trends in, 47, 50

Cancer pain. See Pain

Cancer patient(s)
  acceptance of disease, 470
  accepting responsibility to recover, 303, 342
  attitudinal profile of, 339
  autonomy of, 64, 65
  biochemical profile of, 338, 340
  biomechanical profile of, 338, 340
  biomedical profiles of, 336, 338
  change in attitude toward life of, 461–463
  change in priorities of, 461, 462
  childhood trauma of, 463, 464

hegemony of, 83, 84
international differences in, 29, 30, 31–44
palliative, 526
potentially curative, 526
relative efficacies of, 57
synergism with nutritional approaches, 101
terminology for, 79
vitamin E and, 237
cultures of, 29, 57–62
ethical, 84
exploitative, 84
in France, 32–34
in Germany, 34–36
in Great Britain, 36, 37
individualized vs. protocol-directed, 60
information sources for, 72–74, 539–544
   computer database searches, 540
   consultants, 542–544
   hospital libraries, 541
   medical school libraries, 541
   public services, 539
intensive experimental, 430
in Japan, 40–43
mainstream, 79. *See also* Cancer therapy(ies), conventional
minerals and, 239–242, 246
multimodal, 102, 111
"no regrets," 525
patient-centered, 13
patient's monitoring of, 74
progress in, 52–54
"quack," 85, 96, 97, 397
"rescue," 40, 58
"secret," 398–402
traditional medicines. *See also* Chinese medicine (traditional)
types of hospitals providing, 59–61
unconventional, 79–81, 82n
   AIDS model and, 88, 89
   case and anecdotal evidence in, 95
   cautions about, 524–527
   Chinese medicine. *See* Chinese medicine (traditional)
   choices in, 79–81, 524–527
   in controlling cancer, 110, 111
   costs of, 108
   debate over, 83–91
   electromagnetic approaches, 104
   esoteric, 104

evaluation of, 106–109
framework for evaluating, 93–111
and functional status, 110
government regulation of, 84, 89
herbal. *See* Herbal remedies
humane approaches, 105
individual "cures" with, 94
lack of scientific studies of, 94
legal sanctions against, 83–87, 89, 90
legitimization of, 85, 90, 91
and life extension, 94
media's role in, 87
New Age movement and, 87
nutritional. *See* Diet(s); Nutritional approaches
physical. *See* Physical therapy(ies)
practitioner of. *See* Practitioners of unconventional therapies
problems of documentaion of, 96
psychic approaches, 104
psychological approaches, 137–190. *See also* Psychological approaches
psychophysiological, 101
and quality of life, 111
quality of service delivery in, 106, 108
risks of, 84
scientific evaluation of, 91
spiritual approaches, 113–135. *See* Spiritual approaches
subcultures of, 80–81
and symptom control, 111
synergism of, 101, 102
terminology for, 79–80, 82n
traditional medicines, 102, 369, 370
treatment centers for, 588–602
typology of, 98–106
using conventional methods, 104
varying quality of, 79
vital quartet of, 102
in United States, 37–40
unorthodox, 79, 80
vitamins, 219–239. *See also* specific vitamins
Cancer therapy specialist(s)
choice of, 63, 65–69
competence of, 61
different views of, 57, 58
Candlelighters Childhood Cancer Foundation, 549

DES, in prostate cancer, 422
Desensitization, 144, 145
Desikachar, 582
Desodification, 600
Destagnation herbal remedies, 383, 384
Destagnation of blood, 386
Detoxification, 252, 253, 256, 266, 298, 324
  of liver, 267
DeVita, Vincent T., Jr., 52, 72–74, 202, 541
de Vries, Marco J., 186–188, 255
Dexamethasone, 480t
Dextropropoxyphene, 480t
Dharmananda, Subhuti, 386
Diagnosis. *See* Cancer diagnosis
Diazepam, 480t
Diet(s). *See also* Nutritional approaches
  anticancer, 100, 250–259
    Block, 250, 342–348
    Gawler, 255–259
    Gerson, 100, 250–252, 261–281
    Hippocrates wheat-grass, 100, 209, 250, 253
    Kelley-Gonzalez, 100
    Kushi's Cancer Prevention Diet, 289, 300, 315
    Livingston-Wheeler, 100, 250, 323, 325
    macrobiotic. *See* Macrobiotics
    overview of, 250–259
    raw foods, 250, 253, 254
  Ayurvedic, 250
  Balanced, 301
  for breast cancer, according to Kushi, 292, 293
  cancer-promoting, 343
  and course of cancer, 197–199
  high-fat, 288. *See also* Fat intake
  Japanese, 286, 310–312
  Livingston-Wheeler, 325
  low-fat, 285
  practical guidelines for, 215
  to prevent micrometastases, 348
  radical therapeutic, 204
  salt-free, 263
  vegetarian. *See* Vegetarian diet
  Western, 288, 312
Diet, Nutrition and Cancer, 200. *See also* National Research Council

Dietary changes
  psychological benefits of, 313
  stress of, 312
Dietary chemoprevention, 221, 222
Dietary fat. *See* Fat intake
Dietary fiber. *See* Fiber
Dietary guidelines (National Research Council), 200, 201
Dietary recommendations
  to maintain weight with cancer, 200, 202, 204–210, 215
  to prevent cancer, 199–202
  silence on, 202–204
Dietary repletion, and tumor growth, 205
Dietary supplements, toxic doses of, 201
Diethylstilbestrol (DES), 422
Dietitians, 571
Digestion, 257
Digestive enzymes, 257, 258
Dignity, 10, 490, 491
Dimethyl sulfoxide, 588
Disability from cancer, 140
Disaster syndrome, 516
Disease
  English concept of, 36
  vs. illness, 19, 20, 484
  as invader, 33
Disfigurement, 140
Dislocation, problem of, 459
Distancing, emotional, 140
Distress, and survival, 159
Divorce, 148, 459, 460, 465
Dobbs, B. Z., 362
Doll, R., 205
"Don't live" messages, 464
Downs, S. E., 367
Doxorubicin (Adriamicin)
  cardiotoxicity of, 101, 235, 238
  and hair loss, 237
  vitamin C and, 235
  vitamin E and, 237
Drug(s)
  illegal, to treat AIDS, 88
  monitoring use of, 89–91
  obtaining patents for, 398, 399
  orphan, 399
Drug abuse, pain medication and, 477
Drug addiction, 444, 449
  to opiates, 147, 477, 485, 486

Hallucinations, near-death, 503, 504, 507
Hallucinogenic stimuli, 505
Haloperidol, 480t
Hanck, 234, 236
Handbook of Psychooncology, 139–143
Hara, Hiroshi, 42, 420
Haraldsson, Erlendur, 503–505
Haramaki, 42
Harner, Michael, 122
Hatha yoga, 121, 581
Hawaii, cancer rates in, 311
Hay fever, 243
Headache, 364
Head and neck cancer
  adjuvant therapy for, 51
  Chinese herbs for, 383
  retinoic acid in, 222
  spontaneous remission of, 184
  vitamin A in, 221
  vitamin C in, 234
Head and neck surgery, acupuncture in, 376–
  378
Heading Toward Omega, 506
Healers, 81, 362–365, 558
  traditional ethnic, 81
  wounded, 124
Healing, 13–25
  affirmations and, 131
  anger and, 16
  attitudinal, 563
  biophysical potential for, 109
  choices in, 25, 529
  circle of, 496
  conditions of, 16–18, 110
  creativity and, 23
  with crystals, 104
  vs. curing, 9, 13, 14, 19, 20, 109
  imagery and, 23
  impediments to, 302–304
  inner work of, 529, 532
  intentional, 128
  patient's participation in, 20–22
  perennial philosophy of, 122
  power of, 14–16
  psychic, 104
  psychosocial context of, 19
  psychospiritual, 99, 109, 110
  psychosynthesis and, 22

religious, 81, 362, 364
role of medicine in, 19, 20
and sense of connection, 126
in shamanism, 122–125
shared, 125
social support and, 468
spiritual. *See* Spiritual healing
spirituality and, 24
Therapeutic Touch in, 362–365
transpersonal, 128–130
types of, 13
without curing, 109
of wounds, 407
yoga and, 121
Healing crises, 253, 527
Healing into Life and Death, 496
Healing power, 14–16
Healing response, to near-death experience,
  15
Healing Yourself, 167
Health care systems
  American, 37–40
  British, 36, 37
  French, 32–34
  German, 34–36
  Japanese, 40–43
Health fraud, 84, 86. *See also* Quackery
Health Maintenance Organizations, 60
Health promotion, intensive, 109
Health promotion movement, 87
Health psychology, 19
Health Resource, The, 543
Health spas, 33, 34, 35
Health Training and Research Center, 607
Hearing ability, prior to unconsciousness,
  15
Hearing impairment, 444
Heart, as seat of soul, 34
Heart damage
  doxorubicin-induced, 101, 235, 238
  vitamin C for, 235
Heart disease, 180, 343
  Ornish approach to, 288
Heart drugs, German view of, 34
Heart infections, 444
Helplessness, learned, 64
Helplessness-hopelessness, 150,
  176

choice of, 65, 74
cultures of cancer therapy at, 59–61
support groups in, 560
Hospital Ernesto Contreras, 595
Hospitalization, in Japan, 43
Hospital libraries, 541
Hotline for cancer information, 71
Hour of Our Death, The, 495
Housing, changes in, 459
Houston, Robert G., 82n, 111n, 419, 420
  on Gerson, 275
  on Revici, 448, 449, 452
How Can I Help?, 524
Howe, Geoffrey, 230
Hoxsey, Harry, 264, 399
Hoxsey, John, 593
Hoxsey herb remedy, 81, 103, 399, 588,
  593
H&R Block, 72, 540
Hsu, Hong-Yen, 385, 386
Humane approaches to cancer, 105
Huxley, Aldous, 116, 117, 121, 285
Hydrazine sulfate, 103, 400, 433–440
  American Cancer Society approval of, 435
  antitumor effects of, 434–437
  for cachexia, 434–437
  clinical trials of, 439, 440
  for lung cancer, 94, 95
  mechanism of, 434
  resources for, 602
  Soviet studies of, 435, 436, 438, 439
Hydrochloric acid, 324
Hydrogen peroxide, vitamin C and, 233
Hydroxyzine, 480t
Hypersensitivity syndromes, 243, 244
Hyperstimulated immunity, 243, 244
Hypertension, 288
Hyperthermia, 95
  juzentaihoto with, 382
Hypnosis and Behavioral Medicine, 146, 171
Hypnosis (hypnotherapy), 80, 99, 171–175
  for bone marrow aspiration, 145
  for fear, 462, 463
  for pain, 474, 482
  and survival, 154, 172, 173
Hypnotic trance, 145
Hypnotizability, 339
Hysterectomies, "birthday," 38

Iatrogenic complications of therapy, 74
Identity problems, 468
Ikemi, Yujiro, 184–186
Illness
  "carrying," 41
  creative role of, 125
  vs. disease, 19, 20
  iatrogenic, 74
Illness and Culture in Contemporary Japan
Illness memoirs, 5, 9
Image of Cancer, 170
Imagery, 9, 99
  aggressive, 166, 174
  assessment technique in, 170
  of cancer cells, 164–166
  for fear, 462, 463
  induction of, 168
  inner advisor, 169
  language of, 163
  methods of, 23
  for nausea and vomiting, 144, 145
  negative, 165
  for pain, 474
  predictive power of, 170, 171
  of problems, 168
  qualities of, 166
  Rossman approach, 167–169
  scoring in, 170
  and self-healing, 167–169
  Simonton approach, 163–167
  spiritual, 98
  visual, 80
Imagery in Healing, 170
Immune function
  acupuncture and, 379
  isolation and, 127
Immune hyperstimulation, 243, 244
Immune response, in malnutrition, 208
Immune system, 408f
  in biopsychosocial medicine, 19
  imagery of, 165
  meditation and, 153
  neurological and psychological connection
    to, 137
Immuno-Augmentative Centre, Ltd., 598,
  604
Immuno-Augmentative Therapy, 107, 399,
  402, 588

Japan
cancer therapy in, 40–43
patient's rights in, 43
Japanese acupuncture, 371
Japanese diet, 286, 310–312
and breast cancer, 346
and stomach cancer, 310
Japanese folk medicine, 41–43
Jeans, Sir James, 501
Jibyo, 41
Jin shin, 577
Jnana yoga, 121
Job-related problems, 459, 468
Johanson, Gary, 509
John Birch Society, 90
Judaism, 119
Jung, Carl C., 22, 124, 126, 163
on death, 493
Juzentaihoto (JT-48, JTT), 381, 382

Kabat-Zinn, Jon, xvii, 565
Kagawa, Toyohiko, 286
Kanpo, 41–43
Kaptchuk, Ted, 371, 374, 375
Karma yoga, 121
Kelley, William D., 576, 588
Kelley-Gonzalez nutritional program, 100
Kelp, 293, 311, 324, 346
Khoshbin, Bijan, 591
Kiecolt-Glaser, Janice R., 127, 148
Kimler, Bruce F., 236
Kindness, loving, 496
Kobasa, S. C., 149
Koch's postulates, 321
Kombu, 293, 346
Kondo, T., 378
Korean War, 484, 528
Koumei, Nakayama, 385, 386
Krebs, Ernst, 603
Krieger, Dolores, 362
Kripalu Center for Yoga and Health, 582
Kübler-Ross, Elisabeth, 496, 511–513
Kung Fu, 373
Kunz, Dora, 362
Kushi, Aveline, 287
Kushi, Lawrence, 205, 287, 299, 313, 344
on chemoprevention, 222

Kushi, Michio
approach to breast cancer, 290–298
analysis of, 295–298
"home cares," 293–295
approach to macrobiotics, 285–304
biography of, 286–288
Kushi Institute, 286, 287, 314, 588
Kushi Institute, The, 573
Kuzmina, E.G., 379

Lack, Sylvia, 508
Lactic acid, 434
Lad, Vasant, 585
Ladner, Hans, 224
Laetrile, 81, 103, 436, 588, 595, 600, 603
cyanide toxicity with, 604
Laminaria, 346
Language of unconscious, 23
Lao-tzu, 299
prayer of, 133
LaPorte, Ron E., 360
Laryngeal cancer
vitamin A in, 221
vitamin C in, 230
Laser acupuncture, 379
Latin patients' response to amputation, 33
Lawlis, Frank, 170, 174
Laying on of hands, 98, 115, 355, 362, 364, 558, 578
Layman, D. K., 356
Lead, 239
Leahy, Dennis, 497
Leanness
and cancer, 359
and estrogen, 357
Learned helplessness, 64
Learning profile of patient, 338, 339
Lechner, Peter, 271
Legalization of complementary therapies, 97
Legal sanctions against unconventional therapies, 83–87, 89, 90
Legumes, 343
Lente insulin, 595
Lentils, 293
Lentinus edodes, 310, 345, 346
Leprosy, 320
Lerner, Max, 3–6, 64, 113

LeShan, Lawrence, 20, 123, 138, 160–163, 444, 461, 610
Letting go, 496, 532
Leukemia, 8
  acute lymphocytic, 49
  antineoplastons for, 414
  caloric intake and, 205
  chemotherapy for, 49, 325
  of childhood, 49, 50
  exercise and, 358
  and hives, 243
  juzentaihoto for, 381
  Livingston vaccine for, 327
  massage technique in, 361
  pain in, 478
  personality factors in, 176
  radiation-induced, food restriction in, 209
  survival in, 49
  in twins, 177
  vitamin C in, 235–237, 246
  zinc and, 241
Leukemia cells, vitamin A and, 220
Leukemia Society of America, 548
Leukoplakia, retinoids and, 221
Leukotrienes, 449
Levamisole, 384
Levine, Ondrea, 496
Levine, Stephen, 496, 497
Levorphanol, 480t
Levy, Sandra, 149
Li, Wen Y., 381
Libido, withdrawal of, 516
Libraries, medical, 72, 73, 526, 541
Library resources, 72–74
Licensing of unconventional practitioners, 84, 86, 90
Liehr, Joachim, 233
Lien, Eric J., 381
Life
  change in attitude toward, 461–463
  fighting for, 15, 339, 531
Life adjustment problems, and pain, 481
Life after death, 489, 503, 530
Life changes, stressful, 148
Life energy. See Energy(ies)
Life expansion, 529
Life extension
  in breast cancer, 154–158
  Chinese medicine for, 379

healing and, 14, 529
hydrazine sulfate and, 437
hypnosis and, 154, 172, 173
multimodal efforts and, 102
psychological approaches to, 152–163
  in malignant melanoma, 158–160
  in metastatic breast cancer, 154–158
  psychotherapy, 160–163
social support and, 141
with unconventional therapies, 94
Life extension hypothesis, 100
Life force. See Prana; Qi
Life recall (flashbacks), 15, 506
Lifestyle changes, 9, 10
Life-threatening experiences, 15
Lindemann, Erich, 514, 515
Ling, Gilbert N., 269
Ling, Guo, 391
Linoleic acid, 346
Lin-Xian province, esophageal cancer in, 231
Lipid(s), 346
  Revici's study of, 444–447, 451
Lipid envelopes, 446, 447
Lipid imbalances, and cancer, 445–447, 451
Lipid peroxidation, 233, 235
Lipkin, Mark, Jr., 31
Liquefactive necrosis of tumors, 448
Listening, 524
  and healing, 17
Literature
  on cancer therapies
    computer databases, 73, 540
    consultants, 542
    medical libraries, 72, 541
  on death and dying, 492–494
Liu, Yongmo, 391
Live cell therapy, 588
Liver
  detoxification of, 267
  French view of, 33
Liver cancer
  herbal therapy for, 383
  Hippocrates program for, 253
  macrobiotics for, 298
Liver function on Gerson therapy, 274
Liver juice, 257, 281n
Liver metastases
  antineoplastons for, 414, 419
  Gerson therapy for, 273

Netherlands, physician-assisted suicide in, 490
Network, social, loss of, 459, 467
Networking, in choice of physician, 66–69
Neuroblastoma, 235, 237
Neurokinesthesia, 341
Neurological disease, qi gong for, 391
Neurological factors, in immunity, 137
Neurological system, in biopsychosocial medicine, 19
Neuromodulators, 379
Neurotransmitters, 379
New Age self-care, 87
New Age theories of cancer, 303
Newbold, Vivien, 306, 307
New Patient Program (Simonton Cancer Center), 569
Newton, Bernauer, 154, 172–174
Ney, Lloyd, 547
Niacin, 271
Nieper, Hans A., 600
Nightingale, Florence, 125
Nightshade vegetables, 346
Niki, Etsuo, 232
Nitrosamines
  vitamin C and, 231
  vitamin E and, 237
Nixon, President Richard M., 87
Non-Hodgkin's lymphoma, 3
  antineoplastons for, 414, 423
  celiac syndrome and, 244
  chemotherapy for, 49
Nonsteroidal anti-inflammatory drugs, 557
Nordenstrom, Bjorn, 104
Norris, Patricia, 172
Northwest Oncology Clinic, 555
Norway, colon cancer in, 48
Novalis, 34
NSAIDS, 557
Nurse, as information resource, 67
Nursing care, for dying patient, 491, 508–510
Nurturance, 360
Nutrient intake, balanced with physical activity, 205
Nutrients. See also Macronutrients; Micronutrients
  deficiencies of, 198
  restriction of, 204–210, 215
    and weight loss, 252–255

scientific view of
  macronutrients, 197–215
  micronutrients, 219–246
  toxic doses of, 201
Nutrient uptake by cancer cells, 207
Nutrition
  and cancer, scientific view of, 197–199
  macronutrients in, 197–215
  micronutrients in, 219–246
  physician training in, 343
Nutritional approaches, 100, 101. See also Diet(s)
  categories of, 199, 200
  to enhance conventional therapies, 101
  greater acceptance of, 95
  macrobiotics. See Macrobiotics
  mixed evidence on, 197–199
  practical guidelines for, 215
  resources for, 571–577
  silence on, 202–204
  synergistic, 101
  unconventional, 197–199. See also under specific therapies
    Block's program, 335–349
    Gawler's program, 255–259
    Gerson diet, 261–281
    Livingston-Wheeler program, 319–332
    macrobiotics, 285–315
    overview of, 250–259
    resources for, 572–577
  vegetarianism. See Vegetarian diet
Nutritional imbalance, 257
Nutritional-metabolic programs, 81, 331
Nutritional repletion, and tumor growth, 205
Nutritional science
  on macronutrients, 197–215
  on micronutrients, 219–246
Nutritional supplements, 81, 250, 347
Nutritional support
  for complications of therapy, 202
  to enhance conventional therapies, 204
Nutritionists, 571
  mainstream, 202–204
Nuts, 325, 326, 343

Obesity, 201
  and breast cancer, 254, 310
  and cancer, 209

benefits of, 125
characterizing, 473, 483
chronic, 475–477
  benign (vs. cancer), 481
  preexisting, 477
  psychosocial consequences of, 476
Commonweal approach to, 483
constructive vs. destructive, 473
control of, 471–487
  acupressure for, 486
  acupuncture for, 372, 376–379, 471, 486, 528
  alternative approaches to, 111, 486, 528
  analgesics for, 478, 479, 480f, 480t. See also Analgesia; Analgesic drugs
  anesthetic blocks, 476
  Chinese medicine for, 103, 471, 486, 528
  choices in, 527, 528
  in drug addicts, 477
  gateway theory on, 473
  Gerson therapy for, 279
  group therapy for, 155, 156
  herbal remedies for, 486
  hypnosis for, 145, 482
  imagery for, 474
  inadequate, 471, 474, 475
  irradiation of bone metastases for, 476
  massage for, 486
  muscle relaxation for, 486
  opiates for, 147, 471, 485
  psychological approaches to, 476, 482
  strategies for, 478
  transcutaneous nerve stimulation (TENS) for, 486
  vitamins for, 326
coping with, 457, 458
disappearance of, at time of death, 506
of dying patient, 477
emotional, 476
etiologic components of, 476
expression of, 473, 474
facts about, 471
fear of, 471, 474, 475
  prophylactic analgesia for, 479
immediate relief of, 478
as indicator of recurrence, 476
intractable, 477
language of, 472, 473

nerve compression and, 478
and personal growth, 458, 484, 528
probability of, 477
psychological approaches to, 471, 481, 482
related to treatment, 476–478
response to, context and, 484, 528
sensory categories of, 473
shifting of, 484
spiritual, 476
spiritual use of, 485
vs. suffering, 19, 20, 476, 477, 484, 528
as teacher, 484, 528
Therapeutic Touch for, 384
"total," 476
type of cancer and, 477
types of (Foley classification), 475–478
understanding, 472
"unsharability" of, 472
Pain killers. See Opiate(s)
Pain medications
  hallucinogenic, 505
  immunodepressive effects of, 478
  underuse of, 475, 527
Pain Questionnaire, McGill, 473
Pain threshold, 478
Panax schinseng (ginseng), 384
Pancreatic cancer, 6
  antineoplastons for, 423, 424
  exercise and, 359
  macrobiotics for, 298, 306, 307–309
  Revici therapy for, 451
  SEER study of, 307–309
  vitamin C in, 230
Pancreatic enzymes, 258
Pancreatin, 267, 268
Papanicolaou (Pap) smear, 48
Paracelsus Klinik, 600
Paracetamol, 480t
Paralysis, 449
Paraneoplastic syndrome, 326
Paranormal abilities, 373, 374
Parapsychology, 500, 502
Parasite, within cancer cell, 321
Parental deprivation, 177, 178
Parenteral feeding, 337
Parents, problems with, 463, 464
Park, Chan H., 235
Parker, Willard, 161

Physician's assistant, as information resource, 67

Physician's Handbook (Livingston), 326, 333

Physician's Handbook of Symptom Relief in Terminal Care, 509

Physics and Philosophy, 501

Physiological healing, 109

Phytates, 347

Phytotherapie, 35

Pickering, George, 125

Pickled foods, 201

Pincus, Lily, 516

Pine Street Chinese Benevolent Association, 583, 584

Pituitary surgery, acupuncture in, 376

Placebo effect, 397

Placebo potential, 107, 108

Placenta, cancer of, 49

Planetree Health Resource Centers, 542

Plant(s)
 anticancer. *See also* Herbal remedies
 immune systems of, 337

Plant compounds, protective, 346, 347

Plant foods. *See* Vegetarian diet

Plant therapy
 in Germany, 35
 in Japan, 42

Pleasures, restriction of, 459

Pledge, patient-physician, 69–71

Pleomorphic microbes, 320

Plescia, Otto, 449

Pleural effusion, 273

Pluralistic medicine, 31, 44, 83–85

Poetry, on death, 492

Political conflict over unconventional therapies, 85–91

Polyporus umbellata, 381

Polysaccharides
 interferon-like, 346
 from seaweed, 310, 311
 Zhuling, 381

Polyunsaturated fats, 211

"Pornography of death," 495

Potassium supplementation, 267–271

Potts, Eve, 65, 71

Poultry, 323, 343

Practical Resources for Cancer Survivors, 561

Practitioners of unconventional therapies

considerations in choosing, 525–527
 ethics of, 96, 97
 evaluation of, 106, 108
 "hero's journey" of, 107
 legal strictures on, 84–86, 90

Prana, 363, 374, 388. *See also* Qi

Prasad, Kedar N., 235, 237, 239

Prather, Hugh, 118

Prayer, 98, 113–115, 127–133
 of Confederate soldier, 132
 Inuit Indian, 133
 intercessionary, 128–130
 of Lao-tzu, 133
 Navajo, 131

Prayer services, 557

Preleukemia, 235

Prenisolone, 480t

Pressure points
 in acupressure, 372
 in reflexology, 362

Prevention. *See* Cancer, prevention of

Prioritizing, after cancer diagnosis, 21, 461

Private-practice oncologists, 60

Problems, psychosocial, and pain, 481

Problems of living with cancer, 458–470
 and community relationships, 459, 463, 467
 in creative life, 460, 468
 and personal relationships, 459, 463–469
 psychological, 459, 481
 relating to childhood, 459, 463, 464
 relating to children, 459, 465
 relating to daily patterns, 459
 relating to disease itself, 459
 relating to finances, 459, 469
 relating to friends, 466–468
 relating to intimate partners, 459, 464
 relating to residence, 459
 work-related, 459, 468

Professional competition, 57, 58

Professional organizations
 providing lists of specialists, 66

Professional training programs, 607–610

Progenitor cryptocides, 321–323, 328, 331, 447

Progressive muscle relaxation. *See* Relaxation

Prophylactic surgery, 37

Prostaglandins, 557

Prostate cancer, 3, 17
  advocacy group for, 547
  affluence and, 205
  antineoplastons for, 422, 423
  dietary factors and, 100
  exercise and, 359
  fat intake and, 210
  fiber and, 213
  French approach to, 33
  Gerson therapy for, 277
  in Hawaii, 311
  hormonal therapy for, 4, 49
  in Japan, 311, 312
  macrobiotics for, 254, 309
  metastatic
    antineoplastons for, 420
    macrobiotics for, 305
    nontoxic therapies in, 214
    raw foods diet in, 253, 254
  survival in, 50
  vitamin A in, 221
  zinc and, 241
Prostate Cancer Report, 547
Prostatectomy, 33
  American view of, 38
  bleeding after, 444
Prostate epithelial cells, vitamin A and,
    220
Prostate hypertrophy, 444
Protease inhibitors, 310, 347
Protein intake, and cancer, 212
Protein restriction, 267
  and cellular immunity, 208
Proust, Marcel, 125
Psalm of David, 133
Psoriasis, 407
Psychiatrists, 558
Psychiatry, consultation-liaison, 139
Psychic abilities, 373, 374
Psychic approaches, 104
Psychic diagnosis of cancer, 104
Psychic power, 131, 134
Psychics, 503
Psychic surgery, 104, 588
Psychoeducational programs, 99
Psychokinesis, 502, 503
Psychological approaches, 137–190
  adjunctive, 80
  goals of, 99, 100

  hypnosis, 171–175. *See also* Hypnosis (hyp-
    notherapy)
  imagery, 163–171. *See also* Imagery
  "legitimization" of, 95
  to life extension, 152–163
  to pain, 471, 476, 481, 482
  personality and social support, 149–152
  psychoneuroimmunology, 137
  psychooncology, 138–143
  psychotherapy, 160–163. *See also* Psycho-
    therapy
  to reduce stress of cancer, 143–146
  and spirituality, 115
  and spontaneous remissions, 183–188
  training in, 607–610
  types of, 80
Psychological counselors, 557, 558
Psychological factors
  in cancer
    "cancer-prone personality," 175–181
    personality type, and recovery, 181–183
    and site of tumor, 175–181
    stress, 146–152
  in Japanese medicine, 41, 42
Psychological problems, 460
Psychological services/support groups, 558–
    569
Psychological suffering, 19, 20, 473, 528
Psychological trauma, 463
Psychology, transpersonal, 22
Psychoneuroimmunology, 19, 137
Psychooncology, 138–143
Psychosocial approaches, 80
Psychosocial consequences of pain, 476
Psychosocial context of healing, 19
Psychosocial-cultural gestalt, 337
Psychosocial factors, in disease, 138
Psychosocial problems, and pain, 481
Psychosocial profiles, 336, 338–340
Psychosocial support, and life extension, 94
Psychospiritual healing process, 109, 110
Psychospiritual perspectives on death/dying,
    495–497
Psychosynthesis, in healing, 22
Psychotherapist(s), 558–560
  inappropriate, 526, 527
Psychotherapy, 80, 99, 142
  to aid shift in consciousness, 462
  and life extension, 160–163

for pain, 482
and shamanism, 123
Psychotropic agents, 480t
Psyllium hydrophilic mucilloid, 213
Public services, 539
Pulse, in diagnosis, 373, 389
Purification, pain and, 121
Pyridoxal cream, in melanoma, 225
Pyridoxine. *See* Vitamin B$_6$
Pyridoxine deficiency, 208

Qi (vital energy), 355, 363, 387–389. *See also* Prana
emission of, 389
obstruction of, 386
Qi gong, 101, 355, 373, 374, 387–393
for cancer, 390–393
external vs. internal, 389
"new," 391, 392
resources for, 583
for side effects of conventional therapies, 391–393
Qi meridians, 373, 388
Qi-related phenomena, 373, 374
"Quack Busters," 86, 87, 89, 90 351
Quackery, 85, 397
"Quack" stereotypes, 96, 97
Quality of care
monitoring of, 74, 75
in patient decision making, 63 65
Quality of life
American view of, 39
British view of, 37
Chinese herbs and, 382
German view of, 36
with Gerson therapy, 279
healing and, 15
on Livingston program, 328–330
meditation and, 153
in terminal care, 510
unconventional therapies and, 111
vitamin C and, 227
Quality of service delivery, evaluation of, 106, 108
Quantum forces, 445
Quercetin, 595
Quinn, Janet F., 363
Quinoa, 345

R. A. Bloch Cancer Foundation, 72, 540
Radial artery, in diagnosis, 373
Radiation
ionizing, 347
from television, 294, 297
Radiation burns, 444, 449
Radiation-induced free radicals, 232
Radiation therapist(s)
choice of, 63, 65–69
view of cancer therapies, 57, 58
Radiation therapy
benefits of, 49
for breast cancer, 49
caloric restriction during, 209
for cervical cancer, 49
Chinese herbs with, 383
effect on fatty acids, 449
for Hodgkin's disease, 49
imagery in, 164
Livingston on, 325
pyridoxine with, 224
qi gong with, 391–393
side effects of, Chinese medicine for, 103, 369, 375, 379, 392, 393
for testicular cancer, 49
vitamins with, 198, 234
Radical surgical procedures, cultural attitudes toward, 32, 33, 36, 37–39
Radioactive strontium, 311
Raja yoga, 121
Random number generator, 502
Raucheisen, M. L., 364
Raw foods diet, 250, 253, 254, 325
Rebalancing, in Therapeutic Touch, 363
Rebirth, at time of death, 508
Recalled by Life, 9, 305
Recall of life experiences (flashbacks), 15, 506
Recollections of Death, 507
Recovery, factors in, 302–304
Rectal cancer
caloric intake and, 205
exercise and, 359
fiber and, 212
hydrazine sulfate for, 439
meditation and, 153
spontaneous remission of, 185
vitamin A in, 221
vitamin C in, 230
Recuperative powers, 14

Skin rash, gluten-induced, 244

Sleep deprivation, and pain threshold, 478

Smith, Elaine M., 52

Smoked foods, 202

Smoking, 323
  and cancer risk, 201, 215
  exercise and, 358, 359
  and lung cancer, 51, 53, 201
  synergism with fat intake, 211

Smoking prevention, 51, 52

Snow, Rachel, 358

Social consequences of pain, 476

Social context of healing, 19

Social networks, loss of, 459, 467

Social policies in American medicine, 38

Social support, 141. *See also* Support groups
  in breast cancer, 157
  to reduce stress, 149
  and spontaneous remission, 188
  and survival, 157

Social workers, 558

Sodium, elimination of, 600

Sodium ascorbate. *See* Vitamin C

sodium nitrite, 231

Sodium-potassium balance, 267–271

Sodium restriction, 263, 267, 268

Sodium selenite, 240

Soft tissue tumors
  antineoplastons for, 414

Soldiers' pain, 484, 528

Solomon, Raychel, 575

Somatoscope, 597

Soul
  safeguarding, 109, 122
  seat of, 34, 42

Soup, 325
  anticancer, 263
  miso, 293, 310

Soviet medicine, pain control in, 378

Soybean paste, 310

Soybean products, 347

Soy products, 345

Sparks, T. F., 154

Spas, health, 33, 34, 35

Speckhart, Vincent, 327, 328

Spiegel, David, 141, 154–158, 279, 309

Spinal alignment, 365, 366

Spinal metastases, 365
  physical therapies and, 577–579

Spirit
  definition of, 114
  survival of, 500–508
  as unifying force, 134

Spiritual approaches, 98
  training in, 607–610

Spiritual counselors, 557, 558

Spiritual energies, 109, 115, 127

Spiritual healing, 81
  definition of, 114
  Reiki, 10

Spiritual imagery, 98

Spirituality
  definition of, 114, 115
  divisiveness of, 134
  and healing, 24, 113
  and perennial philosophy, 116
  and psychological therapies, 115
  vs. religion, 113, 115

Spiritual midwife, 123

Spiritual pain, 476

Spiritual paths, 117, 118

Spiritual quest, 116

Spiritual revival, 134

Spiritual texts, Hindu, 120

Spiritual traditions, 116–118

Spiritual use of pain, 485

Splenic extract, 324

Spontaneous remissions, 183–188

Spontaneous Remissions: An Annotated Bibliography, 183

Spouse
  death of, 459, 460
  problems related to, 459, 460, 464

Sprue, celiac, 244

Squamous cell carcinoma
  beta-carotene in, 221
  Chinese herbs for, 383

Squash, 347

Stages of dying
  Kübler-Ross on, 511–513
  Lindeman on, 514, 515
  Shneidman on, 513

Stagnation of blood, herbal remedies for, 383, 384, 386

Stanway, Andrew, 82n

Transplantation, bone marrow. *See* Bone marrow transplantation
Trauma, childhood, 463, 464
Treating Cancer with Chinese Herbs, 385
Treatment of Cancer by Integrated Chinese-Western Methods, The, 386
Trials of therapy. *See* Clinical trials
Triglycerides, 446
Trust, in practitioner, 523, 525
Truth-telling, 339
Tryptophan metabolism disorders, 224
Tsuda, Hideaki, 420–422, 424
Tubercle bacillus, 222, 320, 328
Tuberculosis
  pulmonary, 263, 320
  of skin, 263
Tumor(s), anabolic vs. catabolic, 445, 446, 450
Tumor embolus, 148
Tumor growth
  dietary repletion and, 205
  nutrition and, 204
  stress and, 146–148
  vitamin C and, 233, 234
Tumorigenesis
  fat intake and, 211
  Kushi's theory of, 290, 291
Tumor mitosis, in melanoma, 151
Tumor necrosis, liquefactive, selenium and, 448
Tumor regression, meditation and, 153
Tumosterone, 601
Tung oil, 446
"Turning point," cancer as, 461–463, 529
Twins, leukemia in, 177
Type A behavior pattern, 180
Type C behavior pattern, 180, 181
Tyrosine restriction, 208

Ullman, Dana, 586
Unconscious, language of, 23
Unconventional cancer therapies. *See* Cancer therapy(ies), unconventional
Unconventional Cancer Treatments (OTA), 98, 525, 587, 588
Underfeeding, 204–210, 215
Unschuld, Paul, 371
Uremic poisoning, 505

Uric acid, 232
Urinary peptides, in antineoplastons, 399, 406
Urine
  odor of, with antineoplastons, 419
  surface tension of, 449
Usua, Mikao, 579
Uterine cancer
  acupuncture in, 379
  personality factors in, 176, 182
  pyridoxine in, 224
  qi gong for, 391
  vitamin C in, 229, 233
Uterine fibroids, 42
Uterus, removal of, 38

Vaccine(s)
  autogenous, 319, 323, 324, 327, 328, 604
  BCG, 324, 328
  Maruyama, 328
Values, transformation of, 21
van Baalen, Daan C., 186–188, 255
Veach, Virginia, 483
Vedanta, 286
Vega Study Center, 570, 573, 588
Vegetable juices, 223, 257, 267, 325, 326
Vegetable oils, 346
Vegetables, 201, 325, 326, 343, 345, 346
  carotenoids in, 221
  fiber in, 212, 215
  nightshade family, 346
  sea, 293, 296, 345, 346
  and stomach cancer, 310
  vitamin C in, 230
Vegetarian diet, 81, 251, 252, 267, 305, 346, 347
  benefits of, 313
  and breast cancer, 309
  Burton's view of, 403
  and estrogen excretion, 309
  in Livingston program, 323
  in macrobiotics, 285, 288
Vegetarianism, in Great Britain, 37
Ventafridda, Vittorio, 478
Vertigo, 444
Vietnam War, 484, 528
Vinegar baths, 324
Viniyoga, 582